# Amino Acids as
# Chemical Transmitters

# NATO ADVANCED STUDY INSTITUTES SERIES

A series of edited volumes comprising multifaceted studies of contemporary scientific issues by some of the best scientific minds in the world, assembled in cooperation with NATO Scientific Affairs Division.

**Series A: Life Sciences**

*Recent Volumes in this Series*

The series is published by an international board of publishers in conjunction with NATO Scientific Affairs Division

| | | |
|---|---|---|
| A | Life Sciences | Plenum Publishing Corporation |
| B | Physics | New York and London |
| C | Mathematical and Physical Sciences | D. Reidel Publishing Company Dordrecht and Boston |
| D | Behavioral and Social Sciences | Sijthoff International Publishing Company Leiden |
| E | Applied Sciences | Noordhoff International Publishing Leiden |

# Amino Acids as Chemical Transmitters

Edited by
## Frode Fonnum
*Norwegian Defense Research Establishment*
*Kjeller, Norway*

**PLENUM PRESS • NEW YORK AND LONDON**
Published in cooperation with NATO Scientific Affairs Division

Library of Congress Cataloging in Publication Data

Nato Advanced Study Institute on Amino Acids as Chemical Transmitters, Oslo, Norway, 1977.
    Amino acids as chemical transmitters.

    (NATO advanced study institutes series: Series A, Life sciences; v. 16)
    Includes index.
    1. Neurotransmitters–Congresses. 2. Amino acids–Congresses. I. Fonnum, Frode, 1937-    II. Title. III. Series.
QP364.7.N37 1977              599'.01'88                78-2362
ISBN 0-306-35616-3

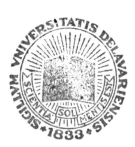
Proceedings of the NATO Advanced Study Institute on Amino Acids as Chemical Transmitters held in Oslo, Norway, August 14–21, 1977

© 1978 Plenum Press, New York
A Division of Plenum Publishing Corporation
227 West 17th Street, New York, N.Y. 10011

Printed in the United States of America

PREFACE

This volume represents the proceedings of a NATO Advanced
Study Institute on Amino Acids as Chemical Transmitters, which
took place at Spåtind Hotel in Norway, August 14-21, 1977.  The
meeting is related to two previous meetings on metabolic compartmentation in the brain.  The first of these meetings took place at
Rockefeller Foundation, Bellagio, Italy, July 11-16, 1971 and the
proceedings, Metabolic Compartmentation in Brain, were edited by
R. Balazs and J.E. Cremer and published by Macmillan in 1973.  The
second meeting was an Advanced Study Institute on Metabolic Compartmentation and Neurotransmission Relation to Brain Structure
and Function, which was held in Oxford, September 1-8, 1974.  The
proceedings were edited by S. Berl, D.D. Clarke and D. Schneider
and published as Volume 6 of the NATO ASI Life Science series by
Plenum Press.

The object of the present meeting was to review and discuss
the present status of amino acids as chemical transmitters.  Several
issues such as electrophysiological response, localization, synthesis, release and receptor binding of transmitter candidates were
discussed.  The possible morphological correlates to these functions were also reviewed.  During the meeting 24 leading papers
were given.  In addition, several of the participants presented
important new findings during the discussion.  Some of these have
been included as short reports.

The main financial support was obtained from NATO, Scientific
Affairs Division.  But additional support was recieved from the
Norwegian Research Council for Science and the Humanities and the
following firms: A/S Apothekernes Laboratorium for Specialpraepara-
ter, CIBA-Geigy AG, F. Hoffmann-La Roche and Co. AG, Nyegaard and Co.
A/S, Åge Randmael A/S, and Synthelabo Group Ltd.

F. Fonnum
Oslo, October 1977

CONTENTS


PART I: MORPHOLOGY

PART II: ELECTROPHYSIOLOGY AND NEUROPHARMACOLOGY

## PART III: LOCALIZATION

## PART IV: THE VISUAL SYSTEM

# MORPHOLOGICAL CORRELATES FOR TRANSMITTER SYNTHESIS, TRANSPORT, RELEASE, UPTAKE AND CATABOLISM: A STUDY OF SEROTONIN NEURONS IN THE NUCLEUS PARAGIGANTOCELLULARIS LATERALIS

Victoria Chan-Palay

Department of Neurobiology
Harvard Medical School
Boston, Massachusetts 02115, USA

The aim of this report is to gather available evidence from the literature and to provide fresh evidence from new experiments for the morphological intraneuronal correlates for transmitter synthesis, packaging, transport, uptake, and metabolism in the mammalian central nervous system. A large body of literature is available for the catecholamines (norepinephrine and dopamine) and gamma-amino butyric acid and they have been the subject of recent extensive reviews (Bloom, 1973; Roberts et al., 1976). The present report will explore the indoleamine-serotonin systems. The pathways for the biosynthesis and catabolism of serotonin (5HT) and related indoleamines are well known and aptly discussed by Cooper et al., 1974, pp. 175-199. The essential steps are summarized in Table 1. The essential amino acid tryptophan is converted enzymatically by tryptophan hydroxylase, the rate limiting enzyme, to 5-hydroxytryptophan which undergoes decarboxylation to form 5-hydroxytryptamine or serotonin (5HT). These initial steps represent the synthesis of 5HT; once formed, 5HT is stored, transported or released by the indoleamine neuron in the course of its activity. 5HT is metabolized by monoamine oxidases in the presence of aldehyde dehydrogenase to form 5-hydroxyindole acetic acid. This report will review the findings of several pertinent studies using cytochemical or immunological methods in order to discover the intracellular organelles in indoleamine neurons which relate to the synthesis, transport, uptake, and catabolism of 5HT.

The initial approach for studying 5HT neurons at the cellular level has been through the Falck-Hillarp fluorescence technique. Dahlström and Fuxe (1964) pioneered the mapping of 5HT neuronal cell bodies in the brain stem by this method, after pretreatment of

TABLE 1. PATHWAYS IN SYNTHESIS AND CATABOLISM OF 5HT

```
TRYPTOPHAN
    │ tryptophan hydroxylase          ┌─────────────┐
    ▼                                 │  Synthesis  │
5-HYDROXYTRYPTOPHAN                   └─────────────┘
    │ amino                                  │
    │ acid                            ┌──────▼──────┐
    │ decarboxylase                   │  Transport  │
    ▼                                 │  Storage    │
5-HYDROXYTRYPTAMINE                   │  Release    │
    │ monoamine                       │  Uptake     │
    │ oxidase and                     └─────────────┘
    │ aldehyde                               │
    │ dehydroxylase                   ┌──────▼──────┐
    ▼                                 │  Catabolism │
5-HYDROXYINDOLE ACETIC ACID          └─────────────┘
```

the animals with monoamine oxidase inhibitors. These authors referred to the groups of yellow, transiently fluorescent neurons as groups $B_1$ to $B_9$, roughly divided as follows: $B_1$, the nucleus raphe pallidus and neighboring cells groups; $B_2$, the raphe obscurus; $B_3$, the raphe magnus, nucleus paragigantocellularis lateralis and a few other cells; $B_4$, the area postrema; $B_5$, the raphe pontis and other neurons; $B_6$, neurons beneath the floor of the fourth ventricle; $B_7$, raphe dorsalis and the caudal portion of the Edinger-Westphal nucleus; $B_8$, the median raphe, raphe linearis and neurons in the neighboring reticular formation; $B_9$, the neurons within and around the medial lemniscus. The major problem with the fluorescence methods for 5HT is their insensitivity for the display of most terminal axonal fields. Nevertheless, the method remains a potent tool for revelation of neuronal cell bodies that contain endogenous 5HT. Numerous attempts have been made to enhance the induction of 5HT fluorescence, and some increase in fluorescence can be achieved by pharmacological manipulation with monoamine oxidase inhibitors to reduce 5HT catabolism — reserpine has been given to reduce amine release, tryptophan has been given to increase availability of precursor in order to increase synthesis, or analogs such as 6-hydroxytryptamine have been administered in order to load the axonal plexuses with fluorescent products.

Another approach to the cellular display of 5HT neurons is the application of immunocytochemistry at the light and electron micro-scopic levels. In a series of recent studies Pickel and her collaborators (Joh et al., 1975; Pickel et al., 1976; Pickel et al., 1977) raised antibodies against the enzyme tryptophan hydroxylase and then used these for the immunocytochemical localization of serotonin neurons in the raphe nucleus and their axonal processes

in the locus coeruleus.  The location of the enzyme was detected by
means of the unlabeled primary antibody-peroxidase antiperoxidase
method (Sternberger, 1974).  These investigators demonstrated that
tryptophan hydroxylase is localized (1) to membranes of the endoplasmic reticulum and Golgi apparatus in the cell body, (2) to
microtubules in the dendrites and axon and (3) to the surface
membranes of small vesicles and large granular vesicles (LGV) in
axonal varicosities.  They suggested that the association of this
enzyme (which catalyzes the initial and probably rate-limiting step
in the biosynthesis of 5HT) with the endoplasmic reticulum and the
Golgi apparatus represents the site of 5HT synthesis and its
association with microtubules indicates the mode of transport of
this transmitter.

Another way to display monoamine cells and their terminals is
to take advantage of their selective uptake systems for extracellular transmitter and to use autoradiography after the administration
of exogenous labeled transmitter.  Labeled $^3$H-5HT can be administered by intraventricular pulse injection (Aghajanian et al., 1966;
Fuxe and Ungerstedt, 1968; Bloom et al., 1972), by continuous
intraventricular infusion (Chan-Palay, 1975, 1977a), by local
instillation (Mouren-Mathieu et al., 1976), or by topical application (Descarries et al., 1975).  Such injections are known to
produce selective labeling of 5HT neurons and axons because of the
high affinity, saturable stereospecific uptake system that 5HT
neurons exhibit in biochemical experiments.  Morphological data
obtained from endogenous fluorescence studies and autoradiography
after injections with exogenous $^3$H-5HT (Fuxe et al., 1968) indicate
that comparable structures are demonstrated by the two techniques.


SEROTONIN NEURONS IN THE NUCLEUS PARAGIGANTOCELLULARIS LATERALIS

The 5HT neurons in this nucleus of the medullary reticular
formation were recognized as part of a group of yellow fluorescent
neurons designated B$_3$ by Dahlström and Fuxe (1964) in their studies
with the Falck-Hillarp method.  Electrical stimulation of the PGCL
facilitated the firing of raphe pontis and median raphe neurons,
presumably by serotoninergic mechanisms (Couch, 1970), a finding
which suggests  that these two groups of 5HT neurons are linked.
Lesions placed in the PGCL followed by an intraventricular pulse
injection of $^3$H-5HT resulted in degenerating synaptic terminals in
the raphe pontis, and supported the suggestion that these two 5HT
neuron groups interact (Bloom et al., 1972).

Recently the autoradiographic mapping of indoleamine neurons
in the brains of the rhesus monkey (Chan-Palay, 1977a) and the rat
(Chan-Palay, 1977b) have shown that certain neurons in the caudal
PGCL selectively take up $^3$H-5HT and lie in a neuropil having numerous
5HT axonal terminals.

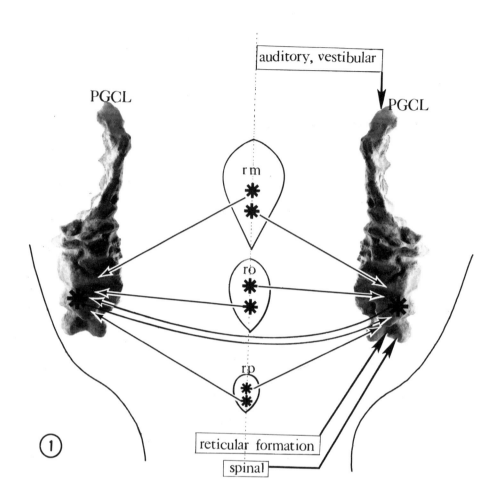

FIGURE 1. A summary of the major inputs to the PGCL nucleus. These
include auditory, vestibular, reticular, and spinal inputs, and
inputs from the indoleamine neuron-containing nuclei – the raphe
magnus (rm), raphe obscurus (ro), raphe pallidus (rp), and the
caudal PGCL of the other side of the brain. Modified from Andrezik,
Chan-Palay, and Palay, 1977, Fig. 7.


    The entire PGCL nucleus in the rat has been carefully defined
and reconstructed from serial sections of the brain by Andrezik et
al., 1977. A model of the nucleus is reproduced in Figure 1. The

TABLE 2. SOURCES OF INDOLEAMINE AFFERENTS TO PGCL

| | |
|---|---|
| N. raphe pallidus | 2+ |
| N. raphe obscurus | + |
| N. raphe magnus | 3+ |
| N. paragigantocellularis lateralis, contralateral | + |

PGCL begins at the level of the rostral magnocellular reticular nucleus at a point approximately at the level of the rostral third of the inferior olivary nucleus. Caudally, where most of the 5HT neurons are found, the PGCL is bounded on its medial aspect by the ventral portion of the nucleus gigantocellularis and laterally by the lateral reticular nucleus and the parvocellular reticular nucleus. The rostral portion of the PGCL abuts dorsally on the nucleus gigantocellularis and the nucleus ambiguus. Laterally it abuts on the motor nucleus of the facial nerve. The caudal, serotonin-containing part of the PGCL measures 1.1 mm at its widest and occupies a large area of the ventral brain stem. It attenuates more rostrally as the model in Figure 1 displays.

In order to facilitate further study of this system of neurons, one needs to know their anatomical connections with other parts of the brain. Retrograde transport of horseradish peroxidase (HRP) injected into the nucleus would allow the mapping of sources of its afferents or inputs, thus providing some indication of such connections. Minute injections of HRP were injected precisely into separate parts of the PGCL, and neurons throughout the brain and spinal cord labeled by HRP after retrograde transport were recorded (Andrezik and Chan-Palay, 1977; Andrezik et al., 1977). These studies demonstrated that the PGCL receives multiple connections from the spinal cord, numerous nuclei of the reticular formation in the pons and medulla, the vestibular nuclei, and several nuclei of the auditory system. In addition, the caudal PGCL in which the 5HT neurons lie, is connected with the PGCL of the other side of the brain, as well as with three other raphe nuclei. These are the raphe obscurus, the raphe magnus and the raphe pallidus, all three of which also contain populations of 5HT neurons (see Dahlström and Fuxe, 1964; Chan-Palay, 1977a, 1977b). Thus, the PGCL is linked to numerous centers in the brain and has possible direct connections with other serotoninergic cell groups in the raphe. These data are summarized in Table 2 and Figure 1. The remainder of this report will be concerned with presentation of fresh evidence from a study of the 5HT neurons of the caudal PGCL with fluorescence microscopy and by autoradiography after intraventricular infusions of $^3$H-5HT.

## Materials and Methods

The fluorescence microscopic data was obtained from the brains of three rats (Sprague-Dawley, 250 g body weight) pretreated with Clorgyline (May and Baker, 100 mg/100 g body weight), a monoamine oxidase inhibitor. The animals were anesthetized with ether. The tissues were frozen, lyophilized and treated with formaldehyde vapors according to the Falck-Hillarp technique. Paraffin sections 10μm thick of this tissue at intervals of 100μm were obtained from the medulla and examined (Figs. 2a,c).

Autoradiograms of comparable regions in the medulla were obtained from the brains of six normal rats (Sprague-Dawley, 200 g body weight) pretreated with Clorgyline. These animals were anesthetized with 35% chloral hydrate and $^3$H-5HT was continuously infused into the lateral ventricle for three hours. Selective uptake of 5HT in these animals was enhanced by the use of a competitive binding paradigm with $^3$H-5HT and cold norepinephrine (NE), in which both substances were infused simultaneously, the latter in 10 times greater concentration than the former. $^3$H-5HT creatinine sulphate (New England Nuclear, 24 Ci/mmol specific activity) at a concentration of $10^{-5}$M together with NE at $10^{-4}$M was freshly prepared with sterile 0.9% saline, filtered through a millipore sieve, and introduced in a total volume of 500μl over three hours. At regular intervals small aliquots of CSF were removed in order to prevent increased intracranial pressure. At the end of the infusion, the animal was perfused with 1% glutaraldehyde and 1% formaldehyde in 0.12M phosphate buffer. High resolution light microscopic autoradiograms were prepared from material postfixed in osmium tetroxide and embedded in epoxy resin, sectioned at 4μm, coated with Kodak NTB-2 emulsion, and exposed for 3 to 4 weeks prior to development and light staining with toluidine blue (see Fig. 2b).

The electron microscope studies reported here were made on material obtained from three adult rhesus monkeys (Macaca mulatta). They were tranquilized with Sernalyn (Biocentric Labs, 0.05ml/kg body weight) and maintained on 1% sodium pentobarbital i.v., and pretreated with Nialamide (monoamine oxidase inhibitor, 100mg/kg body weight), 2 hours prior to the experiment. Intraventricular infusions with $^3$H-5HT creatinine sulphate (Amersham Searle, specific activity 16-18 Ci/mM) at a concentration of $10^{-5}$M or $10^{-6}$M were continued for 3 hours for a total of approximately 3000μl of diluted tracer. Possible increased intracranial pressure was relieved by a lumbar puncture at L4/L5. Fixation of the brain was obtained by vascular perfusion with 1% glutaraldehyde/1% formaldehyde mixtures followed by 3% glutaraldehyde/3% formaldehyde, and the brains were removed, postfixed in osmium tetroxide, and embedded in epoxy resin (Palay and Chan-Palay, 1974, pp.328-329). High resolution light and electron microscopic autoradiography was performed on tissues from the medulla at the level of the caudal PGCL. Serial sections of the entire block were prepared, mounted on slides, dried overnight, and

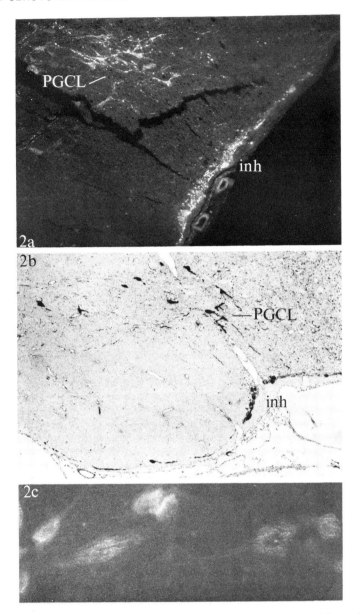

FIGURES 2a,b.Comparison between Falck-Hillarp preparation showing neurons of the PGCL and nucleus interfascicularis hypoglossi (inh) with endogenous 5HT fluorescence (Fig. 2a) and an autoradiogram showing the corresponding neurons after uptake of $^{3}$H-5HT from a continuous intraventricular infusion (Fig. 2b). Rat, X 350.
FIGURE 2c. Higher magnification of several 5HT fluorescent neurons from the PGCL of the rat showing the reticular, non-granular disposition of the fluoresence. Rat, Falck-Hillarp method, X 2,100.

dipped in NTB-2 emulsion. The sections were exposed for 6 months, developed in D19, and stained with 1% toluidine blue (see Figs. 3a, b). After study of these preparations, oriented regions were selected from the same areas and electron microscope autoradiograms were prepared. The celloidin film stripping method was used with Ilford L4 emulsion, exposures of up to 14 months followed by rapid development (20-30 secs) in a physical developer, paraphenylene-diamine. (See Chan-Palay, 1977a, pp. 503-511 for details on all these methods.) A total of six separate specimens, one from the caudal PGCL of each side of the brains of the 3 rhesus monkeys, were examined in the electron microscope. From each specimen, at least forty adjacent serial sections, each approximately 700Å to 1000Å thick, and spanning a total of 2.8µm to 4.0µm of tissue, were prepared as autoradiograms. From this material, every labeled struc-ture was photographed in the electron microscope. The micrographs were collated so that micrographs of identified adjacent or nonadja-cent serial sections could be assembled for reconstruction of indi-vidual labeled axonal boutons. The aim of this lengthy project was to determine whether synaptic junctions were present or absent in identified, serially sectioned 5HT labeled boutons.

Comparison of 5HT Neurons in the PGCL of Rat by
Fluorescence and Autoradiographic Methods (Figs. 2a,b).

The 5HT neurons of the ventral medulla have been demonstrated to have precisely the same appearance, location and disposition in fluorescence preparations from the Falck-Hillarp technique (Fig. 2a) as in autoradiograms after intraventricular administration of $^3$H-5HT (Fig. 2b). The caudal PGCL contains several hundred conspicuous neurons with large somata measuring 20-25µm by 25-40µm, with short dendrites that extend in and around the nucleus. Other neighboring neurons such as the interfascicular nucleus of the hypoglossal nerve which are also known to contain 5HT from previous studies (Dahlström and Fuxe, 1964; Chan-Palay, 1977a,b) are fluorescent and label by autoradiography as well. The significant difference between the two types of preparations - fluorescence demonstrating endogenous 5HT and autoradiography demonstrating 5HT uptake mechanisms - is that few 5HT axon terminals visible by the former method are readily demonstrable by the latter method. This discrepancy represents a limitation of the fluorescence methods for 5HT axon detection and does not indicate non-specificity in the autoradiographic method.

A closer examination of suitable fluorescent PGCL neurons indicates that the fluorescent material has a diffuse, reticulated disposition throughout the cell body and is axially oriented in dendrites. It is brighter in the somatic cytoplasm than in the dendrites. The fluorescent material does not appear to be granular (see Fig. 2c). These observations suggest that the endogenous 5HT lies in the smooth and rough endoplasmic reticulum and the Golgi apparatus of the cell body and in axially oriented structures such as on filaments and microtubules and smooth endoplasmic reticulum in the dendrites.

### Cytology of 5HT Neurons in the PGCL of Rhesus Monkey

In the rhesus monkey, the caudal PGCL on each side of the brain contains approximately 300 neurons that are labeled by $^3$H-5HT. They are distinctive, large neurons with fusiform perikarya (30-35µm by 45-50µm) with stout, long dendrites that issue from the ends of the cell. They occur individually or in small clusters of 3 to 5. In the autoradiograms the perikaryon and dendrites are heavily labeled, and in any single section segments of labeled dendrites up to 300µm long may be observed (see Figs. 3a,b). These labeled processes occur in between other elements of the heavily myelinated neuropil in and around the nucleus; other labeled structures, probably varicosities of preterminal axons and terminals boutons, are also present (see Figs. 3a,b).

Within the labeled cells, silver grains are present over the nucleus and nucleoli as well (Fig. 3b) with heavier concentrations over the latter. High resolution electron microscope autoradiography was used to study the precise locations of label over the various cellular organelles of serotoninergic neurons. Labeled neurons displayed silver grains over their perikarya, dendrites, and parent axons, and most heavily over their axonal varicosities. In the electron microscopic autoradiograms, silver grains were localized to certain organelles. The discreteness of the localization of these grains was enhanced by lengthy exposures (up to 14 months) of the thin sections followed by brief development (up to 30 secs) in a low sensitivity physical developer. In almost all cases, these procedures resulted in discrete labeling of organelles with a few silver grains and little background. The illustrations given here are taken from this material. In a few cases, shorter exposures of 2 to 4 months were used with physical development of 60 secs. Material developed in more sensitive developers such as Microdol-X were used only for test examination because of the higher background and poorer localization of silver grains to individual cellular organelles.

Electron microscope autoradiograms of indoleamine neurons show heavily labeled nucleoli and lightly labeled nuclei. The perikaryal cytoplasm is labeled with silver grains over several organelles:

(a) The Golgi apparatus, which elaborately encircles the nucleus is accompanied by numerous vesicles, particularly on its maturing face. These vesicular profiles are of various types: (i) round, 800-1000 Å in diameter, with a dense homogeneously dark center separated by an 80-100 Å clear rim from the membrane; (ii) elliptical, 1200-1500 Å by 900 Å, with a dense content as described in (i);

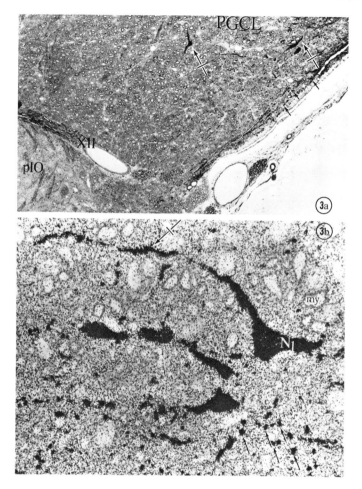

FIGURE 3a. Low magnification autoradiogram in the region of the PGCL
in the rhesus monkey after intraventricular infusion of $^3$H-5HT.
Several labeled neurons and a few labeled dendrites are indicated
by crossed arrows and segments of labeled axons with small arrows.
In the vicinity, the principal nucleus of the inferior olive (pIO)
and the hypoglossal nerve (XII) are indicated. Rhesus monkey. 1µm
epoxy-embedded material counterstained with toluidine blue. X125.

FIGURE 3b. Higher magnification autoradiogram from a nonadjacent
serial section in the PGCL in the rhesus monkey.  Portions of
several labeled neurons are shown, one of which ($N_1$) has labeled
nucleus, nucleolus, and long dendrites (crossed arrow).  Other
small clumps of silver grains suggestive of labeled axons or boutons
(small arrows) are present in the neuropil amongst numerous large
myelinated axons that are not labeled (my).  3H-5HT. Rhesus monkey.
1µm epoxy-embedded material counterstained with toluidine blue. X620.

(iii) round, 400-600 Å in diameter, usually clear but sometimes having a granular floccular content; (iv) granular and agranular vesicles of various sizes budding from the Golgi membranes. When present silver grains are usually not directly over the Golgi lamellae, but are adjacent to them, over large granular vesicles or over smaller granular and agranular vesicles (see Figs. 4a, 4b, 5a, 5b). These observations suggest that the transmitter molecule or a labeled metabolite has been incorporated into vesicular packets by the Golgi apparatus.

(b) Tubular profiles of the smooth endoplasmic reticulum and microtubules (Figs. 5a, 6b), suggesting that these organelles may be involved in the nonvesicular binding and transport of $^3$H-5HT or a labeled metabolite.

(c) Mitochondria (Fig. 5b), probably indicating the presence of $^3$H-5HT or a metabolite during metabolism by monoamine oxidases.

d) Multivesicular profiles (Fig. 5c) and tubular profiles with dense material suggesting that they too are involved in the packaging, transport and recycling of $^3$H-5HT.

In dendrites, the silver grains lie over the smooth endoplasmic reticulum, microtubules, and large dense core vesicles (Figs. 6a,b). Rarely a lysosome (Fig. 6c) or an alveolate vesicle (Fig. 6d) is also labeled.

The main axons of indoleamine neurons are myelinated fibers. Numerous examples of labeled large caliber axons, 3-5μm in diameter, with sheaths consisting of 8-12 myelin lamellae were observed (Figs. 7a-7c). Within these axons, silver grains are found over microtubules, the smooth endoplasmic reticulum, and occasional dense core vesicles.

Organization of the Neuropil. Labeled 5HT neurons in the PGCL display numerous axosomatic contacts upon their surfaces. These can be readily divided into two types: 1) synapses with non-indoleamine, unlabeled axonal boutons and 2) synapses with indole-amine-containing, labeled boutons (illustrated schematically in Figs. 8a,b). The labeled dendrites of 5HT neurons in the PGCL are also recipients of these two types of synapses (illustrated schematically in Figs. 9a,b). Electron micrographs of these two types of synaptic contacts are given in Fig. 10a, which shows a 5HT labeled dendrite receiving an unlabeled synaptic bouton, and in Fig. 10b which shows both axon and dendrite containing 5HT.

Indoleamine Axon Terminals. Of all the processes of serotonin neurons, the axonal terminals are the most heavily labeled by silver grains. Numerous profiles of axonal boutons are labeled after $^3$H-5HT administration. These boutons can be classified according to several

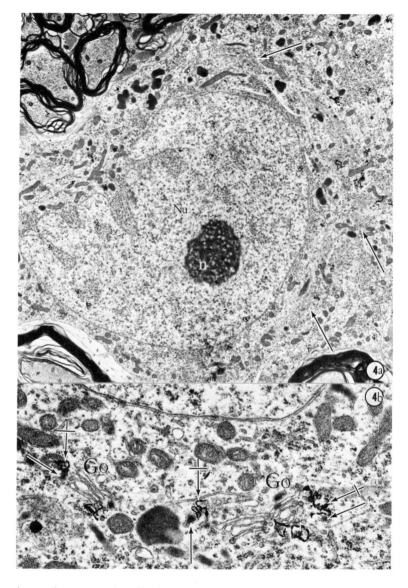

FIGURE 4a,b (Opposite). (4a) This PGCL cell is marked by silver
grains over various perikaryal organelles, the Golgi apparatus
(arrows), and over the lobulated nucleus (Nu) and nucleolus (n).
(4b) The Golgi apparatus in a PGCL 5HT neuron. Silver grains (crossed
arrows) are over large granular vesicles (900 Å with granular or
black content), and small, clear or agranular vesicles (arrows) at
the periphery and maturing face of the Golgi apparatus. Rhesus monkey,
³H-5HT, exposure 14 mos, physical development 40 sec, poststained
in lead citrate. 4a) X9,600; 4b) X32,000.

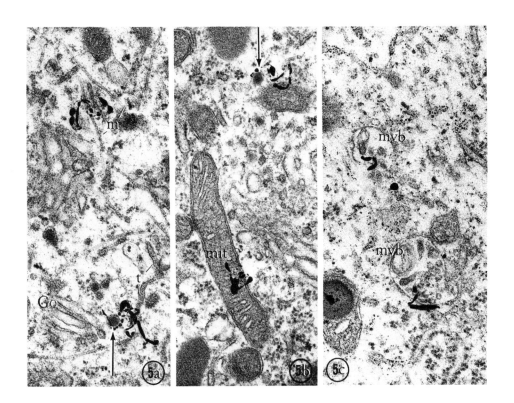

FIGURE 5a-c. Labeled organelles in 5HT neurons involved in the packaging, transport, and metabolism of 3H-5HT. (5a) Note the large
granular vesicle (arrow) at the periphery of a stack of Golgi lamellae and the tubular reticulum (t), and microtubules (m), labeled by
silver grains. X65,000. (5b) Mitochondria (mit) and a nearby large
granular vesicle (arrow) labeled by silver grains. X55,000. (5c) Two
profiles of multivesicular bodies with clear or granular content
labelec by silver grains. X70,000. Rhesus monkey, 3H-5HT, exposure
14 mos, physical development 40 sec, poststained in lead citrate.

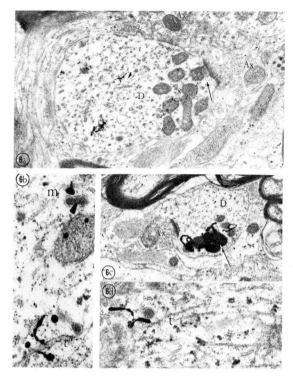

FIGURE 6a. The dendrite of an indoleamine neuron. The dendrite (D) which contains numerous profiles of microtubules and tubular reticulum is labeled by silver grains. The dendrite is surrounded by several axons (Ax), one of which synapses with it. The indoleamine dendrite bears a row of subsynaptic dense granules (arrow) as well as a large knot of filamentous dense material flanked by numerous mitochondria. Similar subsynaptic specializations have been described in the cerebellar nuclei of monkeys (Chan-Palay, 1977, pp. 168-178). $^3$H-5HT, rhesus monkey, exposure 14 mos, physical development 40 sec, poststained in lead citrate. X28,000.

FIGURE 6b. This dendrite of an indoleamine neuron contains labeled microtubules (m), large granular vesicles and the tubular reticulum (t). Rhesus monkey, $^3$H-5HT, exposure 14 mos, physical development 40 sec, poststained in lead citrate. X72,000.

FIGURE 6c. A rare labeled lysosome within a dendrite (D) of an indoleamine neuron, which receives a synapse from an unlabeled axon (Ax). Rhesus monkey, $^3$H-5HT, physical development 40 sec, poststained in lead citrate. X30,000.

FIGURE 6d. Labeled microtubule (t) and large granular alveolate vesicle in the dendrite of an indoleamine neuron. Rhesus monkey, $^3$H-5HT, exposure 14 mos, physical development 40 sec, poststained in lead citrate. X70,000.

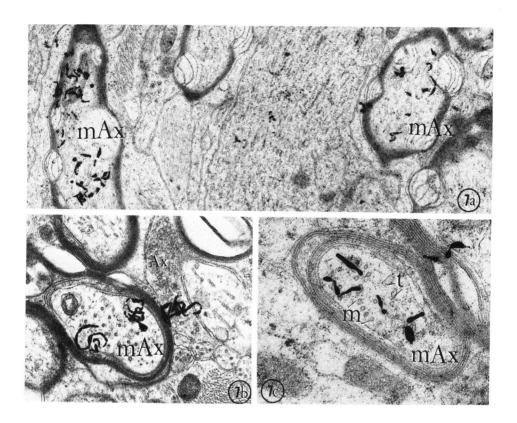

FIGURE 7a-c. Segments of myelinated parent axons (mAx) of indoleamine PGCL neurons labeled by intraventricular infusions of $^3$H-5HT
(7a). These axons (mAx) have approximately a dozen layers of myelin
per sheath and contain microtubules (m̲), tubular reticulum (t̲), and
occasional large granular vesicles (7b,7c). Rhesus monkey, 3H̅-5HT,
exposure 14 mos, physical development 40 sec, poststained in lead
citrate. X25,000; 30,000; 50,000.

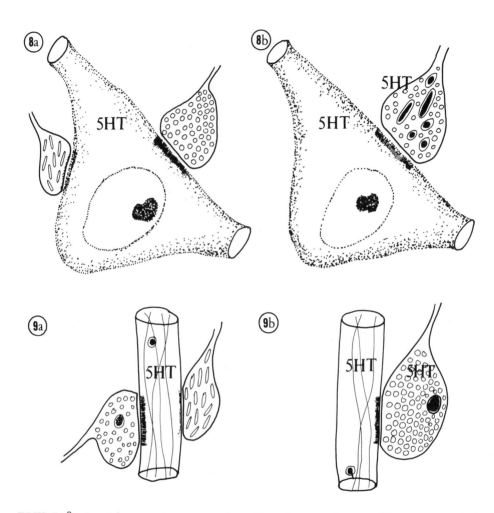

FIGURE 8a,b. Diagram to summarize the observed <u>synaptic</u> arrangements
on indoleamine neuronal perikarya: (a) 5HT neuron as the recipient
of non-5HT axon terminals with various axoplasmic morphology;
(b) 5HT neuron as the recipient of a 5HT axon terminal.

FIGURE 9a,b. Diagram to summarize the observed synaptic arrangements
on indoleamine dendrites: (a) 5HT dendrite as the recipient of
non-5HT axon terminals of differing morphology; (b) 5HT dendrite
as the recipient of 5HT axon terminal.

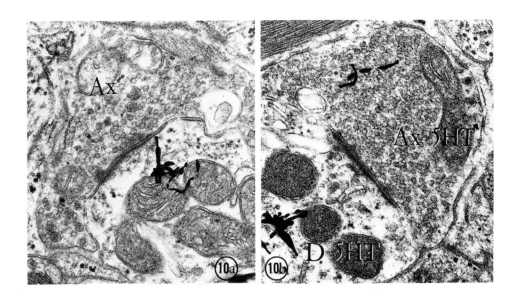

FIGURE 10a.   Labeled dendrite postsynaptic to a non-indoleamine
synaptic axon terminal (Ax).  The axon contains numerous small
clear, granular, and large granular vesicles and engages in a Gray's
type 1 synaptic junction.  Rhesus monkey, [3]H-5HT, PGCL, exposure 14
mos, physical development 40 sec. X22,000.

FIGURE 10b. Indoleamine axon (Ax-5HT) presynaptic to a dendrite of
an indoleamine PGCL neuron (D-5HT). The axon bears numerous small
clear vesicles and only occasional large granular vesicles.
The synapse is Gray's type 1. Rhesus monkey, PGCL, [3]H-5HT, exposure
14 mos, physical development 40 sec. X48,000.


criteria: (a) their overall size; (b) their axoplasmic morphology,
e.g., synaptic vesicle populations, matrix density; (c) the presence
of synaptic junctions, e.g., axosomatic, axodendritic, axo-axonic,
or serial synapses;(d) the identification of the postsynaptic
element; (e) the lack of morphologically identifiable synaptic
junctions on axonal boutons through two to seven serial thin sections, each approximately 700 Å - 1000 Å thick; (f) their frequency
of occurrence in the neuropil; (g) the amount of autoradiographic
label over the terminal.  This scheme was devised and used for the
classification of indoleamine axons in the cerebellum labeled by
intraventricular infusions of [3]H-5HT (see Chan-Palay, 1975; 1977b,
Table 15-2) and in the paratrigeminal nucleus (Chan-Palay, 1977c).
These studies indicated that various axons with different axoplasmic
and labeling characteristics were distinguishable with synaptic or
nonsynaptic relationships.  In the present study, a total of 1200

electron micrographs of labeled structures in the PGCL were collected
from autoradiograms of the serial sections prepared as described in
the Methods section.  In this collection each of 168 axonal boutons
could be recognized in at least two serial sections.  Of these, 141
bore structures that could be identified as synaptic junctions,
while the remaining 27 did not.  These data suggest that in the PGCL
neuropil, axonal boutons can be either synaptic or nonsynaptic.
Within the limits of the sampling procedure described, the counts
indicate that approximately 84% of these boutons bear synapses and
16% do not.

Synaptic Boutons (Figs. 11a-e; 12a-d; summarized in Table 3).
A number of morphologically different synaptic varicosities were
observed.  The majority of these were presynaptic elements (Figs.
11a-e); however, a few were involved in more complex, axo-axonic
relations (Figs. 12a-c).  Figure 11a shows a small (1μm) labeled
bouton with small, clear, round synaptic vesicles (diameter approximately 450 Å) in a Gray's 1 synaptic contact with a non-5HT dendrite.

Figure 11b shows an axonal bouton (0.8μm in size) which contains
pleomorphic synaptic vesicles in a light axoplasmic matrix.  There
are small, clear vesicles measuring 360 Å in diameter, some approximately 450 Å with small dense dots, others which are tiny tubular
profiles 200 Å across, and a few large granular vesicles approximately 800 Å in diameter with black cores 500 Å in diameter.  This
axon is seen in opposition with an unlabeled dendrite at an atypical
symmetrical Gray's type 2 junction.

Figure 11c provides a comparison between two different varieties
of indoleamine axons.  The axon in the lower left contains numerous
small, agranular vesicles and several other large 900 Å granular
vesicles with variably dense cores.  It is lightly labeled and makes
a long synaptic contact of the Gray's 1 variety with a non-indole-
aminergic unlabeled dendrite.  The second axon in the upper center
of this figure is approximately 1μm across, unusually heavily
labeled, and contains a pleomorphic population of small agranular
vesicles and several round (900 Å) and elliptical (1300 Å) large
granular ones with variably dense cores.

Figures 11d and 11e  are illustrations from non-adjacent serial
sections through a labeled indoleamine axon terminal which partially
envelopes a dendritic spinous process with which it makes a pronounced Gray's type 1 synapse.  The varicosity is 2-3μm long and
contains a population of small pleomorphic clear synaptic vesicles
near the synaptic junction.  Numerous large granular vesicles are
more peripherally situated; some are round (700 Å to 900 Å), others
are elliptical (about 1300 Å by 900 Å), and all have variably dense
centers with a clear rim of approximately 100 Å between core and
vesicular membrane.

Apart from these simple synaptic arrangements in which the
indoleamine axons are presynaptic, the PGCL neuropil contains other

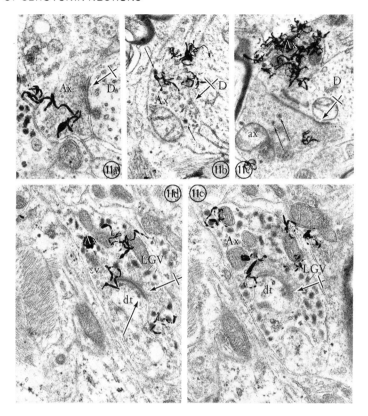

FIGURE 11a-c. Indoleamine axons of heterogeneous axoplasmic morphology in axodendritic synapses.  (11a) The labeled axonal bouton (Ax)
bears numerous small 450 Å clear vesicles in a dark matrix and has
a Gray's type 1 synapse (crossed arrow) with the dendrite (D).
X54,000.  (11b) The labeled axon (Ax) bears a pleomorphic population
of clear and granular vesicles and a few        (Continued Opposite)
(Fig. 11b, Continued) large granular vesicles (small arrows) with
black centers.  It synapses through an atypical Gray's type 2
junction (crossed arrows) with a dendrite (D). X48,000. (11c) Two
labeled axons of different axoplasmic description in the vicinity
of a dendrite (D). The dendrite is in synapse (crossed arrow) with
one of these axons (ax), containing round clear vesicles and large
granular vesicles (arrows) and light autoradiographic label. The
second axon (Ax) is heavily labeled but lacks a visible synaptic
junction.  Rhesus monkey, $^3$H-5HT, PGCL. X25,000.

FIGURE 11d,e. Indoleamine axodendritic synapse in serial sections.
These two sections show a large indoleamine axonal varicosity (Ax),
containing small clear vesicles (sv) and numerous round and elliptical large granular vesicles (LGV), in synapse (crossed arrows)
with a dendritic thorn (dt).A row of dense granules is present in the
immediate subsynaptic region (arrow).Rhesus monkey, $^3$H-5HT, X31,000.

labeled axons which engage in more complex and unusual relationships, such as axo-axonic and reciprocal synapses. Figures 12a and 12b are non-adjacent serial sections through two large axonal boutons, which are approximately 3µm long and are closely entwined with one another. The axons have contrasting axoplasmic morphology; that on the left is unlabeled and contains numerous small clear, small granular, and large granular vesicles in a dark matrix. The one on the right is labeled and contains a conspicuous population of large granular vesicles of round and elliptical outline, varying from 1000 Å to 3000 Å in size. A few smaller tubular or agranular vesicular profiles are also visible. The two axons communicate one with the other via an axo-axonic synapse, with the 5HT axon most probably as the postsynaptic element. Another indoleamine axon of similar morphology is shown in Figure 12c. In all three illustrations, indoleamine axons appear to be in axo-axonic contact with non-indoleamine ones, a circumstance which suggests that some form of presynaptic interaction may occur via 5HT as the neural mediator.

Figure 12d shows two labeled profiles, one axonic (right) and the other dendritic (center), in synaptic contact. An unlabeled axon (left) is also in synapse with the central dendritic process. The labeled axon contains small clear 400 Å to 500 Å vesicles with an occasional 900 Å granular vesicle and the junction is Gray's type 1. This micrograph and that in Figure 10b show that interactions between 5HT axons and 5HT dendrites occur, i.e., synapses between neural elements that utilize the same transmitter.

Nonsynaptic Axonal Boutons. (Figs. 13a-c, summarized in Table 3) Besides these classical synaptic arrangements and the more complicated variations of axo-axonic relations between one or more indoleamine axon and axons of other transmitter content, the neuropil of the PGCL contains labeled axons that do not exhibit morphologically identifiable synaptic contacts. These constitute approximately 16% of the 5HT bouton population. These axons have features that distinguish them from the others. They are small caliber axons, usually no thicker than 0.1µm to 0.2µm in their intervaricose portions, and up to 1.0µm in the varicosities. Many of these labeled axons are scattered throughout the neuropil, but are most readily recognized in the subpial regions of the ventral medulla. Despite their diminutive size these axons are heavily labeled, particularly in their intervaricose regions (Figures 13a,b). In these segments the axons contain several microtubules and small tubular membranous profiles in a dark axoplasmic matrix. The tubular profiles are approximately 200 Å wide and 600 Å long with either clear or dense content (Figures 13a,b). Larger 900 Å vesicles are also found occasionally (Figure 13c).

Table 3 summarizes the six classes of $^3$H-5HT labeled axon terminals in the neuropil of the PGCL according to the sizes and shapes of their varicosities, their synaptic vesicle populations, density of axoplasmic matrix, style of synaptic junction, post-

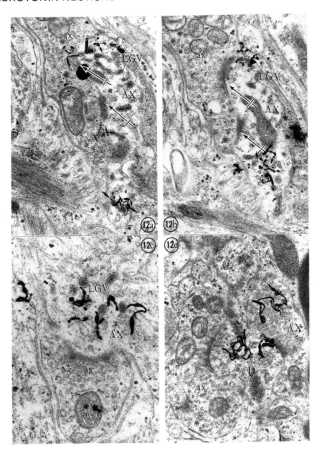

FIGURE 12a,b. Serial sections through an axo-axonic synapse involving an indoleamine axon.  The labeled axon (AX) contains numerous
large·elliptical and round granular vesicles (LGV) in a light axoplasmic matrix.  It synapses through a small Gray's type 1 junctional
complex (crossed arrows) with another axon (ax), which is not labeled
and contains numerous small clear vesicles and a few large granular
vesicles in a dark axoplasmic matrix.  Rhesus monkey, PGCL, $^3$H-5HT.
X40,000.

FIGURE 12c. Possible axo-axonic synapse between a labeled indole-
aminergic axon (AX) containing numerous large granular vesicles
(LGV) and another axon (ax). Rhesus monkey, PGCL, $^3$H-5HT. X50,000.

FIGURE 12d. Complex synaptic relationships between three neuronal
elements in the PGCL neuropil. Two of these processes are labeled
by $^3$H-5HT, one of these is an axon (AX) which synapses through a
clear Gray's 1 junction with the second process (D) which is probably a dendrite.  The third element (ax) is an unlabeled axon which
also synapses upon neural process (D) through a Gray's type 1
synapse.  Rhesus monkey, PGCL. X45,000.

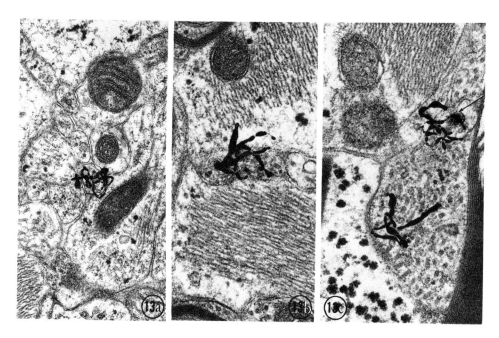

FIGURE 13a-c. Nonsynaptic axonal boutons in the PGCL labeled by uptake of $^3$H-5HT. These axons share a typical morphology: they are thin in the non-varicose segments, heavily labeled, and contain very small tubular profiles about 200 Å in diameter filled with a dense content (Figs. 13a,b). In the varicosities (Fig. 13c) there are many more tubular profiles of similar description mixed with an occasional large granular vesicle (arrow). Rhesus monkey, $^3$H-5HT. 13a) X35,000; 13b) X45,000; 13c) X50,000.

TABLE 3.  Summary of six classes of axon terminals in the PGCL labeled by autoradiography after intraventricular infusions of tritiated serotonin.  Sizes and shapes of axonal varicosities and their synaptic vesicles are diagrammed and tabulated.  Density of axoplasmic matrix, style of synaptic junctional complex, postsynaptic sites, incidence at these sites compared to total number of labeled axons, and the relative density of autoradiographic grains are specified for each category of bouton.

| Appearance | Synaptic Vesicles | | | Matrix | Junction | Receptive sites | Incidence (- - 6+) | Grains (0 - 4+) |
| | small | large granular | tubular | | | | | |
|---|---|---|---|---|---|---|---|---|
| SYNAPTIC 1μm | numerous, round clear, 450Å | occasional, 900Å variably dense | | moderate | Gray's 1 | dendrites | 2+ | 1+ |
| 0.8μm | round, granular 360Å  dense dot, 170Å | occasional, 800Å variably dense cores | occasional, 200Å granular, dense dot, 100Å | light | Gray's 2 | dendrites | 2+ | 2+ |
| 2.3μm | clear, pleomorphic | numerous, variably dense core  700Å, core 500Å  1250Å, core1000Å | | light | Gray's 1 | dendrites | 3+ | 2+ |
| 1μm | round, clear, 400Å | occasional, 900Å | | dark | Gray's 1 | dendrites | 1+ | 4+ |
| 3μm | | numerous 1000-3000Å variably dense core | | light | Gray's 1 | axons (postsynaptic) | 2+ | 2+ |
| NONSYNAPTIC 1μm | | occasional, 900Å variably dense | numerous, clear 200Å x 600Å  granular, 200Å x 600Å dense dot,170Å | dark | nonsynaptic | nonsynaptic | 3+ | 2+ |

synaptic sites, the incidence or frequency of occurrence at these sites compared to the total number of labeled neruons, and the relative density of autoradiographic gains. It is obvious from the data presented that there are demonstrably different types of 5HT axons in the neuropil. The heterogeneity of the axonal population is not surprising since it may reflect the multiple origins of 5HT axons in the PGCL. There are connections between PGCL neurons of the two sides of the brain, there are fibers from the several raphe nuclei, and there are also the axons of the 5HT neurons intrinsic to the PGCL. A comparable situation exists in the cerebellum (see Chan-Palay, 1975, 1977a), where at least six different classes of 5HT axon terminals were found and in which at least five raphe sources of 5HT axons were demonstrated. Moreover, heterogeneity in axoplasmic contents of 5HT neurons appears to be the general rule rather than the exception. Other regions of the brain such as the paratrigeminal nucleus (Chan-Palay, 1977c), the nucleus coeruleus (Pickel et al., 1977), and the caudate nucleus (Calas et al., 1976) also appear to have heterogeneous populations of 5HT axons.

In the PGCL the 5HT axonal boutons are to a large extent synaptic, but a small proportion of them bear no morphologically identifiable synaptic junctions and have been termed nonsynaptic. This dichotomous organization has been described for 5HT terminals elsewhere in the brain; in the cerebellum (Chan-Palay, 1975, 1977a, b); in the cerebral cortex (Descarries et al., 1975); in the caudate nucleus (Tennyson et al., 1974; Calas et al., 1976); in the locus coeruleus (Pickel et al., 1977; Léger and Descarries, 1976) and in the paratrigeminal nucleus of the medulla (Chan-Palay, 1977c). Nowhere are the nonsynaptic 5HT axons better displayed than in the ventricular, supraependymal, and leptomeningeal plexuses (Chan-Palay, 1976), where it has been suggested that upon neural activity these axons release their transmitter directly into the cerebrospinal fluid, and then take it up again (see discussion, Chan-Palay, 1977a, pg. 418-422). Thus, 5HT may be involved in two modes of action, (1) the synaptic or specific afferent contact mode, and (2) a nonsynaptic, neurohumoral mode of neural mediation.

Morphological Correlates. The cytological examination of labeled indoleamine neurons in the PGCL demonstrates that the $^3$H-5HT accumulated under the influence of monoamine oxidase inhibitors is sequestered in the neuron in specific organelles. The most important of these is the Golgi apparatus, which appears to be involved in packaging and delivering vesicular products in which are incorporated $^3$H-5HT or a labeled metabolite. Besides the Golgi apparatus, the smooth endoplasmic reticulum, and microtubules are also likely to be involved in transport of $^3$H-5HT in bound or metabolized form, and multivesicular bodies and alveolate vesicles may be involved in the recycling of $^3$H-5HT. Mitochondria are the major sites of catabolism of $^3$H-5HT and therefore are commonly labeled in auto-

TABLE 4. INTRACELLULAR ORGANELLES FOR THE
SEQUESTRATION OF 5HT NEURONS OF MAMMALIAN CNS.

| Method | Functional Mechanism | Cell Body | Dendrites | Axons |
|---|---|---|---|---|
| Fluores. (LM) | endogenous 5HT storage synthesis transport | reticular (non-granular) | + | + |
| Immunocytochem. (EM) | tryptophan hydroxylase synthesis transport | (rf. Joh et al., 1975, raphe neurons) endoplasmic ret. Golgi app. | microtubules | microtubules |
| | | rf. Pickel et al., 1977, locus coeruleus) | | LGV small ves. tubular ves. |
| Autoradio. (EM) | $^3$H-tryptophan synthesis transport | (rf. Chan-Palay, 1977a) | + | + |
| Autoradio. (EM) | $^3$H-5HT uptake storage breakdown transport | nucleus nucleolus Golgi apparatus and vesicles smooth end. ret. mitochondria multivesicular bod. lysosomes microtubules | smooth e.r. mitochondria microtubules | LGV small ves. smooth e.r. mitochondria microtubules filaments |

radiograms. The reasons for sequestration of radioisotope over the nucleus and nucleolus of the indoleamine neuron remain obscure.

The axonal terminals appear to be the greatest reservoir for sequestration of $^3$H-5HT or its labeled metabolites. This is not surprising since the terminals are probably the sites of greatest activity in synthesis, transport, storage, release and uptake of 5HT. These observations suggest that not only do axon terminals have the machinery for uptake of $^3$H-5HT but that the parent axon, cell soma, and dendrites have it as well, and this may account in part for the considerable amounts of radioactive label observed throughout the cell. Nonetheless, there must be a significant amount of intracellular translocation of the $^3$H-5HT and other labeled metabolites via dendritic, axoplasmic, retrograde and anterograde transport.

These findings on the various intracellular organelles for the sequestration of 5HT, along with those of others cited earlier from the literature, are summarized in Table 4, and schematically

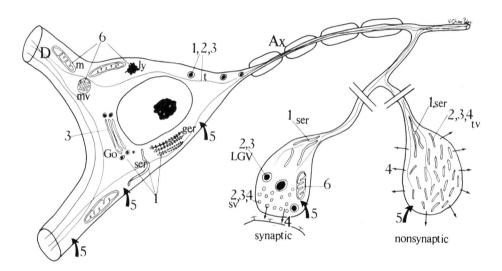

FIGURE 14. Schematic diagram summarizing the intracellular organelles in indoleamine neurons involved in 5HT synthesis (1), transport (2), storage (3), release (4), uptake (5) and catabolism (6). A 5HT neuron is shown with its dendrites (D), soma, axon in myelinated (Ax) and unmyelinated portions with synaptic and nonsynaptic boutons. The intracellular organelles associated with these processes are indicated: Golgi apparatus (Go), lysosomes (ly), mitochondria (m), microtubules (t), multivesicular bodies (mv), smooth endoplasmic reticulum (ser), granular endoplasmic reticulum (ger), tubular vesicles (tv), small vesicles (sv), and large granular vesicles (LGV).

represented in Figure 14. The evidence from fluorescence, immuno-cytochemical, and autoradiographic studies shows that 5HT is syn-thesized and packaged for transport and release in the smooth endo-plasmic reticulum, rough endoplasmic reticulum and Golgi apparatus, stored and transported in large granular vesicles, multivesicular bodies and on microtubules and filaments to peripheral dendritic and axonal processes. How much 5HT is in soluble form in the cytosol is not known. Release presumably takes place at synaptic and nonsynaptic terminals; uptake principally at the terminals and at dendrites and the cell body as well. Synthesis and packaging of transmitter probably occurs in the axon terminals as well as elsewhere in the smooth endoplasmic reticulum. Catabolism of 5HT is demonstrably associated with the mitochondria throughout the cell and its processes, and probably also involves multivesicular bodies, lysosomes, and the cytosol.

The Role of Synaptic Vesicles. In the cell body, generally only large granular vesicles are found, usually labeled by $^3$H-5HT uptake. However, the total number of somatic large granular vesicles is usually small and they are as a rule inconspicuous. Their presence cannot be used as a hallmark for 5HT neurons since similar vesicles in comparable numbers exist in non-indoleamine-containing cells as well. In the 5HT axonal boutons, there is a remarkable variety of vesicle populations: small pleomorphic, clear or granular, large granular, large granular alveolate, and small tubular profiles. The nonsynaptic boutons are generally associated with the unusual small tubular profiles. The synaptic boutons have a large number of different synaptic vesicle morphologies (see Summary in Table 3). Regardless of the presence or absence of the morphology of the small vesicles, all these axons contain LGV. This can be exclusively LGV or there may be a small number of smaller vesicles scattered in the axoplasm. Seemingly, LGV may be the only consistent feature in all 5HT axons; however, even they vary in morphology, size, and content from one 5HT axon to another. Presum-ably all vesicular forms have something to do with 5HT storage, transport, release and uptake, but their precise roles remain to be elucidated.

In summary, this report has explored and presented new evidence concerning the cytological correlates for synthesis, packaging, transport, uptake, and catabolism of 5HT. The 5HT system has been selected as only one example of several transmitters which can be submitted to this type of cytological, cytochemical, immunological, and cytopharmacological scrutiny. The glutamate, gamma-amino butyric acid, norepinephrine, and dopamine systems can be fruitfully examined in a similar fashion.

## ACKNOWLEDGEMENTS

Supported in part by US Public Health Service Grants NS 10536 and NS 03659 and Training Grant NS 05591 from the National Institute of Neurological and Communicative Disorders and Stroke. It is a pleasure to thank Mr. H. Cook for photographic assistance, and Ms. T. Van Itallie, J. Hilsz, J. Parsons and J. Smith for their invaluable help in this work. I am grateful to Dr. J. Andrezik for the use of his model reconstruction of the PGCL nucleus for Figure 1; to Dr. G. Jonsson, Karolinska Institute for the use of Figures 2a,c from our collaborative unpublished data, and to May and Baker for the Clorgyline.

## REFERENCES

Aghajanian, G.K., Bloom, F.E., Lovell, R.A., Sheard, M.H., and Freedman, D.X., 1966, The uptake of 5-hydroxytryptamine-$^3$H from the cerebral ventricles: autoradiographic localization, Biochem. Pharm. 15:1401-1403.

Andrezik, J.A., and Chan-Palay, V., 1977, The nucleus paragigantocellularis lateralis (PGCL): Definition and afferents, Anat. Rec. 184:524-525.

Andrezik, J.A., Chan-Palay, V., and Palay, S.L., 1977, The nucleus paragigantocellularis lateralis in Rat. Its morphology and afferents as demonstrated by retrograde transport of horseradish peroxidase, Exptl. Brain Res., in press.

Bloom, F.E., 1973, Ultrastructural identification of catecholamine-containing central synaptic terminals, J. Histochem. Cytochem. 21:333-348.

Bloom,F.E., Hoffer, B.J., Siggins, G.R., Barker, J.L., and Nicoll, R.A., 1972, Effects of serotonin on central neurons: Microiontophoretic administration. Fed. Proc. 31:97-106.

Calas, A., Besson, M.J., Gaughy, G., Alonso, G., Glowinski, J., and Cheramy, A., 1976, Radioautographic study of in vivo incorporation of $^3$H-monoamines in the cat caudate nucleus: identification of serotoninergic fibers. Brain Res. 118:1-13.

Chan-Palay, V., 1975, Fine structure of labelled axons in the cerebellar cortex and nuclei of rodents and primates after intraventricular infusions with tritiated serotonin. Anat. Embryol. 148:235-265.

Chan-Palay, V., 1976, Serotonin axons in the supra-and subependymal plexuses and in the leptomeninges; their roles in local alterations of cerebrospinal fluid and vasomotor activity, Brain Res. 102:103-130.

Chan-Palay, V., 1977a, "Cerebellar Dentate Nucleus; Organization, Cytology and Transmitters", Springer Verlag, Berlin, Heidelberg, New York.

Chan-Palay, V., 1977b, Demonstration of indoleamine neurons and
    their processes in the rat brain and their loss in chronic diet-
    induced thiamine deficiency, J. comp. Neurol., in press.
Chan-Palay, V., 1977c, The paratrigeminal nucleus.  II. Identifica-
    tion and interrelations of catecholamine, indoleamine axons
    and Substance P immunoreactive cells in the neuropil,
    J. Neurocytol., in press.
Cooper, J.R., Bloom, F.E., and Roth, R.H., 1974, "The Biochemical
    Basis of Neuropharmacology", pp. 175-201, Oxford University
    Press, New York.
Couch,J.R., 1970, Responses of neurons in the raphe nuclei to sero-
    tonin, norepinephrine and acetylcholine and their correlation
    with an excitatory synaptic input.  Brain Res. 19:137-150.
Dahlström, A., and Fuxe, K., 1964, Evidence for the existence of
    monoamine-containing neurons in the central nervous system.
    I. Demonstration of monoamines in the cell bodies of brain stem
    neurons.  Acta physiol. scand., Vol. 62, Suppl. 232:3-56.
Descarries, L., Beaudet, A., and Watkins, K.C., 1975, Serotonin
    nerve terminals in adult rat neocortex, Brain Res. 100:563-588.
Fuxe, K., and Ungerstedt, U., 1968, Histochemical studies on the
    distribution of catecholamines and 5-hydroxytryptamine after
    intraventricular injections, Histochemie 13:16-28.
Fuxe, K., Hökfelt, T., Ritzén, M., and Ungerstedt, U., 1968, Studies
    on uptake of intraventricularly administered  tritiated nora-
    drenaline and 5-hydroxytryptamine with combined fluorescence
    histochemical and autoradiographic techniques, Histochemie
    16:186-194.
Joh, T.H., Shikimi, T., Pickel, V.M., Reis, D.J., 1975, Brain
    tryptophan hydroxylase: purification of production of antibodies
    to, and cellular and ultrastructural localization in serotonergic
    neurons of rat midbrain, Proc. Natl. Acad. Sci. USA  72:3575-3579.
Léger, L., and Descarries, L., 1976, The serotonin innervation of
    rat locus coeruleus: axon terminals with a special type of pre-
    synaptic organelle, Soc. Neuroscience (Abstract).
Mouren-Mathieu, A.M., Léger, L., and Descarries, L., 1976, Radio-
    autographic visualization of central monoamine neurons after
    local instillation of tritiated serotonin and norepinephrine in
    adult cat, Soc. Neuroscience Abstracts, Vol. II, Part 1, pg. 497.
Pickel, V.M., Joh, T.H., and Reis, D.J., 1976, Monoamine synthesizing
    enzymes in central dopaminergic, noradrenergic and serotonergic
    neurons.  Immunocytochemical localization by light and electron
    microscopy.  J. Histochem. Cytochem. 24:792-806.
Pickel, V.M., Joh, T.H., and Reis, D.J., 1977, A serotonergic
    innervation of noradrenergic neurons in nucleus locus coeruleus:
    demonstration by immunocytochemical localization of the trans-
    mitter specific enzymes tyrosine and tryptophan hydroxylase,
    Brain Res., in press.
Robert, E., Chase, T.N., and Tower, D.B., 1976, "GABA in Nervous
    System Function", Kroc Foundation Series, Vol. 5, Raven Press,
    New York.

Sternberger, L., 1974, "Immunocytochemistry", Foundations of Immun-
    ology Series, (A. Osler and L. Weiss, eds)., pg. 171, Prentice
    Hall Inc., New Jersey.
Tennyson, V.M., Heikkila, R., Mytilineou, C., Cote, L., and Cohen,
    G., 1974, 5-hydroxydopamine 'tagged' neuronal boutons in rabbit
    neostriatum: interrelationship between vesicles and axonal
    membranes, Brain Res. 82:341-348.

# COMMENTS ON THE MORPHOLOGY OF INHIBITORY AXONS

Fred Walberg

Anatomical Institute, University of Oslo

Karl Johansgt. 47, Oslo 1, Norway

This review will deal with experimental studies made in our and other laboratories concerning the morphology of Purkinje axon terminals and other boutons using GABA as their transmitter.

Our own studies started with experiments on cats where ablations were made of various parts of the cerebellar cortex, and where the ensuing fiber degeneration in the vestibular and cerebellar nuclei was studied with silver techniques, especially the modifications of Nauta and Fink-Heimer.

These early light microscopical findings (Walberg et al., 1958) show that the Purkinje cell axons were distributed to the dorsal region only of the lateral and the adjacent part of the descending vestibular nuclei. What at that time was thought to be the degenerating boutons appeared to make contact with all types of cells with the great majority of the synapses on giant cells. However, later investigations have shown that interpretation of findings within silver stained sections studied in the light microscope must be made with great caution, especially since degenerating fiber systems vary greatly in their affinity to silver (see Walberg, 1971, 1972 for references).

The observations made in the light microscope of the operated animals revealed a similar localized distribution of the Purkinje cell axons within the cerebellar nuclei (Walberg and Jansen, 1964). Subsequent studies by other authors and in various species have given further details in the very precise terminal distribution of these fibers (Eager, 1966, 1969; Courville et al., 1973; Haikes, 1975a,b, 1976; Courville and Diakiw, 1976).

What are then the ultrastructural characteristics of the
Purkinje axon boutons in the cat in the nuclei here mentioned?

Let us first consider the ultrastructure of normal boutons in
the vestibular nuclei, especially the lateral vestibular nucleus
(the nucleus of Deiters). Our electronmicroscopical analysis of
this nucleus (Mugnaini et al., 1967) revealed that there are great
variations as to the morphology of the axonal knobs. All the
different types of boutons are in synaptic contact with neuronal
perikarya, dendritic trunks, small dendrites or dendritic spines,
and do not show any specific preference in distribution as regards postsynaptic structures. Of particular interest is that some
boutons form synapses both with dendrites and perikarya. In such
instances the bouton to body synapse may resemble Gray's type 1,
while the other may have an appearance like type 2.

The ultrastructural features of the boutons in the cerebellar
nuclei of the cat are largely similar. In an extensive study
Angaut and Sotelo (1973) have described three boutontypes, medium
sized, large and climbing-like. The most common type is the medium
sized bouton, and more than 87% of the total population belong to
this type. Most of the medium sized boutons have round vesicles,
some have flattened or pleomorphic shapes. The active zones of the
medium sized boutons are, however, not related to the shape of the
vesicular population. Medium sized boutons can have an active zone
of type 1 on one side and of type 2 on the other side, while the
synaptic vesicles are of the round variety. Other boutons with
flattened vesicles can show synapses of type 1. Thus, arrangement
found in the cerebellar nuclei of the cat is similar to that found
in the vestibular nuclei in the same species (Mugnaini et al.,
1967).

No identification of the Purkinje axon terminals was made in
the above mentioned ultrastructural studies of normal cats. Such
an identification has, however, been attempted in the rat by Chan-
Palay (1973). Of the six classes of boutons observed in the cerebellar nuclei of this animal, the most numerous belongs to the
axons of the Purkinje cell. 98% of the vesicles in these boutons
were said to be elliptical, and the synaptic junction of an intermediate type.

A secure identification of the Purkinje axon boutons can be
made in animals where tracer techniques are used. However, before
referring to such investigations, a brief survey will be given of
the microchemical investigations indicating that GABA is the putative transmitter of the Purkinje cells. In these studies (Fonnum
et al, 1970) we compared the activity of glutamate decarboxylase
(GAD) with the distribution of the Purkinje axon terminals in the
cat. Corresponding to the morphological finding that the Purkinje

cells axons terminate in the dorsal, but not in the ventral part
of the lateral vestibular nucleus, the level of GAD was more than
two times higher (per dry weight) in the dorsal than in the ventral
part. When Purkinje cells in the vermis in the anterior cerebellar
lobe were destroyed, 50 to 70% of the GAD activity was lost dorsally,
whereas it was unaltered in the ventral part of the lateral vestibular nucleus. Destruction of the Purkinje cells in the left cerebellar hemisphere that send their axons to the left nucleus interpositus, resulted in a 70% loss of activity in the left, but not in
the right nucleus interpositus where the activity was similar to
that found in unoperated animals. Similar conclusions with somewhat different techniques have been made by Obata (1969), Okada and
Shimada (1976), and Otsuka et al., (1971).

Turning now to the experiments made with tracer techniques, injections of tritiated leucine into the left paramedian lobule and
adjacent part of the vermis of the cat permitted an identification
of Purkinje axon boutons in the cerebellar nuclei (Walberg et al.,
1976). In this study synaptic vesicles with width to length ratios
from 1:1 were classified as round, those with ratios 1:1,1 - 1:1,7
as elliptical, all others as flat. This classification is similar
to that used by Chan-Palay (1973) in the above mentioned study in
the rat.

Our analysis revealed that Purkinje axon boutons have a pleomorphic vesicle population. The test for skewness shows, furthermore, that the boutons fall in two groups with rather homogeneous
vesicle populations. The first group consists of 78% of the
boutons, the other of 8% of the boutons.[1]

The frequency histogram made from the main group of boutons
(78%) shows that the majority of the synaptic vesicles in this group
has a ratio from 1:1,1 - 1:1,7, the smallest average diameter of
the vesicles being 340 Å, the largest average diameter 440 Å. Such
vesicles therefore belong to the category elliptical. Flattened
vesicles with a ratio above 1:1,7 (smallest average diameter 250 Å,
largest average diameter 500 Å) are few compared to the round or
slightly ovoid type of vesicle.

The frequency histogram of the round vesicle profiles (ratio
1:1) shows that the majority of the round vesicles have a size from
340 - 400 Å, and that therefore the round vesicles are not crosscut

---

[1]  The group constituting 8% of the boutons has synaptic vesicles
of the round type. Whether this means that the boutons of this
group belong to a separate population of Purkinje cells is not
known.

profiles of cylindrical synaptic vesicles. We were, however, not
able to show whether some of the "round" vesicles actually are
elliptical or disc-shaped structures seen from above, since stereo-
scopical studies of the type made by Gray and Willis (1968) and
Dennison (1971) were not performed. However, it should in this
context be stressed that Chan-Palay (1973) on her material from
normal rats with a solution differing from ours, but with almost
similar tonicity, shows a frequency histogram for the ellipticity
of synaptical vesicles almost similar to ours.

Do the findings made by Chan-Palay (1973) on normal rats and
our investigation with tracer techniques on cats support the theory
that excitatory boutons have synaptic vesicles of the round type,
and that inhibitory boutons have flattened vesicles (Uchizono, 1965)?
If definitions as round, elliptical and cylindrical are used, the
authors who use such expressions should clearly give the criteria
they base their definitions on. Furthermore, they should make statistical analyses of the type made by Chan-Palay (1973) and by Walberg
et al., (1976). Referring to our own findings, round means vesicles
with a ratio 1:1, elliptical vesicles with a ratio 1:1,1 - 1:1,7,
cylindrical vesicles with ratios above 1:1,7. With this definition
the large majority of synaptic vesicles in the Purkinje axon terminals (73%) in the main type of boutons in the cat (78% of all boutons
measured) are elliptical. Cylindrical vesicles represent 19% of the
vesicle population, round vesicles 8% of the total population. If
slightly ovoid vesicles (ratio up to 1:1,3) are included in the
category round, then the number of "round" vesicles in the boutons
increases to 14%. Vesicles with ratios up to 1:1,3 are usually by
morphologists called round.

Another factor making generalizations impossible is the observation that flattening of vesicles is a result of the osmolarity of
the buffer solution used in the fixative or during processing of the
tissue (Bodian, 1970; Valdivia, 1971; Korneliussen, 1972). Direct
comparisons of the results obtained in various laboratories can
therefore scarcely be made. Referring to this difficulty, it has
recently been stressed that vesicle size rather than shape in the
crayfish stretch receptor organs should be emphasized as the important parameter (Tisdale and Makajima, 1976).

Roberts and coworkers have with immunocytochemical methods
likewise shown that generalizations are hazardous. In their elegant
investigations GAD was in rats localized both light and electron
microscopically. McLaughlin et al., (1975) observed in the spinal
cord GAD-containing boutons presynaptic to dendrites and cell bodies
in the dorsal and ventral horns, a finding compatible with the assumption that GABA boutons may mediate postsynaptic inhibition of
spinal interneurons and motoneurons. GAD-positive boutons presynaptic other boutons were also observed in the dorsal horn and motor

nuclei, a finding in agreement with the suggestion that GABA may be the transmitter mediating synaptic inhibition via axoaxonal synapses in the spinal cord. Of great interest was that several of the labelled boutons had predominantly round synaptic vesicles, and that some of them showed symmetrical, others asymmetrical synaptic contacts. From these findings it was concluded that the vesicle shape and the morphology of synaptic contacts not per se necessarily indicate synaptic action, and that these features not necessarily are related to the type of synaptic transmitter or its synthesizing enzyme.

In a subsequent publication the immuno-peroxidase method was applied to the substantia nigra (Ribak et al., 1976). Large amounts of the GAD-positive reaction product was present throughout this region. Most of the boutons were positive, and established axodendritic and axosomatic synapses. Symmetric as well as asymmetric synaptic junctions were found, with the former being the most frequent type. The authors counted and categorized 60 different GAD-positive boutons in random electron micrographs from substantia nigra. Their data show that about 85% of GAD-positive terminals form symmetric synaptic junctions, approximately 15% form asymmetric junctions. The authors conclude that there is need for caution when students want to speculate upon functional aspects of synapses solely on the basis of their ultrastructural characteristics. An equally restrictive attitude has recently been taken by Duncal et al., (1970), who made a thorough investigation of vesicle shape and size in the cerebellar nuclei of normal hamsters. They conclude that in the hamster's cerebellum size and shape of synaptic vesicles do not allow for a distinction between excitatory and inhibitory synapses.

Let me also recall that as concerns the study of the ultrastructural distribution of acetylcholinesterase, McDonald and Rasmussen (1971) from studies of the cochlear nuclei conclude that boutons with cholinesterase activity can have round or flattened vesicles, and that the shape of synaptic vesicles in boutons cannot be used as a parameter "which is useful in predicting if nerve endings will have histochemical evidence of AChE activity". (Loc.cit. p. 16). Similar conclusions are reached by Westrum and Broderson (1976), who studied the spinal trigeminal nucleus. Furthermore, Ritter and coworkers (1974) made the same statement after a study of the hippocampal region.

The recent observation by Kuffler (1977) should likewise be recalled. In the cardiac ganglion of vertebrates the same transmitter, acetylcholine, acting on two different types of chemo-receptors, has two distinct effects on the postsynaptic membrane. Acetylcholine can therefore evoke excitation and inhibition in individual neurons, another finding warning against generalizations.

## REFERENCES

Angaut, P., and Sotelo, C., 1973, The fine structure of the cerebellar central nuclei in the cat II. Synaptic organization, Exp. Brain Res., 16:431-454.

Bodian, D., 1970, An electron microscopic characterization of classes of synaptic vesicles by means of controlled aldehyde fixation, J. Cell Biol., 44:115-124.

Chan-Palay, V., 1973, On the identification of the afferent axon terminals in the nucleus lateralis of the cerebellum. An electron microscope study, Z. Anat. Entwickl.-Gesch., 142: 149-186.

Courville, J., and Diakiw, N., 1976, Cerebellar corticonuclear projection in the cat. The vermis of the anterior and posterior lobes, Brain Res., 110:1-20.

Courville, J., Diakiw, N., and Brodal, A., 1973, Cerebellar corticonuclear projection in the cat. The paramedian lobule. An experimental study with silver methods, Brain Res., 50: 25-45.

Dennison, M.E., 1971, Electron stereoscopy as a means of classifying synaptic vesicles, J. Cell Sci., 8:525-539.

Duncan, D., Morales, R., and Benignus, V.A., 1970, Shapes and sizes of synaptic vesicles in the cerebellum of the Syrian hamster-cortex and deep nuclei, Anat. Rec., 168:1-8.

Eager, R.P., 1966, Patterns and mode of termination of cerebellar corticonuclear pathways in the monkey (Macaca mulatta), J. comp. Neurol., 126:551-566.

Eager, R.P., 1969, Modes of termination of Purkinje cell axons in the cerebellum of the cat, in "Neurobiology of Cerebellar Evolution and Development" (R. Llinas, ed.) pp. 585-601, American Medical Association. Education & Research Foundation, Chicago.

Fonnum, F., Storm-Mathisen, J., and Walberg, F., 1970, Glutamate decarboxylase in inhibitory neurons. A study of the enzyme in Purkinje cell axons and boutons in the cat, Brain Res., 20:259-275.

Gray, E.G., and Willis, R.A., 1968, Problems of electron stereoscopy of biological tissues. J. Cell. Sci., 3:309-326.

Haines, D.E., 1975a, Cerebellar corticovestibular fibers of the posterior lobe in a prosimian primate, the lesser bushbaby (Galago senegalensis), J. comp. Neurol., 160:363-398.

Haines, D.E., 1975b, Cerebellar cortical efferents of the posterior lobe vermis in a prosimian primate (Galago) and the tree shrew (Tupaia), J. comp. Neurol., 163:21-40.

Haines, D.E., 1976, Cerebellar corticonuclear and corticovestibular fibers of the anterior lobe vermis in a prosimian primate (Galago senegalensis). J. comp. Neurol., 170:67-96.

Korneliussen, H., 1972, Elongated profiles of synaptic vesicles in motor endplates. Morphological effects of fixative variations, J. Neurocytol., 1:279-296.

Kuffler, S.W., 1977, Synaptic excitation and inhibition, XXVIIth
    Int. Congr. of Phys. Sciences.
McDonald, D.M., and Rasmussen, G.L., 1971, Ultrastructural charac-
    teristics of synaptic endings in the cochlear nucleus having
    acetylcholinesterase activity, Brain Res., 28:1-18.
McLaughlin, B.J., Barber, R., Saito, K., Roberts, E., and Wu, J.Y.,
    1975, Immunocytochemical localization of glutamate decar-
    boxylase in rat spinal cord, J. comp. Neurol., 164:305-322.
Mugnaini, E., Walberg, F., and Hauglie-Hanssen, E., 1967, Observa-
    tions on the fine structure of the lateral vestibular nucleus
    (Deiters' nucleus) in the cat, Exp. Brain Res., 4:146-186.
Obata, K., 1969, Gamma-aminobutyric acid in Purkinje cells and
    motoneurones. Experientia 25:1283.
Okada, Y., and Shimada, C., 1976, Gamma-aminobutyric acid (GABA)
    concentration in a single neuron - localization of GABA in
    Deiters' neuron, Brain Res., 107:658-662.
Otsuka, M., Obata, K., Miyata, Y., and Tanaka, Y., 1971, Measure-
    ment of aminobutyric acid in isolated nerve cells of cat central
    nervous system, J. Neurochem., 18:287-295.
Ribak, C.E., Vaughn, J.E., Saito, K., Barber, R., and Roberts, E.,
    1976, Immunocytochemical localization of glutamate decarbocy-
    lase in rat substantia nigra, Brain Res., 116:287-298.
Ritter, J., Wenzel, J., Daniel, H., and Duwe, G., 1974, Zur elektron-
    mikroskopischen Darstellung von Acetylcholinesterase in
    Neuronen und Synapsen des Zentralen und peripheren Nervensys-
    tems, Acta histochem., 49:176-203.
Tisdale, A.D. and Nakajima, Y., 1976, Fine structures of synaptic
    vesicles in two types of nerve terminals in crayfish stretch
    receptor organs: influence of fixation methods, J. comp. Neurol.,
    165:369-386.
Uchizono, K., 1965, Characteristics of excitatory and inhibitory
    synapses in the central nervous system of the cat, Nature 207:
    242-243.
Valdivia, O., 1971, Methods of fixation and the morphology of syn-
    aptic vesicles, J. comp. Neurol., 142:257-274.
Walberg, F., 1971, Does silver impregnate normal and degenerating
    boutons?  A study based on light and electron microscopical
    observations of the inferior olive, Brain Res., 31:47-65.
Walberg, F., 1972, Further studies of silver impregnation of normal
    and degenerating boutons.  A light and electron microscopical
    investigation of a filamentous degenerating system, Brain Res.,
    36:353-369.
Walberg, F., Bowsher, D., and Brodal, A., 1958, The termination of
    primary vestibular fibers in the vestibular nuclei in the cat.
    An experimental study with silver methods.  J. comp. Neurol.,
    110:391-419.
Walberg, F., and Jansen, J., 1964, Cerebellar corticonuclear projec-
    tion studied experimentally with silver impregnation methods,
    J. Hirnforsch., 6:338-354.

Walberg, F., Holländer, H., and Grofová, I., 1976, An autoradiographic identification of Purkinje axon terminals in the cat,
J. Neurocytol., 5:157-169.
Westrum, L.E., and Broderson, S.H., 1976, Acetylcholinesterase
activity of synaptic structures in the spinal trigeminal
nucleus, J. Neurocytol., 5:551-563.

# ULTRASTRUCTURAL ANALYSIS OF AXO-DENDRITIC INITIAL COLLATERAL TERMINALS OF A FELINE SPINOCERVICAL TRACT NEURONE, STAINED INTRACELLULARLY WITH HORSERADISH PEROXIDASE

Jonas Rastad

Department of Anatomy, University of Uppsala

Box 571, S-751 23 Uppsala, Sweden

The introduction of intracellular staining methods in neuro-biology has provided possibilities for extensive light and electron microscopical studies of single neurones. Intracellular administration of horseradish peroxidase (Jankowska et al., 1976; Snow et al., 1976) has, in this respect, proven superior to other intracellular stains, since the enzyme rapidly distributes in neuronal processes visualizing both dendritic and axonal arborizations, including terminals of initial axon collaterals (Cullheim and Kellerth, 1976; Rastad, 1976; Rastad et al., in press). Thus ultrastructural investigations of initial axon collaterals of lumbar feline spinocervical tract (SCT) cells have demonstrated boutons with axo-dendritic, axo-somatic and axo-axonal synapses (Rastad, 1976; Rastad et al., in press) situated in the same or neighbouring segments of the spinal cord. The purposes of the present study were to investigate the appearance of axo-dendritic initial collateral terminals of a feline spinocervical tract cell, stained intracellularly with horseradish peroxidase (HRP), and to quantitatively analyse the extent of ultrastructural differences between terminals originating from one functionally characterized neurone.

The general method of intracellular staining of SCT cells with HRP has been described elsewhere (Jankowska et al., 1976; Rastad et al., in press). It is, however, important to emphasize the processes, which particularly affect the present results. The cat was thus transcardially perfused with a 3 litre mixture of 2 % glutaraldehyde and 1 % formaldehyde in 0.15M sodium cacodylate buffer. The appropriate part of the lumbar enlargement was dissected out and kept in the same fixative, as used for the perfusion, for about 7 h, before a 3 h rinse in 0.15M sodium cacodylate buffer. Transverse sections, about 80-120 µm thick, were cut by means of a tissue sectioner and incubated for peroxidase reaction (Grahman and Karnovsky 1966). After a brief rinse in 0.15M sodium cacodylate buffer, the sections were post-fixated for 15-20 min in a 1 % solution of osmium tetroxide in 0.15M sodium cacodylate buffer. They were then dehydrated and embedded in Epon 812. The method of embedding has been described elsewhere (Rastad et al., in press). The sections were placed between transparent acetate foils and allowed to polymerize. Stained structures were photographed in the light microscope and camera lucida drawings were made. Consecutive drawings of the cell and its processes were matched together. Sections containing stained profiles of interest for ultrastructural analysis were then "re-embedded" (Holländer, 1970) and cut in ultrathin serial sections.

The series of ultrathin sections were systematically investigated for histochemically stained structures. A stained axo-dendritic terminal was defined as an enlarged neuronal profile containing the enzyme reaction product, accumulated synaptic vesicles and exhibiting a synaptic contact with a dendrite. The series of sections through a stained bouton was searched for that with the maximal length of direct apposition, without intervenient profiles, between the terminal and its postsynaptic structure. When a terminal showed synaptic contacts with more than one neuronal profile, the section was used which demonstrated the longest of these apposition lengths. A terminal was thus defined as axo-dendritic if its longest apposition length was in contact with a dendrite. The section with the maximal apposition length was also used for the analyses of the bouton area densities of synaptic vesicles and mitochondria as well as for measurements of the sizes of synaptic vesicles.

Out of the total number of 92 axo-dendritic terminals a group of 25 were sampled at random. Estimations of the area densities of synaptic vesicles and mitochondria were made in each of these terminals. The calculations were made using the principle of point-counting (Weibel and Elias, 1967) on electron micrographs of total magnifications of about 95000x. The point sampling screen had points, 15 mm apart, evenly distributed in a quadratic pattern. The area densities of vesicles and mitochondria were estimated by dividing the number of points falling on these structures by the total number of points falling on the bouton.

The size of the synaptic vesicles of the 25 terminals was measured at magnifications of 120000-180000x. The longest and shortest perpendicular diameters of all distinguishable and non-overlapping synaptic vesicles were calculated. The ratio of the diameters of each vesicle was estimated by dividing the longest diameter by the shortest (Chan-Palay, 1973).

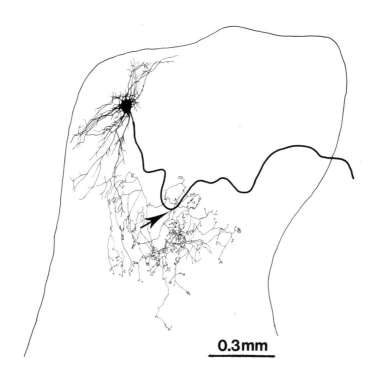

0.3mm

FIGURE 1.Schematic reconstruction of the dendritic and initial collateral arborizations of the SCT cell. The neurone was stained with
a micropipette with a tip diameter of 2 µm, filled with a 25 % solution of HRP (type II) dissolved in 0.2M sodium hydroxide. The cell
was injected by a constant depolarizing current of 10 nA, applied
for 28 min.Arrow points at the start of the collateral. 60x.

The cell body of the investigated SCT cell was situated in the
medial part of lamina III (Rexed, 1954) of the rostral end of segment
L 7 (Fig. 1). It had perpendicular diameters of 51x41 µm, as measured
on electron micrographs through the centre of the nucleolus. The
neurone showed no apparent ultrastructural damage (Jankowska et al.,
1976) following impalement of the electrode and administration of
the HRP.

The axon left the soma from its ventro-lateral aspect and showed
one initial collateral emerging at a distance of about 580 µm from
the cell body. The collateral branched extensively in laminae IV-VI
and some branches coursed among ventrally directed dendrites (Fig. 1).
The total length of all traced collateral branches amounted to about
10900 µm, and they were situated in a rostro-caudal domain of the

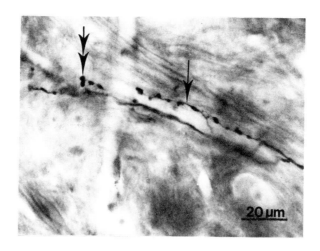

FIGURE 2: Light micrograph of stained collateral boutons (double
arrow). The terminals are aligned along a profile ultrastructurally
identified as a dendrite. The terminals are mainly boutons of
passage, connected by thin terminal axons (single arrow). 700x.


spinal cord of about 1000 μm. The collateral showed, by light
microscopy, a total of 274 terminal enlargements. These terminals
were mostly arranged in spherical groups of 3-12 terminals.
However, on one occasion, 26 boutons were seen aligned along a
profile (Fig. 2), which, in the electron microscope, proved as a
large dendrite. The ultrastructural appearance of the enzyme
reaction product in neuronal somata and prosesses has been described
elsewhere (Cullheim and Kellerth, 1976; Jankowska et al., 1976;
Rastad et al., in press).

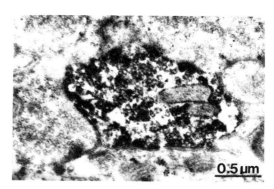

FIGURE 3. Electron micrograph of a stained axo-dendritic bouton.
28000x.

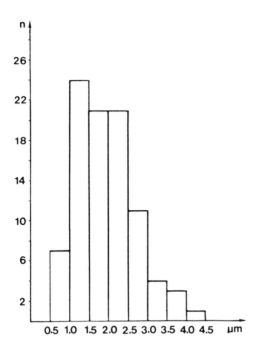

FIGURE 4. The distribution of the maximal apposition lengths of 92 axo-dendritic terminals, mean = 1.9 μm, SEM = 0.07.

A total of 92 axo-dendritic terminals was ultrastructurally analysed. They were seen in synaptic contact with dendrites (Fig. 3) with diameter ranges of 7.5 μm to 0.9 μm. The synaptic clefts showed a mean thickness of 29 nm (n=17), as measured in their widest parts, and the postsynaptic membrane thickenings were inconspicuous (Fig. 3). The synaptic clefts of heavily labelled terminals sometimes appeared to contain the enzyme reaction product. No precipitate was, in these regions, found elsewhere in the extracellular space. Such terminals were not included in the present investigation, as the enzyme reaction product concealed too much of the fine structure of the terminals.

The distribution of the maximal apposition lengths of the 92 terminals is shown in Fig. 4. They ranged from 4.3 μm to 0.8 μm with a mean value of 1.9 μm. The area densities of synaptic vesicles and mitochondria were analysed in the randomized group of terminals and showed mean values of 25 % and 19 %, respectively (Fig. 5).

A total of 1800 synaptic vesicles was analysed for length and width. All vesicles were devoid of dense cores. The distribution of maximal diameters and diameter ratios of the investigated vesicles

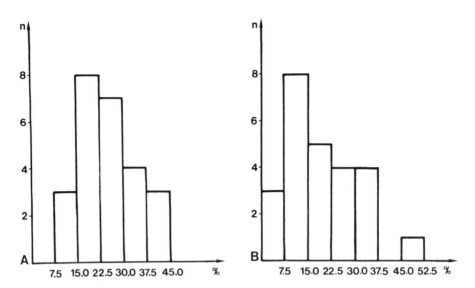

FIGURE 5. The distribution of the area densities of synaptic
vesicles (A) and mitochondria (B) of 25 axo-dendritic terminals.
Synaptic vesicles: mean = 25.1 %, SEM = 1.85. Mitochondria: mean =
18.7 %, SEM = 2.12.

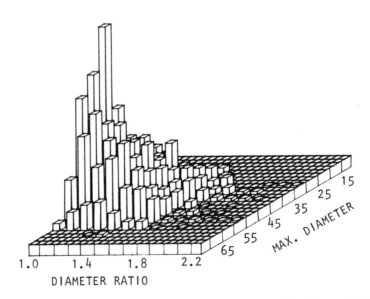

FIGURE 6. The two dimensional frequency-distribution of the maximal
diameters and diameter ratios of 1800 synaptic vesicles of 25 terminals. The highest single staple represents 125 vesicles.

is shown in Fig. 6. The number of measured vesicles per bouton varied between 20 to 178 (mean=72). Vesicles exhibiting diameter ratios of 1.0 were, in the investigated projection, regarded as round (Dennison, 1971; Chan-Palay, 1973; Walberg et al., 1976). These round vesicles constituted about 21 % of the total population. Their diameters showed extreme values of 61 and 20 nm and an average of 43 nm. The largest group of vesicles (about 76 %) had diameter ratios of 1.1 - 1.7. These were designated as elliptical (Chan-Palay, 1973), and showed a largest average diameter of 46 nm and a smallest of 36 nm. About 3 % of the vesicles showed diameter ratios of 1.8 - 2.3 and were regarded as flat (Chan-Palay, 1973). This group showed  mean  longest and shortest diameters of 44 nm and 24 nm, respectively.

The longest diameter of each vesicle was used for one-way analyses of variance, which were performed within the three classes of diameter ratios. None of these groups showed significant variations (p $<0.05$) between  the terminals.

The method of intracellular staining with HRP is unique in the respect that it provides possibilities for morphological analysis of populations of axon terminals originating from a single functionally identified neuron. When investigating the ultra-structural differences between such terminals it is important to emphasize some aspects of the technique.

The ultrastructural identification of stained boutons primarely depends on the presence of the enzyme reaction product. This precipitate partly conceals the bouton ultrastructure and thus reduces the possibilities for discrimination of terminals on the basis of their fine structure, as the appearance and arrangement of axoplasmic matrix, microtubules, neurofilaments as well as pre- and intersynaptic characteristics (Palay and Chan-Palay, 1973; Chan-Palay, 1973). The number of boutons available for investigations mainly relies on the extent of the light microscopical visualization of the collateral ramifications. This might be incomplete, since some branches, in reconstructions of axon collaterals (cf. Fig. 1 and Rastad et al., in press), lack terminal enlargements. This could be due to the complexity of collateral ramifications, making exact matching of consecutive drawings somewhat difficult, or to uneven cellular distribution of the administered HRP. The latter might occur since the amount of enzyme reaction product differs in stained terminals. It has also been assumed that weakly stained boutons  remain undetected by light microscopy (Rastad et al., in press). In addition, it appears as if the  substrate migration is limited within sections, since sometimes stained main axons of motoneurones (S. Cullheim, personal communication) and SCT-cells (J. Rastad, unpublished observations), in transversing a section, only are visualized in its superficial parts.

The results of the present investigation concerning the distribution of the apposition lengths of the axo-dendritic terminals suggest that the forms or sizes of their apposition surfaces differ in appearance from botuon to bouton. Interestingly, preliminary results have indicated statistically significant differences between the maximal apposition lengths of axo-dendritic and axo-somatic terminals of this SCT neurone. The area densities of mitochondria showed a wide range. Due to the procedure of sampling of the areas of these measurements, with an over-representation of organellas close to the post-synaptic structure, this large variation does not have to imply equally large variations in the actual volume densities of mitochondria. The study of single synaptic vesicles indicates the presence of different vesicular forms and sizes. The analyses of variance suggest small differences in the vesicular populations of the different boutons.

The investigated neuron was subjected to several hours of artificial stimulation both prior to, during and after the enzyme administration. This has been shown to alter the bouton fine structure in several ways (for references see Cohen, 1973). Accordingly, a depletion and an increased flattening of synaptic vesicles (Korneliussen et al., 1972), an increase in bouton apposition lengths (Pysh and Wiley, 1972) and a decrease in areas of axon terminals (Fifkova and Van Harreveld, 1977) have been reported. Thus the interpretation of the present results of vesicular area densities and sizes is complex. In addition, increased flattening of synaptic vesicles has been observed as a result of many preparatory steps (Walberg, 1966; Bodian, 1970; Valdivia, 1971; Korneliussen, 1972), of which some were used in the present investigation.

The demonstration of locally ramifying initial collaterals of SCT neurones indicates that these cells may not only be involved in forwarding information to supraspinal centres (for references see Brown, 1973), but also in mediating various spinal reflexes (see Rastad et al., in press). Conclusions, about the possible functional significance of such reflex activity, will have to await future studies. It is, however, interesting to note that preliminary investigations have shown satisfactorily stained and preserved SCT neurones, lacking initial collaterals arising from the first millimeters of the stem axon.

## ACKNOWLEDGEMENTS

The author is greatly indebted to Dr S. Griph for valuable advice concerning the statistical evaluation of the material. This study was supported by the Swedish Medical Research Council (project no B78-12X-02710-10A).

REFERENCES

Bodian, D., 1970, An electron microscopic characterization of classes of synaptic vesicles by means of controlled aldehyde fixation, J.Cell Biol. 44:115-124.

Brown, A.G., 1973, Ascending and long spinal pathways: dorsal columns, spinocervical tract and spinothalamic tract, in "Handbook of Sensory Physiology. Somatosensory System," Vol.II (A. Iggo, ed.), Springer Verlag, Heidelberg, pp. 315-338.

Chan-Palay, V., 1973, On the identification of the afferent axon terminals in the nucleus lateralis of the cerebellum. An electron microscope study, Z.Anat.Entwickl.-Gesch. 142:149-186.

Cohen, L.B., 1973, Changes in neuron structure during action potential propagation and synaptic transmission, Physiol.Rev. 53:373-418.

Cullheim, S., and Kellerth, J.-O., 1976, Combined light and electron microscopic tracing of neurons, including axons and synaptic terminals, after intracellular injection of horseradish peroxidase. Neurosci.Lett. 2:307-313.

Dennison, M.E., 1971, Electron stereoscopy as a means of classifying synaptic vesicles, J.Cell Sci. 8:525-539.

Fifková, E., and Van Harreveld, A., 1977, Long-lasting morphological changes in dendritic spines of dentate granular cells following stimulation of the entorhinal area, J.Neurocytol. 6:211-230.

Graham, R.C., and Karnovsky, M.J., 1966, The early stage of absorption of injected horseradish peroxidase in the proximal tubules of mouse kidney: ultrastructural cytochemistry by a new technique, J.Histochem.Cytochem. 14:291-302.

Holländer, H., 1970, The section embedding (SE) technique. A new method for the combined light microscopic and electron microscopic examination of central nervous tissue, Brain Res. 20:39-47.

Jankowska, E., Rastad, J., and Westman, J., 1976, Intracellular application of horseradish peroxidase and its light and electron microscopical appearance in spinocervical tract cells, Brain Res. 105:557-562.

Korneliussen, H., 1972, Elongated profiles of synaptic vesicles in motor endplates. Morphological effects of fixative variations, J.Neurocytol. 1:279-296.

Korneliussen, H., Barstad, J.A.B., and Lilleheil, G., 1972, Vesicle hypothesis: effect of nerve stimulation on synaptic vesicles of motor endplates, Experientia, 28:1055-1057.

Palay, S.L., and Chan-Palay, V., 1973, Cerebellar cortex, cytology and organization, Springer Verlag, Heidelberg.

Pysh, J.J., and Wiley, R.G., 1972, Morphologic alterations of synapses in electrically stimulated superior cervical ganglia of the cat, Science, 176:191-193.

Rastad, J., 1976, An ultrastructural study of axon collateral arborization of spinocervical tract cells intracellularly stained with horseradish peroxidase, J.Ultrastr.Res., 57:219.

Rastad, J., Jankowska, E., and Westman, J., Arborization of initial
    axon collaterals of spinocervical tract cells stained intra-
    cellularly with horseradish peroxidase, Brain Res. In press.
Rexed, B., 1954, A cytoarchitectonic atlas of the spinal cord in
    the cat, J.Comp.Neurol. 100:297-380.
Snow, P.J., Rose, P.K., and Brown, A.G., 1976, Tracing axons and
    axon collaterals of spinal neurons using intracellular injection
    of horseradish peroxidase, Science 191:312-313.
Valdivia, O., 1971, Methods of fixation and the morphology of
    synaptic vesicles, J.Comp.Neurol. 142:257-274.
Walberg, F., 1966, Elongated vesicles in terminal boutons of the
    central nervous system, a result of aldehyde fixation. Acta
    Anat. 65:224-235.
Walberg, F., Holländer, H., and Grofová, I., 1976, An autoradio-
    graphic identification of Purkinje axon terminals in the cat,
    J.Neurocytol. 5:157-169.
Weibel, E.R., and Elias, H., 1967, Introduction to stereologic
    principles, in "Quantitative Methods in Morphology," (E.R.
    Weibel, H.Elias, eds.), Springer Verlag, Heidelberg.

# ELECTRON CYTOCHEMISTRY OF GABA—TRANSAMINASE IN RAT CEREBELLAR CORTEX, AND EVIDENCE FOR MULTIMOLECULAR FORMS OF THE ENZYME

J.C. Hyde

Department of Anatomy, The London Hospital Medical

College, Turner Street, London E1 2AD, England

GABA-transaminase (GABA-T) can be localized histochemically in the CNS using the technique described by Van Gelder (1965) and adaptations thereof (Hyde and Robinson, 1976). Recently, this technique has been improved so that GABA-T can be localized at both light and electron microscopic levels in the same tissue preparations, and increased resolution of enzyme sites is achieved (Hyde and Robinson, 1976a).

For enzyme cytochemistry the CNS is perfused with 200 ml of a fixative consisting of 2% (v/v) formaldehyde and 2% (v/v) glutaraldehyde in 0.1M phosphate buffer, pH 7.4. Small blocks (1mm$^3$) of perfused nervous tissue are incubated in the following medium:

```
Tris-maleate buffer 0.1M, pH 7.6
GABA and α—ketoglutarate (disodium salt):      5.0  mg/ml
NAD⁺:                                           1.0  mg/ml
Nitro—blue tetrazolium:                         1.0  mg/ml
Sodium malonate:                                3.0  mg/ml
Sodium cyanide:                                 0.05 mg/ml
Phenozine methosulphate:                        0.05 mg/ml
Sodium chloride:                                7.2  mg/ml
Magnesium chloride:                             1.02 mg/ml
Triton X—100:                                   0.5% (v/v)
```

The tissues are washed in isotonic saline, fixed again in formaldehyde/glutaraldehyde (2%/2%), and then in 2% (w/v) osmium tetroxide, dehydrated and finally embedded in Araldite resin. Thin sections (2µm) are cut for light microscopy, or ultrathin sections (silver—gold) for electron microscopy. Methods can be found in more detail in Hyde and Robinson, 1976a.

GABA-T activity is seen as a blue formazan precipitate in
light microscopic studies, or as an electron dense precipitate in
electron microscopic studies. Formazan precipitation can be
completely inhibited by the addition of 5 µg/ml amino-oxyacetic
acid as GABA-T inhibitor, (Wallach, 1961) or by the absence of
GABA from the incubation medium.

Light microscopy of cerebellar cortex stained for GABA-T
activity (Fig.1) shows that in the upper molecular layer the
enzyme is localized in small nerve cell bodies identified as
stellate nerve cells by their morphology and position. GABA-T is
also found in filamentous processes, thought to be processes of
Bergmann glial cells, running from the Purkinje cell layer to the
pial surface, in basket nerve cells, in the pericellular baskets
at the base of Purkinje cells, and in glial cell bodies which
surround Purkinje nerve cells.

Electron microscopy supports the light microscope findings
and shows that the localization of GABA-T is mitochondrial, thus
substantiating earlier biochemical studies (for example,
Salganicoff and DeRobertis, 1965). Electron microscopy shows that
GABA-T is found within mitochondria of stellate nerve cells (Fig.2),
of basket nerve cells (Fig.3), of basket cell axons in the
Purkinje cell pericellular basket (Fig.4), and of astrocytic
glial cells (Fig.5), probably Bergmann glia, immediately adjacent
to Purkinje cell bodies.

What is the overall function of GABA-T in nerve and glial
cells in the cerebellar cortex?

Does glial cell GABA-T degrade neurotransmitter GABA which has
been taken up into their cell bodies?

Why is GABA-T found in pre-synaptic processes of probable
GABA neurones in the cerebellar cortex, for example, basket cell
axon terminals in the Purkinje cell pericellular basket?

---

The micron marker in Fig.1 is equivalent to 25µm, in Fig.2-5, 1µm.
Fig.1  stellate nerve cell(s); basket nerve cells(b); Bergmann
fibres (large arrows); Purkinje pericellular basket (large arrow-
heads); Purkinje cells(p); glial cells (small arrowheads).
Fig.2  stellate nerve cell(St); mitochondria (m-arrowheads).
Fig.3  basket nerve cell(BC); mitochondria (m-arrowheads).
Fig.4  Purkinje nerve cell(PC); basket cell axons (asterisk);
mitochondria (small arrowheads). This preparation was stained
with alkaline lead citrate for 30 seconds to increase contrast.

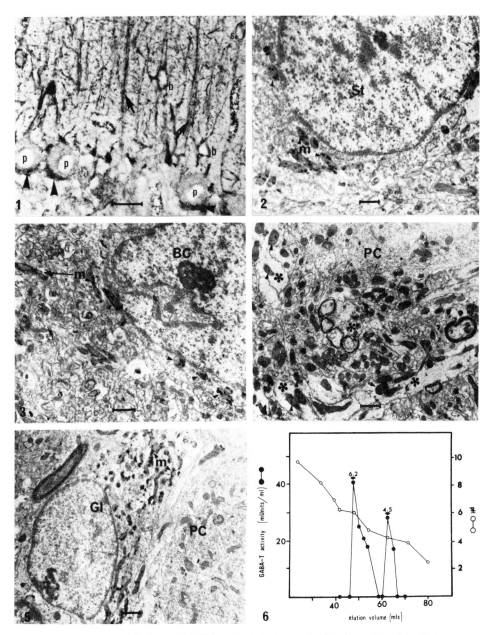

Fig.5 Bergmann glial cell(Gl); Purkinje cell(PC); mitochondria
(m-arrowheads).
Fig.6 Elution profile of GABA-T multimolecular forms on a pH 3-9
"Ampholine" isoelectricfocusing gradient.  Open circles represent
the pH gradient, monitored at 10°C, closed circles represent
GABA-T activity in mUnits/ml of elution volume.
The isoelectric points of the two forms of GABA-T are pH 6.2
and 4.5.

The answers to these questions are as yet unknown, although the presence of GABA-T in Bergmann glia might indicate that these cells degrade GABA taken up from inhibitory basket cell/Purkinje cell synapses. They could also act as insulators at these synapses, removing and degrading "free" GABA which may be present, since the use of GABA as a chemical transmitter in the cerebellar cortex is widespread.

GABA-T in pre-synaptic sites (basket cell axons, for example) could act as a regulator of GABA levels in these areas, although this role is traditionally given to glutamate decarboxylase, the enzyme which synthesizes GABA.

To obtain more information about the possible role of GABA-T in nervous tissues, we have carried out a preliminary examination of the occurrence of multimolecular forms of the enzyme in brain using isoelectricfocusing, since the GABA-T's in glial and neuronal compartments could be different protein species, with unsimilar physico-chemical properties. Therefore a technique allowing us to study and purify these proteins is required.

Whole rat brain (20% w/v) was homogenized in 1% (w/v) glycine at $4^{\circ}$C, containing dithiothreitol (1mM), pyridoxal phosphate (0.2mM), EDTA (0.1mM) and Triton X-100 (0.2% v/v). The homogenate was frozen and thawed twice, filtered through glass wool and centrifuged at 100,000g on an MSE Superspeed 60 ultracentrifuge. The membrane free supernatant was treated with solid ammonium sulphate as described by Schousboe et al (1973), to give a protein fraction precipitating between 40 and 80% ammonium sulphate saturation. The precipitate was recovered by centrifugation at 20,000g, dissolved in 1% glycine containing dithiothreitol, pyridoxal phosphate and EDTA and dialysed against an excess of the same buffer to remove the ammonium sulphate. The dialysed protein fraction was subjected to column isoelectricfocusing in an LKB 440 ml column using a final concentration of 1% (v/v) "Ampholine" carrier ampholytes having a pH range 3-9, in a glycerol gradient at $10^{\circ}$C. The period of focusing was 72 h at a final potential of 650 V, 5mA. After focusing the column was eluted at 120 ml/h and 2 ml fractions collected into nitrogen gas-filled tubes. The pH of each fraction was monitored at $10^{\circ}$C and GABA-T activity assayed by a spectrophotometric modification of the method of Pitts et al (1965). A duplicate assay was carried out in the presence of 50µM amino-oxyacetic acid, when no GABA-T activity could be detected.

After assay, two enzyme peaks were found, with isoelectric points of pH 6.2 and 4.5 at $10^{\circ}$C. (Units of enzyme activity are µmoles of NADH produced /minute at $37^{\circ}$C, pH 8.6).

The existence of two multimolecular forms of GABA-T, as

shown by isoelectricfocusing, is in agreement with Tardy et al (1976), who separated GABA-T from brain into two separate species using DEAE-cellulose chromatography. Schousboe et al (1973) found only one form of GABA-T, which was purified 1200-fold. However, in the latter case the GABA-T was prepared from a brain mitochondrial fraction and not from whole brain homogenates, which might explain the discrepancy between results.

Thus two forms of GABA-T exist. It should therefore be possible to determine the cellular origin of each of these forms and to study their properties, by isolating GABA-T from glial- and neuronal-enriched cell preparations. Furthermore, antibodies to each form of the enzyme could be prepared in order to establish their roles via biochemical and ultrastructural studies.

## ACKNOWLEDGEMENTS

Part of this work was supported by a Wellcome Trust Grant. I would like to thank the ASI and the Wellcome Trust who provided me with financial assistance towards this conference.

## REFERENCES

1. Van Gelder, N.M. J.Neurochem. 12: 231-237, 1965
2. Hyde, J.C., and Robinson, N. Histochemistry 46: 261-268, 1976.
3. Hyde, J.C., and Robinson, N. Histochemistry 49: 51-65, 1976a.
4. Wallach, D.P. Biochem. Pharmacol. 5: 323-331, 1961
5. Salganicoff, L., and DeRobertis, E. J.Neurochem. 12: 287-309, 1965.
6. Schousboe, A., Wu, J-Y, and Roberts, E. Biochemistry 12: 2868-2873, 1973.
7. Pitts, F.N., Quick, C., and Robins, E. J.Neurochem. 12: 93-101, 1965.
8. Tardy, M., Rolland, B., Adeline, J., and Gonnard, P. J.Neurochem. 27: 1285-1286, 1976.

# PRE- AND NON-SYNAPTIC ACTIVITIES OF GABA AND RELATED AMINO ACIDS

# IN THE MAMMALIAN NERVOUS SYSTEM

David R. Curtis

Department of Pharmacology

Australian National University, Canberra, Australia

The importance of GABA as an inhibitory transmitter in the mammalian brain and spinal cord is well recognized, especially in relation to hyperpolarizing postsynaptic inhibition which involves an increase in the membrane conductance and potential of neurones.

The inhibition by micro-electrophoretic GABA of a number of different types of central neurone, and the reduction by GABA antagonists, such as picrotoxinin and bicuculline, of synaptically evoked inhibitions, have revealed some of the "gabergic" pathways within the cerebral cortex, deeper nuclei, hippocampal cortex, cerebellum, brain stem and spinal cord (Curtis and Johnston, 1974a). Furthermore, neurochemical and histochemical analyses have been made of the cellular, and even the synaptic, distribution of GABA and its related enzymes in certain regions of the CNS. Investigational difficulties, however, complicate all of these studies, and although the list of pathways is impressive for which acceptable evidence is available for the function of GABA as a transmitter (see Curtis, 1975), more detailed information is required in many instances to establish firmly the role of this amino acid at particular inhibitory synapses.

Many aspects of amino acid neurotransmission will be covered in other papers of this volume, and this paper reviews pre- and non-synaptic effects of GABA, effects which might be considered either as non-physiological artifacts or as vital to the role of GABA in the central nervous system. Presynaptic functional effects of GABA are of course well established in crustacean peripheral nervous systems (Dudel and Kuffler, 1961; Gerschenfeld, 1973; Dudel and Hatt, 1976). The depolarization by GABA of peripheral sensory

and autonomic ganglion cells in mammals, however, might possibly
be rejected as important to the physiological role of this amino
acid, whereas depolarization of afferent terminals within the
spinal cord and dorsal column relay nuclei could well underlie the
phenomenon of "presynaptic" inhibition.

## AUTONOMIC AND SENSORY GANGLIA

The levels of GABA, L-glutamate-1-carboxylase (GAD) and
4-aminobutyrate-2-oxoglutarate aminotransferase (GABA-T) within
mammalian autonomic and dorsal root ganglia are low, relative to
those in areas of the CNS considered to be rich in GABA-releasing
terminals. Results from a variety of sources are listed in Table I.

Both types of tissue take up exogenous GABA, largely into
glial satellite cells, by high affinity processes which differ
in some respects from those found in brain (Bowery and Brown, 1972;
Young et al., 1973; Schon and Kelly, 1974a,b; Iversen and Kelly,
1975). The metabolism of GABA is predominantly glial in location
(Minchin and Beart, 1975), and the concentration of GABA within
glia of the rat superior cervical ganglion has been estimated as
0.5-1 mM (Bowery et al., 1976; Bertilsson et al., 1976), a figure
which can be compared with a value of 58 mM estimated for Purkinje
cell terminals within Deiters' nucleus (Fonnum and Walberg, 1973).

Exogenous GABA can be released by "stimuli" such as a raised
extracellular potassium concentration (Bowery and Brown, 1972;
Minchin and Iversen, 1974), electrical stimulation of autonomic
ganglia or presynaptic nerve trunks (Bowery and Brown, 1974b), and
by certain GABA analogues which are substrates for the glial carrier
process (Bowery et al., 1976). Inhibition of the transport process
enhanced the effect of exogenous GABA on ganglion cells (Brown and
Galvan, 1977).

A number of investigators have reported that GABA, and some
GABA analogues, depolarize neurones in autonomic and sensory
ganglia. The initial studies of de Groat and his colleagues
established that systemic (intra-arterial, intravenous) GABA
depolarized the cat superior cervical ganglion, the rabbit inferior
mesenteric ganglion and the cat pelvic ganglion (de Groat, 1966,
1970; de Groat et al., 1971). The depolarization, recorded
between the surface of ganglia and postsynaptic nerve trunks, was
accompanied by depression of the muscarinic but not of the nicotinic
firing of ganglion cells, and was reduced by picrotoxin and bicuculline, substances which alone had complex effects on ganglionic
transmission (see also de Groat and Lalley, 1973), but not by
strychnine. Glycine was inactive, and GABA was the most effective
of the analogues tested, including 3-aminopropane sulphonic acid
and β-hydroxy-GABA. Depolarization still occurred after chronic

TABLE I

APPROXIMATE LEVELS OF GABA, GAD, GABA-T IN MAMMALIAN TISSUES

| | Dorsal Root Ganglion | Spinal Dorsal Horn | Spinal Roots | Superior Cervical Ganglion | Deiters' Nucleus |
|---|---|---|---|---|---|
| GABA μmol/g | <0.06[a] 0.5[c] 0.5[d] | >2[b] 9.7[d] | 0.1[e] | (0.3 mmol/g protein; cerebral cortex, 14)[f] | 1.8[a] |
| GAD μmol $CO_2$/h/g | 1.7[c] 0.2–0.4[g] | 7[h] 13[i] | 0.8[c] 3–4[i] | 0.2–1.5[g] | 16[j] |
| GABA–T μmol succinate/h/g | 3.4[c] | 14[i] | 2.5[c] 1[i] | 20[k] | |

a   Otsuka *et al.*, 1971; cat     g   Kanazawa *et al.*, 1976; rat

b   Miyata and Otsuka, 1972; cat     h   Kelly *et al.*, 1973; rat

c   Beart *et al.*, 1974; rat     i   Graham and Aprison, 1969; cat

d   Berger *et al.*, 1977; rabbit     j   Fonnum *et al.*, 1970; cat

e   Graham *et al.*, 1967; cat     k   Salvador and Albers, 1959; monkey

f   Bertilsson and Costa, 1976; rat

preganglionic denervation of the cat superior cervical ganglion
(de Groat, 1970).

   Subsequent investigators have used the superfused desheathed
rat superior cervical ganglion *in vitro*, a preparation which has
permitted a more accurate estimate of effective GABA and antagonist
concentrations, a more detailed analysis of GABA receptors, and a
study of the ionic mechanism of depolarization (Bowery and Brown,
1974a; Adams and Brown, 1975). The threshold concentration for
GABA was approximately 1 µM, changes in membrane potential were
recorded indirectly by surface electrodes, and the response to
GABA was not impaired by preganglionic nerve degeneration.

   Of a large series of GABA analogues the molar potencies of
only 3-aminopropane sulphonic acid and trans-4-aminocrotonic
acid exceeded or equalled that of GABA (Bowery and Brown, 1974a;
Bowery and Jones, 1976). Although these results, and especially
those obtained with imidazole acetic acid and 4-aminotetrolic
acid, suggest that ganglionic GABA receptors differ from those on
spinal interneurones in the cat, the two types of investigation
cannot be related on a quantitative basis since in the cord amino
acids were administered micro-electrophoretically (Beart *et al.*,
1971; Johnston *et al.*, 1975).

   Reversible antagonism of amino acid depolarization was
demonstrated using bicuculline ($IC_{50}$: 14 µM), picrotoxin (37 µM),
tetramethylenedisulphotetramine (Bowery *et al.*, 1975), and
"isopropyl bicyclophosphate" (Bowery *et al.*, 1976), in concentrations having relatively little effect on the depolarization of
ganglion cells by carbamylcholine. Strychine was a relatively
weak and unspecific GABA antagonist, and depolarization by GABA
was not influenced by concentrations of hyoscine and hexamethonium
in combination which blocked responses to carbamylcholine. Ganglia
were not depolarized by either L-glutamic acid or glycine at
concentrations of 10 mM (see also de Groat, 1966).

   The depolarization of cultured rat superior cervical ganglia
by GABA was shown to be accompanied by an increased membrane
conductance (Obata, 1974), and a subsequent detailed analysis, in
which intracellular recording from superior cervical ganglia
*in vitro* was combined with alteration of the extracellular concentration of chloride ions, indicated that GABA increased the membrane
permeability to chloride ions which were apparently at equilibrium
at a potential less depolarized than that of the resting membrane
(Adams and Brown, 1975). A similar mechanism had been proposed
for the depolarization by GABA of both ganglion cells and presynaptic fibres in bullfrog paravertebral sympathetic ganglia
*in vitro* (Koketsu *et al.*, 1974), effects also blocked by picrotoxin.
A reduced release of acetylcholine from presynaptic fibres in

these ganglia as a consequence of depolarization by GABA was proposed as an explanation of reduced nicotinic transmission by the amino acid.

The effect of GABA on sensory ganglia, which are generally considered not to contain synapses, appears to be similar to that on autonomic neurones. Ramón y Cajal (1911) described afferent fibres to sensory ganglia, fibres which were regarded as of sympathetic origin. Complex perineuronal complexes of fibres have been described, some of which originate from intraganglionic neurones and some from sympathetic ganglia, together with contacts between neurones and terminals which contain neither vesicles nor mitochondria (Milokhin and Reshetnikov, 1971). In another study of rat ganglia, however, no synapses were observed (Zenka and Högl, 1976).

Depolarization, recorded between the body of the ganglion and the sectioned end of afferent fibres, was first described by de Groat (de Groat, 1972; de Groat *et al.*, 1972) using the nodose ganglion and lumbar dorsal root ganglia of cats *in situ*. Amino acids were administered intra-arterially or intravenously; by the former route threshold doses for GABA were of the order of 0.05-2 μg (nodose) and 2.5-20 μg/kg (lumbar). For lumbar dorsal root ganglia, 3-aminopropane sulphonic acid was equal in potency to GABA; β-alanine and δ-amino-*n*-valeric acid were much less potent. Relatively large amounts of L-glutamate, L-aspartate, DL-homocysteate and glycine were inactive. Bicuculline and picrotoxin, but not strychnine, reduced the depolarizing action of GABA. Relatively large doses of GABA (50 or 100 mg/kg, intravenous) also depolarize dorsal root ganglia in the cat, recording from dorsal root filaments sectioned centrally near the cord (Levy, 1975). Although depolarization of axons was considered possible, these doses of GABA did not depolarize ventral root filaments also sectioned near the cord.

The depolarization by GABA of cultured rat dorsal root ganglion cells (Obata, 1974; Lawson *et al.*, 1976), rat lumbar dorsal root ganglion cells *in vivo* (Feltz and Rasminsky, 1974; electrophoretic GABA) and bullfrog dorsal root ganglia *in vitro* (Nishi *et al.*, 1974), is accompanied by an increased membrane conductance. The effects of altering extracellular ion concentrations suggest that GABA enhances chloride permeability in the latter tissue (Nishi *et al.*, 1974). This was confirmed in a subsequent intracellular investigation of rat ganglia *in vivo* (Deschenes *et al.*, 1976), in which the responses of ganglion cells to GABA was biphasic, an initial transient peak depolarization falling to a plateau level. Furthermore, evidence was found for an associated increase in extracellular potassium ion activity, possibly a consequence of glial uptake of GABA (Deschenes and Feltz, 1976).

Further knowledge of the GABA receptor on ganglion cells requires additional studies of the effects of topical or electro-phoretic GABA analogues: 3-aminopropane sulphonic acid is apparently as effective as GABA, imidazole acetic acid is weak, and both L-glutamate and β(p-chlorophenyl)-GABA are inactive (P. Feltz - unpublished). As with autonomic ganglia, glial amino acid uptake may contribute to the apparent relative potencies of GABA analogues. L-Glutamate is inactive when administered electrophoretically near cultured dorsal root ganglion cells (Ransom and Nelson, 1975; Lawson *et al.*, 1976).

The depolarization of autonomic and sensory ganglia by GABA may be produced by an increase in membrane permeability to chloride ions. Such a change in membrane permeability appears also to account for the *hyperpolarization* by GABA of central neurones (see Krnjević, 1974), and hence the *intracellular* concentration of chloride ions in the peripheral ganglia seems to be maintained at a higher level than that of centrally located neurones. An inwardly directed chloride pump, maintaining intracellular levels greater than those expected from an equilibrium distribution, has been postulated (de Groat, 1972, Nishi *et al.*, 1974; Adams and Brown, 1975). The distribution of ions within the rabbit superior cervical ganglion suggests that the equilibrium potential for chloride ions may be approximately 30 mV less depolarized than the resting membrane potential (Woodward *et al.*, 1969). This figure was based on an indirectly estimated intracellular chloride concentration of 23.5 mM, some 13.5 mM higher than that predicted for the passive distribution of chloride across a membrane having a resting potential of -70 mV (see Adams and Brown, 1975). Further-more, the figure is substantially higher than the 17.5 mM estimated for desheathed cat sciatic nerves (Krnjević, 1955), a value possibly representative of dorsal root fibres and ganglion cells. All of these estimates, however, may be in error because of technical difficulties, and direct measurements are required of the intracellular chloride ion activity in autonomic and sensory ganglion neurones.

The fact remains, however, that both types of cell are depolarized by GABA, whereas neurones within the brain and spinal cord are hyperpolarized. Since the effects of GABA on the ganglion cells of different types of afferent fibre have yet to be determined, and the extent to which changes in the membrane potential of ganglion cell bodies influence transmission through ganglia remains uncertain, it is difficult to assess the functional significance of the presence of GABA receptors on sensory ganglia. Within autonomic ganglia, changes in cell body excitability, and in the ability of presynaptic terminals to release transmitter, may be functionally important. There are a number of reports of the effects of systemically administered GABA on autonomic functions in

different animal species (Elliott and Hobbiger, 1959; Stanton and
Woodhouse, 1960; Stanton, 1963; Srimal and Bhargava, 1966), and, in
the absence of evidence for synaptic release within ganglia, it is
possible that circulating GABA may modulate ganglionic transmission.
Brown and Galvan (1977) suggest that uptake may be significant in
maintaining low extraneuronal concentrations of GABA since plasma
levels (2-4 µM; Crowshaw *et al.*, 1967) may exceed threshold concentrations at which GABA depolarizes autonomic ganglia *in vitro*.

Another modulating influence on autonomic and sensory ganglion
cells may be the release of GABA from glia as a consequence of
raised extracellular potassium levels produced by activity of the
neurones (Minchin and Iversen, 1974; Deschenes and Feltz, 1976).
It remains to be determined, however, whether significant changes
in extracellular potassium concentration occur within ganglia under
*in vivo* conditions, where sustained synchronous discharge of more
than a few ganglion cells seems unlikely.

A relationship between synaptic activity and GABA in the rat
superior cervical ganglion was also suggested by recent measurements, after microwave fixation, of GABA levels under a variety of
conditions (Bertilsson *et al.*, 1976). Control levels (approx.
0.3 mmol/g protein) were quadrupled by pretreatment of the animals
with amino-oxyacetic acid, and were reduced by either pretreatment
with a nicotinic ganglionic blocking agent, chronic section of the
preganglionic fibres or prior administration of the anaesthetic
urethane. These manoeuvres produced no significant changes in the
level of glutamic acid in the ganglia.

Several investigations using isolated ganglia may be relevant
to a relationship between the central effects of pentobarbitone and
GABA-mediated synaptic inhibition. Nicoll (1975a) found that pentobarbitone (>200 µM) depolarized frog dorsal root ganglion cells and
increased membrane conductance; an action similar to that of GABA
was proposed. Pentobarbitone (>80 µM) also depolarized the isolated
rat superior cervical ganglion (Bowery and Dray, 1976). The threshold concentration for GABA in this latter investigation was 1 µM,
responses to pentobarbitone were less susceptible to antagonism by
bicuculline methochloride than were those to GABA, and pentobarbitone reduced the effectiveness of bicuculline methochloride as a
GABA antagonist.

## SPINAL PRESYNAPTIC FIBRES AND TERMINALS

### Methods of Investigation

The effects of GABA, and other substances, on primary
afferent fibres and terminals within the cord or dorsal column
relay nuclei are not so readily determined as those upon ganglion

cells. Prolonged intracellular recording with well maintained
membrane potentials is rarely possible (Eccles and Krnjević, 1959),
and extracellular ion levels cannot be altered sufficiently under
*in vivo* conditions to provide very specific information regarding
the participation of particular ions in producing alterations of
membrane potential.

Changes in the polarization of primary afferents can be
determined indirectly by recording potentials from the surface of
the cord or relay nuclei, from dorsal root fibres, from within the
tissue with extra- or intra-cellular microelectrodes, or by
measuring excitability changes of fibres using the technique
introduced by Wall (1958). In this latter procedure, glass or
insulated metal micro-electrodes are first used as recording
electrodes to locate sites where afferents terminate, and are then
used as extracellular monopolar microstimulating electrodes.
Antidromically conducted impulses are recorded peripherally from
the appropriate afferent fibres, and changes in fibre excitability
are determined from the size of just-threshold negative electrical
pulses, usually of duration 0.1-0.3 msec. Enhanced fibre
excitability is generally accepted as an indication of fibre
depolarization; although decreased excitability does not necessarily indicate hyperpolarization.

Although systemically or topically administered drugs may
modify terminal excitability, the exact site of action of the
added compounds, and the relationship of their effects to
synaptically evoked events, are difficult to determine. It has
been possible to study the effects of micro-electrophoretically
administered amino acids and other compounds on terminal
excitability, although the conditions for these experiments seem
more exacting than those for recording intracellularly from spinal
interneurones.

Since the concentrations of substances ejected micro-
electrophoretically are highest near pipette orifices (Curtis,
1976), it is important when using this method of administering
amino acids to measure excitability changes of only those terminals
and fibres which are close to the drug-ejecting pipettes
(Sverdlov and Kozhechkin, 1975). Analyses of such microstimulating
techniques suggest that fibres and terminals with electrical
thresholds less than 1 µA lie within 75 µm of the electrode (0.1
µA, 30 µm; Jankowska and Roberts, 1972; Roberts and Smith, 1973;
see also Katz and Miledi, 1965; Stoney *et al.*, 1968; Ranck, 1975;
Bagshaw and Evans, 1976). Single fibres or terminals in the cord
can usually be stimulated with threshold pulses of 0.4-1 µA, and
are identified as to type by the conduction velocity and peripheral
destination of the antidromically conducted impulses.

Since it is not possible to make use of either visual methods (McMahon and Kuffler, 1971) or the technique of recording extra-cellular synaptic potentials (del Castillo and Katz, 1956; Hubbard and Schmidt, 1963; Katz and Miledi, 1965) to locate synaptic sites, the nature of the structures stimulated - myelinated fibre, unmyelinated fibre, node of Ranvier or presynaptic terminal - cannot be determined. The unmyelinated portion, and possibly even the terminals, of the fastest conducting fibres might be expected to have the lowest electrical thresholds, and sensitivity to GABA and bicuculline methochloride appears to be located at or near terminals (see below). Standard electrophysiological methods can be used to place the electrodes close to neurones upon which particular types of fibre terminate, regions in which small diphasic positive-negative presynaptic action potentials can occasionally be recorded (Brooks and Eccles, 1947), thus increasing the chance of stimulating the terminal region.

In view of the relatively small size of primary afferent terminals (Conradi, 1969a; McLaughlin, 1972a; Réthelyi, 1977), the maintenance of a constant distance between them and the stimulating electrode (1-2 μm in diameter) is a serious problem with single fibre microstimulation, and movement of the electrodes over distances as small as 5-10 μm results in considerable alterations of the electrical threshold of single fibres and in their sensitivity to ejected amino acids. A secondary problem is that ejected compounds *per se* may alter the conductance of the medium between the electrode and the fibre, so altering the apparent excitatory effectiveness of the stimulating pulse. Such an effect may be reduced by "balancing" the current used to administer pharmacologically active ions with the simultaneous ejection of inert ions (Na, Cl) of opposite polarity.

Axo-axonic Synapses

The morphology and histochemistry of afferent fibre terminals, and especially of those involved in axo-axonic synapses, are very relevant to discussion of the involvement of GABA in the synaptic depolarization of primary afferent fibres (PAD).

Within lamina IX of the ventral horn of the cat, the terminals of primary afferent fibres, presumably group Ia muscle afferents, are relatively large structures (M boutons, 4-7 μm in length, 1-3 μm diameter) which contain spherical vesicles and form asymmetrical synaptic complexes located mainly on proximal dendrites of motoneurones (Conradi, 1969a,b; McLaughlin, 1972a,b; see also Kuno *et al.*, and Iles, 1976). These structures, which degenerate after dorsal root section, form less than 1% of the total population of terminals within this region, and are them-selves opposed by a number of smaller boutons which contain vesicles

of irregular shape (P boutons, Conradi, 1969a,b; McLaughlin, 1972b;
see also Bodian, 1966). These latter boutons also oppose the
dendritic membrane of motoneurones, but there appears to be some
disagreement as to whether the P-M and P-motoneurone contacts can
be considered as synaptic on the morphological evidence (Conradi,
1969b; McLaughlin, 1972b). To some extent this difficulty may have
arisen because of preconceived ideas regarding the *functional*
differences between boutons having spherical and pleomorphic
vesicles. Vesicle shape, as demonstrated in aldehyde-fixed tissues
(Bodian, 1970; Valdivia, 1971; Uchizono, 1975), most probably
depends on vesicle *content* rather than primarily on bouton function,
and pleomorphic vesicles have been described at other synapses for
which there is acceptable evidence that GABA is the transmitter.

It is thus important that GAD has recently been localized
immunocytochemically within boutons, containing pleomorphic
flattened vesicles, which contact both dendrites and larger
terminals which in turn synapse with motoneurone dendrites in the
ventral horn of the rat (McLaughlin *et al.*, 1975). Although
further investigation is needed of the assumed interneuronal origin
of GAD-containing terminals within this and other regions of the
spinal cord, there appears to be reasonable morphological support
for a role of GABA in axo-dendritic and axo-axonic transmission
involving motoneurones.

Levels of GABA (Miyata and Otsuka, 1972; Berger *et al.*, 1977)
and GAD (Kelly *et al.*, 1973; McLaughlin *et al.*, 1975; Tappaz *et
al.*, 1976) are high in the dorsal horn of the cord, especially in
laminae I - III, a region which contains numerous axo-axonic
synapses (Ralston, 1968; Réthelyi and Szentágothai, 1969).
Morphologically, the presynaptic components of these dorsal horn
synaptic complexes (or glomeruli) were considered to be axon
terminals of intraspinal interneurones, containing "unusually
large, spheroid and somewhat irregular" vesicles (Réthelyi and
Szentágothai, 1969). The postsynaptic elements were considered to
be terminals of the larger primary afferent fibres, presumably of
cutaneous origin, which contain spherical vesicles and also form
axodendritic synapses with spinal interneurones. The involvement
of small non-myelinated afferent fibres in these complexes is
uncertain, although a more recent study suggests that these are
the only type of afferent terminating in the substantia gelatinosa
(lamina II) with extensive axonal arborizations and multiple,
including *en passant*, terminal enlargements (Réthelyi, 1977; see
also La Motte, 1977). Further investigation seems warranted of
the origins of various types of dorsal horn axonal terminal
(see also Ralston, 1968; Coimbra *et al.*, 1974; Beal and Fox, 1976).
Similar axo-axonal, axo-dendritic complexes occur in the substantia
gelatinosa of the spinal trigeminal nucleus (Kerr, 1970; Westrum

and Black, 1971; Gobel, 1975), and the presynaptic elements of the axo-axonal synapses generally contain pleomorphic vesicles.

Again it is very significant that in the dorsal horn of the rat, GAD has been demonstrated immunocytochemically in terminals presynaptic to dendrites, cell bodies and, in laminae II and III, to other boutons (McLaughlin *et al.*, 1975). The presynaptic GAD-containing terminal of these axo-axonic synapses contains flattened or pleomorphic vesicles, the junctions are of the symmetrical type, and the postsynaptic elements usually contain spherical vesicles and make asymmetrical synaptic contacts with other structures. After the intraspinal injection of tritiated GABA in cats, Ljungdahl and Hökfelt (1973) have demonstrated autoradiographically that the amino acid is taken up into terminals, some of which make axo-axonic contacts with larger boutons which in turn synapse with dendrites.

Within the cuneate nucleus, the large terminals of dorsal column fibres form axodendritic synapses with relay neurones. In addition, these terminals are postsynaptic in axo-axonic synapses to small boutons, most probably of interneurones, which appear to contain pleomorphic vesicles and are also presynaptic to dendrites with which the larger terminals synapse (Walberg, 1965, 1966; see also Rustioni and Sotelo, 1974). In the lateral geniculate nucleus, however, the terminals of optic nerve fibres, which synapse within glomeruli with dendritic protrusions of geniculate neurones, are *presynaptic* at axo-axonic synapses on the terminals of Golgi type 2 neurones. These Golgi terminals, which contain pleomorphic vesicles, also synapse with geniculate dendrites (Szentágothai, 1970; Famiglietti and Peters, 1972; Lieberman and Webster, 1975).

In summary, therefore, if flattened pleomorphic vesicles and the presence of GAD can be considered characteristic of GABA-releasing terminals, there is good evidence in the cat and rat for the participation of this amino acid at axo-axonic synapses upon terminals of group Ia spinal afferents and of spinal afferents of as yet undetermined type terminating in the superficial laminae of the dorsal horn. GABA may also be the transmitter of terminals containing pleomorphic vesicles in dorsal column nuclei. The arrangement within the lateral geniculate nucleus is of opposite "polarity" to that required for afferent fibre depolarization. It is possible, however, that the depolarization of optic nerve terminals by impulses in a variety of afferent pathways to the lateral geniculate nucleus may be related to elevated extracellular potassium ion levels rather than to a synaptically active transmitter (Singer and Lux, 1973).

On morphological grounds, Ramon-Moliner (1977) has recently

proposed a non-synaptic inhibitory effect of GABA from granule to
mitral and tufted neurones in the olfactory bulb. In the rat, GAD
is located within the soma and dendrites of granule and periglom-
erular cells (Ribak *et al.*, 1977).

Within the amphibian spinal cord, a preparation used for
numerous studies of the effects of amino acids on primary
afferents, most dorsal root fibres appear to terminate dorsally,
and the distribution of axo-axonic synapses has not been
described (Corvaja and Pellegrini, 1975). The uptake of [$^3$H]GABA,
demonstrated radio-autographically, was found to be maximal in the
dorsal horn of the frog cord and not altered by chronic dorsal
root section. The amino acid thus appears to be associated with
spinal interneurones rather than with primary afferents (Glusman,
1975). In the ventral horn, primary afferents synapse upon fine
dendrites of motoneurones, and the terminals are postsynaptic to
boutons of presumably interneuronal origin which also form
axodendritic synapses (Glusman *et al.*, 1976).

### Terminal Polarization and Transmitter Release

Before considering the evidence that amino acids do influence
primary afferent fibres, and terminals, it is convenient to mention
the relationship between terminal polarization and transmitter
release. The basic mechanism proposed for "presynaptic" inhibition
is reduced effectiveness of excitatory transmission as a consequence
of diminished transmitter release following the activation of axo-
axonic synapses. In both the spinal cord and dorsal column nuclei,
primary afferent depolarization (PAD) accompanies reduced
excitatory effectiveness, and hence axo-axonic synapses in these
regions appear to be depolarizing in nature (Eccles *et al.*, 1963b).

Since an essential factor in the release of transmitter from
synaptic terminals is depolarization of the membrane (Hubbard,
1970), the amount released per impulse might be expected to be
influenced by the presynaptic membrane potential. Changes in the
amplitude of the action potential invading the terminal region may
be important, as well as more direct effects on the release mechanism and the amount of transmitter available for release. Direct
polarization of the presynaptic terminal of the giant synapse in
the squid stellate ganglion has suggested an approximately 10 fold
change in the amplitude of the postsynaptic potential for a 10-30
mV change in that of the presynaptic action potential: a 30%
reduction in the latter almost abolishing transmission (Hagiwara
and Tasaki, 1958; Takeuchi and Takeuchi, 1962; Miledi and Slater,
1966; Katz and Miledi, 1967; Gage, 1967; see also Katz and Miledi,
1971; Erulkar and Weight, 1977). The effect of polarization of
presynaptic terminals has also been studied at the synapse between

Müller axons and spinal interneurones in the lamprey: small changes in action potential amplitude had little or no effect on transmitter release, the process apparently being saturated at presynaptic depolarizations of the order of 100 mV (Martin and Ringham, 1975).

The passage of electrical currents in a dorso-ventral direction across the cat spinal cord *in vivo*, which alters the membrane potential and excitability of intraspinal primary afferent fibres, also appears to modify transmitter release from terminals on motoneurones - presynaptic depolarization depressing excitatory action (Eccles *et al*., 1962). Changes in transmitter release greater than that resulting from "passive" depolarization of the terminal membrane might be expected if the change in membrane potential be generated by an increase in membrane conductance (see Eccles *et al*., 1963b).

## Amphibian Spinal Cord

Because of the technical difficulties associated with investigation of the pharmacology of mammalian primary afferent terminals *in vivo* many investigators have made use of the isolated, hemisected, amphibian spinal cord, recording potentials from dorsal and ventral roots and measuring excitability changes of intraspinal fibres (Eccles, 1946; Schmidt, 1963; Tebēcis and Phillis, 1969; Davidoff, 1972a; Barker and Nicoll, 1973). The isolated hemisected cord of immature rats has also been used (Otsuka and Konishi, 1976). Primary afferents in the amphibian can be depolarized synaptically by stimulating ventral or dorsal roots, or descending tracts, or by adding amino acids to the bathing solution. The ionic concentration of the medium can be changed, and the addition of procaine or tetrodotoxin, or elevation of the magnesium concentration permits a distinction to be made between direct amino acid effects on terminals and fibres and those relayed synaptically.

There is general agreement that amphibian primary afferent terminals are depolarized by GABA, and that this effect, as well as PAD generated synaptically by stimulating dorsal or ventral roots, is blocked by GABA antagonists such as picrotoxin and bicuculline, but not by strychnine (Schmidt, 1963; Grinnel, 1966; Tebēcis and Phillis, 1969; Davidoff, 1972a; Barker and Nicoll, 1973; Barker *et al*., 1975a,b). A site of action at terminals was suggested by the failure of GABA to depolarize dorsal roots sectioned just within the cord (Barker and Nicoll, 1973). Enhanced permeability to chloride ions has been proposed as the mechanism of action of GABA (Nishi *et al*., 1974; Kudo *et al*., 1975; Otsuka and Konishi, 1976; but see also Barker and Nicoll, 1973).

Close structural analogues have effects similar to that of
GABA, including β-alanine, taurine, 3-aminopropane sulphonic
acid, δ-aminolevulinic acid, imidazole acetic acid and (+)-*trans*-
3-aminocyclopentane carboxylic acid, whereas the effects of
glycine are variable, terminal hyperpolarization occasionally
being reported, and not blocked either by strychnine or by GABA
antagonists (Schmidt, 1963; Tebēcis and Phillis, 1969; Davidoff,
1972a; Barker and Nicoll, 1973; Barker *et al*., 1975a; Nicoll,
1976, 1977).

Amphibian terminals are also depolarized by L-glutamate and
L-aspartate, effects generally not found to be blocked by GABA
antagonists (Tebēcis and Phillis, 1969; Davidoff, 1972a; Barker
and Nicoll, 1973; Barker *et al*., 1975a). In addition to
bicuculline and picrotoxin, penicillin-G (Davidoff, 1972c),
(+)-tubocurarine (Nicoll, 1975b) and pentylenetetrazol (Nicoll
and Padjen, 1976) have been reported to block the depolarization
of afferents by GABA. Other substances found to depolarize
amphibian terminals include pentobarbitone, an effect blocked by
picrotoxin and bicuculline (Nicoll, 1975a), and diphenylhydantoin
(Davidoff, 1972b).

## Mammalian Spinal Cord

Eccles *et al*. (1963a) first reported that GABA (and 3-amino-
propanesulphonic acid), applied directly to the exposed spinal
cord of the cat in concentrations of 10-20 mM, produced changes in
potentials recorded from dorsal roots which were consistent with
a central depolarizing action. This conclusion was compatible with
the finding, reported in the same paper, that intravenous picrotoxin
blocked synaptically evoked dorsal root potentials and the
associated long latency and duration inhibition of spinal monosynaptic reflexes. At that time (1963) picrotoxin was known to be
an antagonist of the inhibitory action of GABA at a variety of
crustacean synapses (see Curtis, 1963). Subsequent studies have
demonstrated that picrotoxin is also an antagonist of many types
of GABA-mediated postsynaptic inhibition in the mammalian CNS,
and that these are also blocked by other substances which have
been shown to antagonize the inhibitory action of GABA (Curtis and
Johnston, 1974a,b).

Few studies since 1963 have depended on topical administration
of GABA to central neurones, largely because of the relatively
high concentrations of this and other amino acids required, and the
difficulty of either localizing the site or determining the mode
of action of compounds so administered. Topical GABA (10 mM)
increased the excitability of afferent fibres terminating in the
cuneate nucleus of the cat, an effect reversed by intravenous

picrotoxin (Galindo, 1969). A more extensive investigation in the
rat demonstrated enhanced excitability of afferent terminals in the
cuneate nucleus by GABA (10 mM) and L-glutamate (10 mM), but not by
L-aspartate (10 mM), and a decrease by glycine (Davidson and Southwick, 1971). The finding that GABA, but not L-glutamate, also reduced the depolarization of terminals induced by afferent volleys
that simultaneously inhibited transmission of sensory information
through the nucleus (see Schmidt, 1971), in conjunction with observations of the reduction by picrotoxin and bicuculline, but not by
strychnine, of both this prolonged inhibition and terminal depolarization (Banna and Jabbur, 1969; Davidson and Southwick, 1971),
suggested that synaptically released GABA may have at least two
effects in the dorsal column relay nuclei. GABA reduces the
excitability of cuneate relay neurones (Galindo *et al.*, 1967), an
effect blocked by picrotoxin and bicuculline (Galindo, 1969; Kelly
and Renaud, 1973a,b), and hence is associated with "postsynaptic"
inhibition. Additionally, the depolarization of afferent terminals
suggested a role for GABA in "presynaptic" inhibition. The importance of GABA in both of these processes which reduced transmission
through the cuneate nucleus was strengthened by their reduction when
GABA levels in the nucleus were depleted by intravenous administration of semicarbazide (Banna and Jabbur, 1971; Banna, 1973). Further
studies in which the rat cuneate nucleus was superfused with
solutions containing altered ion concentrations suggested that the
synaptic depolarization of afferent terminals involved an efflux of
chloride ions (Davidson and Simpson, 1976).

In the cat spinal cord, systemically administered picrotoxin
(Eccles *et al.*, 1963a) and bicuculline (Curtis *et al.*, 1971) reduce
the prolonged inhibition of spinal monosynaptic reflexes, and the
associated depolarization of primary afferent terminals, induced by
volleys in muscle and cutaneous fibres, whether the depolarization
be determined by recording dorsal root potentials or more directly
by measuring changes in terminal excitability (see Levy and Anderson,
1972). Furthermore, reduction of the levels of GABA in the spinal
cord of the cat by prior intravenous semicarbazide reduced both the
inhibition of reflexes and PAD (Bell and Anderson, 1972). There
appear to be both phasic and tonic components in presynaptic depolarization by GABA, since the hyperpolarization of afferent terminals,
recorded either as positive dorsal root potentials (Mendell, 1972),
or decreased excitability of intraspinal terminals (Willis *et al.*,
1976), in response to afferent volleys, is also blocked by GABA
antagonists (Levy and Anderson, 1974). There is evidence that
transmitters other than GABA may also be effective at some spinal
axo-axonic synapses (Repkin *et al.*, 1976).

The transient depression of extensor monosynaptic reflexes and
the facilitation of flexor monosynaptic reflexes, in spinal but not
decerebrate cats by GABA administered intravenously in doses

exceeding 0.3 mg/kg (Kuno, 1961; see also Kuno and Muneoka, 1961)
are difficult to interpret in terms of effects on either neurones
or afferent fibres. When administered, however, in somewhat massive
doses (50-100 mg/kg intravenously; 5-10 mg intra-arterially) to high
spinal decerebrate cats, GABA depolarized lumbar dorsal root fibres,
as determined by recording from dorsal root filaments (Levy, 1975).
A direct effect on terminals was proposed since this action of GABA
was blocked by prior intravenous bicuculline (but not by picrotoxin)
and by tetrodotoxin administered intravenously, in doses adequate to
suppress synaptically evoked dorsal root potentials. Depolarization
of dorsal roots by L-glutamate (100 mg/kg) and glycine (100 mg/kg)
was considered to be secondary to hypotension. Under the conditions
of these experiments it is apparent that sufficient GABA penetrated
the blood-brain-barrier to depolarize spinal primary afferent
terminals, and, as mentioned earlier, also dorsal root ganglia.

The effects of amino acids on intraspinal afferent fibres have
been observed more directly using micro-electrophoretic administration in conjunction with measurement of fibre excitability. As
discussed above, such tests have been carried out only in the ventral
and dorsal horns, and the cuneate nucleus, where particular types of
muscle and cutaneous fibre are known to terminate. Actions on fibres
other than at the terminals, although unlikely, have yet to be
excluded. In the original study of Curtis and Ryall (1966), for
example, GABA, DL-homocysteate and L-glutamate, were found to modify
the excitability of cutaneous and muscle afferent terminals only when
there was simultaneous reduction of postsynaptic potentials generated by impulses in the same fibres. Hence the sensitivity of
afferent fibres to these amino acids appeared to be restricted to the
vicinity of the terminals. In contrast, electrophoretic procaine,
as might be expected, reduced the excitability of muscle afferents
coursing through the dorsal horn.

In this particular study, threshold stimulating current pulses
(0.2 msec) were of the order of 0.8-3 µA, and changes in terminal
excitability were assessed from the number of fibres which responded
to pulses of increasing magnitude, to a maximum of approximately
12 µA. Both DL-homocysteate and L-glutamate reversibly increased
terminal excitability, whereas GABA was considered to *reduce* it
(Curtis and Ryall, 1966). In the light of more recent experiments,
a re-evaluation of these results has indicated the significance of
the reported observations that "occasionally the excitability at or
near the threshold value was apparently unaltered or even increased
by GABA", and that excitability changes "particularly at or near the
threshold stimulus intensity, were often irreversible". Considerable
difficulty was experienced in maintaining stable recording and
stimulating conditions in these earlier experiments.

In a subsequent study in the cat cuneate nucleus, Galindo
(1969) illustrated that electrophoretic GABA reduced the electrical

excibability of cutaneous afferent fibre terminals (stimulating current not specified), and that this effect was blocked by intra-venous picrotoxin. Glycine was reported to be ineffective. In a later study of spinal muscle afferent terminals, and using the number of fibres stimulated by a pulse (0.2 msec) of constant but unspecified amplitude (less than 1.5 times threshold), Sverdlov and Kozhechkin (1975) observed that electrophoretic glycine reversibly depressed excitability whereas GABA enhanced it.

In all of these investigations, one barrel of a glass multi-barrel assembly was used as a stimulating electrode, and no compar-isons were made between electrophoretic GABA and synaptically evoked terminal depolarization. More recently, in the dorsal horn of the cat, and using a platinum wire stimulating micro-electrode attached to a three-barrel glass micropipette, Gmelin and Cerletti (1976) report in a preliminary publication that GABA increased the elect-rical excitability of the terminal region of *single* cutaneous fibres by approximately the same amount (22% compared with 28%) as that produced synaptically by stimulating other cutaneous fibres peripherally. Furthermore, this synaptic PAD could be reversibly blocked by electrophoretic bicuculline methochloride. These results have recently been confirmed, and, in addition, the terminals of cutaneous fibres have been shown to be depolarized by L-glutamate (D.R. Curtis, P.M. Headley and D. Lodge - unpublished).

This type of experiment, in which the excitability of a single fibre is measured, has also been carried out in motonuclei of the cat using group Ia extensor muscle afferents, excited with current pulses (0.3 msec) not exceeding 2 µA, passed through the centre barrel of seven barrel glass micropipettes (Curtis *et al.*, 1977). When currents used to eject GABA (0.2 M, pH 3; 0.5 M, pH 5.5) did not exceed 60 nA, fibres having electrical thresholds greater than 1 µA were usually unaffected, whereas those with thresholds less than this were reversibly depolarized, as indicated by a reduced electrical threshold. Decreases in threshold (increased excitability) by as much as 30% were observed with fibres excited by pulses of less than 0.5 µA. In general these depolarizing effects were relatively slow in onset, maximum changes in excita-bility occurring as long as 30-60 sec after the onset of the electrophoretic currents. Recovery times were of similar duration, and, with some fibres, the relatively large change of excitability produced initially by GABA was not maintained, but faded to a reduced plateau level.

Tetanic stimulation (4 volleys at 320 Hz, 1.2-3 x threshold) of flexor muscle afferents 30-140 msec earlier also enhanced terminal excitability, by as much as 30% at optimal intervals of 30-50 msec. This synaptic PAD was reduced in magnitude during depolarization of the terminals by GABA, an observation

consistent with the generation of both depolarizations by increases
in membrane conductance which may be similar.  Furthermore, electrophoretic bicuculline methochloride, which alone had no consistent
effects on fibre excitability, reversibly reduced both the
depolarization induced by GABA and that produced synaptically.  As
in the dorsal horn, the effectiveness of this GABA antagonist in
reducing synaptic PAD was a further indication of the proximity
of the tip of the micropipette to structures associated with the
depolarization of afferent terminals.

Muscle afferent terminals were also depolarized by acidic
amino acids (L-glutamate, L-aspartate and DL-homocysteate).  This
effect, which was not diminished during concomitant synaptic
depolarization, was not reduced by bicuculline methochloride.

In these most recent experiments neither glycine (0.2 M,
0.5 M; pH 3) nor strychnine (10 mM in 165 mM NaCl) had consistent
effects on terminal excitability, and strychnine did not reduce
synaptic PAD.  Both muscimol and 3-aminopropanesulphonic acid were
more potent than GABA in depolarizing terminals, whereas $\beta$(p-chlorophenyl)GABA, which is not a GABA agonist at receptors on spinal
neurones (Curtis $et$ $al$., 1974), neither mimicked nor reduced the
depolarization of terminals by GABA yet reduced synaptically
evoked depolarization.  Although such an effect, which was
relatively slow in onset, may indicate a diminution of the synaptic
release of GABA at axo-axonic synapses, systemically administered
$\beta$-(p-chlorophenyl)GABA reduces both PAD and spinal monosynaptic
reflexes.  This substance may thus reduce PAD by interfering with
the synaptic excitation of spinal interneurones associated with
the generation of PAD.  In contrast, pentobarbitone (20 mM, 50 mM),
which also reduced synaptic depolarization, depolarized group Ia
terminals, GABA-like effects which may account both for anaesthesia
and the potentiation by systemically administered barbiturates of
prolonged spinal inhibition and synaptic PAD (see Eccles $et$ $al$.,
1963a; Schmidt, 1971).

(-)-Nipecotic acid, a cyclic GABA analogue which inhibits the
cellular uptake of GABA by brain and spinal tissue (Krogsgaard-
Larsen and Johnston, 1975), and increases the inhibitory effectiveness of electrophoretic GABA on spinal neurones (Curtis $et$ $al$.,
1976), depolarized terminals and increased depolarization induced
by GABA.  In a number of experiments, however, (-)-nipecotic acid
(0.2 M, pH 3) did not enhance the submaximal synaptic depolarization of these terminals.

These investigations thus provide evidence that GABA
depolarizes muscle and cutaneous afferent terminals in the cat
spinal cord, and suggest that this effect is related to the
depolarization generated by impulses in other afferent fibres,

presumably at axo-axonic synapses.   Preliminary observations
(D.R. Curtis and D. Lodge - unpublished) indicate that when the
excitability of single ventral horn terminals cannot be increased
by more than 5-10% by flexor muscle afferent impulses, then the
terminals, although of relatively low electrical threshold, are
not particularly sensitive to GABA.   Observations of this type may
indicate that the fibres were electrically excited at nodes rather
than at terminals, but further investigation will be necessary to
correlate the depolarizing effects of GABA on different types of
afferent fibre with changes in excitability induced by impulses
in various muscle and cutaneous afferent pathways.

    Further studies are also needed of the mechanism by which
GABA (and glutamate) depolarize afferent terminals, and of the
nature of the membrane receptors involved.   Unless there are clear
differences between GABA receptors on spinal neurones and
afferent terminals, however, it will be difficult to determine
whether terminal depolarization by GABA actually reduces the
amount of excitatory transmitter released by afferent impulses.
The postsynaptic excitability of spinal motoneurones, interneurones and Renshaw cells is reduced by GABA, and synaptic
inhibitions of the cells have been demonstrated which are unlikely
to be produced solely by effects on presynaptic terminals, and
which are sensitive to bicuculline and picrotoxin (Kellerth and
Szumski, 1966; Cook and Cangiano, 1972; Game and Lodge, 1975;
Curtis et al., 1976; Lodge et al., 1977; see also Carlen, Yaari
and Werman, 1977).

PAD and Potassium

    Elevation of the concentration of potassium ions in the extra-
cellular medium has been proposed as a possible contributing
factor to the depolarization of primary afferent terminals by
sensory volleys (Barron and Matthews, 1938; Curtis et al., 1971;
Bruggencate et al., 1974; Krnjević and Morris, 1975; Křiž et al.,
1975; Lothman and Somjen, 1975).   The contribution of changes
resulting from impulses in afferent fibres (Barron and Matthews,
1938) may be minimal: PAD is blocked by antagonists of GABA which
presumably do not interfere with conduction in these fibres, and
the abolition by elevated magnesium ion concentrations of synaptic
activity in the isolated frog spinal cord reduced to the same
extent synaptically induced PAD and changes in extracellular
potassium activity (Syková and Vyklický, 1977).

    Alterations in potassium levels are thus presumably largely
the consequence of neuronal synaptic and action potentials.
Electrophoretically administered potassium ions depolarize spinal
afferent terminals (D.R. Curtis and D. Lodge - unpublished), and

the bicuculline-sensitive synaptic depolarization of these
structures by GABA could be indirect, involving localized elevation
of the potassium concentration, particularly within glial-
enveloped glomeruli, as a consequence of GABA-induced modification
of postsynaptic membrane conductances. The importance of such a
mechanism, although difficult to investigate, may be relatively
minor since afferent terminal excitibility is not influenced by
glycine, an amino acid which hyperpolarizes spinal neurones by
the same mechanism as does GABA. On the other hand, glycine-
releasing inhibitory terminals, located predominantly on cell
bodies, are probably not closely associated with the boutons of
primary afferent fibres, and hence changes in extracellular ion
levels resulting from the electrophoretic administration of glycine
may not influence afferent terminals. The depolarization of
terminals by acidic amino acids, however, may well be indirect,
and a consequence of changes in extracellular ion concentrations
resulting from the excitation of neurones.


CONCLUSIONS

Within the mammalian spinal cord and dorsal column nuclei
there are interneurones which release GABA at two types of
synapse, which may involve a common presynaptic element:
(a) Axo-dendritic (or somatic), which results in an increase in
postsynaptic membrane conductance and potential of neurones, and
hence *hyperpolarizing* "postsynaptic" inhibition.
(b) Axo-axonic, which results in the *depolarization* of (postsynaptic) presynaptic terminals and reduced release of transmitter by afferent impulses, and hence "presynaptic" inhibition
of synaptic transmission.

Both of these actions of GABA may involve an increase in
the permeability of the "postsynaptic" membrane to chloride ions,
the polarity of the resultant change in membrane potential being
determined by the electrochemical gradient of these ions across
the membrane.

The currently available evidence indicates that both actions
of GABA contribute to inhibitions of the discharge of motoneurones,
interneurones and dorsal column relay neurones, inhibitions which
are of relatively long latency and prolonged duration, and which
are produced by impulses in segmental, intersegmental, ascending
and descending afferent fibres. Thus, GABA is an important spinal
inhibitory transmitter, in addition to glycine which is the
transmitter of relatively short latency and duration postsynaptic
inhibitions (Curtis and Johnston, 1974a; Krnjević, 1974; Aprison
*et al.*, 1975).

There seems to be little justification in using the
adjective "presynaptic" alone when referring to these GABA-mediated
inhibitions, especially as the relative contributions of pre- and
postsynaptic mechanisms are unknown, and possibly terms such as
"prolonged", or "bicuculline (picrotoxinin)-sensitive", or even
"GABA-mediated" may be preferable.

The possibility that depolarization by GABA at axo-axonic
synapses may modify the release of transmitter not only from
primary afferent fibres but also from the terminals of excitatory
and inhibitory interneurones adds further complexity to the role
of this amino acid in the nervous system.

The functional significance of the depolarization by GABA
of neurones in peripheral and sensory ganglia remains to be
determined.  Unlike spinal afferent terminals, and virtually
all central neurones, these peripheral neurones appear to be
insensitive to acidic amino acids.

## REFERENCES

Adams, P.R., and Brown, D.A., 1975, Actions of γ-aminobutyric acid
    on sympathetic ganglion cells, *J. Physiol. (London)* 250:
    85-120.
Aprison, M.H., Daly, E.C., Shank, R.P., and Mc Bride, W.J., 1975,
    Neurochemical evidence for glycine as a transmitter and
    model for its intrasynaptosomal compartmentation, *in*
    "Metabolic Compartmentation and Neurotransmission," (S. Berl,
    D.D. Clark and D. Schneider, eds), pp. 37-63, Plenum Press,
    New York.
Bagshaw, E.V., and Evans, M.H. 1976, Measurement of current spread
    from microelectrodes when stimulating within the nervous
    system, *Exp. Brain Res.* 25:391-400.
Banna, N.R., 1973, Antagonistic effects of semicarbazide and
    pyridoxine on cuneate presynaptic inhibition, *Brain Res.*
    56:249-258.
Banna, N.R., and Jabbur, S.J., 1969, Pharmacological studies on
    inhibition in the cuneate nucleus of the cat, *Int. J.
    Neuropharmac.* 8:299-307.
Banna, N.R., and Jabbur, S.J., 1971, The effects of depleting
    GABA on cuneate presynaptic inhibition, *Brain Res.* 33:
    530-532.
Barker, J.L., and Nicoll, R.A., 1973, The pharmacology and ionic
    dependency of amino acid responses in the frog spinal cord,
    *J. Physiol. (London)* 228:259-277.
Barker, J.L., Nicoll, R.A., and Padjen, A., 1975a, Studies on
    convulsants in the isolated frog spinal cord.  I. Antagonism
    of amino acid responses, *J. Physiol. (London)* 245: 521-536.

Barker, J.L., Nicoll, R.A., and Padjen, A., 1975b, Studies on convulsants in the isolated frog spinal cord. II. Effects of root potentials. *J. Physiol. (London)* 245:537-548.

Barron, D.H., and Matthews, B.H.C., 1938, The interpretation of potential changes in the spinal cord, *J. Physiol. (London)* 92:276-321.

Beal, J.A., and Fox, C.A., 1976, Afferent fibres in the substantia gelatinosa of the adult monkey (*Macaca mulatta*): a Golgi study, *J. comp. Neurol.*, 168:113-143.

Beart, P.M., Curtis, D.R., and Johnston, G.A.R., 1971, 4-Amino-tetrolic acid: a new conformationally-restricted analogue of γ-aminobutyric acid, *Nature (London) New Biol.*, 234:80-81.

Beart, P.M., Kelly, J.S., and Schon, F., 1974, γ-Aminobutyric acid in the rat peripheral nervous system, pineal and posterior pituitary, *Biochem. Soc. Trans.* 2:266-268.

Bell, J.A., and Anderson, E.G., 1972, The influence of semi-carbazide-induced depletion of γ-aminobutyric acid on presynaptic inhibition, *Brain Res.* 43:161-169.

Berger, S.J., Carter, J.G., and Lowry, O.H., 1977, The distribution of glycine, GABA, glutamate and aspartate in rabbit spinal cord, cerebellum and hippocampus, *J. Neurochem.* 28:149-158.

Bertilsson, L., and Costa, E., 1976, Mass fragmentographic quantitation of glutamic acid and γ-aminobutyric acid in cerebellar nuclei and sympathetic ganglia of rats, *J. Chromatog.* 118:395-402.

Bertilsson, L., Suria, A., and Costa, E., 1976, γ-Aminobutyric acid in rat superior cervical ganglion, *Nature (London)* 260:541-542.

Bodian, D., 1966, Synaptic types on spinal motoneuron: an electron microscopic study, *Johns Hopkins Hosp. Bull.* 119:16-45.

Bodian, D., 1970, An electron microscopic characterization of classes of synaptic vesicles by means of controlled aldehyde fixation, *J. cell Biol.* 44:115-124.

Bowery, N.G., and Brown, D.A., 1972, γ-Aminobutyric acid uptake by sympathetic ganglia, *Nature (London) New Biol.* 238:89-91.

Bowery, N.G., and Brown, D.A., 1974a, Depolarizing actions of γ-aminobutyric acid and related compounds on rat superior cervical ganglia *in vitro*, *Br. J. Pharmacol.* 50:205-218.

Bowery, N.G., and Brown, D.A., 1974b, On the release of accumulated [3H]-γ-aminobutyric (GABA) from isolated rat superior cervical ganglia, *Br. J. Pharmacol.* 52:436-437P.

Bowery, N.G., Brown, D.A., and Collins, J.F., 1975, Tetramethylene-disulphotetramine: an inhibitor of γ-aminobutyric acid induced depolarization of the isolated superior cervical ganglion of the rat, *Br. J. Pharmacol.* 53:422-424.

Bowery, N.G., Brown, D.A., Collins, G.G.S., Galvan, M., Marsh, S., and Yamini, G., 1976, Indirect effects of amino-acids on sympathetic ganglion cells mediated through the release of γ-aminobutyric acid from glial cells, *Br. J. Pharmacol.* 57:73-91.

Bowery N.G., Collins, J.F., and Hill, R.G., 1976, Bicyclic phos-
    phorus esters that are potent convulsants and GABA antagonists,
    *Nature (London)* 261:601-603.
Bowery, N.G., and Dray, A., 1976, Barbiturate reversal of amino acid
    antagonism produced by convulsant agents, *Nature (London)* 264:
    276-278.
Bowery, N.G., and Jones, G.P., 1976, A comparison of γ-aminobutyric
    acid and the semi-rigid analogues 4-aminotetrolic acid, 4-amino-
    crotonic acid and imidazole-4-acetic acid on the isolated
    superior cervical ganglion of the rat, *Br. J. Pharmacol.* 56:
    323-330.
Brooks, C. McC., and Eccles, J.C., 1947, Electrical investigation
    of the monosynaptic pathway through the spinal cord,
    *J. Neurophysiol.* 10:251-274.
Brown, D.A., and Galvan, M., 1977, Influence of neuroglial transport
    on the action of γ-aminobutyric acid on mammalian ganglion
    cells, *Br. J. Pharmacol.* 59:373-378.
Bruggencate, G. ten., Lux, H.D., and Liebl, L., 1974, Possible
    relationships between extracellular potassium activity and
    presynaptic inhibition in the spinal cord of the cat,
    *Pflügers Archiv.* 349:301-317.
Carlen, P.L., Yaari, Y., and Werman, R., 1977, Measurement of moto-
    neurone membrane properties during postsynaptic and presynaptic
    inhibition in the cat spinal cord. *Proc. int. Union Physiol.*
    *Sci.* 13:118.
Coimbra, A., Sodré-Borges, B.P., and Magalhães, M.M., 1974, The
    substantia gelatinosa Rolandi of the rat. Fine structure cyto-
    chemistry (acid phosphatase) and changes after dorsal root
    section, *J. Neurocytology*, 3:199-217.
Conradi, S., 1969a, Ultrastructure and distribution of neuronal and
    glial elements on the motoneuron surface in the lumbosacral
    spinal cord of the adult cat, *Acta physiol. scand. Suppl.* 332:
    5-48.
Conradi, S., 1969b, Ultrastructure of dorsal root boutons on lumbo-
    sacral motoneurons of the adult cat, as revealed by dorsal root
    section, *Acta physiol. scand. Suppl.* 332:85-111.
Cook. W.A. Jr., and Cangiano, A., 1972, Presynaptic and postsynaptic
    inhibition of spinal motoneurones, *J. Neurophysiol.* 35:389-403.
Corvaja, N., and Pellegrini, M., 1975, Ultrastructure of dorsal root
    projections in the toad spinal cord. An experimental neuro-
    anatomical study following transection of dorsal root, *Arch.*
    *ital. Biol.* 113:122-149.
Crowshaw, K., Jessup, S.J., and Ramwell, P.W., 1967, Thin-layer
    chromatography of 1-dimethylaminonaphthalen-5-sulphonyl
    derivatives of amino acids present in superfusates of cat
    cerebral cortex, *Biochem. J.* 103:79-85.
Curtis, D.R., 1963, The pharmacology of central and peripheral
    inhibition, *Pharmac. Rev.* 15:333-364.
Curtis, D.R., 1975, Gamma-aminobutyric and glutamic acids as
    mammalian central transmitters, *in* "Metabolic Compartmentation

and Neurotransmission" (S. Berl, D.D. Clarke and D. Schneider, eds.), pp. 11-36, Plenum Press, New York.

Curtis, D.R., 1976, The use of transmitter antagonists in micro-electrophoretic investigations of central synaptic transmission, *in* "Drugs and Central Synaptic Transmission", (P.B. Bradley and B.N. Dhawan, eds), pp. 7-35, Macmillan, London.

Curtis, D.R., Duggan, A.W., Felix, D., and Johnston, G.A.R., 1971, Bicuculline, an antagonist of GABA and synaptic inhibiton in the spinal cord, *Brain Res.* 32:69-96.

Curtis, D.R., Game, C.J.A., Johnston, G.A.R., and McCulloch, R.M., 1974, Central effects of β-(*p*-chlorophenyl)-γ-aminobutyric acid, *Brain Res.* 70:493-499.

Curtis, D.R., Game, C.J.A., and Lodge, D., 1976, The *in vivo* inactivation of GABA and other inhibitory amino acids in the cat nervous system, *Exp. Brain Res.* 25:413-428.

Curtis, D.R., Game, C.J.A., Lodge, D., and McCulloch, R.M., 1976, A pharmacological study of Renshaw cell inhibition, *J. Physiol. (London)* 258:227-242.

Curtis, D.R., and Johnston, G.A.R., 1974a, Amino acid transmitters in the mammalian central nervous system, *Ergebn. Physiol.* 69:97-188.

Curtis, D.R., and Johnston, G.A.R., 1974b, Convulsant alkaloids, *in* "Neuropoisons", (L.L. Simpson and D.R. Curtis, eds.), pp. 207-248, Plenum Press, New York.

Curtis, D.R., Lodge, D., and Brand, S.J., 1977, GABA and spinal afferent terminal excitability in the cat, *Brain Res.* 130: 360-363.

Curtis, D.R., and Ryall, R.W., 1966, Pharmacological studies upon spinal presynaptic fibres, *Exp. Brain Res.* 1:195-204.

Davidoff, R.A., 1972a, The effects of bicuculline on the isolated spinal cord of the frog, *Expl. Neurol.* 35:179-193.

Davidoff, R.A., 1972b, Diphenylhydantoin increases spinal presyn-aptic inhibition, *Amer. Neurol. Assoc. Trans.* 97:193-196.

Davidoff, R.A., 1972c, Penicillin and presynaptic inhibition in the amphibian spinal cord, *Brain Res.* 36:218-222.

Davidson, N., and Simpson, H.K.L., 1976, Concerning the ionic basis of presynaptic inhibition, *Experientia* 32:348-349.

Davidson, N., and Southwick, C.A.P., 1971, Amino acids and presynaptic inhibition in the rat cuneate nucleus, *J. Physiol. (London)* 219:689-708.

de Groat, W.C., 1966, The action of GABA and related amino acids on a sympathetic ganglion, *Proc. Aust. Physiol. Soc. 9th Meeting,* 15.

de Groat, W.C., 1970, The actions of γ-aminobutyric acid and related amino acids on mammalian autonomic ganglia, *J. Pharmacol. exp. Ther.* 172:384-396.

de Groat, W.C., 1972, GABA-depolarization of a sensory ganglion: antagonism by picrotoxin and bicuculline, *Brain Res.* 38: 429-432.

de Groat, W.C., and Lalley, P.M., 1973, Interaction between picro-
    toxin and 5-hydroxytryptamine in the superior cervical
    ganglion of the cat, *Br. J. Pharmacol.* 48:233-244.
de Groat, W.C., Lalley, P.M., and Block, M., 1971, The effects of
    bicuculline and GABA on the superior cervical ganglion of
    the cat, *Brain Res.* 25:665-668.
de Groat, W.C., Lalley, P.M., and Saum, W.R., 1972, Depolarization
    of dorsal root ganglia in the cat by GABA and related amino
    acids: antagonism by picrotoxin and bicuculline, *Brain Res.*
    44, 273-277.
del Castillo, J., and Katz, B., 1956, Localization of active spots
    within the neuro-muscular junction of the frog, *J. Physiol.*
    *(London)* 132:630-649.
Deschenes, M., and Feltz, P., 1976, GABA-induced rise of extra-
    cellular potassium in rat dorsal root ganglia: an electro-
    physiological study *in vivo*, *Brain Res.* 118:494-499.
Deschenes, M., Feltz, P., and Lamour, Y., 1976, A model for an
    estimate *in vivo* of the ionic basis of presynaptic inhibition:
    an intracellular analysis of the GABA-induced depolarization
    in rat dorsal root ganglia, *Brain Res.* 118:486-493.
Dudel, J., and Hatt, H., 1976, Four types of GABA receptors in
    crayfish leg muscles characterized by desensitization and
    specific antagonist. *Pflügers Archiv.* 364:217-222.
Dudel, J., and Kuffler, S.W., 1961, Presynaptic inhibition at the
    crayfish neuromuscular junction, *J. Physiol. (London)* 155:
    543-562.
Eccles, J.C., 1946, Synaptic potentials of motoneurones,
    *J. Neurophysiol.* 9:87-120.
Eccles, J.C., Kostyuk, P.G., and Schmidt, R.F., 1962, The effect
    of electric polarization of the spinal cord on central
    afferent fibres and on their excitatory synaptic action,
    *J. Physiol. (London)* 162:138-150.
Eccles, J.C., and Krnjević, K., 1959, Potential changes recorded
    inside primary afferent fibres within the spinal cord,
    *J. Physiol. (London)* 149:250-273.
Eccles, J.C., Schmidt, R.F., and Willis, W.D., 1963a, Pharmaco-
    logical studies on presynaptic inhibition, *J. Physiol.*
    *(London)* 168:500-530.
Eccles, J.C., Schmidt, R.F., and Willis, W.D., 1963b, The mode of
    operation of the synaptic mechanism producing presynaptic
    inhibition, *J. Neurophysiol.* 26:523-538.
Elliott, K.A.C., and Hobbiger, F., 1959, Gamma-aminobutyric acid;
    circulatory and respiratory effects in different species; re-
    investigation of the anti-strychnine action in mice,
    *J. Physiol. (London)* 146:70-84.
Erulkar, S.D., and Weight, F.F., 1977, Extracellular potassium and
    transmitter release at the giant synapse of squid, *J. Physiol.*
    *(London)* 266: 209-218.

Famiglietti, E.V. Jr., and Peters, A., 1972, The synaptic glomerulus
    and the intrinsic neuron in the dorsal lateral geniculate
    nucleus of the cat, *J. comp. Neurol.* 144:285-334.
Feltz, P., and Rasminsky, M., 1974, A model for the mode of action
    of GABA on primary afferent terminals: depolarizing effects of
    GABA applied iontophoretically to neurones of mammalian dorsal
    root ganglia, *Neuropharmacology* 13:553-563.
Fonnum, F., Storm-Mathisen, J., and Walberg, F., 1970, Glutamate
    decarboxylase in inhibitory neurons.  A study of the enzyme
    in Purkinje cell axons and boutons in the cat, *Brain Res.* 20:
    259-275.
Fonnum, F., and Walberg, F., 1973, An estimation of the concentra-
    tion of γ-aminobutyric acid and glutamate decarboxylase in
    the inhibitory Purkinje axon terminals in the cat, *Brain Res.*
    54:115-127.
Gage, P.W., 1967, Depolarization and excitation-secretion coupling
    in presynaptic terminals, *Fedn Proc.* 26:1627-1632.
Galindo, A., 1969, GABA-picrotoxin interaction in the mammalian
    central nervous system, *Brain Res.* 14:763-767.
Galindo, A., Krnjević, K., and Schwartz, S., 1967, Micro-
    iontophoretic studies on neurones in the cuneate nucleus,
    *J. Physiol. (London)* 192:359-377.
Game, C.J.A., and Lodge, D., 1975, The pharmacology of the
    inhibition of dorsal horn neurones by impulses in myelinated
    cutaneous afferents in the cat, *Exp. Brain Res.* 23:75-84.
Gerschenfeld, H.M., 1973, Chemical transmission in invertebrate
    central nervous systems and neuromuscular junctions, *Physiol.
    Rev.* 53:1-119.
Glusman, S., 1975, Correlation between the topographical
    distribution of [$^3$H]GABA uptake and primary afferent
    depolarization in the frog spinal cord, *Brain Res.* 88:109-114.
Glusman, S., Vazquez, G., and Rudomin, P., 1976, Ultrastructural
    observations in the frog spinal cord in relation to the
    generation of primary afferent depolarization, *Neurosci.
    Lett.* 2:137-145.
Gmelin, G., and Cerletti, A., 1976, Electrophoretic studies on
    presynaptic inhibition in the mammalian spinal cord,
    *Experientia* 32:756.
Gobel, S., 1975, Golgi studies of the substantia gelatinosa
    neurons in the spinal trigeminal nucleus, *J. comp. Neurol.*
    162:397-416.
Graham, L.T., Jr., and Aprison, M.H., 1969, Distribution of some
    enzymes associated with the metabolism of glutamate, aspartate,
    γ-aminobutyrate and glutamine in cat spinal cord, *J. Neurochem.*
    16:559-566.
Graham, L.T., Jr., Shank, R.P., Werman, R., and Aprison, M.H.,
    1967, Distribution of some synaptic transmitter suspects in
    cat spinal cord: glutamic acid, aspartic acid, γ-aminobutyric
    acid, glycine and glutamine, *J. Neurochem.* 14: 465-472.

Grinnell, A.D., 1966, A study of the interaction between moto-
    neurones in the frog spinal cord, *J. Physiol. (London)* 182:
    612-648.
Hagiwara, S., and Tasaki, I., 1958, A study of the mechanism of
    impulse transmission across the giant synapse of the squid,
    *J. Physiol. (London)* 143:114-137.
Hubbard, J.I., 1970, Mechanism of transmitter release, *in*
    "Progress in Biophysics and Molecular Biology", Vol. 21,
    (J.A.V. Butler and D. Noble, eds.), pp. 33-124, Pergamon
    Press, Oxford.
Hubbard, J.I., and Schmidt, R.F., 1963, An electrophysiological
    investigation of mammalian motor nerve terminals, *J. Physiol.
    (London)* 166:145-167.
Iles, J.F., 1976, Central terminations of muscle afferents on
    motoneurones in the cat spinal cord, *J. Physiol. (London)* 262:
    91-117.
Iversen, L.L., and Kelly, J.S., 1975, Uptake and metabolism of
    γ-aminobutyric acid by neurones and glial cells, *Biochem.
    Pharmacol.* 24:933-938.
Jankowska, E., and Roberts, W.J., 1972, An electrophysiological
    demonstration of the axonal projections of single spinal
    interneurones in the cat, *J. Physiol. (London)* 222:597-622.
Johnston, G.A.R., Curtis, D.R., Game, C.J.A., McCulloch, R.M.,
    and Twitchin, B., 1975, *Cis* and *trans*-4-aminocrotonic acid as
    GABA analogues of restricted conformation, *J. Neurochem.* 24:
    157-160.
Kanazawa, I., Iversen, L.L., and Kelly, J.S., 1976, Glutamate
    decarboxylase activity in the rat posterior pituitary, pineal
    gland, dorsal root ganglion and superior cervical ganglion,
    *J. Neurochem.* 27:1267-1269.
Katz, B., and Miledi, R., 1965, Propagation of electric activity in
    motor nerve terminals, *Proc. R. Soc. B.* 161:453-482.
Katz, B., and Miledi, R., 1967, A study of synaptic transmission
    in the absence of nerve impulses. *J. Physiol. (London)* 192:
    407-436.
Katz, B., and Miledi, R., 1971, The effect of prolonged
    depolarization on synaptic transfer in the stellate
    ganglion of the squid, *J. Physiol. (London)* 216:503-512.
Kellerth, J.-O., and Szumski,A.J., 1966, Effects of picrotoxin on
    stretch-activated postsynaptic inhibitions in spinal moto-
    neurones, *Acta physiol. scand.* 66:146-156.
Kelly, J.S., Gottesfeld,Z., and Schon, F., 1973, Reduction in GAD
    I activity from the dorsal lateral region of the deafferented
    rat spinal cord, *Brain Res.* 62:581-586.
Kelly, J.S., and Renaud, L.P., 1973a, On the pharmacology of
    γ-aminobutyric acid receptors on the cuneo-thalamic relay
    cells of the cat, *Br. J. Pharmacol.* 48:369-386.
Kelly, J.S., and Renaud, L.P., 1973b, On the pharmacology of
    ascending, descending and recurrent postsynaptic inhibition of

the cuneo-thalamic relay cells in the cat, *Br. J. Pharmacol.*
48:396-408.

Kerr, F.W.L., 1970, The organization of primary afferents in the
subnucleus caudalis of the trigeminal: a light and electron
microscopic study of degeneration, *Brain Res.* 23:147-165.

Koketsu, K., Shoji, T., and Yamamoto, K., 1974, Effects of GABA on
presynaptic nerve terminals in bullfrog *(Rana catesbiana)*
sympathetic ganglia, *Experientia* 30:382-383.

Kříž, N., Syková, R., and Vyklický, L., 1975, Extracellular
potassium changes in the spinal cord of the cat and their
relation to slow potentials, active transport and impulse
transmission, *J. Physiol. (London)* 249:167-182.

Krnjević, K., 1955, The distribution of Na and K in cat nerves
*J. Physiol. (London)* 128:473-488.

Krnjević, K., 1974, Chemical nature of synaptic transmission in
vertebrates, *Physiol. Rev.* 54:418-540.

Krnjević, K., and Morris, M.E., 1975, Correlation between extracellular focal potentials and $K^+$ potentials evoked by primary
afferent activity, *Can. J. Physiol. Pharmacol.* 53:912-922.

Krogsgaard-Larsen, P., and Johnston, G.A.R., 1975, Inhibition of
GABA uptake in rat brain slices by nipecotic acid, various
isoxazoles and related compounds, *J. Neurochem.* 25:797-802.

Kudo, Y., Abe, N., Goto, S., and Fukuda, H., 1975, The chloride-
dependent depression by GABA in the frog spinal cord,
*Eur. J. Pharmacol.* 32:251-259.

Kuno, M., 1961, Site of action of systemic gamma-aminobutyric acid
in the spinal cord, *Jap. J. Physiol.* 11:304-318.

Kuno, M., and Muneoka, A., 1961, Effects of long chain omega-amino
acids on the spinal cord, *Proc. Jap. Acad.* 37:398-401.

Kuno, M., Munoz-Martinez, E.J., and Randić, M., 1973, Synaptic
action on Clarke's column neurones in relation to afferent
terminal size, *J. Physiol. (London)* 228:343-360.

LaMotte, C., 1977, Distribution of the tract of Lissauer and
the dorsal root fibers in the primate spinal cord, *J. comp.
Neurol.* 172:529-562.

Lawson, S.N., Biscoe, T.J., and Headley, P.M., 1976, The effect of
electrophoretically applied GABA on cultured dissociated
spinal cord and sensory ganglion neurones in the rat,
*Brain Res.* 117, 493-497.

Levy, R.A., 1975, The effect of intravenously administered γ-aminobutyric acid on afferent fiber polarization, *Brain Res.* 92:
21-34.

Levy, R.A., and Anderson, E.G., 1972, The effect of the GABA
antagonists bicuculline and picrotoxin on primary afferent
terminal excitability, *Brain Res.* 43:171-180.

Levy, R.A., and Anderson, E.G., 1974, The role of γ-aminobutyric
acid as a mediator of positive dorsal root potentials, *Brain
Res.* 76:71-82.

Ljungdahl, Å., and Hökfelt, T., 1973, Autoradiographic uptake
    patterns of [³H]GABA and [³H]glycine in central nervous
    tissues with special reference to the cat spinal cord, *Brain
    Res.* 62:587-595.
Lodge, D., Curtis, D.R., and Brand, S.J., 1977, A pharmacological
    study of the inhibition of ventral group Ia-excited spinal
    interneurones, *Exp. Brain Res.* 29:97-105.
Lothman, E,W., and Somjen, G.G., 1975, Extracellular potassium
    activity, intracellular and extracellular potential responses
    in the spinal cord, *J. Physiol. (London)* 252:115-136.
McLaughlin, B.J., 1972a, The fine structure of neurons and
    synapses in the motor nuclei of the cat spinal cord, *J. comp.
    Neurol.* 144:429-460.
McLaughlin, B.J., 1972b, Dorsal root projections to the motor
    nuclei in the cat spinal cord, *J. comp. Neurol.* 144:461-474.
McLaughlin, B.J., Barber, R., Saito, K., Roberts, E., and Wu, J.Y.,
    1975, Immunocytochemical localization of glutamate
    decarboxylase in rat spinal cord, *J. comp. Neurol.* 164:305-322.
McMahan, U.J., and Kuffler, S.W., 1971, Visual identification of
    synaptic boutons on living ganglion cells and of varicosities
    in postganglionic axons in the heart of the frog, *Proc. R. Soc.
    B.* 177:485-508.
Martin, A.R., and Ringham, G.L., 1975, Synaptic transfer at a
    vertebrate central nervous system synapse, *J. Physiol. (London)*
    251:409-426.
Mendell, L., 1972, Properties and distribution of peripherally
    evoked presynaptic hyperpolarization in cat lumbar spinal cord,
    *J. Physiol. (London)* 226:769-792.
Miledi, R., and Slater, C.R., 1966, The action of calcium on neuronal
    synapses in the squid, *J. Physiol. (London)* 184:473-498.
Milokhin, A.A., and Reshetnikov, S.S., 1972, Morphology of receptor
    innervation of spinal ganglia, *Neurosci. Behav. Physiol.* 5:
    93-103.
Minchin, M.C.W., and Beart, P.M., 1975, Compartmentation of amino
    acid metabolism in the rat dorsal root ganglion; a metabolic
    and autoradiographic study, *Brain Res.* 83:437-449.
Minchin, M.C.W., and Iversen, L.L., 1974, Releasee of [³H]gamma-
    aminobutyric acid from glial cells in rat dorsal root ganglia,
    *J. Neurochem.* 23,533-540.
Miyata, Y., and Otsuka, M., 1972, Distribution of γ-aminobutyric
    acid in cat spinal cord and the alteration produced by local
    ischaemia, *J. Neurochem.* 19:1833-1834.
Miyata, Y., and Otsuka, M., 1975, Quantitative histochemistry of
    γ-aminobutyric acid in cat spinal cord with special reference
    to presynaptic inhibition, *J. Neurochem.* 25:239-244.
Nicoll, R.A., 1975a, Presynaptic action of barbiturates in the
    frog spinal cord, *Proc. Natl. Acad. Sci. U.S.A.* 72:1460-1463.

Nicoll, R.A., 1975b, The action of acetylcholine antagonists on
    amino acid responses in the frog spinal cord *in vitro*,
    *Br. J. Pharmacol.* 55:449-458.

Nicoll, R.A., 1976, The interaction of porphyrin precursors with
    GABA receptors in the isolated frog spinal cord, *Life Sci.
    Oxford* 19:521-526.

Nicoll, R.A., 1977, The effect of conformationally restricted
    amino acid analogues on the frog spinal cord *in vitro*,
    *Br. J. Pharmacol.* 59:303-309.

Nicoll, R.A., and Padjen, A., 1976, Pentylenetetrazol: an
    antagonist of GABA at primary afferents of the isolated frog
    spinal cord, *Neuropharmacology* 15:69-71.

Nishi, S., Minota, S., and Karczmar, A.G., 1974, Primary afferent
    neurones: the ionic mechanism of GABA-mediated depolarization,
    *Neuropharmacology* 13:215-219.

Obata, K., 1974, Transmitter sensitivities of some nerve and
    muscle cells in culture, *Brain Res.* 73:71-88.

Otsuka, M., and Konishi, S., 1976, GABA in the spinal cord, *in*
    "GABA in Nervous System Function," Vol. 5, (E. Roberts,
    T.N. Chase and D.B. Tower, eds.), pp. 197-202, Raven Press,
    New York.

Otsuka, M., Obata, K., Miyata, Y., and Tanaka, Y., 1971,
    Measurement of γ-aminobutyric acid in isolated nerve cells of
    cat central nervous system, *J. Neurochem.* 18:287-295.

Ralston, H.J., 1968, Dorsal root projections to dorsal horn
    neurons in the cat spinal cord, *J. comp. Neurol.* 132:303-330.

Ramon-Moliner, E., 1977, Reciprocal synapses of the olfactory bulb:
    questioning the evidence, *Brain Res.* 128:1-20.

Ramon y Cajal, S., 1911, "Histologie du Systeme Nerveux de l'Homme
    et des Vertebres," Vol. 2, pp. 442-452, Maloine, Paris.

Ranck, J.B., 1975, Which elements are excited in electrical
    stimulation of mammalian central nervous system, a review,
    *Brain Res.* 98:417-440.

Ransom, R., and Nelson, P.G., 1975, Neuropharmacological responses
    from nerve cells in tissue culture, *in* "Handbook of Psycho-
    pharmacology," Vol. 2, (L.L. Iversen, S.D. Iversen and S.H.
    Snyder, eds.), pp. 101-127, Plenum Press, New York, London.

Repkin, A.H., Wolf, P., and Anderson, E.G., 1976, Non-GABA
    mediated primary afferent depolarization, *Brain Res.* 117:147-
    152.

Réthelyi, M., 1977, Preterminal and terminal axon arborization in
    the substantia gelatinosa of cat's spinal cord, *J. comp.
    Neurol.* 172:511-528.

Réthelyi, M., and Szentágothai, J., 1969, The large synaptic
    complexes of the substantia gelatinosa, *Exp. Brain Res.* 7:
    258-274.

Ribak, C.W., Vaughn, K., Saito, K., Barber, R., and Roberts, E.,
    1977, Glutamate decarboxylase localization in neurons of the
    olfactory bulb, *Brain Res.* 126:1-18.

Roberts, W.J., and Smith, D.O., 1973, Analysis of threshold currents
    during microstimulation of fibres in the spinal cord, *Acta
    physiol. scand.* 89:384-394.
Rustioni, A., and Sotelo, C., 1974, Some effects of chronic
    deafferentation on the ultrastructure of the nucleus
    gracilis of the cat, *Brain Res.* 73:527-533.
Salvador, R.A., and Albers, R.W., 1959, The distribution of
    glutamic-γ-aminobutyric transaminase in the nervous system of
    the Rhesus monkey, *J. biol. Chem.* 234:922-925.
Schmidt, R.F., 1963, Pharmacological studies on the primary
    afferent depolarization of the toad spinal cord, *Pflügers
    Archiv.* 277:325-346.
Schmidt, R.F., 1971, Presynaptic inhibition in the vertebrate
    central nervous system, *Ergebn. Physiol.* 63:20-101.
Schon, F., and Kelly, J.S., 1974a, Autoradiographic localisation
    of [$^3$H]GABA and [$^3$H]glutamate over satellite glial cells,
    *Brain Res.* 66:275-288.
Schon, F., and Kelly, J.S., 1974b, The characterisation of [$^3$H]GABA
    uptake into the satellite glial cells of rat sensory ganglia,
    *Brain Res.* 66:289-300.
Singer, W., and Lux, H.D., 1973, Presynaptic depolarization and
    extracellular potassium in the cat lateral geniculate
    nucleus, *Brain Res.* 64:17-33.
Srimal, R.C., and Bhargava, K.P., 1966, Peripheral neural effects
    of gamma aminobutyric acid, *Arch. int. Pharmacodyn. Ther.*
    164:444-450.
Stanton, H.C., 1964, Mode of action of gamma-aminobutyric acid on
    the cardiovascular system, *Arch. int. Pharmacodyn. Ther.* 143:
    195-204.
Stanton, H.C., and Woodhouse, F.H., 1960, The effect of gamma-*n*-
    butyric acid and some related compounds on the cardiovascular
    system of anaesthetized dogs, *J. Pharmacol.* 128:233-242.
Stoney, S.D., Jr., Thompson, W.D., and Asanuma, H., 1968, Excitation
    of pyramidal tract cells by intracortical microstimulation:
    effective extent of stimulating current, *J. Neurophysiol.* 31:
    659-669.
Sverdlov, Yu.S., and Kozhechkin, S.N., 1975, Effects of glycine and
    gamma-aminobutyric acid on excitability of central terminals
    of primary afferent fibres, *Neurophysiol. USSR*, 7:388-394.
Syková, E., and Vyklický, L., 1977, Changes of extracellular
    potassium activity in isolated spinal cord of frog under high
    Mg$^{2+}$ concentrations, *Neurosci. Lett.* 4:161-165.
Szentágothai, J., 1970, Glomerular synapses, complex synaptic
    arrangements, and their operational significance, *in* "The
    Neurosciences: Second Study Program", (F.O. Schmitt, ed.),
    pp. 427-443, The Rockefeller University Press, New York.
Takeuchi, A., and Takeuchi, N., 1962, Electrical changes in pre-
    and postsynaptic axons of the giant synapse of *Loligo*,
    *J. gen. Physiol.* 45:1181-1193.

Tappaz, M.L., Zivin, J.A., and Kopin, I.J., 1976, Intraspinal glutamic decarboxylase distribution after transection of the cord at the thoracic level, *Brain Res.* 111:220-223.

Tebēcis, A.K., and Phillis, J.W., 1969, The use of convulsants in studying possible functions of amino acids in the toad spinal cord, *Comp. Biochem. Physiol.* 28:1303-1315.

Uchizono, K., 1975, "Excitation and Inhibition. Synaptic Morphology" Igaku Shoin Ltd., Tokyo.

Valdivia, O., 1971, Methods of fixation and the morphology of synaptic vesicles, *J. comp. Neurol.* 142:257-274.

Walberg, F., 1965, Axoaxonic contacts in the cuneate nucleus, probable basis for presynaptic depolarization, *Expl. Neurol.* 13:218-231.

Walberg, F., 1966, The fine structure of the cuneate nucleus in normal cats and following interruption of afferent fibres. An electron microscopic study with particular reference to findings made in Glees and Nauta sections, *Exp. Brain Res.* 2:107-128.

Wall, P.D., 1958, Excitability changes in afferent fibre terminations and their relation to slow potentials, *J. Physiol. (London)* 142:1-21.

Westrum, L.E., and Black, R.G., 1971, Fine structural aspects of the synaptic organization of the spinal trigeminal nucleus (pars interpolaris) of the cat, *Brain Res.* 25:265-287.

Willis, W.D., Núñez, R., and Rudomin, P., 1976, Excitability changes of terminal arborization of single Ia and Ib afferent fibers produced by muscle and cutaneous conditioning volleys, *J. Neurophysiol.* 39:1150-1159.

Woodward, J.K., Bianchi, C.P., and Erulkar, S.D., 1969, Electrolyte distribution in rabbit cervical ganglion, *J. Neurochem.* 16: 289-299.

Young, J.A.C., Brown, D.A., Kelly, J.S., and Schon, F., 1973, Autoradiographic localization of sites of [3H]γ-aminobutyric acid accumulation in peripheral autonomic ganglia, *Brain Res.* 63:479-486.

Zenker, W., and Hogl, E., 1976, The prebifurcation section of the axon of the rat spinal ganglion cell, *Cell Tiss. Res.* 165: 345-363.

# QUANTITATIVE STUDIES OF IONTOPHORETICALLY-
# APPLIED EXCITATORY AMINO ACIDS

A. Nistri and J.F. MacDonald

Anaesthesia Research, McGill University

3655 Drummond St., Montreal H3G 1Y6

When relative potencies of a group of agonists are compared, it is customary to derive these values from dose-response curves. This is not simple when dealing with excitatory substances applied iontophoretically to in vivo central neurones. In fact the actual dose used is unknown and a number of problems regarding the properties of the iontophoretic electrode greatly complicate this matter (Kelly et al., 1975). We describe here some methods to obtain dose-response relations for iontophoretically-applied excitatory amino acids on interneurones of the cat spinal cord. The experimental set-up has been previously described (MacDonald and Nistri, 1977). These dose response relations were obtained with quisqualate, a very active glutamate agonist; similar results were found with glutamate, aspartate or ibotenate. "Doses" were expressed as total charge applied (current x ejection time; nC) to allow comparisons between drugs which had to be ejected for different times (for a given substance the ejection time was kept constant). Within the current range used, approximately constant firing rates (plateau response) were achieved near the end of the ejection period. Such plateau responses probably represent an equilibrium drug distribution in the receptive area. The simplest way of obtaining dose-response relations was the sequential method (Fig. la) where varying currents were applied as shown by the tracings above this plot. In Fig. 1B a cumulative method was used: increasingly larger currents, without interdose rest (see corresponding tracings), were given. This plot was very similar to that of Fig. la, although with the

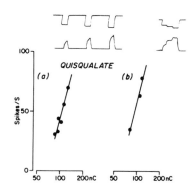

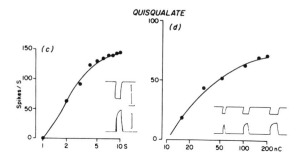

Fig. 1.    Different methods of obtaining dose-response
relations.    Some original tracings (currents, top; spike
activity, bottom) are shown above (a) & (b) & beside (c) &
(d).    In (c) calibration bars (also  valid for all the
other tracings):  current 15 nA; time (horizontal bar)
10 s; response 100 spikes/s.   Abscissa (log scale): nC
for (a), (b) and (d).   Ordinate:
spikes/s.   Same neurone for each method.

cumulative method the risk of depolarization block was
high.   Fig. 1c shows another type of cumulative dose-
response plot (see Kelly et al., 1975) where a single
large response was plotted against elapsed time (calibrations in Fig. 1c  also apply to all the other tracings).
This plot differs from the previous ones and resembles
that of Fig. 1d where a fixed dose was applied for varying periods.   To check for a linear relationship between
drug release and current, we constructed dose-response
plots with the increment method (Katz and Thesleff, 1957).
Currents were alternatively applied to 2 different quisqualate barrels of the  same electrode to evoke matching
responses.   The simultaneous application of both currents
was arbitrarily taken as a dose-unit.   The procedure is

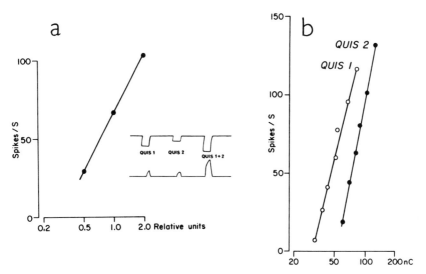

Fig. 2a: Increment method for dose-response relation
to quisqualate (QUIS). The inset shows tracings of some
responses used (calibrations as in Fig. 1c).
Fig. 2b: Sequential dose-response plots obtained from
two different barrels (both containing quisqualate, QUIS).
Responses of Fig. 2a and b are from the same neurone used
for Fig. 1.

then repeated for higher units. This plot (Fig. 2a) confirms a linear proportionality between release and current.
Figure 2b shows that sequential dose-response relations
obtained from different barrels of the same electrode
have similar shapes and slopes. Furthermore, varying
retaining currents (5-20 nA) did not alter the shape and
slope of the dose-response lines. A relatively long
(10 s) application of quisqualate might produce responses
with variable contributions from distant neuronal regions
and thus give spurious quantitative results. This was
checked on the same neurones (Fig. 3) by comparing the
sequential dose-response plot (10 s applications, open
circles, right) with a similar plot achieved with 50 ms
applications (closed circles, left). Obviously different
nC ranges were used but very similar slopes were observed.
With very small currents (outside the range used for
these plots) responses did not reach a plateau within
10 s ejection time, suggesting that diffusion might have
been a limiting factor. However, with higher currents
plateau responses were achieved before the termination

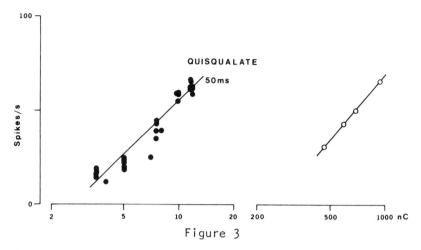

Figure 3

of the current ejection and were not influenced by longer
applications. Figure 4 shows that 10 s (open circles)
or 20 s (filled circles) applications gave a dose-response
relation in which all the points fell on the same line.

Sequential plots were deemed the most useful to
calculate potencies. In practice this was done by comparing approximately parallel log-dose response lines
for different substances (Fig. 5). A fixed response
(50 spikes/s) corresponding to a submaximal firing level
was chosen; the charge of each drug needed to achieve
this response was taken to express the appropriate potency values (usually expressed as ratios to a reference
drug, e.g. glutamate). With this method we found quisqualate and N-methyl-D-aspartate 8 and 4 times more
potent than glutamate respectively whereas aspartate

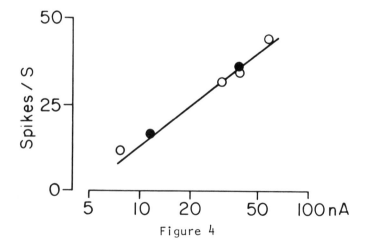

Figure 4

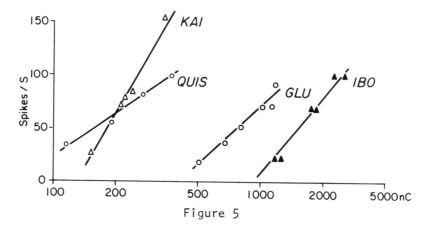

Figure 5

and ibotenate were equipotent (or slightly less potent) to glutamate. A reliable comparison was more difficult when a drug (e.g. kainate) gave a plot clearly non-parallel to the reference drug. Kainate responses also had additional features such as a long latency followed by abrupt onset, no plateau and a long "tail".

In conclusion, the present method allowed calculations of agonist potencies; however, the transport number of each drug ought to me measured (if possible) to ensure that varying ionic mobilities do not significantly contribute to apparently different drug potencies.

## REFERENCES

Katz, B. and Thesleff, S. 1957. A study of the "desensitization" produced by acetylcholine at the motor endplate. J. Physiol. (Lond.), 138, 63-80.

Kelly, J.S., Simmonds, M.A. and Straughan, D.W. 1975. Microelectrode techniques, in "Methods in Brain Research" (P.B. Bradley, ed.), pp. 333-377, Wiley Press, London.

MacDonald, J.F. and Nistri, A. 1977. Actions of microiontophoretically-applied ibotenate on cat spinal interneurones. Can. J. Physiol. Pharmacol., 55, 965-967.

# INTERACTIONS OF CENTRAL DEPRESSANTS WITH AMINO ACIDS AND THEIR ANTAGONISTS

A. Dray and N.G. Bowery

Departments of Pharmacology, School of Pharmacy,
29/39 Brunswick Sq. London WC1N 1AX & St. Thomas's
Hospital Medical School, London SE1 7EH, U.K.

Since their introduction over 70 years ago, barbiturates have been invaluable therapeutic and experimental agents. While they possess a wide spectrum of pharmacological actions e.g. hypnotic, anaesthetic, anticonvulsant, their precise mechanism and site/s of action remains obscure. A multitude of actions on synaptic processes have however been proposed. Thus _in vitro_ and _in vivo_ studies suggest actions on cell metabolism (see Sharpless 1970) neurotransmitter synthesis (Richter & Crossland, 1949; Anderson & Bonnycastle, 1960; Corrodi et al, 1966) release (Mitchell, 1963; Phillis & Chong, 1965; Phillis 1968; Cutler & Dudzinski, 1974) and inactivation (Cutler et al, 1974). More specifically they have been suggested to affect a number of post-synaptic processes, for example, they modify the actions of putative excitatory neurotransmitters acetylcholine and glutamate (see Bradley & Dray, 1973). Perhaps of greater significance, barbiturates have been shown to increase the duration of central pre-and post-synaptic inhibition at spinal and supra-spinal sites (Eccles et al, 1963; 1971; Nicoll et al, 1975), processes considered to be mediated by GABA. Although a direct action on post-synaptic GABA receptors may account for these effects (Nicoll, 1975) other interactions with post-synaptic events triggered by GABA e.g. ionic conductance changes, may also be involved (Ransom & Barker, 1976).

In a series of _in vitro_ and _in vivo_ experiments we have examined the effects of barbiturates and a number of other central depressant drugs on the actions of inhibitory amino acids, particularly GABA and glycine. During this study we observed that barbiturates and other hypnotics prevented or reversed the actions of convulsant amino acid antagonists (Bowery & Dray, 1976).

93

The in vitro experiments were made on the isolated superfused
rat superior cervical ganglion preparation (Bowery & Brown, 1974;
Brown & Marsh, 1975) in which the activation of GABA receptors
produces a dose-dependent depolarizing surface potential. Pentobarbitone also depolarized the ganglion (threshold 100 - 300 μM)
but was some 100 times less potent than GABA and its actions were
much more prolonged. Bicuculline methochloride (BMC) reversibly
antagonised the effect of both agents but the responses to pentobarbitone were clearly less susceptible. At concentrations
(4 - 80 μM) too low to depolarize the ganglion pentobarbitone
produced inconsistent effects on the responses to low doses of
GABA. In some experiments potentiation was seen and in others
GABA responses were unchanged. However, at higher GABA concentrations (i.e. > ED50), pentobarbitone produced a marked reduction
of GABA responses. On the other hand, in the presence of BMC
sufficient to produce  a marked antagonism of GABA responses, the
addition of pentobarbitone (5 - 80 μM) into the superfusate
displaced the GABA dose-response curve back towards the control.
An apparent reversal of the BMC antagonism had occurred. A similar
interaction occurred if the pentobarbitone superfusion preceded
that of BMC. In this situation the expected decrease of GABA
responses by BMC did not occur. Such interactions were also
demonstrable with other GABA mimetics e.g. muscimol and 3-amino-
propane sulphonic acid. In addition the antagonism of GABA by a
number of other antagonists, picrotoxin, tetramethylenedisulphotetramine, isopropyl bicyclophosphate was also prevented or
reversed by pentobarbitone. As with BMC there was an interdependence
between the concentration of antagonist and that of pentobarbitone.
Of particular interest was the observation that pentobarbitone
readily reversed the non-selective antagonism of GABA by strychnine
but did not modify the additional depression of matching carbachol
responses. Moreover, pentobarbitone did not affect the depression
of carbachol responses by hexamethonium.

The reversal of BMC antagonism was observed with a number of
other barbiturates. Thiopentone and amylobarbitone were of similar
activity to pentobarbitone; quinal barbitone was 2 - 3 times more
potent but the anticonvulsants phenobarbitone and mephobarbitone
were less active than pentobarbitone. A number of other hypnotics
shared BMC reversal properties e.g. benzodiazepines, glutethimide,
chloral hydrate but other classes of drug were also effective e.g.
haloperidol, promethazine, amitriptyline. In contrast, antidepres-
sants of the monoamine oxidase inhibitor class, tranylcypromine
and iproniazid were ineffective and so was the neuroleptic tri-
fluoperazine.

The benzodiazepines were of particular interest since they
appeared to be active at concentrations lower than any of the
barbiturates. However, in contrast to the barbiturates, they
could never fully reverse the effect of BMC. Figure 1 shows

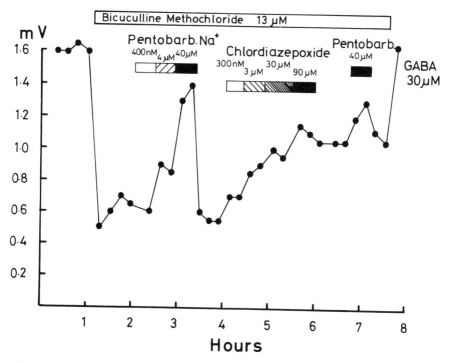

Fig. 1: Reversal by pentobarbitone and chlordiazepoxide of GABA antagonism produced by bicuculline methochloride in an isolated superior cervical ganglion of the rat. Each dot represents the magnitude of a single response to GABA (30 μM) (ordinate : milli volts) applied for 1 min. The abscissa is time in hours. Bicuculline methochloride (13 μM) was continuously superfused over the tissue during the period indicated by the open horizontal bar. Pentobarbitone and chlordiazepoxide were applied in increasing concentrations (0.4 - 40 μM and 0.3 - 90 μM respectively) during the periods shown by the hatched/closed horizontal bars. Note (i) the dose-dependent increase in the response to GABA in the presence of either pentobarbitone or chlordiazepoxide (ii) the threshold concentration for chlordiazepoxide was lower than for pentobarbitone although the latter produced a greater enhancement at higher concentrations (iii) the more rapid offset of the action of pentobarbitone.

the comparative effects of increasing concentrations of pento-barbitone and chlordiazepoxide. The threshold concentrations of pentobarbitone was 0.4 - 4 μM whereas 0.3 μM chlordiazepoxide produced some enhancement of the GABA response. However, whereas 40 μM pentobarbitone produced 80% reversal, even 90 μM chlordiaze-

poxide produced less than 60% reversal. The effect of chlordiazepoxide also differed in time course to pentobarbitone. Thus the
partial reversal of BMC by chlordiazepoxide often lasted for hours
whereas that to pentobarbitone was quite rapid in offset (Fig. 1).
Additionally prior superfusion of the ganglion with chlordiazepoxide
appeared to reduce the effect of subsequent superfusion with BMC.

It was unlikely that the reversal of BMC antagonism could be
attributed to potentiation of GABA per se. Experiments with
nipecotic acid, which inhibits GABA transport into neurones and
glia (Krogsgaard-Larsen & Johnston, 1975; Johnston et al, 1976;
Bowery et al, 1976) showed that this compound potentiated the
response to a low dose of GABA (3 μM) (see Brown & Galvan, 1977).
In the presence of BMC the resulting GABA antagonism was the same
as that obtained in the absence of nipecotic acid and only when
pentobarbitone was introduced was there any reversal of the BMC
effect.

The in vivo experiments were performed on urethane anaesthetised
rats. Multibarrelled micropipettes were used to record extracellular
activity from single brain stem neurones and to administer substances
by electrophoresis. As shown in Figure 2, when BMC selectively
antagonised the inhibition of spontaneous neuronal firing produced
by GABA, the concurrent administration of pentobarbitone from
the same electrode partially or completely reversed this antagonism.
The reversal could be overcome by increasing the expulsion of BMC.
Reversal was unaccompanied by spike changes or depression of background firing. When pentobarbitone was administered to the same
neurones in the absence of BMC, inconsistent effects were observed.
Thus the responses to GABA or glycine were unaffected in most cells
(5 of 8 cells) but slightly potentiated (one cell) or reduced in
others (2 cells). Direct depression of neuronal firing by pentobarbitone was only observed with high ejecting currents (100 - 150
μA). When additional reduction of glycine responses were produced
by BMC, pentobarbitone always reversed this antagonism sooner than
that of GABA.

Strychnine was also tested on neurones where pentobarbitone
had already been shown to reverse BMC effects (Figure 2). The
concurrent administration of pentobarbitone reversed strychnine
antagonism of glycine in one third of the neurones tested.
Moreover, pentobarbitone always readily reversed any non-selective
block of GABA by strychnine (Figure 2). Though the in vitro
experiments showed that quinalbarbitone was more active than
pentobarbitone, this was not evident in vivo. Quinalbarbitone
ejected electrophoretically exhibited the same spectrum of
activity as pentobarbitone in the brain stem experiments.
Benzodiazepines were less able to reverse the effects of
BMC. Chlordiazepoxide restored the effects of GABA in 50% of
cells tested. However, unlike the reversal seen with barbiturates,

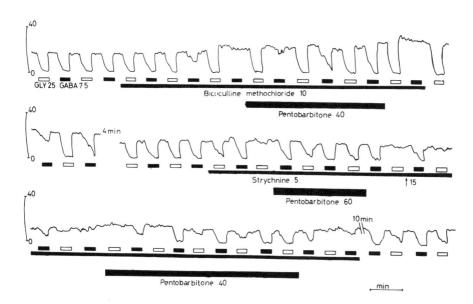

Figure 2: The continuous ratemeter record (firing frequency in
Hz against time in minutes) of a spontaneous brain stem neurone
shows reproducible depression by glycine and GABA. The top trace
shows that the continuous administration of bicuculline methochloride selectively reduced the responses to GABA. The additional
continuous administration of pentobarbitone restored the response
to GABA without producing any significant effect on background
firing rate. Shortly after the cessation of pentobarbitone
administration the GABA response was again completely blocked by
bicuculline. After complete recovery of the responses to GABA a
continuous administration of strychnine (5 nA) selectively reduced
the glycine response (middle trace continuation of top trace). An
additional administration of pentobarbitone restored the glycine
response which was again blocked after the pentobarbitone current
was switched off. Increasing the ejecting current of strychnine
to 15 nA (at arrow) produced additional antagonism of the GABA
response. A repeated administration of pentobarbitone rapidly
restored the GABA response and also that of glycine. Responses
to both GABA and glycine were blocked after pentobarbitone was
switched off, and recovered some 10 min after the strychnine
administration was stopped. In all records the horizontal bars
indicate the duration of drug ejection and the ejecting currents
are indicated in nA.

this effect with chlordiazepoxide was only partial (20 - 40%
reversal) a finding which concurs with the in vitro studies.
Flurazepam could not be shown to reverse BMC antagonism and
both benzodiazepines   had additional actions on spontaneous
firing and in the responses to GABA or glycine.

    In studies with intravenous infusions of barbiturates (0.4 -
3 mg/Kg) thiopentone, hexobarbitone and pentobarbitone produced
short-lasting (2 - 7 mins) reversal of BMC antagonism of GABA
responses. Intravenous clonazepam (100 μg/Kg) only partially
restored GABA responses, but this effect was extremely prolonged
(2 hours).
    Clearly, barbiturates and other central depressants have a
number of actions on post-synaptic membranes. The hypnotic and
anaesthetic properties of barbiturates have been considered to
result in part from an interaction with central inhibitory
processes mediated by GABA (Nicoll et al, 1975). Our data
suggests that barbiturates may also interact with parts of the
post-synaptic membrane which is indirectly associated with
inhibitory amino-acid receptors. Thus barbiturates reverse the
effects of the convulsant amino-acid antagonists BMC and strychnine
at concentrations which have no obvious direct effect and at which
no significant modification of GABA, glycine or other agonist
responses are observed. This interaction was more easily demonstrated with BMC than with strychnine possibly because of the different
binding affinity of these substances to their site of action
(Zukin et al, 1974; Young & Snyder, 1974).

    A tentative explanation to account for these observations
assumes that amino acids and their antagonists bind to the cell
surface at different sites. Thus when an antagonist is present
it prevents access of the amino-acid to its receptor, not because
of preferential binding to the receptor but by occluding or
distorting it. Barbiturates may have affinity for the antagonist
binding site and could therefore displace the antagonist without
affect the receptor. The possibility of differences in agonist
and antagonist sites has been suggested by Young & Snyder (1974)
in the case of glycine and strychnine. As yet there is little
evidence of separate sites for BMC and GABA, although the results
described by Collins & Cryer elsewhere in this symposium would
support this possibility. Briefly, using the [3]H-GABA binding
assay of Snyder and his coworkers (Zukin et al, 1974), Collins &
Cryer have been able to show that although pentobarbitone does not
interfere with [3]H GABA binding (in confirmation of results previously obtained by Zukin et al, 1974) it will prevent BMC from
displacing [3]H GABA. The [3]H GABA normally displaced by BMC is
considered by Snyder to be that fraction binding to receptors.
Möhler & Okada (1977), on the other hand, have recently described
specific binding of [3]H-bicuculline methiodide (BMI) to synaptosomal membranes prepared from cerebellar cortex. They reported

that pentobarbitone in common with many other drugs, did not interfere with the binding of BMI.

An interesting feature of these binding studies is the apparent lack of GABA-mimetic activity attributed to pentobarbitone in intact preparations (Nicoll, 1975). Other, more recognised GABA-mimetics e.g. 3-aminopropane sulphonic acid and imidazole acetic acid displace $^3$H GABA and $^3$H-BMI from specific binding sites, but pentobarbitone does not.

While our observations do not indicate that barbiturates produce their hypnotic effects by interacting with endogenous substances which mask amino acid receptors, they may suggest a mechanism to explain their efficacy in acute convulsant poisoning. Moreover, it could be reasoned that the effects of barbiturates on various conductance mechanisms e.g. $Na^+$ $Ca^{++}$ $K^+$ (Blaustein, 1968; 1976; Sato et al, 1967) and maybe $Cl^-$ does not require an interaction with neurotransmitter receptors but an effect on closely associated parts of the membrane linked to it and the ionophore.

REFERENCES

Anderson, E.G. & Bonnycastle, D.D., 1960, A study of the central
    depressant action of pentobarbital, phenobarbital and die-
    thylether in relationship to increases in brain 5-hydroxy-
    tryptamine, J. Pharmac. exp. Ther., 130:138-143.
Blaustein, M.P., 1968, Barbiturates block $Na^+$ and $K^+$ conductance
    increases in voltage clamped lobster axons, J. Gen Physiol.,
    51:293-307.
Blaustein, M.P., 1976, Barbiturates block calcium uptake by stimu-
    lated and potassium-depolarized rat sympathetic ganglia,
    J. Pharmc. expå Ther., 196:80-86.
Bowery, N.G. & Brown, D.A., 1974, Depolarizing actions of γ-amino-
    butyric acid and related compounds on rat superior cervical
    ganglia in vitro, Br. J. Pharmac., 50:205-218.
Bowery, N.G. & Dray, A., 1976, Barbiturate reversal of amino acid
    antagonism produced by convulsant agents, Nature (London),
    264:276-278.
Bowery, N.G., Jones, G.P. & Neal, M.J., 1976, Selective inhibition
    of neuronal GABA uptake by  cis-1,3-aminocyclohexane carboxylic
    acid, Nature (London), 264:281-284.
Bradley, P.B. & Dray, A., 1973, Modification of the responses of
    brain stem neurones to transmitter substances by anaesthetic
    agents, Br. J. Pharmac., 48:212-224.
Brown, D.A. & Marsh, S., 1975, A very simple method for recording
    ganglion depolarization, J. Physiol. (London), 246:24-26P.
Brown, D.A. & Galvan, M., 1977, Influence of neuroglial transport
    on the action of γ-aminobutyric acid on mammalian ganglion
    cells, Br. J. Pharmac., 59:373-378.
Collins, J.F. & Cryer, G., 1978, A study of the GABA receptor using
    $^3$H-bicuculline methobromide, This symposium.
Corrodi, H., Fuxe, K. & Hökfelt, T., 1966, The effect of barbiturates
    on the activity of the catecholamine neurones in the rat brain,
    J. Pharm. Pharmac., 18:556-558.
Cutler, R.W.P. & Dudzinski, D.S., 1974, Effect of pentobarbital on
    uptake and release of $^3$H-GABA and $^{14}$C-glutamate by brain
    slices, Brain Res., 67:546-548.
Cutler, R.W.P., Markowitz, D. & Dudzinski, D.S., 1974, The effect
    of barbiturates on $^3$H GABA transport in rat cerebral cortex
    slices, Brain Res., 81:189-197.
Eccles, J.C., Schmidt, R. & Willis, W.D., 1963, Pharmacological
    studies on presynaptic inhibition, J. Physiol (London),
    168:500-530.
Eccles, J.C., Faber, D.S. & Táboriková, H., 1971, The action of a
    parallel fiber volley on the antidromic invasion of Purkyne
    cells of cat cerebellum, Brain Res., 25:335-356.
Johnston, G.A.R., Krogsgaard-Larsen, P., Stephanson, A.L. &
    Twitchin, B., 1976, Inhibition of the uptake of GABA and
    related amino acids in rat brain slices by the optical isomers

of nipecotic acid, J. Neurochem., 26:1029-1032.

Krogsgaard-Larsen, P. & Johnston, G.A.R., 1975, Inhibition of GABA uptake in rat brain slices by nipecotic acid, various isoxazoles and related compounds, J. Neurochem., 25:797-802.

Mitchell, J.F., 1963, The spontaneous and evoked release of acetylcholine from the cerebral cortex, J. Physiol., London, 165:98-116.

Möhler, H. & Okada, T., 1977, GABA receptor binding with [3]H(+) bicuculline methiodide in rat CNS, Nature, London, 267:65-67.

Nicoll, R.A., 1975, Pentobarbital: action on frog motoneurons, Brain Res., 96:119-123.

Nicoll, R.A., Eccles, J.C., Oshima, T. & Rubia, F., 1975, Prolongation of hippocampal inhibitory postsynaptic potentials by barbiturates, Nature, London, 258:625-627.

Phillis, J.W., 1968, Acetylcholine release from the cerebral and cerebellar cortices: its role in cortical arousal, Brain Res., 7:378-389.

Phillis, J.W. & Chong, G.C., 1965, Acetylcholine release from the cerebral and cerebellar cortices: its role in cortical arousal, Nature, London, 207:1253-1255.

Ransom, B.R. & Barker, J.L., 1976, Pentobartital selectively enhances GABA-mediated post-synaptic inhibition in tissue cultured mouse spinal neurones, Brain Res., 114:530-535.

Richter, D. & Crossland, J., 1949, Variation in acetylcholine content of the brain with physiological state, Am. J. Physiol., 159:247-255.

Sato, M., Austin, G.M. & Yai, H., 1967, Increase in permeability of the postsynaptic membrane to potassium produced by 'Nembutal', Nature, London, 215:1506-1508.

Sharpless, S.K., 1970, The barbiturates in 'The pharmacological basis of therapeutics' (Goodman, L.S. & Gilman, A., ed.), MacMillan, London & Toronto.

Young, A.B. & Snyder, S.H., 1974, Strychnine binding in rat spinal cord membranes associated with the synaptic glycine receptor: cooperativity of glycine interactions, Molec. Pharmac. 10:790-809.

Zukin, S.R., Young, A.B., & Snyder, S.H., 1974, Gamma-aminobutyric acid binding to receptor sites in the rat central nervous system, Proc. Nat. Acad. Sci. U.S.A., 71:4802-4807.

CRITICAL EVALUATION OF THE USE OF RADIOAUTOGRAPHY AS A TOOL IN THE

LOCALIZATION OF AMINO ACIDS IN THE MAMMALIAN CENTRAL NERVOUS

SYSTEM

J.S. Kelly and Fabienne Weitsch-Dick[*]

MRC Neurochemical Pharmacology Unit
Dept. of Pharmacology, Medical School, Hills Road
Cambridge, U.K.

In this chapter we describe a method for analyzing the
distribution of silver grains over electron microscopic autoradiographs by comparing the frequency with which silver grains formed
clusters of 0,1,2,3,4 or more silver grains over the tissue which
is thought to accumulate the label most avidly with that which
occurred over the rest of the tissue present on the autoradiograph.
Since in a large number of studies with GABA and $\beta$-alanine in
various regions of the brain the frequency with which the different
sizes of clusters occurred over both areas of the electron microscopic autoradiographs was as predicted by the Poisson's theorem
it appears that the increase in clusters over the more densely
labelled tissue is the natural consequence of a random process
involving rare events. It therefore, follows that the clusters
over nerve terminals are unlikely to be the result of an all or
none phenomenon and that a fairly careful analysis is required to
determine the probability with which each cluster size will be
over the tissue which is presumed to accumulate the label most
avidly. In this study, for instance, the probability that a
single silver grain would lie over the tissue which accumulated
the label most avidly was only rarely better than 2:1. However,
the probability increased progressively as the number of silver
grains in the cluster and the probability that a cluster containing 3 grains would lie over the more densely labelled tissue was
always better than 13:1. Fortunately it is possible that the

[*]Present address: I.N.S.E.R.M. U-106, Histologie Normale et
Pathologique du Systeme Nerveux,
Centre Medico-Chirurgical Foch,
42 Rue Desbassayns de Richemont
92150 Suresnes, France.

Poisson distribution of silver grains over both the tissue
thought to take up the radioactivity most avidly and the rest of
the tissue present on the autoradiograph can be calculated from
the mean densities of silver grains per unit area and the number
of unit areas occupied by each of the tissues thus avoiding the
more detailed analysis carried out by the authors.

The original electron miscroscopic autoradiographic findings
of Bloom and Iversen (1971) and Iversen and Bloom (1972) were
particularly convincing since almost every part of these authors'
work was heavily supported by a wealth of biochemical findings
that did not involve the use of radioautography. For instance,
Iversen and Bloom (1972) showed that the uptake of $^3$H-GABA into
slices of cerebral cortex described in earlier biochemical
experiments (Iversen and Johnston 1971) led to a 8.2 fold increase
in the silver grain density over all nerve terminals as oppose to
the rest of the tissue present on the autoradiographs. In this
instance, the rest of the tissue included glial cell fragments,
neuronal perikarya, dendrites, myelineated axons, unmyelineated
axons and the space between the tissue islands. However, it
should be mentioned that there was an appreciable amount of background radioactivity over these tissues and only two thirds of
the silver grains lay over identified nerve terminals. However,
this background radioactivity was relatively unimportant since
the vast bulk of the label was restricted to the nerve terminals
which occupied less than 23% of the tissue area. In addition,
since the bulk of the label was restricted to approximately 27%
of the nerve terminals the density of silver grains over the
nerve terminals that were considered to be specifically labelled
was therefore 30 times greater than that over the rest of the
present on the tissues autoradiographs. Of course, the concentration of the bulk of the silver grains (71%) over a small percentage of the nerve terminals which occupied approximately 6.2% of
the tissue area made it envitable that the silver grains would
appear to cluster over the labelled nerve terminals. Although
Iversen and Bloom claimed that this clustering of the silver
grains over a small but constant percentage of the nerve terminals
regardless of the period of autoradiographic exposure was reminiscent of an all or none process, their finding that the number of
silver grains over the individual nerve terminals varied between 1
and greater than 5 made this proposal highly unlikely. Indeed,
we have now shown that Iversen and Bloom's (1972) suggestion that
the percentage of nerve terminals that are labelled does not
alter as the number of silver grains per nerve terminal is
increased by extending the autoradiographic exposure period is
probably erroneous. As shown in Fig. 2, at greater autoradiographic exposure periods than those tested by Iversen and Bloom,
the percentage of labelled as opposed to unlabelled nerve

terminals continues to increase as the number of silver grains. It should be noted however, that we were only able to count the number of silver grains over the more densely labelled nerve terminals by using the more precise phenidon method of development developed by Lettre and Paweletz (1966). After exposure of 10-20 days the percentage of nerve terminals labelled by this method and the number of silver grains per terminal was little different from that observed by Iversen and Bloom (1972). In keeping with the view that exposure to low concentrations of $^3$H-GABA will only label a specific population of nerve terminals our results show that although greater exposure periods increases the number of silver grains per autoradiograph neither the percentage of nerve terminals considered to be specifically labelled or indeed the ratio by which the mean density of silver grains over the nerve terminals thought to be specifically labelled exceeded that over the rest of the tissue present on the autoradiographs was unaltered.

Iversen and Bloom (1972) (Fig. 3 in their paper) also reported that the increase in the number of silver grains over the labelled nerve terminals associated with a 20 as opposed to a 10 day exposure period was accompanied by a shift to the right of the histograms which showed the frequency with which nerve terminals containing 1,2,3,4 and 5 silver grains occurred. This finding also suggests that the clustering is quite coincidental and simply a feature of the high density of silver grains over the labelled nerve terminals. For instance in Fig. 1, their data (filled bars on the histogram) is shown to be little different from the open histograms which show the frequency with which clusters of 1,2,3, 4 and 5 silver grains would be expected to occur if the number silver grains over each nerve terminal resulted from a random process similar to that predicted by Poisson's theorem.

Poisson's theorem states that if the <u>mean</u> number of silver grains per unit area is m, then the chance p of observing any particular number x (0,1,2,3, etc) over a nerve terminal is

$$P_x = \frac{m^x}{x!} e^{-m}$$

For a sufficiently large number of observations N, the value $N_{px}$ should come close to the actually observed number of squares or terminals which contain x silver grains. Thus if we know the mean number m of silver grains per unit area we can calculate the number of terminal squares containing clusters of 0,1,2,3 ... x silver grains by the means of Poisson's theorem which predicts

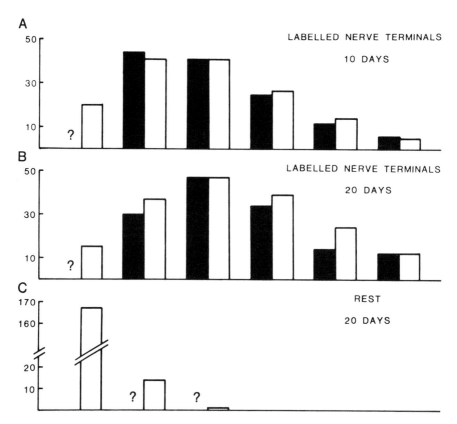

Fig. 1.  Histograms to show the observed and theoretical distribution of silver grain clusters over electron microscopic
autoradiographs of cerebral cortex slices incubated with $^3$H-GABA.
The filled bars in A and B were drawn from the data of Iversen
and Bloom (1972) (Fig. 3) and show the frequency with which
clusters of 1,2,3,4 or 5 grains occurred over the labelled nerve
terminals after autoradiographic exposure periods of 10 and 20 days
respectively.  The total number of labelled nerve terminals was
151 and 182 at 10 and 20 days respectively.  The theoretical
histograms were calculated using the Poisson's theorem on the
basis that in A N=151 and m=2.0 and B N=182 and m=2.5.  In C it is
assumed that the labelling over an area of the rest of tissue on
the autoradiograph equal to that covered by 182 nerve terminals
after 20 days autoradiographic exposure would be 1/30th of that
over the nerve terminals and therefore N would be equal to 182
and m=0.083.

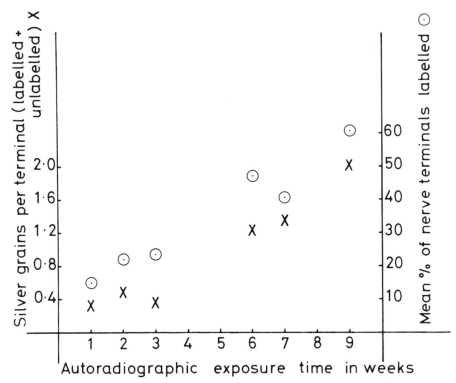

Fig. 2.    Graph from the unpublished observations of Kelly and
Weitsch-Dick to show the way in which the mean number of silver
grains and the % of nerve terminals that are labelled on electron
microscopic autoradiographs of cerebral cortex slices incubated
with $^3$H-GABA (final concentration 5μM) increase with the length
of the autoradiographic exposure period.  Even although the
development of the silver grains was by the phenidon  method of
Lettre and Paweletz (1966) the results obtained after about 10 and
20 days exposure were similar to that of Iversen and Bloom (1972).


that the clusters of silver grain distributed as follows:

$$n_0 = Ne^{-m}$$

$$n_1 = mn_0$$

$$n_2 = \frac{m}{2} n_1$$

$$n_3 = \frac{m}{3} n_2$$

$$n_x = \frac{m}{x} n_{x-1}$$

The theoretical histograms in A are based on their observations that the mean density of silver grains over the 151 labelled nerve terminals was 2 and in B the corresponding values 182 and 2.5 respectively. In the absence of any experimental data about the distribution of silver grains over the rest of the tissue in C I have attempted to plot the clustering that might be expected to occur over the background by assuming that the labelling over an area of background similar in size to that of the nerve terminals would be 1/30th of that over a nerve terminal (see earlier). Under these circumstances Poisson's theorem would predict that a similar area of background would contain 14 single silver grains and that at least one region the size of a nerve terminal would contain a cluster of two silver grains.

If for the moment we accept that the silver grains over the nerve terminals are not distributed in the all or none fashion suggested by Iversen and Bloom (1972) but as predicted by Poisson's theorem then these authors estimate of GABAnergic nerve terminal density in the cerebral cortex may need revision. For instance, the theoretical histograms in Fig. 1 for autoradiographic exposures of 10 days, calculated from Poisson's theorem predict that approximately 20 of the unlabelled terminals would in all probability have contained as much radioactivity as the labelled terminals and should therefore have been considered as GABAnergic. On the other hand the same theorem also predicts that approximately 10 of the nerve terminals labelled with a single silver grain contained levels of radioactivity which are no greater than over the rest of the tissue present in the autoradiographs. Equally predictable was the observation that the number of labelled as apposed to unlabelled nerve terminals would increase as an increase in the period of autoradiographic exposure led to an increase in the total number of silver grains over the entire electron microscopic autoradiograph. In addition there would be a decrease in the number of unlabelled terminals which would in all probability contain the same level of radioactivity as the labelled terminals. In other words, the prediction of Iversen and Bloom (1972) was fairly exact since the number of unlabelled nerve terminals likely to contain the same level of radioactivity as the labelled terminals only slightly exceeded the number of terminals labelled by a single grain which in all probability contained only background levels of radioactivity.

The theorem also predicts however, that only by selecting conditions which lead to autoradiographs in which the mean density of silver grains over the nerve terminals is rather less than one will autoradiographs be obtained in which the background labelling over the rest of the tissue is vanishingly small. However, the penalty for this approach will be that the number of nerve terminals unlabelled by silver grains which will contain the same

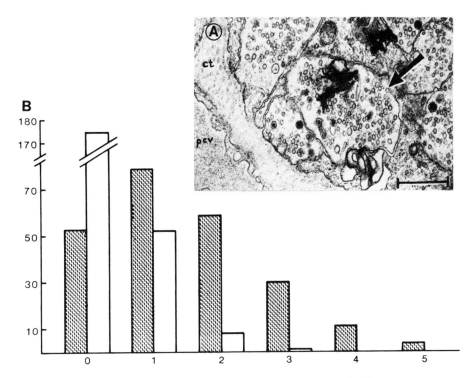

Fig. 3. Electron microscopic autoradiograph and histograms to show the distribution of silver grains over the rat median eminence following the injection of [3]H-dopamine. In A the electron microscopic autoradiograph from the paper of Cuello and Iversen (1973) show a labelled nerve terminal (arrow) in the vicinity of a portal capillary vessel (pcV) in the external layer of the rat median eminence; ct = connective tissue space. Calibration bar = 0.5μM.

The theoretical histograms in B were drawn by trial and error using the Poisson's theorem until they matched the data of Iversen and Cuello (1972) which showed 17% of 239 synaptic terminals or varicosities to be labelled specifically with 3 silver grains or more. The hatched histograms show the probable distribution of silver grains over the nerve terminals thought to take up the label specifically and the open histograms the probable distribution of silver grains over the rest of the tissue which included unlabelled nerve terminals and terminals labelled with less than 3 grains.

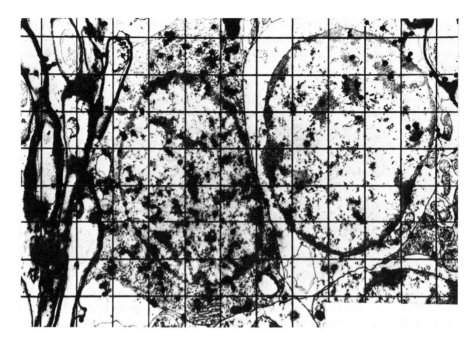

Fig. 4.    Electron microscopic autoradiograph from the deep
granular layer of a rat cerebellar follium following the microinjection of $^3$H-β-alanine.  The density of silver grains over the
glial cell (gl) was five times greater than that over the closely
apposed granule cell and the rest of the tissue of the autoradiograph.  To assist the analysis described in the text the autoradiograph has been divided into an array of squares O.9μm intervals.
Exposure time = 4 weeks; calibration = lμm.

level of radioactivity as the labelled nerve terminals will be
approximately eleven times greater than those labelled with a
single silver grain.

    This analysis is also useful in another way, since regardless
of whether Poisson's theorem is truely applicable to this type
of data inspection of the histograms obtained experimentally show
the probability with which a single grain will lie over a nerve
terminal as oppose to the rest of the tissue in Fig. lA to be
only 2.6:1 (37 and 14).  For a similar area containing 2 grains
the probability rises to 47:1 and at greater grain densities
becomes infinite.  Of course, looking back I am intrigued by the
way in which Iversen and Bloom (1972) clearly recognized the
importance of the clusters.  Indeed, one might go further and
suggest that from the very beginning Iversen and Bloom

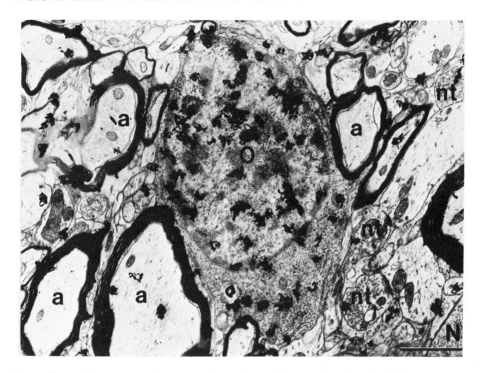

Fig. 5.    Electron microscopic autoradiograph of a labelled
oligodendrocyte in the rat cuneate nucleus after a micro-injection
of $^3$H-β-alanine.   The high density of silver grains (eleven fold)
over the satellite oligodendrocyte (O) as apposed to the rest of
the tissue containing an adjacent neurone (N) is further exagger-
ated by the use of the conventional Kodak D19B developer.

intuitively recognized the significance of the clusters and thus
Cuello and Iversen (1973) stated that "labelled axons were defined
as those in which the terminal profiles contained 3 or more
silver grains".  Since they do not state how they arrived at this
number one can only summarize that they noticed clusters of one
and two silver grains over structures other than nerve terminals.

     Since they examined 236 synaptic profiles and found 41 of
these terminals to contain 3 or more silver grains we can by
trial and error draw a series of histograms based on Poisson's
theorem in which one will show the frequency with which the nerve
terminals must have been labelled with 1,2,3,4,5 and 6 silver
grains (Fig. 1D, hatched histogram).  Much in the same way a
second histogram can be drawn to show the probable distribution
of silver grains over the rest of the tissue on the autoradiograph
which would fit their observation that clusters of less than 3
grains never occurred over the nerve terminal considered to be

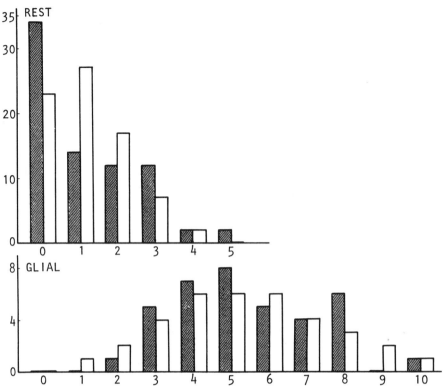

Fig. 6.    Histograms to show the observed and theoretical
distribution of silver grains over the glial cells and the rest
of the tissue shown in Fig. 4.  As described in the text the
histograms were constructed by counting the silver grains in each
square and incrementing the appropriate bin of one or other
histogram depending on whether or not the tissue in the square
belonged predominantly to the glial cell or the rest of the tissue
of the autoradiograph.  The distribution shown in the theoretical
histograms (clear) was calculated from Poisson's theorem in the
basis that the mean density of silver grains over the 37 squares
which lay over the glial cell was 5.43 (i.e. N=37 and m=5.43).
The mean density of silver grains over the 76 squares which lay
rest of the tissue was 1.21 i.e. N=76 and m=-.21.)

labelled specifically.  It is interesting to note that such a
distribution can only be drawn by assuming that the number of
silver grains over the rest of the tissue was 1/5th that over the
nerve terminals thought to be specifically labelled.  However,
under these circumstances approximately 1 in 2.2 of the nerve
terminals labelled with 1 or 2 grains would have in all probability
contained the same level of radioactivity as those labelled with
3 or more grains.  However, histograms drawn on the assumption

that there was an even greater differential uptake of radioactivity into the specifically labelled population of nerve
terminals as apposed to the rest of the tissue make it even more
likely that nerve terminals labelled by one or two grains belonged to the same population of nerve terminals which were labelled
with three or more grains.

Since all these difficulties appear to be an unavoidable
result of the way in which silver grains are distributed over
the tissues which take up the radioactivity most avidly it is
even more frustrating to report that the new immunohistochemical
techniques now under development may well lead to the all or none
deposition of the reaction product over the specifically labelled
terminals.  For instance Roberts and his colleagues (McLaughun
et al 1974 and 1975) using an antibody against GAD now appear to
have shown at a number of locations that the reaction product is
deposited specifically over the nerve terminals thought on a
number of other grounds to be GABAnergic.  Since apart from some
reservations about antigenic specificity and the inability of the
antigen to penetrate the tissue these authors only discuss the
significance of false negatives I must assume these authors also
share my view that this technique leads to all or none labelling.
On the other hand, the statistical process I have described which
determines the distribution of silver grains over the specifically
labelled nerve terminals in the autoradiographs ensures that
whenever there is a significant degree of labelling over the
rest of tissue present in the autoradiograph the ability of the
tissue under a single silver grain to accumulate the label will
be in doubt and that when the labelling is restricted to a few
sparse grains over the tissue thought to take up the label most
avidly there will be a large number of unlabelled nerve terminals
able to take up the label equally well.

Many of the difficulties described above have been examined
in some detail using electron microscopic autoradiographs prepared
by Dick and myself by micro-injecting GABA analogues into certain
regions of the central nervous system and preparing the animals
15-30 mins later by fixation with 5% glutaraldehyde (Kelly and
Dick, 1976).  Not only does this method result in good tissue
preservation which allows the nature of tissue under each silver
grain to be determined but as shown in Fig. 4 the development of
the autoradiographic activity by the phenidon  method of Lettre
and Paweletz (1966) the distribution of silver grains can be
determined with great precision.

As predicted by the in vitro results of Schon and Kelly (1974)
the injection of $^3$H-$\beta$-alanine leads in Fig. 4 predominantly to the
labelling of a glial cell which in this instance lies satellite
to a granule cell which is not thought to take up the radioactivity.

However, closer inspection of the labelling over the granule cell
leads to a number of difficulties since not only are there a
considerable number of silver grains over the granule cell but in
places where they are clustered, the density appears to equal
that over certain areas of the glial cell. From what I have said
earlier there appears to be two alternatives to this dilemma.
The first is to discard this section and to ensure that on the
next autoradiograph that almost all of the radioactivity overlies
the glial cell either by using a less radioactive part of the
tissue block or a shorter autoradiographic exposure period. In
addition, the apparent differential labelling can be enhanced by
using the standard developer which produces larger more conspicuous silver grains (Fig. 5). A better approach however is to
carry out a proper analysis of the silver grain distribution and
in this way to determine the probability with which silver grains
will lie over glial cells as appose to other structures present
on the autoradiograph.

As shown in Fig. 4 a detailed analysis involves the division
of the electron microscopic autoradiograph into an array of
squares each approximately $1 \mu m^2$. For each square in turn the
silver grains are counted and the appropriate bin of one of two
histograms (Fig. 6) incremented depending on the number of silver
grains over the square and whether the tissue in the square is
predominantly glial or tissue belonging to the rest of the electron
microscopic autoradiograph. Where possible adjacent squares which
contain equal parts of both tissues are rationalised as two new
squares and the appropriate bins of the histograms incremented.
In Fig. 6 the scales of histograms take into account the difference
in area between the glial cell and the rest of the autoradiograph.
The density of silver grains over the glial cell is approximately
4.6 times greater than that over the rest of the tissue which has
a mean silver grain density of approximately 1.2 silver grains
per square. The two experimental histograms shown in Fig. 6
approximate to a second set of theoretical histograms calculated
for each area and the appropriate mean density of silver grains
using Poisson's theorem. Apart from a single square, squares
containing 0,1 and 2 silver grains never lay over the glial cell
and on all but two occasions squares containing 4 or more silver
grains occurred only over glial cells. The remaining 10 squares
containing 3 silver grains were distributed equally over both
tissues. In other words the probability that a glial cell will
underly a single silver grain evoked by specific β-alanine uptake
is only of the order of 4.5:1 and that this probability increases
progressively as the number of silver grains in a square increases
until squares which contain as many as 4 silver grains and above
have a probability of 13:1 of overlying a glial cell. In order to
confirm that the correspondence between the observed distribution
and that calculated from Poisson's theorem is not a chance

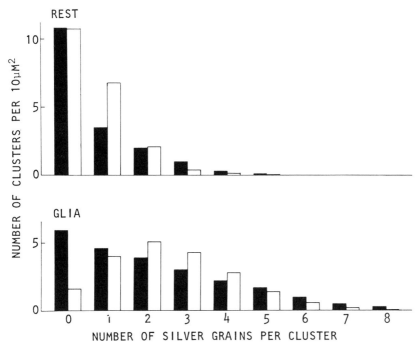

Fig. 7.    Distribution of silver grains over 7 electron microscopic
autoradiographs of the rat cerebral cortex following the microinjection of ³H-β-alanine.    Analysis was by the method described
in the legend of Fig. 4 and necessitated the construction of an
array of squares.    The histograms in this figure obtained from 7
electron microscopic autoradiographs should be compared with that
in Fig. 6 which was obtained from the single microscopic autoradiographs shown in Fig. 4.

finding on a single electron microscope autoradiograph, Fig. 7
shows two histograms constructed in a similar way from 7 more
electron microscopic autoradiographs in which each of the columns
of the histogram has been corrected to show the number of clusters
of that particular size which would overly 10μm² of either the
glial cells or the rest of the tissue present on the autoradiographs.

     Unfortunately, this form of analysis is rather tedious and
when applied to small structures such as nerve terminals
involves the preparation of numerous large prints or the construction of arrays of very small squares.    Even then one is forced
rather arbitarily to assign squares which contain more than one
tissue to one histogram or another.    However, in Figs. 8,9,10 and 11

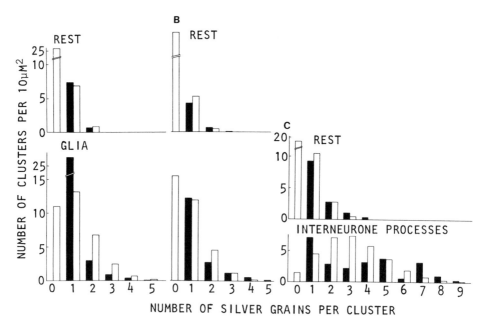

Fig. 8.    Histograms to show the observed and theoretical distribution of silver grain clusters over electron microscopic autoradiographs following the microinjection of $^3$H-β-alanine into three
different regions of the rat brain.   The observed distributions
were calculated by simply counting the individual silver grains
and the clusters of silver grains over the glial cells and the
rest of tissue present on the autoradiographs. In clusters the
silver grains touched and the assignment of a cluster to one or
other histogram depended on the tissues which underlay the apparent
geometric centre of the cluster.   The histograms were normalized
to take account of the differences in tissue areas.   The areas of
each tissue were determined by the use of an array of points as
described by Haug (1971).   The theoretical distributions (open
histograms) were calculated according to Poisson's theorem.

In **A** the analysis was from 5 electron microscopic autoradiographs of the rat cerebral cortex in which the area of the glial
was 415μm$^2$ and the rest of the tissue 988μm$^2$.   On each electron
micrographs the average number of silver grains over the glia was
36 and the rest 5.

In B the analysis was from 6 electron microscopic autoradiographs from the cuneate nucleus in which the surface area  of the
glia was 682μm$^2$ and the rest 1844μm$^2$.   On each electron micrograph
the average number of silver grains over the glia was 27 and the
rest 6.

In C the analysis was from seven electron microscopic autoradiographs of the rat cerebellar cortex in which the surface area
of the glia was 674μm$^2$ and the rest 1682μm$^2$.   On each electron
micrograph the average number of silver grains over the glia was
55.0 and over the rest 12.0.

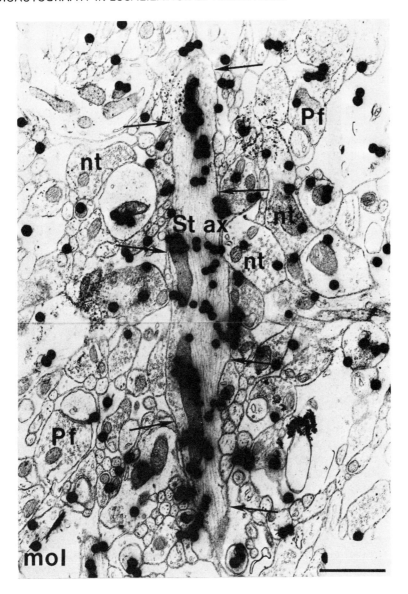

Fig. 9. Electron microscopic autoradiograph to show the distribution of silver grains over stellate cell processes in the molecular layer of a cat cerebellar folium following the microinjection of [3]H-GABA. The density of silver grains over a stellate cell axon (St ax) identified by its core of neurofilaments, its longitudinally oriented mitochondria and the presence of ellipsoidal vesicles is nine times higher than that over the adjacent parallel fibres (Pf) and nerve terminals (nt) filled with round vesicles. Exposure time = 8 weeks; calibration = 1μm.

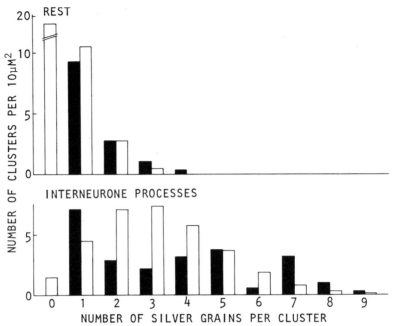

Fig. 10.     Histograms to show the observed and theoretical
(open bars) distribution of silver grain clusters over the inter-
neurone process on the molecular layer of the cat cerebellar
thought to take up the radioactivity most avidly following the
microinjection of $^3$H-GABA and the rest of the tissue present in
the autoradiographs from an analysis of 7 electron microscopic
autoradiographs, similar to that shown in Fig. 9.   The surface
area of the interneuronal processes was $31\mu m^2$ and that the rest
of the tissue $212\mu m^2$.   On each micrograph the average number of
silver grains over the interneuronal processes was 81 and over
the rest 28.


are shown histograms taken from electron microscopic autoradiographs of glial cells of the cerebellar cortex and the cuneate
nucleus and interneuronal processes and Golgi cell axons in the
cerebellum in which the distribution of silver grains was analysed
simply by counting the size and number of silver clusters over
each tissue.    Clearly over the less densely labelled tissue the
observed distribution of clusters is almost identical to that
predicted by the Poisson theorem.    However, where the silver grain
density is greater the excess of single grain clusters can often
be reconciled with the paucity of clusters in the other columns.
However, this is of little importance since from each pair of
histograms a minimum number of silver grains can be determined
which divides the clusters which predominantly lie over the tissue

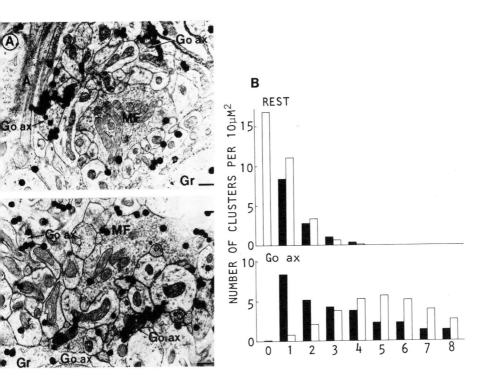

Fig. 11.    Electron microscopic autoradiographs and histograms to
show the density of silver grains over the glomeruli and the
granular layer of the cat cerebellar cortex following the microinjection of [3]H-GABA.

     In A the clusters of silver grains are concentrated over the
small Golgi cell axons (Go ax, arrows) which lie adjacent to the
large unlabelled mossy fibres (MF) both of which form synaptic
contacts with the granule cell dendrites.   The surrounding granule
cells (Gr) are themselves unlabelled.   The density of silver grains
over the Golgi axon terminals was ten times greater than over the
mossy fibres.   Exposure time = 60 days; calibration = 0.5μm.

     In B histograms to show the observed and theoretical (open
bar) distribution of silver grain clusters 0,1,2,3,4 and more over
the Golgi axon terminals (Go) as apposed to the rest of the tissue
present in the autoradiograph analysis 7 electron micrographs.   The
surface area of the Golgi axon terminals was 34.4μm$^2$ and the rest
193μm$^2$.   On each micrograph the average number of silver grains
over the Golgi axons and terminals was 219 and over the rest 22.

thought to take up the radioactivity most avidly from those over
the rest of the tissue present on the autoradiographs. Again
these histograms show only too clearly that little significance
can be placed on the distribution of single silver grains over a
particular tissue. Perhaps more importantly I believe that this
series of histogram suggests that on many occasions the analysis
can be simplified still further and the minimum size of silver
grain clusters which will lie predominantly over the tissue which
takes  up the radioactivity most avidly, determined fairly
accurately by simply using Poisson's theorem to construct theoretical histograms which show the most likely distributions of silver
grain clusters over the tissue under study over the rest of tissue
present on the autoradiographs.

## ACKNOWLEDGEMENT

F.W.-D. is grateful to the Wellcome Trust for financial support.

## REFERENCES

Cuello, A.C., and Iversen, L.L., 1973, Localization of tritiated
    dopamine in the median eminence of the rat hypothalamus by
    electron microscope autoradiography. Brain Research, 63:
    474-478.

Haug, H., 1971, Stereological methods on the analysis of neuronal
    parameters in the central nervous system. J. Microsc. 95:
    165-180.

Iversen, L.L., and Bloom, F.E., 1972, Studies of the uptake of
    $^3$H-GABA and  $^3$H glycine in slices and homogenates of rat
    brain and spinal cord by electron microscopic autoradio-
    graphy. Brain Research 41: 131-143.

Iversen, L.L., and Johnston, G.A.R., 1971, GABA uptake in rat
    central nervous system: comparison of uptake in slices and
    homogenates and the effects of some inhibitors. J. Neurochem.,
    18: 1939-1950.

Kelly, J.S., and Dick, Fabienne, 1976, Differential labeling of
    glial cells and GABA-inhibitory interneurones and nerve
    terminals following the microinjection of $[\beta-^3H]$ alanine,
    $[^3H]$DABA and $[^3H]$GABA into single folia of the cerebellum.
    Cold Spring Harbor Symposia, XL: 93-106.

Lettre, H., and Paweletz, N., 1966, Problems der electronenmik-
    roskopischen autoradiographie. Naturwissenschaften 11: 268.

McLaughlin, B.J., Wood, J.G., Saito, K., Barber, R., Vaughn, J.E.,
    Roberts, E., and Wu, J.-Y. 1974, The fine structural
    localization of glutamate decarboxylase in synaptic terminals
    of rodent cerebellum. Brain Research 76: 377-391.

McLaughlin, B.J., Wood, J.G., Saito, K., Roberts, E., and Wu, J.-Y. 1975, The fine structural localization of glutamate decar-boxylase in developing axonal processes and presynaptic terminals of roden cerebellum. Brain Research 85: 355-371.

Schon, F., and Kelly, J.S., 1975, Selective uptake of $[^3H]\beta$-alanine by glia: association with the glial uptake system for GABA. Brain Research 86: 243-257.

# TRANSMITTERS IN THE BASAL GANGLIA

P. L. McGeer, E. G. McGeer and  T. Hattori

Kinsmen Laboratory of Neurological Research, Department

of Psychiatry, University of B.C., Vancouver, B.C.

The basal ganglia govern the extrapyramidal system. Unfortunately neither term is precisely defined. Here we shall include in the basal ganglia the caudate, putamen, external globus pallidus, internal globus pallidus' (entopeduncular nucleus), subthalamic nucleus and substantia nigra. The caudate and putamen together will be referred to as the NCP. Certain subcortical nuclei, such as the nucleus accumbens and amygdala, which are more concerned with functioning of the limbic system, will not be discussed. The motor functioning associated with the basal ganglia seems to include the establishment of peripheral motor tone, the initiation and gross control of movement, and postural adjustments associated with balance.

The pathways of the basal ganglia, as they are known today, are shown in Fig. 1. For simplicity, the Figure has been divided into input (1A), processing (1B), and output (1C) systems. Pathways 1 to 4 represent the main inflow into the chief processing centers in the caudate and putamen. They include (Fig. 1A): 1) the cortico-striatal, 2) the nigro-striatal, 3) the thalamo-striatal and 4) the raphe-striatal.

Little is known about processing within the caudate and putamen. However, pathways leaving the caudate and putamen have been identified. These include (Fig. 1B): 5) neostriato-pallidal, 6) neostriato-nigral, 7) pallido-subthalamic-pallidal and 8) pallido-nigral.

Output from the basal ganglia complex to affect other systems include (Fig. 1C): 9) nigro-thalamic, 10) nigro-brain stem, 11) pallido-thalamic, 12) pallido-habenula and 13) pallido-tegmental.

Still other pathways, such as the cortico-nigral and nigro-

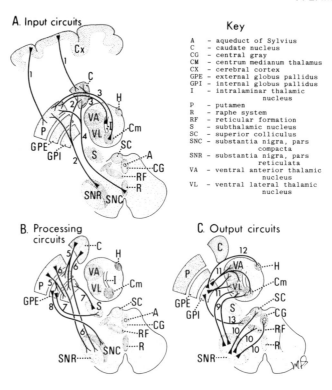

**A. Input circuits**

**Key**

A   – aqueduct of Sylvius
C   – caudate nucleus
CG  – central gray
CM  – centrum medianum thalamus
CX  – cerebral cortex
GPE – external globus pallidus
GPI – internal globus pallidus
I   – intralaminar thalamic
        nucleus
P   – putamen
R   – raphe system
RF  – reticular formation
S   – subthalamic nucleus
SC  – superior colliculus
SNC – substantia nigra, pars
        compacta
SNR – substantia nigra, pars
        reticulata
VA  – ventral anterior thalamic
        nucleus
VL  – ventral lateral thalamic
        nucleus

**B. Processing circuits**

**C. Output circuits**

Figure 1. Pathways of the Basal Ganglia

amygdaloid have been reported and further discoveries will unquestionably be made. But even for the more established pathways, much work remains to be done in fingerprinting them biochemically, that is, establishing what transmitter each tract uses.

There are six known or putative neurotransmitters of proven or probable importance in the extrapyramidal system. These are: glutamate (pathway 1), dopamine (pathway 2), serotonin (pathway 4), acetylcholine (internal NCP processing), GABA (pathways 5, 6, 8 and internal NCP processing) and substance P (pathway 6).

## SPECIFIC NEUROTRANSMITTERS

### A. Neurotransmitters Associated with Input Pathways to the NCP

1. Dopamine. The nigro-striatal dopaminergic tract is probably
the best known and most widely studied pathway in the central nervous
system. After the initial histochemical definition of this tract
(Anden, et al., 1964), its dopaminergic nature has been confirmed
by physiological, biochemical, pharmacological and immunohistochemical techniques. This nigro-striatal dopaminergic tract has proved
to be a model system for axonal transport studies. Protein and neurotransmitters have been used for anterograde measurements and horseradish peroxidase for retrograde.

Through the specificity offered by some of these transport
studies, and by use of the selective neurotoxin, 6-hydroxydopamine
(6-OHDA), the morphology of dopaminergic structures has been unequivocally established at the electron microscopic level.

The dopaminergic cells labelled by either horseradish peroxidase
(HRP) retrogradely transported from the NCP (Fig. 2A) or by 6-OHDA-
induced degeneration (Fig. 2B), were concentrated in the zona compacta.
Their nuclei had smooth envelopes with either no indentations or only
one small indentation, while the nuclei of unaffected cells frequently
had many deep nuclear indentations. Such cells were concentrated in
the zona reticulata and recent axonal transport studies suggest they
may project primarily to the thalamus and other areas outside of the
extrapyramidal system.

The dopaminergic nerve endings in the striatum (Fig. 3) are small,
make asymmetrical axospinous contacts and contain mildly pleomorphic
vesicles of 450 to 550 Å diameter. Boutons of this particular morphology account for about 80% of the terminals labelled by [3]H-protein

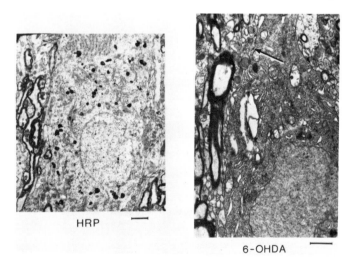

HRP

6-OHDA

Figure 2: Dopamine cells in the substantia nigra of a rat labelled
by HRP or 6-OHDA-induced degeneration. Bar = 2 μm

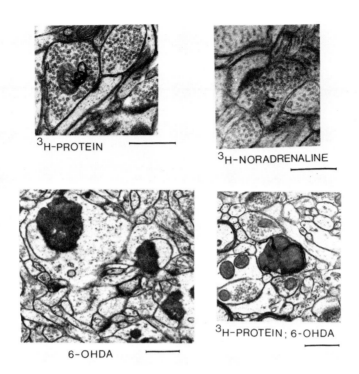

Figure 3: Dopaminergic nerve endings in rat neostriatum labelled by axonal transport and/or selective degeneration. Bar = 1 µm

transported from the nigra (Fig. 3A); the other 20% of labelled terminals may correspond to a second, non-dopaminergic nigro-striatal tract proposed on the basis of physiological studies (Hattori, et al., 1973). Only terminals of this particular morphology are labelled after injections of tritiated noradrenaline into the substantia nigra (Fig. 3B)(McGeer, et al., 1975), and they are preferentially destroyed by intraventricular injections of 6-OHDA (Fig. 3C). Following the injection of $^3$H-leucine into the substantia nigra and 6-OHDA treatment, degeneration of such nerve terminals containing labelled protein has been observed (Fig. 3D)(Hattori, et al., 1973).

Boutons with the "dopaminergic" morphology occupy about 16% of the total bouton area in the caudates of normal rats and much less in 6-OHDA-treated animals.

There are two features of this nigro-striatal dopaminergic path that are worthy of further discussion. The first is the high divergence number, and the second is the vulnerability of these cells to age and disease.

With respect to the divergence number, it has been estimated
that the rat has 3,500 substantia nigral cells with some 500,000
nerve endings in the NCP per cell body. There may be many times that
number of nerve endings per cell body in the human. There are roughly
400,000 dopaminergic neurons in the human substantia nigra at birth
(McGeer, et al., 1976a) and an estimated $2 \times 10^{13}$ boutons of all
types in the neostriatum. If 10-16% of these are dopaminergic, as has
been reported respectively for the cat (Kemp and Powell, 1971), and
rat (Hökfelt and Ungerstedt, 1969), then there would be at least
5,000,000 nerve endings per cell body, some ten times as high as in
the rat.

Figure 4 shows the steady decline of human substantia nigra
cells with age. By age 60, the number has dropped from 400,000 to
an estimated 250,000 (McGeer, et al., 1976a).

In Parkinson's disease (designated by the symbol "P" in the
figure), cell counts range from about 60,000 to 120,000. The symptoms
of the disease are due to the loss in function of these substantia
nigra cells but obviously many cells can disappear before decompen-
sation occurs. The only stigmata may be the shuffling gait and
stooped posture often seen in the very elderly.

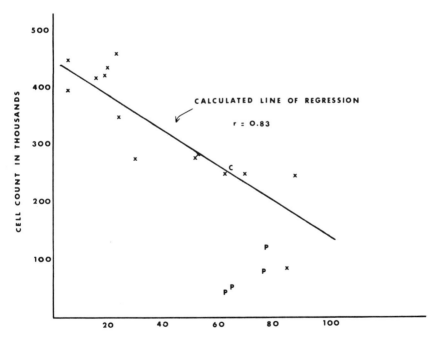

Figure 4: Number of cells in the substantia nigra as a function of
age in humans dying without neurological illness (x's and line),
with Parkinsonism (P's) or Huntington's chorea (C).

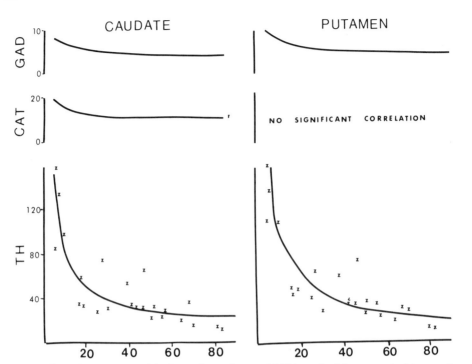

Figure 5: Glutamic acid decarboxylase (GAD), choline acetyltransferase (CAT) and tyrosine hydroxylase (TH) activities as a function of
age in the caudate and putamen of humans dying without neurological
disease. All lines of correlation shown are statistically significant
Individual data shown only for TH.

Of even greater importance than outright cell loss may be a loss
of vitality of the cells. During the period (5-15 years of age) when
melanin pigment begins to accumulate in the dopaminergic cell bodies,
there is a remarkable loss of tyrosine hydroxylase in the neostriatum
where the nerve endings are located (Fig. 5). There is ordinarily a
considerable excess of tyrosine hydroxylase over that required to
synthesize sufficient dopamine, so that the drop may not signify anything beyond a normal physiological adjustment to termination of body
growth. On the other hand, such a severe drop in activity is not
found for other neurotransmitter synthetic enzymes such as choline
acetyltransferase which synthesizes acetylcholine, and glutamic acid
decarboxylase which synthesizes GABA.

2. Glutamate. Chemical evidence for a neurotransmitter role
for glutamate was largely missing until very recent years because

of the lack of any means of differentiating the "transmitter" amino
acid from the larger proportion used for energy metabolism. A major
breakthrough came when Wofsey, et al. (1971) demonstrated high affinity uptake of glutamate and aspartate into a unique population of
synaptosomes from rat brain and spinal tissue. Unfortunately, the
neuronal uptake systems for these two amino acids are so far indistinguishable from one another and also from a high affinity glial
uptake system for the same amino acids. Nevertheless, it is distinct
from the systems accumulating GABA, glycine or dopamine, both on the
basis of competitive uptake and subcellular fractionation studies.

A decrease in the uptake in specific areas after lesions can be
used as presumptive evidence of the existence of major "glutamatergic" or "aspartergic" tracts in mammalian brain. Thus, we have
found that, when the cortex is undercut on one side, a drop of about
40% occurs in high affinity glutamate uptake into the synaptosomal
fraction of the ipsilateral striatum (McGeer, et al., 1977, Table
I). GABA and dopamine uptake are not affected nor are glutamic acid
decarboxylase (GAD) or choline acetyltransferase (CAT) activities.
Divac, et al. (1977) obtained very similar results in rats with
ablated cortices and suggested that the path is bilateral to a small
extent since some drop was also found in glutamate uptake in the
contralateral striatum.

TABLE I.  ACCUMULATION OF GLUTAMATE, GABA OR DOPAMINE, AND GAD AND
          CAT ACTIVITIES IN NEOSTRIATUM ON LESIONED SIDE AS PERCENT
          OF THOSE IN CONTRALATERAL NEOSTRIATUM (MEAN ± S.E.)

| Operation | Accumulation of | | | Activity of | |
|---|---|---|---|---|---|
|  | Glutamate | GABA | Dopamine | CAT | GAD |
| Lobotomy | 59 ± 4%* | 98 ± 4% | 110 ± 20% | 106 ± 8% | 99 ± 8% |
| Thalectomy | 105 ± 3% | 99 ± 6% | 83 ± 20% | 100 ± 4% | 92 ± 9% |
| Both | 58 ± 3%* | | | 96 ± 8% | 109 ± 8% |

* $p < 0.001$ for comparison with controls.

It can be presumed that the pathway is probably glutamatergic
rather than aspartergic on the basis of the relative concentrations
of the amino acids and of so-called receptor binding. The concentrations of glutamate and aspartate are in an almost 6:1 ratio in the
striatum as compared with an approximate 4:1 ratio for whole brain.
Kainic acid binding, which has been reported to be relatively specific for glutamate as compared to aspartate receptors, is higher
in the striatum than in any other brain area (Simon, et al., 1976).

Figure 6 shows autoradiographs of rat neostriatal terminals
labelled by axoplasmic transport following the administration of
tritiated proline to the neocortex. The terminals are presumably
glutamatergic and all show the same morphology with the common

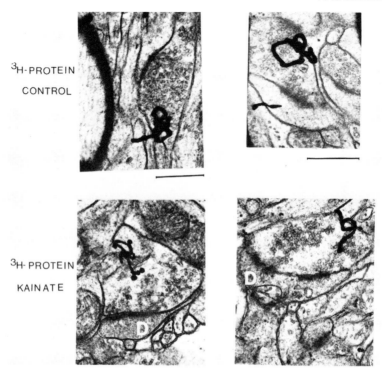

³H-PROTEIN
CONTROL

³H-PROTEIN
KAINATE

Figure 6: Neostriatal boutons labelled by axoplasmic transport from cortex. Bar = 0.5 μm. D's indicate degenerating dendrites.

round vesicles and asymmetric contacts typical of Type I excitatory synapses.

Intra-striatal injections of kainic acid and, to a lesser extent glutamic acid itself, produce striatal cell losses and biochemical changes mimicking those found in Huntington's chorea (Coyle and Schwarcz, 1976; McGeer and McGeer, 1976). On this basis it has been suggested that the cell loss in Huntington's chorea may be due to a genetically determined functional hyperactivity of this glutamatergic tract (McGeer and McGeer, 1976). The excitotoxic effects of small amounts of kainic acid injected into the striatum depend upon the integrity of the cortico-striatal tract (Table II). A possible explanation of these results is that kainic acid acts indirectly and that it is glutamate itself which is the excitotoxic agent.

Further support for this hypothesis is that, following the combination of kainic acid administration into the striatum and ³H-proline into the cortex, there is a highly preferential labelling of nerve endings making contact with degenerating striatal dendrites (Fig. 6). This would be expected if kainic acid were acting indi-

TABLE II. ENZYME LEVELS IN NEOSTRIATA INJECTED WITH 2.5 NMOL OF
          KAINIC ACID AS A PERCENT OF THOSE ON THE CONTRALATERAL
          SIDE (MEAN $\pm$ S.E.)

|         |            | Rats with Lesions of the | |
| Enzyme  | Unlesioned | Cortico-striatal Tract | Thalamus |
|---------|------------|------------------------|----------|
| GAD     | 40 ± 1%    | 96 ± 6%*               | 41 ± 8%  |
| CAT     | 44 ± 3%    | 87 ± 5%*               | 45 ± 9%  |

*Indicates $p < 0.001$ for comparison with data from unlesioned
   rats.

rectly to release glutamate from nerve endings, with the glutamate
then being responsible for the toxic effects at its postsynaptic
receptors.

3. Serotonin. Levels of serotonin and its synthetic enzyme
tryptophan hydroxylase are relatively high in the neostriatum. This
indicates a reasonably prominent, ascending serotonergic tract.
Histofluorescence studies, in combination with 5,6-dihydroxytrypta-
mine (5,6-DHT) administration, suggest that the main source of this
tract is the B9 cell group in the midbrain, with some afferents coming from the B7 and B8 cell groups as well (Fuxe and Johnsson, 1974).
There is also innervation of the substantia nigra and globus pallidus
by ascending serotonin systems.

The probable morphology of the serotonergic synapse in the neostriatum of the rat using glutaraldehyde fixation has been identified
using both p-chloroamphetamine-induced degeneration and labelling by
intraventricularly administered tritiated serotonin (Hattori, et al.,
1976a). Both techniques involved two types of neostriatal nerve endings, indicating that the methods are not absolutely specific. One
type was easily identified as corresponding to the dopaminergic
nerve ending shown in Fig. 3; the other is the presumed serotonergic
nerve ending which is shown in Fig. 7.

On the left in Fig. 7 is a terminal labelled following intraventricular administration of [3]H-serotonin. It is axospinous in
nature, makes a symmetrical contact and contains sparse and somewhat
flattened vesicles. There are always one or more large granulated
vesicles. This type of nerve ending, shown on the right of Fig. 7
as degenerating following p-chloroamphetamine (PCA) treatment, is
preferentially attacked by this serotonergic toxin. About 3-5% of
the total bouton area in the neostriatum is made up of this morphological type.

Further studies will be needed to confirm the extent to which

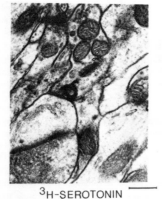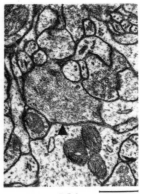

³H-SEROTONIN ————                    PCA ————

Figure 7: Probable Serotonergic Boutons in the Rat Neostriatum.
Arrow points to degenerating bouton. Bar = 0.5 µm

this morphology is duplicated by serotonergic nerve endings in other
areas of brain, as well as to establish the details of the serotonin cell body at the electron microscopic level. So far little can
be said about the physiological role of serotonin pathways to the
basal ganglia.

### B. Neurotransmitters Associated with Processing Pathways within the Basal Ganglia

1. Acetylcholine. The neostriatum contains some of the highest
levels of acetylcholine, choline acetyltransferase (CAT) and acetylcholinesterase of any major structure in the nervous system. The
majority of neurons are small Golgi type II interneurons but large
neurons (Kemp and Powell, 1971), as well as smaller neurons comparable in size to the Golgi type neurons send efferents to caudal
structures (Bunney and Aghajanian, 1976). The probability that
acetylcholine and its synthetic enzyme CAT were contained in interneurons of the neostriatum was originally suggested on the basis
of extensive lesioning studies (McGeer, et al., 1971) which failed
to alter CAT activity in the neostriatum. Support for this conclusion has been derived subsequently from histochemical studies using
a stain for acetylcholinesterase (Lynch, et al., 1972) and from
immunohistochemical studies using a specific antibody for CAT
(McGeer, et al., 1974a). The latter has permitted positive identification of the morphology of the cholinergic cell body (Fig. 8)
and nerve endings (Fig. 9) in the neostriatum (Hattori, et al.,
1976b).

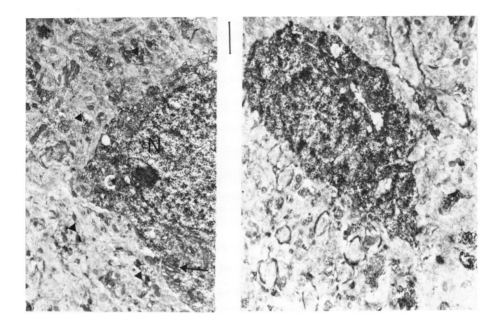

Figure 8: Cholinergic cells in the rat neostriatum stained for CAT by immunohistochemistry. Nucleus (N) is less stained than the cytoplasm (C) and rough endoplasmic reticulum ⟶ . Positive processes (▲) can be seen in surrounding neuropile. Bar = 1 µm

CAT          $^3$H-DFP

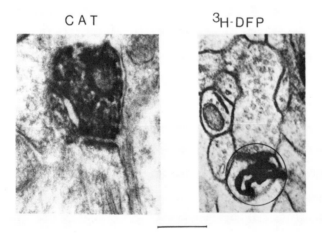

Figure 9: Cholinergic nerve endings in the rat neostriatum stained for CAT by immunohistochemistry (left) or in contact with $^3$H-DFP-labelled receptor (right). Bar = 0.5 µm

Another method of determining cholinergic morphology is via
³H-DFP binding to acetylcholinesterase in cholinoceptive striatal
dendritic spines. A presumed cholinergic bouton is shown (Fig. 9,
right) with the same asymmetrical synaptic contact and common round
vesicles seen in boutons staining for CAT by immunohistochemical
techniques (Fig. 9, left)(Hattori and McGeer, 1974).

Other nuclei of the extrapyramidal system, that is the globus
pallidus, the substantia nigra and the subthalamic nucleus have much
lower CAT activities than are found in the caudate and putamen, but
it should be pointed out that even the relatively low activity of
CAT found in the substantia nigra is comparable in magnitude to the
activity of tyrosine hydroxylase, the key enzyme for the synthesis
of dopamine, found in the NCP. Cholinergic systems in these other
structures can therefore not be discounted, but the anatomy of the
pathways involved is not yet known.

2. GABA. The brain content of GABA is 200-1,000 fold greater
that that of neurotransmitters such as dopamine, noradrenaline,
acetylcholine and serotonin. It is widely and rather evenly distributed, as might be anticipated for a transmitter suspected of being
the inhibitory "workhorse" for interneurons found in almost all
areas of brain. Uptake studies with labelled GABA have suggested that
25-45% of nerve endings, depending on the brain area, may contain
this neurotransmitter (Iversen and Schon, 1973). Some of the highest
levels of GABA and GAD in brain are found in the basal ganglia, particularly in the globus pallidus and substantia nigra, suggesting a
prominent role for this transmitter. At least three pathways of the
basal ganglia utilize GABA.

a) Neostriatal interneurons: The probability that much of the
GABA in the neostriatum is contained in interneurons is suggested
by the small and usually insignificant loss of GABA or GAD following lesions of all known afferents to the neostriatum (McGeer and
McGeer, 1975).

b) Striato-nigral pathway: It has been known for many years
that a prominent striato-nigral path exists with highly preferential
innervation of the pars reticulata. More recently it has been shown
that lesions of the neostriatum or hemitransections anterior to the
globus pallidus will cause some reduction in nigral GAD (Kim, et al.,
1971; Fonnum, et al., 1974). Brownstein, et al. (1977) consider that
the cell bodies of these reticulata afferents originate in the caudal
and lateral aspects of the neostriatum. Since the pathway traverses
the globus pallidus, it has been suggested that there may be some
terminations within the pallidum itself.

c) Pallido-nigral pathway: Compelling evidence in favor of a
descending pallido-nigral GABA-containing pathway came originally

from studies indicating that electrolytic lesions of the globus
pallidus or hemitransections of the brain at the level of the sub-
thalamus led to losses of up to 80% in the GAD activity in the substantia nigra, whereas transections anterior to the globus pallidus
led to much smaller losses in GAD (McGeer, et al., 1974b). The existence of this pathway was established by anterograde axoplasmic flow
studies following injections of [3]H-leucine into the globus pallidus.
Comparative studies were done following similar injections into the
caudate-putamen. Protein labelling of the nigra resulted from both
these injections, there being preferential transport to the zona
compacta following pallidal injections and to the zona reticulata
following NCP injections (Hattori, et al., 1975).

The existence of the pallido-nigral tract has been confirmed
by retrograde transport of HRP (Bunney and Aghajanian, 1976; Grofova,
1975), and the findings relative to GAD duplicated by Brownstein, et
al. (1977).

The morphology of the GABA nerve ending in the substantia nigra
has been clearly defined as a result of immunohistochemical studies
of GAD by Ribak, et al., (1977). The nerve endings make symmetrical
synapses as shown in the upper left picture in Fig. 10. This morphology is in accord with that of nerve endings labelled by axoplasmic
flow of [3]H-protein from the globus pallidus and neostriatum (Fig. 10)
(Hattori, et al., 1975).

3. Substance P. Early bioassay techniques (Pernow, 1953) indicated that substance P occurred largely in gray matter and was particularly concentrated in the basal ganglia, hypothalamus, thalamus
and dorsal root of the spinal cord.

No substantial further progress was made until 1970 when Leeman
and her coworkers isolated from hypothalamic extracts a material
which stimulated salivary secretion when injected into anesthetized
rats. They purified this material, showed its identity in properties
with substance P and identified its unidecapeptide structure (Chang
and Leeman, 1970). The chemical identification and subsequent synthesis of substance P permitted the development of a sensitive and
specific radioimmunoassay as well as an immunohistochemical technique for its localization. Developments in this field are proceeding
rapidly but it is already clear that there is probably a striato-
nigral tract containing substance P which accounts for at least 45-
65% of the substance P in the zona reticulata of the substantia
nigra. This tract appears to come almost entirely from the NCP and
particularly from the anterior portion. This preferential location
of substance P-containing cell soma in the anterior part of the
caudate-putamen is indicated by the results of studies using selective lesions produced either by knife cuts (Brownstein, et al., 1977),
electrolytically (Mroz, et al., 1977) or by intra-striatal injections
of kainic acid (Hong, et al., 1977), a procedure which causes

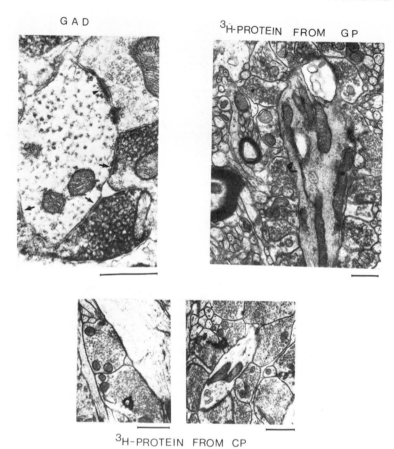

Figure 10: Nerve endings in rat substantia nigra stained for GAD by immunohistochemistry (upper left, courtesy of C.E. Ribak, et al.) or labelled by $^3$H-protein transported from the pallidum (upper right) or neostriatum (bottom). Bar = 0.5 μm

selective destruction of cell soma in the injected area. Additional support for the association of substance P with a striato-nigral tract comes from Kanazawa, et al. (1977), who found decreased levels in the nigra in Huntington's chorea. In this disease there is a loss of neurons in the striatum and particularly in the caudate, and such loss would lead to degeneration of striato-nigral pathways.

Substance P cell bodies have also been reported in the substantia nigra from immunohistochemical studies (Nilsson, et al., 1974; Hokfelt, et al., 1976) but the existence of such cells has not been otherwise confirmed nor is there any evidence available on their

projections. Important work remains to be done in defining the morphological characteristics as well as the exact anatomy of substance
P-containing pathways in the basal ganglia.


### C. Neurotransmitters Involved in Output Pathways from the Basal Ganglia

Unfortunately no definitive evidence yet exists regarding the
neurotransmitters involved in any of the output pathways so far
identified from the globus pallidus and the substantia nigra. In
our hands, lesions of the entopeduncular nucleus cause a loss in
GAD activity in the habenula of about 40% with no change in CAT;
this offers a tentative indication that the tract from the entopeduncular nucleus to the lateral habenula (Nauta, 1974) may have a
GABAnergic component.


## NEURONAL INTERCONNECTIONS IN THE EXTRAPYRAMIDAL SYSTEM

It is clear that many of the tracts, including some very major
ones, in the extrapyramidal system are still not biochemically
finger-printed as to the transmitter which they use. This remains
a major challenge for the biochemical neuroanatomist. Another challenge, however, is posed by the problem of determining the functional
relationships between the various tracts. Some clues may be obtained
from pharmacological studies but definitive evidence can only come
from electron microscopic work, preferably using dual labelling
techniques.

Several laboratories have found that dopamine agonists inhibit
the release of acetylcholine and raise its level in the striatum,
while dopamine antagonists have the converse effects. On the presump-
tion that the dopaminergic input is generally inhibitory, these
results could be explained by a direct dopaminergic innervation of
cholinergic neurons. Such direct innervation was demonstrated at the
electron microscopic level by using 6-OHDA-induced degeneration as a
marker for the dopaminergic nerve endings and the PAP immunohistochemical technique for the cholinergic dendrites. Figure 11 shows
degenerating dopaminergic nerve endings in the neostriatum of a rat
making contact with cholinergic dendrites.

Cholinergic agonists and antagonists generally change GABA
levels in the striatum and substantia nigra in the fashion that
would be expected if there were direct excitatory cholinergic innervation of GABA interneurons and of striato-nigral GABAnergic neurons
(McGeer, et al., 1976b). The smaller effects of dopaminergic agonists
and antagonists on GABA levels were in the same direction and could
be indirectly mediated through the effects upon excitatory cholin-

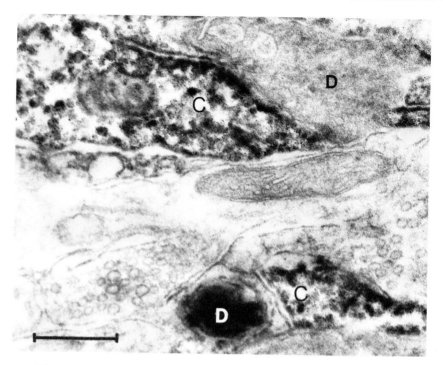

Figure 11: Dopaminergic nerve endings (D) in contact with cholinergic dendrites (C). Bar = 0.5 μm

ergic interneurons. Thus, while the evidence is highly speculative,
it can be postulated that the cholinergic interneurons have a direct
excitatory action on GABAnergic neostriatal neurons.

There are extensive physiological and pharmacological data indicating that there is a very important GABAnergic inhibitory input
upon dopaminergic dendrites in the substantia nigra. Studies of the
substantia nigra following caudate or pallidal injections of tritiated leucine (Hattori, et al., 1975) indicated preferential labelling of the zona reticulata in the case of caudate injections and
of the zona compacta in the case of pallidal injections. Moreover,
following 6-OHDA-induced degeneration of nigral dopaminergic neurons,
terminals labelled by axoplasmic flow from the external pallidum were
seen to make contact with dopaminergic dendrites five times more
frequently than did terminals labelled by axoplasmic flow from the
neostriatum (Fig. 10). Thus, descending GABA neurons from the pallidum innervate dopaminergic dendrites of the substantia nigra.

Other connections are tenuous on the basis of present data but
some speculations are possible. Innervation of both cholinergic and

GABAnergic neurons in the neostriatum by a glutamatergic input from the cortex can be hypothesized on the basis of the marked loss of both CAT and GAD in the neostriatum following injections of small amounts of kainic acid, taken together with the biochemical and electron microscopic evidence previously described that such degeneration is connected with glutamatergic innervation. Moreover, the same tract may innervate substance P neurons descending to the nigra since kainic acid injections into the neostriatum cause losses of substance P in the nigra.

SUMMARY

Figure 12 is a summarizing diagram of a sagittal section of rat brain showing the connections that have been discussed. The nigro-striatal dopaminergic tract (pathway 2 in Fig. 1) is shown innervating cholinergic interneurons in the neostriatum. The raphe-striatal serotonergic tract (pathway 4 in Fig. 1) is drawn without interconnections being shown because information on this point has not yet been developed. The cortico-striatal glutamatergic tract (pathway 1 in Fig. 1) is illustrated innervating cholinergic, GABAnergic and substance P neurons. Cholinergic neurons are shown innervating GABAnergic neurons in the neostriatum. The descending GABA tract from the neostriatum is shown reaching the globus pallidus (pathway 5 in Fig. 1) and the pars reticulata of the substantia nigra (pathway 6 in Fig. 1). The descending GABA tract from the

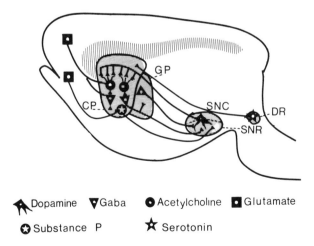

Figure 12: Biochemically "Fingerprinted" Pathways in the Extrapyramidal System and Their Hypothesized Interconnections

globus pallidus (pathway 8 in Fig. 1) is shown making contact with
dopaminergic dendrites of the pars compacta. The descending substance
P tract (also pathway 6 in Fig. 1) reaches the pars reticulata but
the connections there are not known.

Considerable progress has been made in recent years in identifying neurotransmitters, their pathways and their connections. But
it is clear that many of the data are tentative and huge gaps in
our knowledge remain.

## REFERENCES

Anden, N.E., Carlsson, A., Dahlstrom, A., Fuxe, K., Hillarp, N.A.
and Larsson, K. (1964). Life Sci. 3, 523-530.
Brownstein, M.J., Mroz, E.A., Tappaz, M.L. and Leeman, S.E. (1977).
Brain Res., in press.
Bunney, B.S. and Aghajanian, K. (1976). Brain Res. 117, 423-435.
Chang, M.M. and Leeman, S.E. (1970). J. Biol. Chem. 245, 4784-4790.
Coyle, J.T. and Schwarcz, R. (1976). Nature 263, 244-246.
Divac, I., Fonnum, F. and Storm-Mathisen J. (1977). Nature 266,
377-378.
Fonnum, F., Grofova, I., Rinvik, E., Storm-Mathisen, J. and Waldberg,
F. (1974). Brain Res. 71, 77-92.
Fuxe, K. and Johnsson, G. (1974). In "Adv. Biochem. Pharmacol.", vol.
10 (E. Costa, G.L. Gessa and M. Sandler, eds), pp. 1-12. Raven
Press, New York.
Grofova, I. (1975). Brain Res. 91, 286-291.
Hattori, T. and McGeer, P.L. (1974), Exp. Neurol. 45, 541-548.
Hattori, T., Fibiger, H.C., McGeer, P.L. and Maler, L. (1973). Exp.
Neurol. 41, 599-611.
Hattori, T., Fibiger, H.C. and McGeer, P.L. (1975). J. Comp. Neurol.
162, 487-504.
Hattori, T., McGeer, P.L. and McGeer, E.G. (1976a). Neurochem. Res.
1, 451-467.
Hattori, T., Singh, V.K., McGeer, E.G. and McGeer, P.L. (1976b).
Brain Res. 102, 164-173.
Hokfelt, T.H. and Ungerstedt, U. (1969). Acta Physiol. Scand. 76,
415-426.
Hokfelt, T., Meyerson, R. and Nilsson, G. (1976). Brain Res. 104,
181-186.
Hong, J., Yang, H.-Y. T., Racgni, G. and Costa, E. (1977). Brain
Res. 122, 541-544.
Iversen, L.L. and Schon, F.E. (1973). In "New Concepts in Neuro-
transmitter Mechanisms" (A.J. Mandell, ed), pp. 153-193. Plenum
Press, New York.
Kanazawa, I., Bird, E., O'Connell, R. and Powell, D. (1977). Brain
Res. 120, 387-392.
Kemp, J.M. and Powell, T.P.S. (1971). Philos. Trans. R. Soc. Lond.

[Biol. Sci.] 262, 383–401.

Kim, J.S., Bak, I.J., Hassler, R. and Okada, Y. (1971). Exp. Brain Res. 14, 95–104.

Lynch, G.S., Lucas, P.A. and Deadwyler, S.A. (1972). Brain Res. 45, 617–621.

McGeer, E.G. and McGeer, P.L. (1976). Nature 263, 517–519.

McGeer, E.G., Hattori, T. and McGeer, P.L. (1975). Brain Res. 86, 478–482.

McGeer, P.L. and McGeer, E.G. (1975). Brain Res. 91, 331–335.

McGeer, P.L., McGeer, E.G., Fibiger, H.C. and Wickson, V. (1971). Brain Res. 35, 308–314.

McGeer, P.L., McGeer, E.G., Singh, V.K. and Chase, W.H. (1974a). Brain Res. 81, 373–379.

McGeer, P.L., Fibiger, H.C., Maler, L., Hattori, T. and McGeer, E.G. (1974b). In "Advances in Neurology", vol. 5 (F.H. McDowell and A. Barbeau, eds), pp. 153–160. Raven Press, New York.

McGeer, P.L., McGeer, E.G. and Suzuki, J.S. (1976a). Arch. Neurol. 34, 33–35.

McGeer, P.L., Grewaal, D.S. and McGeer, E.G. (1976b). In "Advances in Parkinsonism" (W. Birkmayer and O. Hornykiewicz, eds), pp. 132–140. Editiones Roche, Basle.

McGeer, P.L., McGeer, E.G., Scherer, U. and Singh, K. (1977). Brain Res. 128, 369–373.

Mroz, E.A., Brownstein, M.J. and Leeman, S.E. (1977). Brain Res. 125, 305–311.

Nauta, W.J.H. (1974). J. Comp. Neurol. 156, 19–28.

Nilsson, C., Hokfelt, T. and Pernow, B. (1974). Medical Biology 52, 424–427.

Pernow, B. (1953). Acta Physiol. Scand. Suppl. 105, 1–90.

Ribak, C.E., Vaughn, J.E., Saito, K., Barber, R. and Roberts, E. (1976). Brain Res. 116, 287–298.

Simon, J.R., Contrera, J.F. and Kuhar, M.J. (1976). J. Neurochem. 26, 141–147.

Wofsey, A.R., Kuhar, M.J. and Snyder, S.H. (1971). Proc. Natl. Acad. Sci. USA 68, 1102–1106.

COMMENTS ON LOCALIZATION OF NEUROTRANSMITTERS IN THE BASAL

GANGLIA

F. Fonnum

Norwegian Defence Research Establishment
Division for Toxicology
P O Box 25, N-2007, Kjeller, Norway

The basal ganglia (nucleus caudatus, putamen, globus pallidus, nucleus entopeduncularis) including substantia nigra have received considerable attention because of their importance in the pathogenesis of Huntington's Chorea and Parkinson's syndrome. These regions also contain some of the highest concentrations of putative transmitter candidates in the brain and are therefore very attractive to neurochemists.

The fibre connections between these nuclei have been extensively reviewed (McGeer et al., preceeding Chapter). It is here only necessary to remind ourselves that cells in striatum (nucleus caudatus and putamen) project in a precise topographical way to globus pallidus, nucleus entopeduncularis, to pars reticulata and moderately to the pars compacta of the substantia nigra (Bunney and Aghajanian, 1976; Grofova, 1975; Hajdu et al., 1973; Knook, 1965; Niimi et al., 1970). Further the cells in striatum receive a heavy input from cells localized in the frontal part of cerebral cortex (Webster, 1961; Kemp & Powell, 1971; Buchwald et al., 1973). A projection from cortex to substantia nigra are less certain. (For discussion see Rinvik and Walberg,      ).


Distribution of Neurotransmitter Candidates in unoperated animals

In Table 1 I have tried to summarize our present knowledge on the localization of neurotransmitter candidates in the normal basal ganglia. For simplicity I have when possible selected the average level in striatum as unity. Since there is increasing evidence for a topographical distribution of transmitter candidates

in the rostro-caudal or ventro-dorsal direction of striatum,
data have been given, where available, for both the rostral and
caudal parts of this region.  A very high level of GAD and GABA
are found in substantia nigra, globus pallidus and nucleus
entopeduncularis (Fonnum et al., 1977a).  The highest concentration
of GAD in brain is found in substantia innominata, at a level close
to that of pars reticulata of substantia nigra (Fonnum et al.,
1977b).  In striatum the highest level of GAD is found in the
ventrocaudal part.

The distribution of $Na^+$ independent GABA binding, probably
GABA receptor binding, follow that of GAD activity in the basal
ganglia in the monkey and in the rat.  A much higher level of
GABA receptor binding are, however, found in cerebellar cortex
and to lesser extent in parts of cerebral cortex than in the basal
ganglia (Enna, this volume).  The regional distribution of GABA
receptor binding do therefore not follow the distribution of GAD
and GABA completly.

The concentration of glutamate do not differ greatly in
different parts of the brain.  This is expected since this amino
acid occupies a unique position in brain metabolism.  A high
concentration of a possible marker for glutaminergic nerve
terminals, high affinity uptake of L-glutamate or D-aspartate,
is found in striatum, particularly the rostral part.  The high
affinity uptake of these amino acids are low in the other parts
of the basal ganglia.  The highest concentration of high affinity
uptake of glutamate in brain so far is found in the thalamus
(see below).

Recently several investigators have found very high concentration of peptides like Substance P (Kanazawa and Jessel, 1976;
Hong et al., 1977; Brownstein et al., 1976) and enkephalin (Yang
et al., 1977a) in the basal ganglia.  The highest concentration of
Substance P in brain is found in substantia nigra.  Enkephalin
is present in a very high level in globus pallidus (Yang et al.,
1977b), where it occurs in interneurons (P. Emson, personal
communication).  High levels are also present in striatum (Yang
et al., 1977b).

The level of ChAT, ACh and the muscarinic receptor in striatum
is among the highest in the brain, nucleus interpeduncularis is
the only region having a much higher concentration of ChAT and
ACh (Fonnum et al., 1977b; Yamamura and Snyder, 1974; Cheney et al.,
1976).  Also the turnover of ACh is high in striatum whereas it is
very low in substantia nigra (Mao et al., 1977).  This explains
why the level of ACh itself is not so low in substantia nigra.
On the other side AChE is fairly high in substantia nigra suggesting
that the dopaminergic cells contains AChE.  This may explain why

TABLE 1. DISTRIBUTION OF PUTATIVE NEUROTRANSMITTERS IN BASAL GANGLIA

| | STRIATUM Ant | STRIATUM Post | GLOBUS PALLIDUS | NC. ENTOPEDUNCULARIS | SUBSTANTIA NIGRA Ret | SUBSTANTIA NIGRA Comp |
|---|---|---|---|---|---|---|
| GAD[1] | 0.8 | 1.2 | 2.5 | 2.0 | 5.0 | 3.5 |
| GABA reseptor[2] | | 1.0 | 2.3 | | | 1.4 |
| H.A. GLU[3] | 1.1 | 0.9 | 0.1 | - | | 0.2 |
| Substance P[4] | | 1.0 | 1.5 | | | 7.0 |
| CHAT[1] | 1.0 | 1.0 | 0.4 | 0.2 | 0.1 | 0.1 |
| ACH turnover[5] | | 1.0 | 1.0 | | | 0.1 |
| Dopamine[6,7] | 1.3 | 0.7 | 0.7 | - | 0.1 | 0.1 |
| Noradrenaline[6] | | 0 | 5 | - | 4 | 11 |
| Serotonin[8] | 0.8 | 1.2 | 1.8 | - | 2.0 | 1.8 |
| Enkephalin[9] | | 10 | 76 | - | | - |

[1]Fonnum et al, 1977a; [2]Enna this volume; [3]Divac et al, 1977; [4]Kanazawa & Jessel, 1977; [5]Mao et al, 1977; [6]Versley et al, 1976; [7]Tassin et al, 1976; [8]Palkowitz et al, 1974; [9]Yang et al, 1977.

Shute & Lewis (1963) on the basis of AChE staining wrongly
suggested that the cholinergic input to the striatum was derived
from an area situated near substantia nigra or ventral tegmental
area of Tsai.

Also aromatic amines are well represented in the basal ganglia.
Globus pallidus and substantia nigra have among the highest levels
of noradrenaline in the brain whereas striatum do not contain this
amine (Versteeg et al., 1976). High level of dopamine is localized in striatum, particularly in the rostral part (Tassin et al.,
1976) and in globus pallidus. Parts of the hypothalamus contain
the highest levels of noradrenaline whereas nc. accumbens and
olfactory tubercle contain the highest levels of dopamine
(Versteeg et al., 1976). Serotonin is found in all basal ganglia,
the level in globus pallidus and substantia nigra is among the
highest in the brain (Palkowitz et al., 1974). In striatum most
of serotonin is localized to the posterior part. The highest
level of serotonin in brain is found in the raphe nuclei
(Palkowitz et al., 1974).

## Neurotransmitters in Striato-pallidal, Striato-
## entopeduncular and Striato-nigral Pathways

There is a topographical distribution of striato-pallidal
connections in the rat in a way so that the rostral part of
striatum projects to the rostral part of globus pallidus (Knook,
1965). The transmitter in this pathway have been little investigated. We have therefore made a series of hemitransections of
the brain at various rostro-caudal levels of striatum. The
results show that GAD but not AAD was reduced after these lesions.
The reduction in GAD was dependent upon the position of the lesion
and was always more pronounced in the anterior than the posterior
part (Table 2). The results are therefore consistent with GABA
as a transmitter in the striato-pallidal connections. The
investigation confirms and expands the results from a single
experiment in monkey (Kanazawa & Toyokura, 1974) and in cat
(Fonnum et al., 1974) which have suggested that the striato-
pallidal fibres are GABAergic.

The striato-entopeduncular fibres have been demonstrated in
the rat by degeneration (Knook, 1965) and autoradiographic techniques (Hattori et al., 1973). Oblique hemitransections of the
striatum which involved the anterior part of the tail significantly
reduced the level of GAD in nucleus entopeduncularis, although
to a lesser extent than in globus pallidus. If the lesion also
involved the anterior part of globus pallidus and the caudal part
of striatum, the decrease in GAD was almost complete (Table 2).
The results therefore show that the striato-entopeduncular fibres

are GABAergic.  This is in agreement with electrophysiological
observations (Yoshida et al., 1972) that entopeduncular cells are
monosynaptically inhibited by stimulation of caudate nucleus.  Our
findings do not exclude that some GABA afferents to nucleus entopeduncularis originate in globus pallidus.

TABLE 2
EFFECT OF HEMITRANSECTIONS AT DIFFERENT LEVELS OF THE STRIATUM OR
GAD IN GLOBUS PALLIDUS, NC. ENTOPEDUNCULARIS AND SUBSTANTIA NIGRA

|  | GLOBUS PAL. | NC. ENTOPEDUC. | SUB.NIGRA |
|---|---|---|---|
|  | GAD in percent of unoperated side | | |
| PRECOM. TRANSECT. | 86 | 82 | 55 |
| POSTCOM. TRANSECT. | 31(19-41) | 48(42-51) | 67(62-74) |
| POSTCOM. TRANSECT. +frontal part of globus pallidus | - | 25(12-33) | 20(13-28) |

The results are expressed as mean value with ranges in parenthesis.

      Considerable attention has been paid to the transmitters of
the striato-nigral connections.  Several studies from different
laboratories have demonstrated that in the monkey (Kanazawa and
Toryokura, 1974; Kataoka et al., 1974), cat (Fonnum et al., 1974)
and rat (Kim et al., 1971) the striato-nigral fibres are GABAergic.
It is in this connection of interest to note that striatal
lesions in the cat resulted in a much larger decrease of GAD in pars
reticulata than in pars compacta (caudal part) of substantia
nigra (Fonnum et al., 1974).  The existance of a GABAergic pathway
from striatum to substantia nigra has been refuted by McGeer and
collaborators (McGeer et al., 1971) who have failed to observe
loss of GAD after lesions in striatum, particularly after anterior
hemitransections.  They suggested that the GABAergic projection
to substantia nigra arises in globus pallidus.

      We have reinvestigated the problem of the origin of the GABA-
ergic fibres to nigra in the rat.  When transverse lesions were
made anterior to the commissural connection, then there was no
decrease of GAD in substantia nigra.  Following oblique transections
which included part of the tail of striatum, there was a significant loss of GAD in substantia nigra.  More caudal lesions which
also involved the rostral tip of globus pallidus resulted in a
very large fall in GAD (Table 2).  A similar fall of GAD was
found by Kanazawa et al., (1977) after a large lesion of striatum.

      Recently several studies (Hong et al., 1977; Kanazawa et al.,
1977) have shown a reduction of Substance P in substantia
nigra following striatal lesions.  It seems that

Substance P containing fibres originate in the rostral part of caudate-putamen whereas the majority of GABAergic fibres originate in the caudal part of the region. From our (Fonnum et al., 1974) previous studies on cat, one cannot exclude the possiblility that a proportion of the GABAergic fibres particularly to the caudal part of pars compacta arises from globus pallidus.

Neurotransmitters in the cortico-striatal and cortico-thalamic pathwa

The neostriatum receives a large exitatory projection from the neocortex (Webster, 1961; Kemp & Powell, 1971; Buchwald et al., 1973). A small part of the projection is crossed (Kemp & Powell, 1971). Pharmacological studies have shown that the excitation of striatal neurons after stimulation of cortex may be blocked by glutamate diethylester (Spencer, 1976). Since this component blocks the receptor action of glutamate, the possibility existed that glutamate may be the transmitter of the cortio-striatal fibres.

Evidence is accumulation from studies on cerebellum (Young et al., 1974), hippocampus (Cotman, this volume, Storm-Mathisen, this volume), the visual system (Lund-Karlsen & Fonnum, 1978) and nucleus accumbens (Walaas & Fonnum, 1978) that the high affinity uptakes of L-glutamate of D-aspartate are important markers for nerve terminals using acidic amino acids as chemical transmitters. Only amino acid analysis can, however, differentiate between the two candidates L-glutamate or L-aspartate since D- and L-aspartate and L-glutamate use the same uptake system (Takagaki, this volume; Davies & Johnston, 1976). D-aspartate, which is not metabolised, seems to be the agent of choice for such uptake studies.

In our laboratory (Divac, Fonnum and Storm-Mathisen, 1977; Fonnum, Storm-Mathisen and Divac, 1978) we have shown that ablation of cortex frontal to bregma was accompanied by a significant decrease of the uptakes of both L-glutamate and D-aspartate in the anterior and posterior part of striatum on the lesion side (Table 3). There was also a small decrease on the unoperated side compared to the uptake in the normal animal. The loss of high affinity uptake was slightly more emphasized in the hemidecorticated animal. In the operated animals there were no changes in GABA uptake, GAD activity, ChAT activity or AAD activity, clearly demonstrating that the decrease was not due to any general effect on striatal neurons, but a specific effect caused by destruction of cortical cells which project to striatum. No effect was found after ablation of the occipital cortex which donot project to striatum. Separate studies showed that most of the uptake was confined to the synaptosome fraction and that the reduction was found in this fraction. A similar reduction in high affinity uptake of L-glutamate was found by McGeer et al. (this volume).

In order to differentiate between L-aspartate and L-glutamate as transmittors, we also studied the changes in amino acid level in striatum after hemidecortication. The animals were killed by decapitation and the brain rapidly cooled to near freezing by putting the head in liquid nitrogen for 8 sec. Striatum was rapidly dissected out and homogenized in acetone: 50 mM bicarbonate mixture (1:1). After removal of denaturated proteins, the amino acid content was determined by the dansylation technique using ($^{14}$-C) amino acids as standards (Lund Karlsen & Fonnum, 1977). The results showed a significant fall in L-glutamate but not in any of the other amino acids including aspartate (Fonnum et al., 1978). Similar results have been reported independantly by Kim et al., 1977. The changes in amino acid content and the changes in L-glutamate and D-aspartate high affinity uptake after destruction of the frontal cortex suggest that L-glutamate may be the transmitter of the cortico-striatal fibres.

There is also a heavy projection from cortex, particularly sensory and motor cortex, to the ventral part of thalamus (for review Frigyesi et al., 1972). The projection seems to be completly ipsilateral. The thalamic neurones are excited by aspartate, glutamate and related amino acids (Curtis & Watkins, 1963; McLennan et al., 1968; Tebécis, 1970). There are suggestions that the sensitivity to L-aspartate and L-glutamate varies in the different nuclei so that both may function as transmitter (McLennan et al., 1968; Haldeman et al., 1972).

In our laboratory (Fonnum, Storm-Mathisen and Divac, 1978) we have therefore used the same approach as for the cortico-striatal fibres in order to see if the corticothalamic fibres also are glutamergic. Thalamus was divided into a frontal and caudal part. The results (Table 4) showed that D-asp uptake was more active in unoperated thalamus than in unoperated striatum. The highest uptake activity was confined to the anterior part. After hemidecortication there was a significant decrease in both parts of thalamus. Separate experiments confirmed again that the uptake was mainly localized to the synaptosome fraction and the reduction after lesion was also found in this fraction. Amino acid analysis of the whole of thalamus after lesion showed a significant fall in L-glutamate and a smaller loss in L-aspartate. Further studies will have to differentiate if L-aspartate and L-glutamate are neurotransmitters in different parts of thalamus. The biochemical evidence thus suggest that L-glutamate and perhaps L-aspartate act as neurotransmitters in the cortico-thalamic fibres.

TABLE 3.   UPTAKE OF $(^3H)$-D-ASP (1 μM) IN NEOSTRIATUM AFTER CORTICAL LESIONS ON THE RIGHT SIDE

|                    | n  | ANTERIOR left | ANTERIOR right | POSTERIOR left | POSTERIOR right |
|--------------------|----|---------------|----------------|----------------|-----------------|
|                    |    | per cent of controls |         |                |                 |
| FRONTAL ABLATION   | 5  | $77\pm8$      | $35\pm4$       | $87\pm5$       | $48\pm2$        |
| HEMIDECORTICATION  | 5  | $87\pm6$      | $30\pm3$       | $80\pm4$       | $25\pm2$        |
| OCCIPITAL ABLATION | 7  | $112\pm7$     | $107\pm9$      | $114\pm9$      | $99\pm5$        |
| UNOPERATED CONTROLS (dpm/3min/μg prot) | 12 | $16520\pm430$ | | $14000\pm520$ | |

Mean values $\pm$ SEM

No changes in glutamate decarboxylase, choline acetyltransferase, GABA uptake a aromatic amino acid decarboxylase.

Fonnum, Storm-Mathisen, Divac, 1978

TABLE 4.   UPTAKE OF $(^3H)$-D-ASP IN THALAMUS AFTER RIGHT HEMIDECORTICATION

|                    | N  | ANTERIOR left | ANTERIOR right | POSTERIOR[X] left | POSTERIOR[X] right |
|--------------------|----|---------------|----------------|-------------------|--------------------|
| HEMIDECORTICATION (% of control $\pm$ SEM | 5 | $83\pm5$ | $35\pm5$ | $116\pm20$ | $29\pm8$ |
| CONTROL (dpm/3min/μg prot. $\pm$SEM) | 8 | $39010\pm1460$ | | $21010\pm4090$ | |

Mean values $\pm$ SEM.
X) 25-35% reduction in glutamate decarboxylase and GABA uptake, but not in choline acetyltransferase on both sides.

Fonnum, Storm-Mathisen, Divac, 1978

## REFERENCES

Brownstein, M.Y., Mroz, E.A., Kizer, S., Palkowits, M. and Leeman, S.E., 1976, Regional distribution of substance P in the brain of the rat, Brain Res. 116: 299-305.

Buckwald, D.N., Price, B.D., Vernon, L and Hull, C.D., 1973, Caudate intracellular response to thalamic and central inputs, Exp. Neurol. 38: 311-321.

Bunney, B.S. and Aghajanian, G.K., 1976, The precise localization of nigral afferents in the rat as determined by a retrograde tracing technique, Brain Res. 117: 423-435.

Cheney, D.L., Racagni, G. and Costa, E., 1976, Distribution of acetylcholine and choline acetyltransferase in specific nuclei and tracts of rat brain in "Biology of Cholinergic Function" (Ed. A.M. Goldberg and I. Hanin), pp 655-660.

Curtis, D.R. and Watkins, J.C., 1963, Acidic amino acids with strong excitatory actions on mammalian neurones, J. Physiol. (Lond.) 166: 1-14.

Davies, L.P., and Johnson, G.A.R., 1976, Uptake and release of D- and L-aspartate by rat brain slices, J. Neurochem., 26: 1007-1014.

Divac, I., Fonnum, F. and Storm-Mathisen, J., 1977, High affinity uptake of glutamate in the terminals of cortico-striatal axons, Nature (Lond.), 266: 377-378.

Fonnum, F., Gottesfeld, Z. and Grofová, I., 1977a, Distribution of glutamate decarboxylase, choline acetyltransferase and aromatic amino acid decarboxylase in the basal ganglia of normal and operated rats. Evidence for striato-pallidal, striato-entopeduncular and striato-nigral GABA-ergic fibres, Brain Res. (in press).

Fonnum, F., Walaas, I. and Iversen, E., Localization of GABAergic, cholinergic and aminergic structures in the mesolimbic system (1977b), J. Neurochem., 29: 221-230.

Fonnum, F., Divac, I. and Storm-Mathisen, J., 1978, to be published.

Fonnum, F., Grofova, I., Rinvik, E., Storm-Mathisen, J. and Walberg, F., 1974, Origin and distribution of glutamate decarboxylase in substantia nigra of the cat, Brain Res. 71: 77-92.

Frigyesi, I.L., Rinvik, E., and Yahr, M.D., 1972, Corticothalamic projections and sensorimotor activities, Raven Press, New York, pp 1-584.

Grofova, I., 1975, The identification of striatal and pallidal neurons projecting to substantia nigra. An experimental study by means of retrograde axonal transport of horseradish peroxydase, Brain Res., 91: 286-291.

Hajdu, F., Hassler, R. and Bak, I.J., 1973, Electron microscopic study of the substantia nigra and the strio-nigral projection in the rat, Z. Zellforsch., 146: 207-221.

Haldeman, S., Huffman, R.D., Marshall, K.C., and McLennan, H., 1972, The antagonism of the glutamate-induced and synaptic excitation of thalamic neurones, Brain Res., 39: 419-425.

Hattori, T., McGeer, P.L., Fibiger, H.C. and McGeer, E.G., 1973,
On the source of GABA-containing terminals in the substantia
nigra. Electron microscopic, autoradiographic and biochemical
studies, Brain Res., 54: 103-114.

Hong, J.S., Yang, H.-Y.T., Racagni, G. and Costa, E., 1977,
Projections of substance P containing neurons from neostriatum
to substantia nigra, Brain Res., 122: 541-544.

Kanazawa, I., and Jessel, T., 1976, Post mortem changes and
regional distribution of substance P and the rat and mouse
nervous system., Brain Res., 117: 362-367.

Kanazawa, I. and Toyokura, Y., 1974, Quantitative histochemistry
of -aminobutyric acid (GABA) in the human substantia nigra
and globus pallidus, Confin. Neurol., 36: 273-281.

Kanazawa, I., Emson, P.C. and Cuello, A.C., 1977, Evidence for
the existence of substance P-containing fibres in striato-
nigral and pallido-nigral pathways in rat brain, Brain Res.,
119: 447-453.

Kataoka, K., Bak, I.J., Hassler, R., Kim, J.S. and Wagner, A.,
1974, L-glutamate decarboxylase and cholinacetyltransferase
activity in the substantia nigra and the striatum after
surgical interruption of the strio-nigral fibres of the
baboon, Exp. Brain Res., 19: 217-227.

Kemp, J.M., and Powell, T.P.S., 1971, The site of termination of
afferents fibres in the caudate nucleus. Phil. Trans B,
262: 413-427.

Kim, J.S., Bak, I.J., Hassler, R. and Okada, Y., 1971, Role of
-aminobutyric acid (GABA) in the extrapyramidal motor
system. 2. Some evidence for the existence of a type of
GABA-rich strio-nigral neurons, Exp. Brain Res., 14: 95-104.

Kim, J.S., Hassler, R., Haug, P., and Paik, K.-S., 1977, Effect
of frontal cortex ablation on striatal glutamate acid
level in rat, Brain Res., 132: 370-374.

Lund Karlsen, R. and Fonnum, F., The toxic effect of sodium
glutamate on rat retina: changes in putative transmitters
and their corresponding enzymes, J.Neurochem., 27: 1437-1441.

Lund Karlsen, R., and Fonnum, F., 1978, Evidence for glutamate
as a neurotransmitter in the corticofugal fibres to the
dorsal lateral geniculate body and the superior colliculus
in rats, Brain Res., (in press).

McGeer, P.L., McGeer, E.G., Wada, J.A. and Jung, E., 1971, Effect
of globus pallidus lesions and Parkinson's disease on brain
glutamic acid decarboxylase, Brain Res., 32: 425-431.

McLennan, H., Huffman, R.D., and Marshall, K.C., 1968, Patterns
of excitation of thalamic neurones by amino acids and by
acetylcholine, Nature (Lond.), 219: 387-388.

Niimi, K., Ikeda, T., Kawamura, S. and Inoshita, H., 1970,
Efferent projections of the head of the caudate nucleus
in the cat, Brain Res., 21: 327-343.

Palkowits, M., Saavedra, J.M., and Brownstein, M., 1974, Serotonin content of the rat brain stem nuclei, 80: 237-249.

Shute, C.C.D., and Lewis, P.R., 1963, Cholinesterase containing systems of the brain of the rat, Nature 199: 1160-1164.

Spencer, H.J., 1976, Antagonisin of cortical exitation of striatal neurons by glutamic acid diethylester: evidence for glutamic acid as on excitatory transmitter in the rat striatum, Brain Res., 102: 91-102.

Tassin, J.P., Cheramy, A., Blanc, G., Thierry, A.M. and Glowinski, J., 1976, Topographical distribution of dopaminergic inner-vation and of dopaminergic receptors in the rat striatum. I. Microestimation of ($^3$H) dopamine uptake and dopamine content in microdiscs, Brain Res., 107: 291-301.

Tebécis, A.K., 1970, Effects of monoamines and amino acids on medial geniculate neurons of the cat, Neuropharmacol., 9: 381-390.

Versteeg, D.H.G., van der Gugten, J., de Jong, W., and Palkovits, M., 1976, Regional concentrations of noradrenaline and dopamine in rat brain, Brain Res., 113: 563-574.

Walaas, I., and Fonnum, F., 1978, Localization of neurotransmitters in nucleus accumbens, to be published.

Webster, K.E., Cortico-striate interrelations in the albino rat, J.Anat. (Lond.), 95 (1961) 532-544.

Yang, H.Y.T., Hong, J.S., Fratta, W., and Costa, E., 1977, Distri-bution of enkephalins in rat brain, 6th Int. meet. of the Int. Soc. for Neurochem., (Ed J. Clausen)., p 272.

Yamamura, H.J., and Snyder, S.H., 1974, Muscarinic cholinergic binding in rat brain, Proc. Nat. Acad. Sci., USA., 71: 1725-1729.

Young, A.B., Oster-Granite, M.L., Hermen, R.M., and Snyder, S.H., 1974, Glutamic acid: Selective depletion by viral induced granule cell loss in hamster cerebellum, Brain Res., 73: 1-13.

Yoshida, M., Rabin, A. and Anderson, M., Monosynaptic inhibition of pallidal neurons by axon collaterals of caudato-nigral fibres, Exp. Brain Res., 15: 333-347.

# LOCALIZATION OF TRANSMITTER AMINO ACIDS:  APPLICATION TO HIPPOCAMPUS AND SEPTUM

Jon Storm-Mathisen

Norwegian Defence Research Establishment

Division for Toxicology, N-2007 Kjeller, Norway

The hippocampal formation may be conceived of as a part of the cerebral cortex that is particularly suited for localization studies, owing to its laminar organization.  The main cell bodies, pyramidal and granular cells, are located in discrete layers parallel to the surface of the brain, and the different systems of nerve endings are distributed in bands parallel to these layers. Ten years ago we turned to this structure in order to obtain samples enriched in inhibitory, as opposed to excitatory nerve endings, because at that time Andersen and his associates had developed the concept that the pyramidal and granular cells are inhibited by axo-somatic synapses from basket cells (Andersen et al., 1964), excitatory nerve endings being localized on the dentrites (Andersen et al., 1966).

## γ-AMINOBUTYRIC ACID IN THE HIPPOCAMPAL FORMATION

### Microchemical Measurements of Glutamic Acid Decarboxylase

We adopted the methods developed several years earlier by Lowry (1953) of dissecting samples from freezed dried cryostate sections, and weighing them on a quartz fibre.  These were used for estimating the activity of glutamic acid decarboxylase (GAD), the enzyme synthetizing gamma aminobutyric acid (GABA), which already at that time was an important inhibitory transmitter candidate in brain (Storm-Mathisen and Fonnum, 1971; Storm-Mathisen, 1972). The result indeed showed a peak of activity corresponding to the cellular layers.  An unexpected finding was the high activity also in the outer parts of the molecular layers (see Storm-Mathisen, 1977a for illustration and detailed discussion).  This remains a

155

puzzle, because these layers are not known to contain inhibitory synapses. While the effects of GABA in the molecular layers remain to
be studied, a particular depolarizing action of GABA has been observed in stratum radiatum of CAl (Andersen et al., 1978), in addition
to its usual hyperpolarizing action (Andersen et al., 1978; Segal et
al., 1975). The possibility exists that during strong activation
of this mechanism the membrane resistance could be lowered sufficiently to inhibit the effect of excitatory synapses by shunting their
synaptic current (Andersen et al., 1978). Although stratum radiatum
is the layer with the lowest activity of GAD per unit tissue, it contains a substantial proportion (about 30%) of the total amount of GAD.

In homogenates of the hippocampal formation in isotonic sucrose 75 - 85% of the activity of GAD is particulate (Fonnum, 1972;
Nadler et al., 1974; Storm-Mathisen, 1975) and most of this is found
in "synaptosomes" floating between 1.0 and 1.2 M sucrose (Fonnum,
1973). Although this fraction may contain "gliosomes", such structures are likely to be much less abundant than synaptosomes in the
hippocampal formation, because in this region glial processes
account for a much smaller proportion of the tissue volume than
nerve endings (6% compared to 32%, Nafstad and Blackstad, 1966).
Further, since glial processes are very delicate, they would be
expected to end up in the lighter microsome fractions. Careful
morphological studies of the fractions could possibly shed light
on this problem.

The GAD activity was shown to be localized in structures in-
digenous to the hippocampal formation, since no more than very
small reductions in activity could be induced in any of the zones
by lesions of the various nerve terminal systems. In this investigation, the typical point-to-point organization of the projection systems was exploited, sampling the sites with maximum nerve
degeneration, as judged from adjacent Fink-Heimer preparations
(Storm-Mathisen, 1972). The largest reduction observed, up to
-15% after transaction of fimbria, may possibly be significant,
and the presence of a minor GAD containing pathway here cannot be
absolutely ruled out, but functional changes could well explain
such a small effect. Local lesions were made to destroy basket
cell axons and terminals, and expected reductions (-30% to -55%)
were obtained in GAD with no change in lactate dehydrogenase
(Storm-Mathisen, 1971, and unpublished). However, since the target
areas were very close to the lesions, and since lactate dehydrogenase, may not be an ideal marker to control for direct tissue
damage, these results should be interpreted with caution. (Choline
acetyltransferase, ChAT, and other neurotransmitter markers, are
not useful in so far as the axons containing them pass through the
site of the lesion). Fonnum and Walaas (1978) have recently found
that injection of kainic acid in the hippocampal formation,
destroying a large proportion of the intrahippocampal neurones,
was followed by a 64% loss of GAD with no significant change in

ChAT. This is rather strong evidence for the localization of GAD in intrinsic neurones.

Using an elegant micro-assay, the distribution of GABA has been found to be very similar to that of GAD in the guinea-pig hippocampal formation (Okada and Shimada, 1975). However, in view of more recent results (Tappaz, this volume) the level of GABA measured in the absence of the fast termination of enzyme activity at death, may reflect GAD activity rather than in vivo levels of GABA.

From the results above we may conclude with a fair amount of confidence that GAD is localized in intrinsic structures in the hippocampal formation, and that most of these are nerve endings, some of which belong to the inhibitory basket cells.

Immunohistochemical Visualization of Glutamic Acid
Decarboxylase

After the purification of GAD from brain (Wu et al., 1973), it has been possible to visualize GAD immunohistochemically in the hippocampus (Barber and Saito, 1976). The results confirmed those previously obtained by us, showing elevated concentrations near the cell bodies as well as among the peripheral dendrites. The light microscopic picture suggested that the enzyme was present in nerve endings and intervening axons, concentrated on or close to the cell bodies. Electronmicroscopy showed GAD to be present in nerve terminals, some forming synapses with symmetric thickenings on pyramidal and granular cell somata and dendritic shafts (Ribak et al., 1977). After injection of colchicine to dam up the enzyme in cell bodies, all layers were seen to contain GAD positive interneurones, many of which had the localization and appearance of basket cells (Ribak et al., 1977).

With the GAD immunohistochemical reaction the molecular layers appeared lighter than the cellular layers, in contrast to the situation with GAD measurements. This slight discrepancy could, at least in part, be due to the fact that the immunohistochemical staining reaction in essence is not a quantitative method. Alternatively some of the GAD activity could represent a possible non-neuronal enzyme, not detectable by the immunohistochemical method, which depends on enzyme purified from a nerve terminal preparation. Thus GAD has been demonstrated in non-neuronal tissues, and the enzyme purified from heart appears to differ immunologically from that purified from brain (Wu, 1977).

At this point the so-called "GAD II" is worth mentioning. This $CO_2$-forming activity was once thought to represent a non-neuronal GAD (Haber et al., 1970), but is actually an artifact due to impurities in the substrate $(1-^{14}C)$ glutamic acid (Miller and Martin, 1973). To avoid confusion, the term "GAD II" should be abandoned. This artifact is unlikely to have affected our results, however, since Triton X-100 was used in the assay (compare MacDonnell and Greengard, 1975) and since separate experiments with hippocampal homogenates showed that the production of $CO_2$ was equivalent to the production of GABA and that the activity in the presence of 1 mM amino-oxyacetic acid and 200 mM KCl was 1% of control (Storm-Mathisen and Fonnum, 1971).

## Uptake of γ-Aminobutyric Acid

Like GAD, the high affinity uptake of GABA, measured bio-chemically in the hippocampal formation,is not changed after transection of various afferent pathways (Storm-Mathisen, 1975; see below). To visualize the distribution, we have studied the uptake in hippocampal slices incubated with 1 µM of ($^3$H) GABA 36 000 Ci/mol (Taxt and Storm-Mathisen, in preparation). To avoid problems due to uneven penetration of the labelled substrate, which might obscure the laminar distribution, a whole-mount auto-radiographic technique was adopted (Storm-Mathisen, 1977). Due to the short range of β-particles from $^3$H (Rogers, 1974), this tech-nique displays radioactivity essentially in the superficial 2 µm of the slice. The radioactivity present in the slice prior to fixation was at least 95% GABA, as determined by chromatographic analysis after extraction in ethanol. Fixed and unfixed slices were burned in a Packard sample oxidiser, showing that about 70% of the radioactivity was retained after fixation.

The pictures were essentially identical to those obtained by GAD immunohistochemistry (Barber and Saito, 1976), with respect to neuropil staining. The autoradiographic grains occurred in clus-ters around the cell bodies. In the neuropil layers grains were seen in rows with a random course, probably representing axons, and in small clusters, probably representing nerve endings. Up-take in perikarya was not seen with this technique, probably be-cause these were destroyed by cutting so close to the slice sur-face. Hökfelt and Ljungdahl (1971) and Iversen and Schon (1973) have previously published pictures from restricted parts of the hippocampus showing a similar distribution. These authors used sections from the depth of plastic embedded slices and found labelled perikarya similar to the ones displayed by GAD immuno-histochemistry (Ribak et al., 1977). The uptake activity and pattern was not changed by including β-alanine in the incubation mixture at 1000 times (1 mM) the concentration of GABA. However, the uptake was strongly inhibited, to a similar extent in all layers, by 20 µM (-) nipecotic acid (Johnston et al., 1976) and by

100 μM L(+)-2,4-diaminobutyric acid (Iversen and Kelly, 1975; Lodge et al., 1976). ($^3$H)-L-2,4-diaminobutyric acid (1-2 μM 12 000 Ci/mol) gave a distribution similar to that of GABA, but weaker, whereas there was no significant uptake of ($^3$H)-β-alanine (2 μM, 37 500 Ci/mol). The pattern of uptake was not changed after lesions of the perforant path, the commissural fibres, or axons from CA3/4 pyramidal cells.

These results suggest that the high affinity uptake of GABA occurs into intrinsic neuronal structures, probably the same structures as those containing GAD.

### Release of γ-Aminobutyric Acid

Nadler et al (1977 a,b) have demonstrated that GABA is released in vitro by introduction of Ca$^{++}$ to slices of the hippocampal formation superfused with a depolarizing concentration of K$^+$. Exogenous GABA taken up during preincubation as well as endogenous GABA were released, but the relative proportions of these varied between the regions. The outer dendritic layers of area dentata released GABA as efficiently as the inner samples containing the axo-somatic inhibitory terminals. Lesions of entorhino-dentate or commissural fibres, or removal of granular cells by neonatal X-irradiation did not reduce the release or content of GABA, in agreement with the proposed origination from intrinsic neurones.

## GLUTAMIC ACID AND ASPARTIC ACID IN HIPPOCAMPUS

### High Affinity Uptake as a Marker and the Hippocampal Formation as a Model

The acidic amino acids glutamate (GLU) and aspartate (ASP) have long been important candidates as excitatory transmitters in brain, but localization to definite excitatory neurones is difficult to prove due to the key role of GLU and ASP in general metabolism. The use of high affinity uptake as a marker for neurones possibly releasing these amino acids has been discouraged by reports that GLU is taken up into glia (Hökfelt and Ljungdahl, 1972; Henn et al., 1974; Schon and Kelly, 1974). However, Young et al. (1974) found a 70% reduction in GLU and ASP uptake in cerebella of hamsters deprived of granular cells by neonatal virus infection. Of the endogenous amino acids only GLU was reduced (by 50%). This goes along with biochemical data indicating that GLU and ASP have very similar, or perhaps identical, membrane transport systems (Balcar and Johnston, 1972; Roberts and Watkins, 1975). The only difference reported is that the capacity of lithium to support transport, as a substitute for sodium, appears to be somewhat less poor for ASP than for GLU (Peterson and Ragupathy, 1974; Davies and Johnston,

1976). Thus nerve endings releasing GLU may have the same uptake
system as those releasing ASP. Evidence has been found that D-ASP
travels the same uptake system as L-ASP (Davies and Johnston, 1976).
This has technical advantages since D-ASP is very little metabolized.

The hippocampal formation would seem an ideal region for studying the possible localization of ASP and GLU in excitatory neurones, since this region contains several systems of defined excitatory nerve endings (Andersen et al., 1966; Lömo, 1971): The perforant pathways go from the medial and lateral parts of the entorhinal
area to the outer and the middle zones of the molecular layer of
area dentata, respectively, to excite the dentrites of the granular
cells (Hjorth-Simonsen, 1972; Matthews et al., 1976). The axons of
the granular cells are known as the mossy fibres which have characteristic giant boutons distributed in the hilus fasciae dentatae and
in the stratum lucidum (the mossy fiber layer) in hippocampus CA3,
where they form excitatory synapses with the proximal parts of the
apical dendrites of the pyramidal cells (Blackstad et al., 1970).
Pyramidal cells in CA3 and CA4 give rise to axons with a wide distribution, i.e. in the stratum oriens and radiatum of the hippocampal subfields and in the inner zone of the molecular layer of
area dentata (Gottlieb and Cowan, 1972; Hjorth-Simonsen, 1973;
Zimmer, 1971). Some axons cross over into the contralateral hippocampus and are distributed in the same zones (Blackstad, 1956;
Gottlieb and Cowan, 1973). There are, however, quantitative differences between the distributions on the two sides. It is not known
whether or not a single pyramidal cell can give rise to ramifications in all these locations. CA1 cells excited by CA3 pyramidal
cell axons in turn send their axons to part of the subiculum (Hjorth-
Simonsen, 1973; Swanson and Cowan, 1977). Due to the lamellar organization of the hippocampal formation (Andersen et al., 1971) a
lesion of one or more of the nerve ending systems at a point along
the dorsoventral axis of the hippocampal formation will give rise
to maximum degeneration at approximately the same level as the
lesion. This facilitas sampling by dissection from slices cut
transversely to the dorso-ventral axis of the hippocampal formation
(Storm-Mathisen, 1972, 1977a).

### Ipsilateral and Commissural Axons from Pyramidal
### Cells in CA3 and CA4

The laminar distribution of high affinity uptake of acidic
amino acids was studied in incubated slices using the whole mount
technique (Storm-Mathisen, 1977b), which displays only the surface of the section, directly exposed to the incubating solution
(see above). Various [3]H-labelled amino acids of specific activity
15 800 - 17 800 Ci/mol were used at 1 - 4 µM concentration, except
where stated otherwise (Taxt and Storm-Mathisen, in preparation).

Incubation was for 10 min at 20° in Krebs phosphate solution.
In control experiments with L-ASP and L-GLU 90% and 82 % of the
radioactivity present in the tissue prior to fixation was found to
represent the amino acid added to the incubation mixture. About
50% of the radioactivity was retained after fixation, whether
using L-GLU, L-ASP or D-ASP. The autoradiographic patterns obtained with these amino acids were very similar, as expected from
biochemical data referred to above. The uptake was strongly inhibited in all layers by 20 μM D,L-threo-β-hydroxyaspartic acid or
100 μM L-aspartic acid β-hydroxamate, powerful inhibitors of GLU
uptake in brain tissue (Balcar and Johnston, 1972; Roberts and
Watkins, 1975). Leucine (60 000 Ci/mol, 1 μM) and glycine (9400
Ci/mol, 5 - 12 μM) gave virtually negative autoradiograms.

The uptake activity of GLU, L-ASP and D-ASP was most intense
in stratum radiatum and stratum oriens of hippocampus and in the
inner zone of the molecular layer of area dentata, i.e. in the zones
receiving axon terminals of pyramidal cells in CA3 and CA4. After
interruption of these axons by a lesion in CA3 the uptake was
heavily reduced in the fields mentioned, but not in the outer parts
of the molecular layers of hippocampus and area dentata.

To provide quantitative data and assess the uptake in a different way, samples of stratum oriens and radiatum of CA1 (including
stratum pyramidale, which constitutes a very small proportion  of
the tissue volume) where dissected from fresh hippocampal slices in
the cold and homogenized in buffered sucrose solution to provide
suspensions of nerve ending particles. Samples containing 3 - 10
μg protein where incubated at 25°C for 3 min in 550 μl of Krebs
phosphate solution containing radioactively labelled amino acids at
1 μM concentration (Storm-Mathisen, 1977b; Divac et al., 1977).
This is still in the high affinity range; lower concentrations
should not be used to avoid interference of endogenous amino acids
leaking out from the tissue (Balcar and Johnston, 1975). Blanks
kept at 0°C were deduced. The uptake was linear with time and
the amount of tissue within the range used. The particles were
recovered by membrane filtration or centrifugation, rinsed, dissolved
with Triton X-100 and counted in a Packard liquid scintillation
spectrometer with an absolute activity analyser giving dpm of $^3$H
and $^{14}$C separately.

The uptake of L-GLU and D-ASP was reduced by 80 - 90% in
stratum oriens and radiatum of CA1 after lesions of the axons from
ipsilateral + contralateral pyramidal cells of CA3/4 (compaired to
unoperated and sham-operated controls). Most of this is due to
transection of ipsilateral axons. Interruption of only the contralateral axons resulted in only about 20% loss of D-ASP uptake in
oriens-radiatum of CA1 in the dorsal hippocampus. In a previous
report (Storm-Mathisen, 1977b) a loss of 50% of GLU-uptake in
samples adjacent to a parasagittal transection of the hippocampal

formation was inadvertently referred to as due to loss of contralateral affrents only.  Of necessity, such lesions will also destroy part of the ascending and descending ipsilateral axons, which
course longitudinally for several mm (Hjorth-Simonsen, 1973).
Double reciprocal plots of uptake at 1 - 10 μM D-ASP confirmed
that the reduced uptake activity represented a reduced number of
uptake sites, rather than an increase in the apparent $K_m$ (about
1.4 μM).  The loss of uptake activity was only partial at 3 days
but was complete after 4 to 6 days, and there was no subsequent
change up to 24 days.  There was no loss in GAD activity, or in the
mitochondrial enzyme carnitine acetyltransferase.  It is difficult
to ascribe the large and selective reduction in uptake of GLU and
ASP to secondary changes e.g. in glial cells.  Sections stained to
show cell bodies and the whitish appearence of the zones with degenerated nerve endings suggested the presence of glial hypertrophy,
rather than atrophy.  Fonnum and Walaas (1978) have found that after
partial destruction of intrahippocampal neurones by local injection
of kainic acid a large reduction (50%) occurred in the uptake of
L-GLU with no change in choline acetyltransferase.  (The use of the
contralateral side for control probably contributed to making this
reduction smaller than after the mechanical lesions).  In conclusion, the profound and selective lesion induced reductions in uptake of acid amino acids, suggest very strongly that this uptake
is localized in the terminals and axons of pyramidal cells in
CA3-4.

   To investigate whether the structures also contain elevated
concentrations of GLU or ASP, or both, operated and control animals were killed by microwave irradiation or by decapitation into
liquid nitrogen to avoid post mortem changes in amino acids.  Subsequently 40 μm thick sections were prepared in a cryostate, freeze
dried, dissected and weighed  on a Mettler electronic microbalance.
The amino  acids were extracted with acid acetone and determined by
a double labelling dansyl method.  GLU and ASP both showed about
40% loss in amount per dry weight.  The other amino acids showed
no significant changes (Fonnum and Storm-Mathisen, in preparation).


                        Entorhino-Dentate Axons

   Although the zones containing pyramidal  cell axon terminals
are the highest in GLU and ASP uptake, there is also some uptake
in the other zones, i.e. the molecular layer of hippocampus, and
the outer parts of the molecular layer of fascia dentata.  The
latter contain terminals of the perforant path from area entorhi-
nalis, and had about 1/3 of the GLU uptake activity found in oriens
and radiatum of CA1, when tested in homogenates of dissected
samples.  When both the medial and lateral parts of the perforant
path were transected, inducing degeneration of terminals in both
outer zones of the dentate molecular layer, there was a 40% re-

duction in GLU uptake in these zones based on protein content
(Storm-Mathisen, 1977b). There was no reduction in uptake in the
inner zone of the dentate molecular layer, nor in oriens and radiatum of CA1. While GAD was unchanged in CA1, it was somewhat increased in the perforant path zones. This increase is accounted
for by the reduction in tissue volume occurring here after this
type of lesion (Storm-Mathisen, 1974), which removes a very large
proportion of the synapses (Matthews et al., 1976). Since GAD is
probably localized in intrinsic neurones, it is reasonable to take
the GAD activity as an index of the tissue elements not participa-
ting in the lesion-induced degeneration, and to express the results on the basis on GAD rather than protein. When expressed in
this way GLU uptake was reduced by 52% after perforant path degeneration.

### Electron-Microscopic Autoradiography of Glutamic Acid Uptake, Granular Cell Axons

In collaboration with Leslie Iversen's laboratory in Cambridge
the uptake of $(^3H)$-L-GLU was studied by light- and electron-microscopic autoradiography of incubated slices fixed in glutaraldehyde
and osmiumtetroxide, and embedded in plastic  (Iversen and Storm-
Mathisen, 1976; Storm-Mathisen and Iversen, 1978). The light microscopy showed essentially the same result as that obtained with
whole mounted slices. Electron micrographs were taken systematically to cover the neuropil in stripes of tissue running radially
through the layers of area dentata from fissura hippocampi to hilus
fasciae dentatae. The gross distribution of autoradiographic
grains confirmed that visualized with the light microscope.
Thus the gain densities in the outer and middle zones of the molecular layer were roughly 35% and 60%, respectively, of the grain
density in the inner zone. This had the same grain density as the
hilus. The morphological details were relatively well preserved,
but dendrites were swollen and there was an increased amount of
extracellular space. On the other hand, nerve endings appeared to
be somewhat shrunken. The distribution of grains between tissue
components was similar in the different zones. Nerve endings plus
axons contained nearly 50% of the grains in hilus and in the inner
zone of the molecular layer and somewhat less in the outer and
middle zones, wereas the volume fraction occupied by these structures was about 20%. The relative grain density for nerve endings
plus axons was nearly 3 for the inner zone of the molecular layer
and 2 for the outer two zones, and for the hilus (average grain
density for all tissue components = 1). The values for nerve
endings alone where somewhat higher. Non-axonal structures (dendrites, glia and space) had average grain densities of about 0.5.
The labelling intensity in nerve endings was about 6 times higher
than that in non-axonal structures in the inner part of the molecular layer, and about 3 times higher in the outer two parts of the
molecular layer. In the hilus the value was 6 for small nerve

endings and 5 for mossy fibre terminals (see below).

The labelling of glial elements was only slightly above the
average for all tissue components. However, structures such as
glial lamellae and axons, which are small relative to the half radius, i.e. radius of a circle about a source of disintegration
having 50% probability of containing the resulting autoradiographic
grain (about 0.23 μm in the present material), lose a large proportion of their grains to neighbouring structures (Rogers, 1973).
On the other hand, all structures pick up grains by "cross-firing"
from neighbouring structures. In order to obtain an estimate of
the grain density belonging to small structures, such as glial
lamellae and thin axons, it is therefore necessary to apply statistical analysis, i.e. the hypothetical grain analysis of Blackett
and Parry (1973). Such studies are under way. However, since the
glial lamellae constitute such a small proportion of the tissue
volume in the present material, they would have to have a very high
labelling intensity in order to account for a substantial proportion
of the grains. This does not seem likely from the present data.

The stratum lucidum of CA3 and the hilus fasciae dentatae, which
contain the mossy fibres from the granular cells, were mostly weakly
labelled in whole-mount autoradiograms. However, in light microscope autoradiograms from the depts of plastic embedded slices these
layers contain numerous large clusters of silver grains. These structures, which were not seen in other layers, were suggestive of the
giant mossy fibre nerve endings. Electron microscopy confirmed the
labelling of mossy fibre endings, which are easily identified by
their large size, and characteristic structure, i.e. packed with synaptic vesicles and invaginated by dentritic spinae forming synaptic contacts with asymmetric postsynaptic thickenings (Blackstad
and Kjaerheim, 1961). When labelled, the mossy fibre terminals contained several silver grains, in contrast to the smaller nerve
terminals in the present material. The average labelling intensity
was somewhat less than that of small nerve terminals in hilus and
in the inner molecular layer of fascia dentata, but higher than that
of terminals in the outer layers (see above). Since only some
terminals were labelled, these would contain a higher radioactive
concentration than suggested by the numbers. The actual proportion
of labelled versus unlabelled mossy fibre terminals is hard to know
without making serial sections and/or analyses similar to those
suggested by Kelly (this volume). However, it seems clear that some
terminals had a much higher labelling intensity than others. Some
of the mossy fibre terminals looked damaged, with dark cytoplasm
and irregular outline. Furthermore, they were clearly less frequently labelled in surface autoradiograms of whole mounts than in
autoradiograms from sections through the depth of incubated slices.
This would suggest that the giant mossy fibre terminals could be
more susceptible to damage during the preparation procedure than
the smaller nerve endings. On the other hand, the possibility that

the uptake mechanism for acid amino acids is restricted to a certain population of mossy fibre endings has to be kept open.

The results presented above show that the uptake mechanisms for
GLU and ASP are localized in the axon terminals of 3 known excitatory projections in the hippocampal formation, namely the perforant path, the mossy fibres and the CA3/4 pyramidal cell axons.
The latter also seem to contain high concentrations of endogenous
GLU and ASP (presumably in different populations of neurones).
These results fit very nicely with release experiments on slices
of hippocampus and area dentata (Nadler et al., 1976; Cotman, this
volume. There is some electrophysiological evidence that GLU and ASP
could act as excitatory transmitters in the hippocampal formation
(Schwartzkroin and Andersen, 1975; Spencer et al., 1976; Segal, 1976).

AMINO ACIDS IN SEPTUM AND MAMMILLARY BODY

Efferent connections are known to pass from the hippocampal
formation to inter alia the lateral septum and the mammillary
nuclei (Olpe and McEwen, 1976; Swanson and Cowan, 1977; Meibach and
Siegel, 1977). The source of these projections appears to be
pyramidal cells partly in subiculum, partly in CA1 and CA3. The
projections to the septum is excitatory (DeFrance et al., 1973;
McLennan and Miller, 1974), probably also that to the mammillary
body (MacLean, 1975). The fibres pass through fimbria/fornix and
fornix superior. These fibre tracts were transected bilaterally,
since the projections are partially crossed, and after 9 days
survival the animals were killed and samples of the mammillary
body, and the medial and lateral regions of the septum were prepared from both sides. The septum was dissected from 350 μm
frontal slices according to Koenig and Kippel (1962). The
mammillary bodies were scooped out macroscopically. Animals in
which the skull was opened, but no lesion made, were used as sham
operated controls. The operation reduced the uptake of ($^3$H)-D-ASP
by 2/3 in the lateral septum and by 1/2 in the mammillary body.
The latter figure is probably an underestimate, due to the coarse
dissection of the mammillary body. There was no change in the
medial septum. Uptake of ($^{14}$C) GABA, measured in the same samples
by double labelling, and GAD were not changed. Choline acetyltransferase was hardly changed in medial septum or in the mammillary
body. A 50% increase in the lateral septum could be due to an increased amount of enzyme transported to collaterals of the inter-
rupted septo-hippocampal fibres (Harkmark et al., 1975), or perhaps
to sprouting.

The D-ASP uptake activity in these regions in control animals
was compared to that in oriens and radiatum of CA1. It varied by
almost an order of magnitude between the lowest (medial septum) and
the highest (CA1), and may be indicative of the density of axon
terminals possessing uptake capacity for acidic amino acids. It is
interesting to note that the activities remaining in CA1, lateral

septum and mammillary body after appropriate lesions (see above) are all very similar to the normal activity in the medial septum. GABA uptake and GAD had very similar distributions which differed widely from the distribution of D-ASP uptake. Thus septum was highest and CA1 about 1/3. The similarity of these GABA markers in the medial and lateral parts of the septum and the lack of change after interruption of hippocampo-septal fibres are in agreement with previous findings (Storm-Mathisen, 1972), and consistent with the electrophysiological results of McLennan and Miller (1974) which suggest that inhibitory GABAergic interneurones are operative in both parts of the septum. Choline acetyltransferase showed still a different distribution and was highest in the medial septum, the site of the alleged cholinergic septo-hippocampal neurones. In double labelling experiments the uptake ratio $(^3H)$-D-ASP/$(^{14}C)$-L-GLU was virtually constant $(1.45\pm0.03$, SD, n=22, r=0.997) between CA 1, septum and mammillary body with and without unilateral transection of the hippocampo-septal connection, corroborating the notion that the two uptake activities occur in the same structures.

In conclusion, efferents from the hippocampal formation to the lateral septum and the mammillary body seem to contain uptake activity for acidic amino acids, and could therefore use ASP or GLU as their transmitter.

REFERENCES

Andersen, P., Eccles, J.C. and Löyning, Y., 1964, Location of postsynaptic inhibitory synapses on hippocampal pyramids, J. Neurophysiol., 27:592-607.

Andersen, P., Blackstad, T.W. and Lömo, T., 1966, Location and identification of excitatory synapses on hippocampal pyramidal cells, Exp. Brain Res., 1:236-248.

Andersen, P., Bliss, T.V.P. and Skrede, K.K., 1971, Lamellar organization of hippocampal excitatory pathways, Exp. Brain Res., 13:222-238.

Andersen, P., Bie, B., Ganes, T. and Mosfeldt Laursen, A., 1978, Two mechanisms for effects of GABA on hippocampal pyramidal cells. In: Iontophoresis and Transmitter Mechanisms of the Mammalian Central Nervous System. Eds. R.W. Ryall and J.S. Kelly. North-Holland, Amsterdam, in press.

Balcar, V.J. and Johnston, G.A.R., 1972, The structural specificity of the high affinity uptake of L-glutamate and L-aspartate by rat brain slices, J. Neurochem., 19:2657-2666.

Balcar, V.J. and Johnston, G.A.R., 1975, Liberation of amino acids during the preparation of brain slices, Brain Res., 83:173-175.

Barber, R. and Saito, K., 1976, Light microscopic visualization of GAD and GABA-T in immunocytochemical preparations of rodent CNS. In: GABA in Nervous System Function. Kroc Foundation Series, Vol 5, pp. 113-132. Eds. E. Roberts, T.W. Chase and D.B. Tower. Raven Press, New York.

Blackett, N.M. and Parry, D.M., 1973, A new method for analysing electronmicroscope autoradiographs using hypothetical grain distributions, J. Cell Biol., 57:9-15.

Blackstad, T.W., 1956, Commissural connections of the hippocampal region in the rat, with special reference to their mode of termination, J. comp. Neurol., 205:417-537.

Blackstad, T.W. and Kjærheim, Å., 1961, Special axodendritic synapses in the hippocampal cortex: Electron and light microscopic studies on the layer of mossy fibres, J. comp. Neurol., 117:133-160.

Blackstad, T.W., Brink, K., Hem, J. and Jeune, B., 1970, Distribution of hippocampal mossy fibers in the rat. An experimental study with silver impregnation methods, J. comp. Neurol., 138:433-450.

Davies, L.P. and Johnston, G.A.R., 1976, Uptake and release of D- and L-aspartate by rat brain slices, J. Neurochem., 26:1007-1014.

DeFrance, J.F., Kitai, S.T. and Shimono, T., 1973, Electrophysiological analysis of the hippocampo-septal projections: II. Functional characteristics, Exp. Brain Res., 17:463-478.

Divac, I., Fonnum, F. and Storm-Mathisen, J., 1977, High affinity uptake of glutamate in terminals of corticostriatal axons, Nature, 266:377-378.

Fonnum, F., 1972, Application of microchemical analysis and subcellular fractionation techniques to the study of neurotransmitters in discrete areas of mammalian brain. In: Studies of Neurotransmitters at the synaptic level, Advan. biochem. Psychopharmac., Vol 6, pp. 75-88. Eds. E. Costa, L.L. Iversen and R. Paoletti, Raven Press, New York.

Fonnum, F., 1973, Localization of cholinergic and γ-aminobutyric acid containing pathways in brain. In: Metabolic Compartmentation in the Brain, pp. 245-257. Eds. R Balázs and J.E. Cremer. Macmillan: London.

Fonnum, F. and Walaas, I., 1978, The effect of intrahippocampal injection of kainic acid on neurotransmitter candidates in hippocampus and septum, to be published.

Gottlieb, D.I. and Cowan, W.M., 1972, Evidence for a temporal factor in the occupation of available synaptic sites during the development of the dentate gyrus, Brain Res., 41:452-456.

Gottlieb, D.I. and Cowan, W.M., 1973, Autoradiographic studies of the commissural and ipsilateral association connections of the hippocampus and dentate gyrus of the rat. I. The commissural connections, J. comp. Neurol., 149:393-422.

Haber, B., Kuriyama, K. and Roberts, E., 1970, An anion stimulated L-glutamic acid decarboxylase in non-neural tissues: Occurrence and subcellular localization in mouse kidney and developing chick embryo brain, Biochem. Pharmac., 19:1119-1136.

Harkmark, W., Mellgren, S.I. and Srebro, B., 1975, Acetylcholinesterase histochemistry of the septal region in rat and human: distribution of enzyme activity, Brain Res., 95:281-289.

Henn, F.A., Goldstein, M.N. and Hamberger, A., 1974, Uptake of the neurotransmitter candidate glutamate by glia, Nature, London, 249:663-664.

Hjorth-Simonsen, A., 1972, Projection of the lateral part of the entorhinal area to the hippocampus and fascia dentata, J. comp. Neurol., 146:219-231.

Hjorth-Simonsen, A., 1973, Some intrinsic connections of the hippocampus in the rat: an experimental analysis, J. comp. Neurol., 147:145-162.

Hökfelt, T. and Ljungdahl, Å., 1971, Uptake of ($^3$H) noradrenaline and γ-($^3$H) aminobutyric acid in isolated tissues of rat: an autoradiographic and fluorescence microscopic study. In: Histochemistry of Nervous Transmission, Prog. Brain Res., Vol. 34, pp. 87-102. Ed. E.O. Eränkö. Elsevier, Amsterdam.

Hökfelt, T. and Ljungdahl, Å., 1972, Application of cytochemical techniques to the study of suspected transmitter substances in the nervous system. In: Studies of Neurotransmitters at the Synaptic Level, Advan. Biochem. Psychopharmac., Vol. 6, pp. 1-36. Eds. E. Costa, L.L. Iversen and R. Paoletti. Raven Press, New York.

Iversen, L.L. and Kelly, J.S., 1975, Uptake and metabolism of γ-aminobutyric acid by neurones and glial cells, Biochem. Pharmac., 24:933-938.

Iversen, L.L. and Schon, F.F., 1973, The use of autoradiographic techniques for the identification and mapping of transmitter specific neurones in CNS. In: New Concepts in Neurotransmitter Regulation, pp. 153-193. Ed. A.J. Mandell, Plenum Press, New York.

Iversen, L.L. and Storm-Mathisen, J., 1976, Uptake of ($^3$H) glutamic acid in excitatory nerve endings in the hippocampal formation of the rat, Acta physiol. scand., 96:22A-23A.

Johnston, G.A.R., Krogsgaard-Larsen, P., Stephanson, A.L. and Twitchin, B., 1976, Inhibition of the uptake of GABA and related amino acids in rat brain slices by the optical isomers of nipecotic acid, J. Neurochem., 26:1029-1032.

König, J.F.R. and Klippel, R.A., 1963, The Rat Brain. A Stereotaxic Atlas of the Forebrain and Lower Parts of the Brain Stem, 162 pp., Williams & Wilkins, Baltimore.

Krnjević, K., 1974, Chemical nature of synaptic transmission in vertebrates, Physiol. Rev., 54:418-540.

Krnjević, K. and Schwartz, S., 1967, The action of γ-aminobutyric acid on cortical neurons, Exp. Brain Res., 3:320-326.

Lodge, D., Johnston, G.A.R. and Stephanson, A.L., 1976, The uptake of GABA and β-alanine in slices of cat and rat CNS tissue: regional differences in susceptibility to inhibitors, J. Neurochem., 27:1569-1570.

Lowry, O.H., 1953, The quantitative histochemistry of the brain, J. Histochem. Cytochem., 1:420-428.

Lömo, T., 1971, Patterns of activation in a monosynaptic cortical pathway: the perforant path input to the dentate area of the hippocampal formation, Exp. Brain Res., 12:18-45.

MacDonnell, P. and Greengard, O., 1975, The distribution of glutamate decarboxylase in rat tissues, isotopic vs fluorimetric assays, J. Neurochem., 24:615-618.

MacLean, P.D., 1975, An ongoing analysis of hippocampal inputs and outputs: microelectrode and neuroanatomical findings in squirrel monkey's. In: Isaacson, R.L. and Pribram, K.H., (eds), The Hippocampus, Vol 1, pp. 177-211, Plenum, New York and London.

Matthews, D.A., Cotman, C. and Lynch, G., 1976, An electron microscopic study of lesion-induced synaptogenesis in the dentate gyrus of the adult rat. I. Magnitude and time course of degeneration, Brain Res., 115:1-21.

McLennan, H. and Miller, J.J., 1974, γ-Aminobutyric acid and inhibition in the septal nuclei of the rat, J. Physiol. (London), 237:625-633.

Meibach, R.C. and Siegel, A., 1977, Efferent connections of the hippocampal formation in the rat, Brain Res., 124:197-224.

Miller, L.P. and Martin, D.L., 1973, An artifact in the radiochemical assay of brain mitochondrial glutamate decarboxylase, Life Sci., 13:1023-1032.

Nadler, J.V., Cotman, C.W. and Lynch, G.S., 1974 Subcellular distribution of transmitter-related enzyme activities in discrete areas of the rat dentate gyrus, Brain Res., 79:465-477.

Nadler, J.V., Vaca, K.W., White, W.F., Lynch, G.S. and Cotman, C.W., 1976, Aspartate and glutamate as possible transmitters of excitatory hippocampal afferents, Nature, 260:538-540.

Nadler, J.V., White, W.F., Vaca, K.W. and Cotman, C.W., 1977, Calcium-dependent γ-aminobutyric acid release by interneurons of rat hippocampal regions: lesion-induced plasticity, Brain Res., 131:241-258.

Nadler, J.V., White, W.F., Vaca, K.W., Redburn, D.A. and Cotman, C.W., 1977, Characterization of putative amino acid transmitter release from slices of rat dentate gyrus, J. Neurochem., 29:279-290.

Nafstad, P.H.J. and Blackstad, T.W., 1966, Distribution of mitochondria in pyramidal cells and boutons in hippocampal cortex, Z. Zellforsch. mikrosk. Anat., 73:234-245.

Okada, Y. and Shimada, C., 1975, Distribution of γ-aminobutyric acid (GABA) and glutamate decarboxylase (GAD) activity in the guinea-pig hippocampus - microassay method for the determination of GAD activity, Brain Res., 98:202-206.

Olpe, H.-R. and McEwens, B.S., 1976, Axonal transport in the efferent pathways of the hippocampus: labelling of projection areas after ($^3$H) valine injections, Brain Res., 105:483-495.

Parry, D.M., and Blackett, N.M., 1976, Analysis of electron microscope autoradiographs using the hypothetical gain analysis method, J. Microsc., 106: 117-124.

Peterson, N.A. and Raghupathy, E., 1974, Selective effects of lithium on symaptosomal amino acid transport systems, Biochem. Pharmac., 23:2491-2494.

Ribak, C.E., Vaughn, J.E. and Saito, K., 1977, Immunocytochemical localization of glutamic acid decarboxylase in neuronal somata following colchicine inhibition of axonal transport, Brain Res., in press.

Roberts, P.J. and Watkins, J.C., 1975, Structural requirements for the inhibition for L-glutamate uptake by glia and nerve endings, Brain Res., 85:120-125.

Rogers, A.W., 1973, Techniques of Autoradiography, 372 pp., Elsevier, Amsterdam.

Schon, F. and Kelly, J.S., 1974, Autoradiographic localization of ($^3$H) GABA and ($^3$H) glutamate over satellite glial cells, Brain Res., 66:275-288.

Schwartzkroin, P.A. and Andersen, P., 1975, Glutamic acid sensitivity of dendrites in hippocampal slices in vitro. In: Properties of Dendrites, Advan. Neurol., Vol. 12, pp. 45-51. Ed. G. Kreutzberg, Raven Press, New York.

Schwartzkroin, P.A., Skrede, K.K., Storm, J. and Andersen, P., 1974, Glutamic acid excitation of pyramidal cell dendrites in hippocampal slices, Proc. Intern. Union of Physiological Sciences. 26th International Congress, New Delhi, Vol. 11, p. 391.

Segal, M., 1976, Glutamate antagonists in rat hippocampus., Br. J. Pharmac., 58:341-345.

Segal, M., Sims, K. and Smissman, E., 1975, Characterization of an inhibitory receptor in rat hippocampus: A microiontophoretic study using conformationally restricted amino acid analogues, Br. J. Pharmac., 54:181-188.

Spencer, H.J., Gribkoff, V.K., Cotman, C.W. and Lynch, G.S., 1976, GDEE antagonism of iontophoretic amino acid excitations in the intact hippocampus and in the hippocampal slice preparation, Brain Res., 105:471-481.

Storm-Mathisen, J., 1971, GABA produced in local inhibitory neurones of the hippocampus. In: Third International Meeting of the International Society for Neurochemistry, p. 401. Eds. J. Domonkos, A. Fonyó, I. Huszák and J. Szentágothia. Akadémia Kiadó, Budapest.

Storm-Mathisen, J., 1972, Glutamate decarboxylase in the rat hippocampal region after lesions of the afferent fibre sys-

tems.  Evidence that the enzyme is localized in intrinsic
    neurones, Brain Res., 40:215-235.
Storm-Mathisen, J., 1974, Choline acetyltransferase and acetylcho-
    linesterase in fascia dentata following lesion of the entor-
    hinal afferents., Brain Res., 80:181-197.
Storm-Mathisen, J., 1977a, Localization of transmitter candidates
    in the brain:  The hippocampal formation as a model, Progr.
    Neurobiol., 8:119-181.
Storm-Mathisen, J., 1977b, Glutamic acid and excitatory nerve en-
    dings: reduction of glutamic acid uptake after axotomy,
    Brain Res., 120:379-386.
Storm-Mathisen, J. and Fonnum, F., 1971, Quantitative histochemis-
    try of glutamate decarboxylase in the rat hippocampal region,
    J. Neurochem., 18:1105-1111.
Storm-Mathisen, J. and Iversen, L.L., 1978, Glutamic acid and exci-
    tatory nerve endings: selective uptake of ($^3$H) glutamic acid
    revealed by light- and electronmicroscopic autoradiography,
    to be published.
Swanson, L.W. and Cowan, W.M., 1977, An autoradiographic study of
    the organization of the efferent connections of the hippo-
    campal formation in the rat, J. comp. Neurol., 172:49-84.
Wu, J.-Y., 1977, A comparative study of L-glutamate decarboxylase
    from mouse brain and bovine heart with purified preparations,
    J. Neurochem., 28:1359-1367.
Wu, J.-Y., Matsuda, T. and Roberts, E., 1973, Purification and
    characterization of glutamate decarboxylase from mouse brain,
    J. biol. Chem., 248:3029-3034.
Young, A.B., Oster-Granite, M.L., Herndon, R.M. and Snyder, S.H.,
    1974, Glutamic acid:  Selective depletion by viral induced
    granule cell loss in hamster cerebellum, Brain Res., 73:1-13.
Zimmer, J., 1971, Ipsilateral afferents to the commissural zone of
    the fascia dentata, demonstration in decommissurated rats by
    silver impregnation, J. comp. Neurol., 142:393-416.

# GLUTAMATE CONCENTRATION IN INDIVIDUAL LAYERS OF THE RABBIT HIPPOCAMPUS

Cordula Nitsch[+] and Yasuhiro Okada

Dept. Neurochemistry, Tokyo Metropolitan Institute
for Neurosciences
2-6 Musashidai, Fuchu-shi, Tokyo, Japan

The possible role of L-glutamic acid (GLU) as a neurotransmitter
of the entorhinal pathway (Nadler et al. 1976, Storm-Mathisen 1977),
and of the commissural fibers (Storm-Mathisen 1977), and of the
mossy fibers (Crawford and Connor 1973) is widely discussed. The
regional distribution of a transmitter candidate can enlighten the
role of the substance in question, as for example demonstrated in
the case of GABA (Okada et al. 1971, Okada and Shimada 1975).
Therefore we developed a highly sensitive GLU assay method which
enabled us to measure the GLU content of individual layers of the
three subfields of the hippocampus: regio superior, regio inferior
and dentate gyrus.

The principle of the assay method is a combination of the GLU
assay via production of NADH and the subsequent amplification with
the NADH present using the NAD-cycling procedure described by
Kato et al. 1973. The product of the cycling, malate, is determined fluorometrically after formation of NADH with malate dehydrogenase.

Six adult female rabbits were decapitated. The brains were removed, the hippocampus dissected out and cut perpendicularly to the
longitudinal axis in about 5 mm thick slices which were frozen in
Freon 12 in liquid nitrogen. In a cryotome, 20 µm thick sections
were cut at $-20^\circ$ C, freeze-dried at $-35^\circ$ C under vaccuum, and stored at $-35^\circ$ C. The individual layers of the hippocampus were dissected out under the microscope, using a fine knife. The weight of
the samples was estimated with a quartz fiber balance, weighing in
the range of 0.1 to 0.4 µg. GLU content of the samples was deter-

[+]Present address: Dept. Neurobiology, Max-Planck-Institute for
Brain Research, D-6000 Frankfurt/M.-71, G.F.R.

mined using the oil well technic (Lowry and Passonneau 1972). Details of the procedure will be published elsewhere.

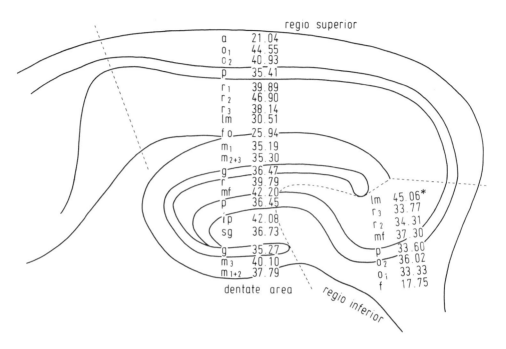

FIGURE 1. Schematic presentation of the GLU distribution in the layers of the rabbit hippocampus. Values are given in mmoles/kg dry weight. For each layer 8 to 11 samples were assayed, the standard deviation never exceeds 10 %.
Nomenclature: a alveus, o stratum oriens, p stratum pyramidale, r stratum radiatum, lm stratum lacunosum moleculare, fo fissura obliterata, m stratum moleculare, g stratum granulare, mf mossy fiber layer, ip infrapyramidal layer, sg subgranular layer, f fimbria. The indices at certain letters indicate the subdivision of the single stratum.
*Only n=3, S.E.M. ± 5.76.

The regional values of the GLU content in the hippocampal regio superior, regio inferior and the dentate area are given in Fig.1.
As already demonstrated for regional areas of the brain (Johnson and Aprison 1971), also in the hippocampus the variation in the GLU concentration is not as large as with other neurotransmitters. This is probably due to the role of GLU as a major metabolite (Balazs et al. 1973). On the basis of the present data alone, it is not possible to determine definitely in which pathway GLU is the specific transmitter. But considering the electrophysio-

logical, neurochemical and morphological data available, as well
as the present finding of a uniform GLU level in the stratum pyramidale and the stratum granulare, one could speculate that those
concentrations higher than in the layers of pure neuronal perikarya are an indication for the possible functional role of GLU
in this area.

The overall highest GLU content is found in the middle of the
stratum radiatum of the regio superior, where a dense termination
of commissural fibers takes place (Raisman et al. 1965). The other
projection fields of the commissural fibers also exhibit a high
GLU level, namely the stratum oriens of CA1, the inner third of
the dentate molecular layer, and the hilus fascia dentata in close
vicinity of the pyramidal cells. Thus, the good correspondence
between the termination of the commissural fibers and the GLU distribution is  strongly supporting the view that this amino acid
could be their transmitter.

In the projection areas of the entorhinal perforant path fibers
we also find some parallels with the regional GLU amount: in the
stratum lacunosum moleculare of the regio inferior which contains
the second highest GLU concentration, and in the dentate gyrus
molecular layer (Hjorth-Simonsen and Jeune 1972). The differences
we found between the inner and the outer blade of the stratum
moleculare remains to be explained on a morphological basis.

It was suggested that the mossy fiber terminals contain GLU as
synaptic transmitter (Crawford and Connor 1973, Storm-Mathisen
1977). The present data neither support nor overrule this concept.
Nevertheless, if GLU should be the transmitter, its comparatively
low concentration in the stratum lucidum of the regio inferior -
the higher GLU content in the corresponding layer of the hilus
dentata could be due to intermingled commissural nerve terminals -
in an area with such densely packed giant boutons (Nitsch and Bak
1974) remains surprising.

## REFERENCES

Balázs, R., Patel, A.J., and Richter, D., 1973, Metabolic compart-
    ments in the brain: their properties and relation to morpho-
    logical structures, in "Metabolic Compartmentation in the
    Brain", (R. Balázs and J.E. Cremer, eds.), pp. 167-184,
    MacMillan Press, London.
Crawford, I.L., and Connor, J.D., 1973, Localization and release
    of glutamic acid in relation to hippocampal mossy fiber path-
    way. Nature (Lond.) 244:442-443.
Hjorth-Simonsen, A., and Jeune, B., 1972, Origin and termination
    of the hippocampal perforant path in the rat studied by silver
    impregnation. J.comp.Neurol. 144:215-231.
Johnson, J.L., and Aprison, M.H., 1971, The distribution of gluta-
    mate and total free amino acids in thirteen specific regions
    of the cat central nervous system. Brain Res. 26:141-148.

Kato, T., Berger, S.J., Carter, J.A., and Lowry, O.H., 1973, An
    enzymatic cycling method for nicotinamide-adenine dinucleotide
    with malic and alcohol dehydrogenases. Anal. Biochem. 53:86-97.
Lowry, O.H., and Passonneau, J.V., 1972, in "A Flexible System of
    Enzymatic Analysis", Academic Press, New York.
Nadler, J.V., Vaca, K.W., White, W.F., Lynch, G.S., and Cotman, C.
    W., 1976, Aspartate and glutamate as possible transmitters of
    excitatory hippocampal afferents. Nature (Lond.) 260:538-540.
Nitsch, C., and Bak, I.J., 1974, Die Moosfaserendigungen des Ammons-
    horns, dargestellt in der Gefrierätztechnik. Verh.Anat.Ges.
    68:319-323.
Okada, Y., Nitsch-Hassler, C., Kim, J.S., Bak, I.J., and Hassler,R.
    1971, Role of $\gamma$-aminobutyric acid (GABA) in the extrapyrami-
    dal motor system.  1. Regional distribution of GABA in rabbit,
    rat, guinea pig and baboon CNS. Exp. Brain Res. 13:514-518.
Okada, Y., and Shimada, C., 1975, Distribution of $\gamma$-aminobutyric
    acid (GABA) and glutamate decarboxylase (GAD) activity in
    the guinea pig hippocampus - microassay method for the deter-
    mination of GAD activity. Brain Res. 98:202-206.
Raisman, G., Cowan, W.M., and Powell, T.P.S., 1965, The extrinsic
    afferent commissural and association fibres of the hippocampus.
    Brain 88:963-996.
Storm-Mathisen, J., 1977, Glutamic acid and excitatory nerve endings
    reduction of glutamic acid uptake after axotomy. Brain Res.,
    120:379-386.

# THE EFFECT OF INTRAHIPPOCAMPAL ADMINISTRATION OF γ-AMINOBUTYRIC ACID (GABA)

Antoni Smialowski

Department of Neuropharmacology Institute of
Pharmacology
Polish Academy of Sciences, Kraków, Poland

Detailed studies have revealed that GABA is present in the intrahippocampal system of basket cells (Storm-Mathisen & Fonnum, 1971). The synaptic endings of these cells are located directly on the cell bodies of the hippocampal pyramidal cells, and thus they play a significant role in regulation of nervous impulses generated in these cells. Microelectrode studies of Segal et al. (1975) have shown a strong inhibitory action of iontophoretic injections of GABA given into hippocampus. This effect was similar for several hippocampal fields tested and, the current necessary to produce inhibition was much lower in the case of GABA than that needed for producing an effect on another hippocampal inhibitory neurotransmitter - noradrenaline (Segal, Bloom, 1974). For GABA a current of 50 nA produced a total, reversible blockade of the activity of hippocampal pyramidal neuron. Other studies of these authors have revealed that GABA was the most potent inhibitory substance among aminoacids tested (β-alanine, glycine), when comparing the electric current necessary to produce half-maximal inhibition.

Previous studies on the role of GABA on the activity of central nervous system or hippocampus have been limited to anesthetized animals. Such an experiment renders impossible determination of the action of GABA under conditions of the normal activity of the animal. Our experiments were thus carried out on non-anesthetized White Danish rabbits (3 - 4 kg) with chronically implanted silver bipolar electrodes, placed in the head of caudate nucleus, basolateral amygdaloid area, dorsal hippocampus and anterior cingular cortex, and with stainless steel cannulas implanted into dorsal hippocampus. The rabits were allowed to recover for at least two weeks following the surgery.

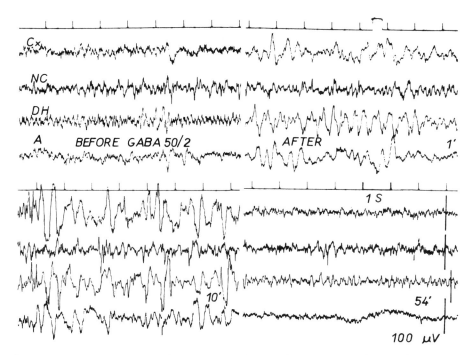

Figure 1.  EEG changes induced by intrahippocampal injection of
           50 µg of GABA.  Abbreviations used:  A-amygdaloid
           complex, Cx - cingular cortex, DH - dorsal hippocampus,
           NC - head of caudate nucleus.

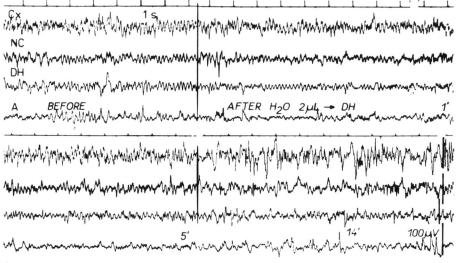

Figure 2.  EEG changes after control injection of solvent (2 µl).
           Explanation as in figure 1.

The experimental sessions were carried out on freely moving rabbits previously adapted to the experimental cage for 30 min. For the next 10 min. the initial EEG was recorded. Thereupon the tested compounds were administered by microsyringe and double-wall cannulas system. The EEG and visual observation were carried out for the following 60 min.

Intrahippocampally administrated GABA, at a dose of 50 µg dissolved in 2 µl of bidistilled water, (pH approx. 6.0) produced disappearance of theta rhytm in the hippocampus and appearance of slow waves in other EEG (Figure 1). Characteristic delta waves appeared 10 - 20 sec after injection of the drug, initially in the hippocampus, and within a few seconds also in other structures. During the period of GABA action (20 - 30 min.) the rabbits became quiet: the spontaneous locomotor activity declined, and the animals mostly lay on the cage floor. After injection of the lower dose the action of GABA was shorter.

Control injections of bidistilled water into the hippocampus (Figur 2) have shown that the solvent produces weak and short-lasting stimulation of behavioral and EEG activity. The group receiving sham injections displayed a similar effect. The control group received water injection because the model studies on the rat (Wolfarth, Boissier, 1976) had shown previously that bidistilled water produced less changes in EEG than injection with polyionic Merle's solution (artificial cerebrospinal fluid), or physiological saline.

Our studies have proved an inhibitory action of intrahippocampally injected GABA. This inhibition appearing initially in the hippocampus caused desynchronization of EEG recordings in other structures and behavioral inhibition. These effects did not appear after control injection of water.

An increase in the activity of inhibitory hippocampal system caused by an elevation of endogenous GABA level results in a depression of activity in the hippocampus itself, and of the other brain structures belonging to limbic and extrapyramidal systems. This indicated the importance of hippocampal GABAergic system in inhibitory mechanisms of the brain.

REFERENCES

Segal, M., and Bloom, F.E., 1974, The action of norepinephrine in
the rat hippocampus I, Iontophoretic studies. Brain Res. 72:
79-97.
Segal, M., Sims, K., and Smissman, E., 1975, Characterization of
an inhibitory receptor in rat hippocampus: A microiontophoretic
study using conformationally restricted amino acids analogues.
Br. J. Pharmacol. 57:181-188.
Storm-Mathisen, J. and Fonnum, F., 1971, Quantitative histochemistry of glutamate decarboxylase in the rat hippocampal region.
J. Neurochem. 18:1105-1111.

NEUROTRANSMITTERS IN THE AMYGDALA: A BRIEF REVIEW

P.C. Emson

MRC Neurochemical Pharmacology Unit
Dept. of Pharmacology
Medical School, Hills Road, Cambridge, England

At a major conference on the amygdala held in 1972
(Elefethriou 1972) the total number of putative transmitters
known to be present in the amygdala was three.  These were noradrenaline, serotonin and acetylcholine (Eidelberg and Woodbury
1972).  Only in the case of the cholinergic system, where acetylcholinesterase staining had been carried out (Shute and Lewis,
1967) was there any data on regional distribution within the
amygdala.  Since this date a number of studies, primarily in the
rat, have examined the distribution of neurotransmitters within
the amygdala.  In this brief review an attempt has been made to
summarize recent data from our laboratory on the amino acid distribution in the rat amygdala and also to present data on the
distribution of putative peptide neurotransmitters within the
amygdala.

## 1.  AMINO ACIDS

The amygdala is closely connected with the hypothalamus with
which it is concerned with a complex range of endocrine and
behavioural functions (Elefethriou 1972).  Anatomical considerations indicate (Egger 1972) that the amygdala may be divided into
the phylogentically older nuclei (medial, cortical and central)
and the more recently evolved nuclei (lateral and basolateral).
The medial, central and cortical nuclei project mainly via the
dorsal route involving the stria terminalis to the supraoptic
nuclei and the hypothalamus.  Whilst the basolateral and lateral
nuclei project to the hypothalamus by the more direct ventral
pathway through the ansa lenticularis.  In support of this
phylogenetic classification of the amygdaloid nuclei, acetylcholinesterase and choline acetyltransferase are associated with

181

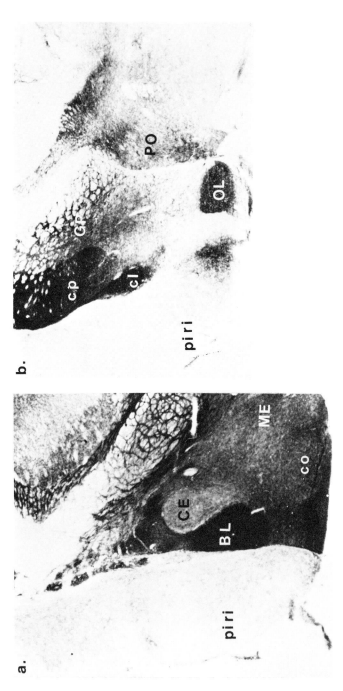

Figure 1a: Coronal section to show the effect of cortical undercutting on the distribution of acetylcholinesterase (AChE) in the amygdala nuclei. Note the depletion of AChE positive material from the piriform cortex and the pile up of AChE positive material in the basolateral and cortical amygdaloid nuclei (x 20). BL, basolateral amygdaloid nucleus, CE, central amygdaloid nucleus, CO, cortical amygdaloid nucleus, ME, medial amygdaloid nucleus and piri, piriform cortex.

Figure 1b: Coronal section to show the position of cuts transecting the ventral amygdofugal pathway (AChE stain) (x 20). CL, claustrum, GP, globus pallidus, CP, caudate putamen, PO, lateral pre-optic area, OL, nucleus of lateral olfactory tract and piri, piriform cortex.

the more recently evolved basolateral and lateral nuclei
(Fig. 1a) and are partially depleted by cuts severing the ventral
pathway (Fig. 1b).  In contrast, glutamic acid decarboxylase
(GAD) (Table I) and γ-aminobutyric acid (GABA) are concentrated
in the phylogenetically older nuclei.  On the basis of this
finding we (Le Gal Le Salle et al, 1977) severed the stria
terminalis tract and measured the GAD content of the amygdala
nuclei and the bed nucleus of the stria terminalis (Table II).
The results showed that there was possibly a small GABA-ergic
projection from the central nucleus to the bed nucleus of the
stria terminalis but that there was no major GABA-ergic projection
to or from the amygdala via the stria terminalis.  Further cuts to
ventral pathway such as in Fig. 1b did not modify the GAD content
of any of the amygdala nuclei (data not significantly different
from Table I) indicating that the majority of GABA within the
amygdala is probably located in intrinsic neurons.

Further work using amino acid analysis (Table III) established
the existence of a small GABA projection from the central amygdaloid nucleus to the bed nucleus of the stria terminalis but showed
no significant change in the amydgala's content of other putative
inhibitory transmitter amino acids such as glycine or taurine.
The central nucleus in common with the other amygdala nuclei has
only a low content of taurine and glycine.

During the course of this investigation we used  fine micro-
knife cuts (0.125mm tungsten wire) to undercut the piriform-
entorhinal cortex area.  The cuts (Fig. 1a) which substantially
deplete the cortex of cholineacetylase and monoamines did not
modify the amino acid content of the undercut cortex (Table IV).
These data indicate that there is no substantial amino acid
projection to this area of cortex, and may suggest that where
large depletions of amino acids occur following undercutting as in
the frontal cortex, this probably reflects neuronal death due to
damage of the vasclature.  In this area of cortex, however, the
blood supply from the cortical surface enters both dorsally and
ventrally so that our knife cuts leave a substantial blood supply
intact.  Although we observed no marked changes in glutamate
content of the piriform cortex or the amygdala, high affinity
uptake studies would be necessary before such a glutamatergic
projection could be ignored (Storm-Mathisen, 1977).

## 2.   SUBSTANCE P AND PEPTIDES IN THE AMYGDALA

The report by Nilsson et al (1974) of a high content of
substance P in the medial and central nuclei of the amygdala
prompted us to confirm this distribution using a sensitive
radioimmunoassay for substance P (Kanazawa and Jessell, 1976).
Substance P is indeed concentrated in the medial and central

TABLE I: REGIONAL DISTRIBUTION OF GLUTAMIC ACIC DECARBOXYLASE AND
γ-AMINOBUTYRIC ACID WITHIN THE AMYGDALOID COMPLEX

| | Glutamic acid decarboxylase μmoles/gram wet wt/h | γ-aminobutyric acid μmoles/gram wet wt |
|---|---|---|
| Piriform cortex | 6.26 ± 0.26 (6) | 1.43 ± 0.04 (6) |
| Anterior amygdala | 4.54 ± 0.27 (4) | 0.87 ± 0.06 (4) |
| Cortico medial nucleus | 10.33 ± 0.23 (4) | 1.97 ± 0.13 (4) |
| Basolateral nucleus | 8.52 ± 0.26 (6) | 1.63 ± 0.11 (4) |
| Central nucleus | 10.26 ± 1.30 (4) | 2.34 ± 0.06 (4) |

TABLE II: GLUTAMIC ACID DECARBOXYLASE ACTIVITY IN THE AMYGDALOID COMPLEX AND BED NUCLEUS OF THE STRIA TERMINALIS AFTER A LESION OF THE STRIA TERMINALIS TRACT

| | GAD ACTIVITY IN PERCENT OF CONTROL SITE |
|---|---|
| Amygdaloid complex | |
| Central nucleus (5) | $76.4 \pm 6.4$* |
| Medial nucleus (6) | $96.8 \pm 6.3$ |
| Nucleus of the lateral olfactory tract (4) | $105.1 \pm 12.5$ |
| Lateral posterior nucleus (5) | $98.4 \pm 4.2$ |
| Cortical nucleus (6) | $90.4 \pm 6.4$ |
| Bed nucleus of the stria terminalis | |
| Rostral (3) | $56.3 \pm 2.9$* |
| Medial-dorsal (4) | $111.0 \pm 10.6$ |
| Medio-ventral (5) | $92.8 \pm 12.9$ |
| Caudal (5) | $78.0 \pm 5.1$ |

TABLE III:  AMINO ACID CONTENT OF THE CENTRAL NUCLEUS AND BED NUCLEUS OF THE
STRIA TERMINALIS AFTER A LESION OF THE STRIA TERMINALIS TRACT

| Amino acid | Central nucleus | | Bed nucleus of stria terminalis | |
|---|---|---|---|---|
| | Lesion side | Control side | Lesion side | Control side |
| Taurine | 0.66 ± 0.24 (4) | 0.78 ± 0.16 (4) | 1.14 ± 0.36 (5) | 1.12 ± 0.29 (5) |
| Aspartic acid | 0.83 ± 0.11 (4) | 0.72 ± 0.11 (4) | 1.33 ± 0.25 (5) | 1.38 ± 0.20 (5) |
| Glutamine | 0.50 ± 0.06 (4) | 0.62 ± 0.08 (4) | 1.38 ± 0.38 (5) | 0.91 ± 0.17 (5) |
| Glutamic acid | 6.14 ± 0.64 (4) | 5.96 ± 0.30 (4) | 5.66 ± 0.97 (5) | 6.77 ± 0.70 (5) |
| Glycine | 0.50 ± 0.03 (4) | 0.48 ± 0.03 (4) | 0.87 ± 0.21 (5) | 0.71 ± 0.09 (5) |
| γ-aminobutyric acid | 2.66 ± 0.16 (4) | 2.53 ± 0.13 (4) | 3.11 ± 1.06*(5) | 4.64 ±0.48 (5) |

Samples were dissected from fresh cold brain sections, frozen on dry ice,
and homogenised in 10% trichloroacetic acid for amino acid analysis.
Amino acid analysis was carried out on a Durham amino acid analyser
with a minimum sensitivity of better than 40 pmoles per sample.

Units are µmoles/gram wet wt.

* denotes significantly different from control side p<0.02 (paired t test)

nuclei of the amygdala (Fig. 2a) and in the bed nucleus of the
stria terminalis (Emson et al, 1978).  No lesion severing any of
the known pathways to or from the amygdala has any effect on the
substance P content of the amygdala.  In particular, cuts inter-
rupting the stria terminalis did not modify the assayable
substance P content of the bed nucleus or the amygdala indicating
there is no significant substance P pathway running in the stria
terminalis.  Substance P positive neuronal cell bodies are found
in the medial amygdala by immunohistochemistry (Hökfelt et al,
1977) consistent with the suggestion that the substance P in the
amygdala is within intrinsic neurones.  However, knife cuts
separating the medial and central nucleus did partially deplete
the central nucleus of substance P (Table V) suggesting a short
substance P containing intra-amygdaloid pathway between the medial
and central nucleus.

TABLE IV:  AMINO ACID CONTENT OF NORMAL
AND UNDERCUT ENTORHINAL CORTEX

| Amino acid | Lesion side | Control side |
|---|---|---|
| Taurine | $5.10 \pm 0.10$ (6) | $5.44 \pm 0.15$ (6) |
| γ-aminobutyric acid | $1.39 \pm 0.05$ (6) | $1.43 \pm 0.04$ (6) |
| Glutamic acid | $6.91 \pm 0.24$ (6) | $6.85 \pm 0.13$ (6) |
| Glutamine | $2.87 \pm 0.31$ (6) | $3.57 \pm 0.61$ (6) |
| Aspartic acid | $1.80 \pm 0.01$ (6) | $1.70 \pm 0.06$ (6) |
| Glycine | $0.44 \pm 0.03$ (6) | $0.40 \pm 0.04$ (6) |

Units are μmoles amino acid per gram.

(From Paxinos and Emson, 1977 unpublished)

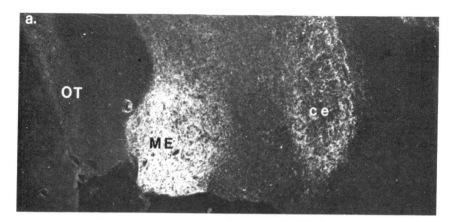

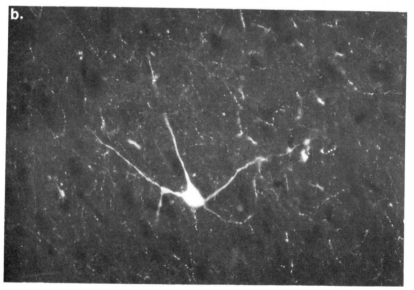

Figure 2a:  Fluorescence micrograph of a horizontal section
stained by the immunohistochemical procedure to demonstrate the
intense substance P immunoreactivity in the medial and central
amygdaloid nucleus (x 100).  CE, central amygdaloid nucleus,
ME, medial amygdaloid nucleus and  OT, optic tract.

Figure 2b:  Immunofluorescence micrograph showing a somatostatin-
positive neuron in the lateral amygdaloid nucleus (x 350).
Photograph by courtesy of Dr T. Hökfelt.

TABLE V:   EFFECTS OF SURGICAL ISOLATION OF THE MEDIAL
           AMYGDALA ("MEDICAL AMYGDALA ISLAND") ON THE
      SUBSTANCE P CONTENT OF THE OTHER AMYGDALOID NUCLEI

| Nucleus | Control animals (pmol/gram) | Operated animals (pmol/gram) |
|---------|-----------------------------|------------------------------|
| Medial | 667. 1 $\pm$ 80.9 | 767.1 $\pm$ 85.2 |
| Central | 208.20 $\pm$ 43.5 | 63.9 $\pm$ 22.2[**] |
| Basolateral | 48. 4 $\pm$  9.62 | 36.0 $\pm$  4.7 |
| Piriform cortex | 53. 2 $\pm$ 11. 8 | 59.5 $\pm$ 15.1 |

Results are the means $\pm$ S.E.M. for a total of six animals.
**Significantly different from other nuclei $p < 0.01$


A number of other putative peptide neurotransmitters
(Otsuka and Takahashi, 1977) have been reported to be localized
within the amygdala (Table VI and Fig. 2b).  Again the majority
of these peptides are located in the phylogenetically older nuclei.
The large number of peptides found in the amygdala approaches
the number found in the hypothalamus and may reflect the interactions between these two areas of the brain.

## 3.   CATECHOLAMINES, 5-HT AND HISTAMINE

Although this review is not primarily concerned with the
amines it should be realised that significant regional distributions of noradrenaline, dopamine, histamine (Ben-Ari et al, 1977)
and 5-HT have been reported from the amygdala.  However, in all
cases the amine containing fibres originate outside the amygdala.
For 5-HT, dopamine, noradrenaline and histamine the ventral
pathway apparently carries the majority of the amine containing
fibres, and only few fibres run with the dorsal stria terminalis
(Lindvall and Björklund, 1974; Ben-Ari et al, 1977; Emson et al,
1978; Azitma, 1978).

## ACKNOWLEDGEMENTS

I am grateful to Dr J.S. Kelly for critically reading this
manuscript and to Dr T. Hökfelt for generously providing the
photograph for Fig. 2b.

TABLE IV:  PUTATIVE PEPTIDE NEUROTRANSMITTERS FOUND IN THE AMYGDALOID COMPLEX

| Peptide | Distribution within the amygdala |
|---|---|
| Substance P | Bed nucleus of stria terminalis, central nucleus and medial nucleus (1,2) |
| Somatostatin | Corticomedial, basal and lateral nuclei (3) |
| Enkephalins | Central nucleus (4) |
| Thyrotropin releasing hormone (TRH) | Distribution unknown (5) |
| Neurotensin | Bed nucleus of stria terminalis and central nucleus (6) |
| Vasoactive intestinal polypeptide (VIP) | Central and medial nuclei (7) |
| Neurophysin | Medial nucleus (8) |

References

1.  Nilsson et al (1975)          5.  Brownstein et al (1974)
2.  Emson et al (1978)            6.  Snyder et al (1977)
3.  Epelbaum et al (1977)         7.  Fuxe et al (1977)
4.  Rossier J. (personal communication)   8.  Swanson L. (1977)

REFERENCES

Azmitia, E., 1978, The serotonin producing neurons of the median
    and dorsal raphe, in "Handbook of Psychopharmacology
    (L.L. Iversen, S.D. Iversen and S.H. Snyder, eds.) (in press).
Ben-Ari,Y., Le Gal La Salle, G., Emson, P., Barbin, G., and
    Garbarg, M., 1977, Neurochemical mapping of transmitter
    candidate systems in the amygdaloid complex and bed nucleus
    of the stria terminalis of the rat, Proc. International
    Physiological Sciences, Vol. XIII, Abst. 177.
Brownstein, M., Palkovitz, M., Saavedra, J., Bassiri, R., and
    Utiger, R., 1974, Thyrotropin releasing hormone in specific
    nuclei of the brain. Science 185: 267-269.
Brownstein, M.J., Palkovitz, M., Saavedra, J.M., and Kizer, J.S.,
    1975, Tryptophan hydroxylase in the rat brain, Brain Research
    97: 163-166.
Conrad, L., Leonard, C., and Pfaff, D., 1974, Connections of the
    median and dorsal raphe nuclei in the rat. An autoradio-
    graphic and degeneration study. J. comp Neurol. 156: 179-206.
Egger, M.D., 1972, Amygdaloid-hypothalamic neurophysiological
    interrelationships, in "The Neurobiology of the Amygdala",
    (B.E. Eleftheriou, ed.), Plenum Press, New York.
Eidelberg, E., and Woodbury, C.M., 1972, Electrical activity in
    the amygdala and its modification by drugs. Possible nature
    of synaptic transmission, a review in "Neurobiology of the
    Amygdala", (B.E. Eleftheriou, ed.), Plenum Press, New York.
Eleftheriou, B.E., 1972, Neurobiology of the amygdala, Plenum
    Press, New York.
Emson, P.C., Paxinos, G., Jessell, T.M., and Cuello, A.C., 1978,
    Substance P in the amygdaloid complex, bed nucleus and stria
    terminalis system of the rat brain, Brain Research
    (submitted for publication).
Emson, P.C., Paxinos, G., and Bjørklund, A., 1978, Effects of
    ventral amygdofugal pathway and stria terminalis lesions on
    the distribution of 5-hydroxytryptamine, dopamine and nora-
    drenaline in the amygdaloid nuclei. A histochemical and
    biochemical study, (in preparation).
Epelbaum, J., Brazeau, J., Tsang, D., Brawer, J., and Martin,
    J.B., 1977, Subcellular distribution of radioimmunoassayable
    somatostatin in rat brain, Brain Research 126: 309-323.
Fuxe, K., Hökfelt, T., Said, S.I., and Mutt, V., 1977, Vasoactive
    intestinal polypeptide and the nervous system: immunohisto-
    chemical evidence for localization in central and peripheral
    neurons particularly intracortical neurons of the cerebral
    cortex, Neuroscience Letters, (in press).
Hökfelt, T., Johansson, O., Kellerth, J.O., Ljungdahl, A.,
    Nilsson, G., Nyards, A., and Pernow, B., 1977, Immunohisto-
    chemical distribution of substance P, in "Substance P"
    (U.S. von Euler and B. Pernow, eds.), Raven Press, New York.

Kanazawa, I., and Jessell, T., 1976, Post mortem changes and regional distribution of substance P in the rat and mouse nervous system, Brain Research 117: 362-367.

Lindvall, O., and Björklund, A., 1974, The organization of the ascending catecholamine neuron systems in the rat brain, Acta Physiol. Scand. Supp. 412.

McGeer, P.L., McGeer, E.G., Scherer, U., and Singh, K., 1977, A glutamatergic corticostriatal pathway, Brain Research 128: 369-373.

Nilson, G., Hökfelt, T., and Pernow, B., 1974, Distribution of substance P-like immunoreactivity in the rat central nervous system as revealed by immunohistochemistry, Med. Biol., 52: 424-427.

Otsuka, M., and Takahashi, T., 1977, Putative peptide neuro-transmitters, in "Annual Review of Pharmacology", Vol. pp 425-439.

Shute, C.C.D., and Lewis, P.R., 1967, The ascending cholinergic reticular system: neocortical olfactory and subcortical projections, Brain 90: 497-520.

Snyder, S.H., Uhl, G.R., and Kuhar, M.J., 1977, Comparative features of enkephalin and neurotensin in the mammalian central nervous system, in Centrally Acting Peptides" (J. Hughes, ed.) Macmillan, (in press).

Storm-Mathisen, J., 1976, Localization of putative neurotransmitters in the hippocampal formation, Experimental Brain Research Suppl. 1: 179-187.

Swanson, L.W., 1977, Immunohistochemical evidence for a neuro-physin-containing autonomic pathway arising in the para-ventricular nucleus of the hypothalamus, Brain Research 128: 346-353.

# GABA MARKERS IN THE HYPOTHALAMUS : TOPOGRAPHICAL DISTRIBUTION

# AND ORIGIN

M.L. Tappaz

Université Claude-Bernard
Département de Médecine Expérimentale
69373 Lyon cedex 2

A few lines of evidence have been gained over the last few years which suggest that γ-aminobutyric acid (GABA) might be involved as a putative inhibitory transmitter in the hypothalamus, a region much less studied than for instance the substantia nigra where such a function appears firmly established. GABA and its biosynthetic enzyme, glutamate decarboxylase (GAD) have been reported to be concentrated in the hypothalamus (Albers and Brady, 1959 ; Fahn and Coté, 1968). Hypothalamic slices present a high affinity GABA uptake system (Hökfelt et al., 1970) and a preferential release of physiologically active amino-acids, including GABA, was produced by electrical stimulation of rat hypothalamic synaptosomes (Edwardson et al., 1972). In some hypothalamic nuclei, inhibitory inputs either from an extrinsic or intrinsic origin were mimicked by GABA application and sensitive to picrotoxin and bicuculine, two drugs assumed to be GABA antagonists (Dreifuss and Matthews, 1972 ; Yagi and Sawaki, 1975). In addition, it has been recently reported that GABA may possibly be involved in the control of the release of hypophysiotropic hormone (Jones et al., 1976 ; Makara and Stark, 1974 ; Mioduszewski et al., 1976 ; Ondo and Pass, 1976 ; Schally et al., 1977).

Anatomical and morphological evidence to support such a role is still scarce. Neuronal cell bodies and processes have been shown to take up exogenous radiolabelled GABA in the hypothalamus (Makara et al., 1975). However the organization of this possible GABAergic network is so far poorly understood due to the lack of a simple and rapid histochemical method such as the histofluorescence technique used for the monoamines. Autoradiography of GABA and GABA analogs (Kelly and Dick, 1976 and this volume) as well as immunohistochemical localization of GAD (McLaughlin et al., 1974 ;

Ribak et al., 1976) have been recently designed. They cannot be considered as routine tools yet and so far, their use has been restricted to regions where strong evidence for GABAergic transmission is already available.

Another approach that we report here to get information about the topographical localization of the GABAergic cells is to quantify GABAergic markers, in our case GABA itself and GAD, in discrete nuclei isolated by microdissection. Biochemical mapping obviously does not provide direct evidence about the cellular localization of the marker, which can be present in cell bodies, axons of passage, nerve terminals or extraneuronal element. Insight into its localization can be indirectly deduced however. For example, a non-uniform distribution suggests that the marker is contained in a restricted population of nerve cells. In addition, valuable information about the origin of the cells containing the putative transmitter can be gained by lesion experiments where decrease of the concentration of the presynaptic marker is expected following the anterograde degeneration of the neurons after lesion of the pathway.

METHODS

Tissue dissection : Nuclei of the hypothalamus and substantia nigra were removed according to Palkovitz's method (Palkovitz et al., 1974). Accuracy of the dissection was histologically checked. In order to prevent post-mortem changes in GABA determination, the rats were killed by exposure to a microwave field, a procedure that inactivated enzymatic processes in less than two seconds (Tappaz et al., 1977).

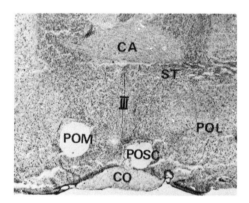

Figure 1. Histological control of the microdissection of hypothalamic nuclei. The medial preoptic (POM) and suprachiasmatic preoptic (POSC) nuclei were removed from unstained frozen slices 300 μm in thickness, using 500 and 300 μm hollow needles respectively. The slices were then sectioned at 30 μm and stained with cresyl violet.

Biochemical assays : GAD was assayed with saturating concentration of pyridoxal phosphate using carboxylabelled glutamate, in such conditions that carbon dioxide and GABA were formed in stoechiometric proportions with less than 10 % excess of carbon dioxide (Tappaz et al, 1977). GABA was measured by an enzymatic cycling microassay (Otsuka et al., 1971).

## DISTRIBUTION OF GAD

In all nuclei examined, except for the median eminence, the GAD activity was higher than in the whole brain. Highest levels were found in the preoptic, anterior and dorsomedial nuclei and lowest in the arcuate, supraoptic nuclei and the median eminence (table 1). Moderate amounts of GAD were measured in the other nuclei. No simple pattern of GAD distribution emerges when the nuclei are separated according to function or anatomical location (figure 2). The reticular part of the substantia nigra remained the richest area with 2-3 times as much activity as most hypothalamic nuclei. Thus, the GAD distribution varies about five-fold between the richest and the poorest regions. This variation is the same order of magnitude as that found for layered structures of

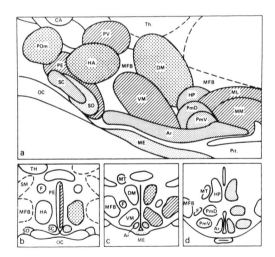

Figure 2. Localization of GAD in nuclei of the hypothalamus. Schematic drawings of a parasagittal section (a) and frontal sections thru the anterior region (b), the tuberal region (c) and premammillary region (d) of the hypothalamus. Concentrations of GAD activity are indicated as follows : light dots < heavy dots < hatches < crossed hatches.
From Tappaz et al., 1977.

TABLE 1:   GAD ACTIVITY IN HYPOTHALAMIC NUCLEI AND SUBSTANTIA NIGRA

| Nucleus | Abbreviation | GAD Activity |
|---|---|---|
| Hypothalamus | | |
| Periventricular zone | | |
| N. Suprachiasmatis (10) | SC | 290±24 |
| N. Periventricularis (16) | PE | 430±14 |
| N. Paraventricularis (16) | PV | 398±23 |
| N. Arcuatus (18) | Ar | 285±12 |
| Median Eminence (16) | ME | 125± 4 |
| N. posterior (12) | HP | 360±17 |
| Medial zone | | |
| N. Preopticus medialis (10 | POM | 590±44 |
| N. Anterior (16) | HA | 498±20 |
| N. ventromedialis, pars (20) lateralis | VM1 | 430±10 |
| N. ventromedialis, pars (10) medialis | VMm | 425±19 |
| N. dorsomedialis (14) | DM | 499±19 |
| N. premammillaris dorsalis (12) | PmD | 331±15 |
| N. premammillaris ventralis (12) | PmV | 327±18 |
| N. mammillaris medialis (12) | MM | 428±10 |
| Lateral zone | | |
| N. preopticus lateralis (14) | POM | 560±32 |
| N. supraopticus (12) | SO | 233±24 |
| Median forebrain bundle (VM level) (14) | MFB | 414±15 |
| N. mammillaris lateralis (12) | ML | 390±14 |
| Substantia Nigra | | |
| Pars reticularis (10) | SNR | 1160±30 |
| Pars compacta (10) | SNC | 480±40 |

The results are mean values (± S.E.M.) for the number of determinations indicated in parentheses expressed in pmoles/h/μg protein. Activity of the whole brain homogenate was 230 ± 16(6). From Tappaz et al., 1977.

the brain (Graham 1973 ; Okada and Shimada 1975 ; Storm-Mathisen and Fonnum 1971). This gradient is larger than for enzymes implicated in general cellular metabolism such as the ATPase (Fahn and Côte 1968). It suggests that GAD is localized in unevenly distributed cells, hence nerve cells. However since the ratio between the highest and poorest regions is lower than for enzymes involved in the biosynthesis of other transmitters, such as the catecholamines (Saavedra et al., 1974), this might indicate that some GAD is localized in glial cells which accounts for a background level. An alternative possibility is that GAD-containing cells may have an extensive distribution in a complex series of local pathways.

## DISTRIBUTION OF GABA

The levels of GABA measured in the various nuclei depended greatly upon the way the rats were killed. When the brain tissue was frozen within three minutes following decapitation, a non uniform distribution of GABA was found with a ten-fold difference between the highest level (Substantia nigra, pars reticularis) and the lowest level (median eminence). However, when the animals were

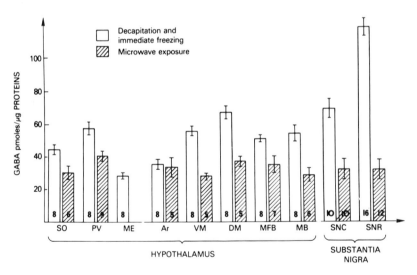

Figure 3. GABA content in hypothalamic nuclei and substantia nigra. The results are mean values for the number of assays indicated (+ S.E.M.). The rats were killed by exposure to microwaves for 2.5 sec. When the animals were decapitated, the brains were quickly removed from the skull and the ventral part of the brain was frozen within 3 min.
From Tappaz et al., 1977.

killed using microwaves, which inactivated enzymatic reactions in
less than two seconds, GABA appeared to be distributed evenly in
all the nuclei (figure 3). Since GABA content and distribution as
well as accuracy of the microdissection were shown to be unaffected by microwave fixation (Tappaz et al., 1977), these values
appear to be the best estimate of endogenous GABA content. The
non-uniform distribution previously reported in frozen hypothalamus (Kimura and Kuriyama, 1975) and confirmed by our own data
results mainly from a large increment in GABA level occuring in
the first minutes following death and represents essentially a
postmortem artefact.

### GAD VERSUS GABA DISTRIBUTION

Our results show that postmortem increases in GABA levels are
directly related to the GAD activity in the various hypothalamic

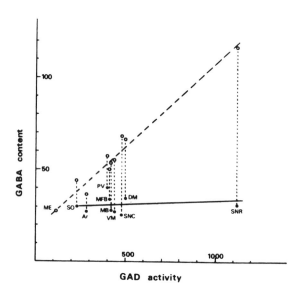

Figure 4. Relationship between GABA level and GAD content in hypothalamus and nigra nuclei. For the determination of GABA levels
the animals were either decapitated and their brain frozen (open
circles), or killed by 2.5 sec exposure to a microwave field
(closed circles). Abbreviations for nuclei are given in Table I.
There is no relationship between GAD and endogenous level of GABA
(r = 0.053), but a significant (p < 0.01) relationship exists
between postmortem level of GABA and GAD (r = 0.980).
From Tappaz et al., 1977.

and substantia nigra nuclei (Figure 4). With the other transmitters there appears to be a close relationship between transmitter level and content of the rate limiting biosynthetic enzymes. For example, in the hypothalamic nuclei, there is a highly significant relationship between levels of noradrenaline and dopamine-$\beta$-hydroxylase (Palkovitz et al., 1974 ; Saavedra et al., 1974). Similarly, in histochemical studies there appears to be a similar localization of catecholamines and their biosynthetic enzyme in cell bodies and terminals.

The lack of topographical overlapping in GAD and GABA distribution at the macroscopic level, suggests that both are not localized in the same elements at the cellular level. There is substantial evidence that GAD is mainly found in neurons. GAD is associated with the synaptosomal fraction of homogenates (Fonnum 1968 ; Salganicoff and De Robertis 1965). Anterograde degeneration following axotomy leads to a large decrease of GAD activity in substantia nigra (Fonnum et al ., 1974 ; Hattori et al., 1973 ; Kataoka et al., 1974) and in cerebellar nuclei (Fonnum et al., 1970). In recent immunohistochemical studies, GAD was visualized in synaptic terminals in the cerebellum (Mc Laughlin et al., 1974) and substantia nigra (Ribak et al., 1976). The gradient in distribution within the hypothalamus also indicates that GABA synthesis occurs mainly in unevenly distributed nerve cells.

In contrast, the uniform distribution of endogenous GABA makes it unlikely that GABA is mainly localized in a restricted population of neurons. In addition, experiments looking at the possible association with neural elements such as synaptosomes, have not provided clear cut results (Mangan and Whittaker, 1966 ; Ryall 1964 ; Weinstein et al., 1963). GABA was assumed to be associated with GAD in nerve cells largely because of the relationships between GABA and GAD content which appears to be a postmortem artefact (Baxter, 1969 ; Fonnum and Walberg, 1973). Taken together these various data led us to the following model of GAD and GABA distribution as a working hypothesis.

GABA synthesis occurs mainly in a restricted population of neuronal cells as reflected by the non uniform distribution of GAD. Since the range of GAD activities is smaller than far most neurotransmitters so far studied, an uniform background GAD activity which minimizes the differences might exist in the glial cells, as shown in glia tissue culture (Schrier and Thompson, 1973). Quantification of this pool is not possible from our study, its highest value would be the lowest values in GAD distribution within the brain nuclei, postulating that in this case the nucleus with the lowest GAD acting is devoid of a GAD-containing nerve cell innervation. A small pool of GABA is postulated to be stored inside the nerve endings. Quantitatively, this pool is not large enough to be reflected in regional differences in discrete nuclei. The main bulk of GABA is stored in a population of cells evenly distributed hence our speculation about a redistribution of GABA in glial

cells, as well as nerve terminals, possess a high affinity uptake
system for GABA (Iversen and Kelly, 1975).

Functionally, the small pool of GABA plays a classical role
of neurotransmitter implicated in a well-defined neuronal circuitry. The best marker for those GABAergic neurons is not GABA
itself, but its biosynthetic enzyme GAD. The large pool represents
GABA taken up by glial cells. This mechanism could be the major
inactivation process and glial cells could represent the principal
site for GABA catabolism. Release of GABA by glial cells as shown
in vitro (Bowery et al., 1976 ; Sellstrom and Hamberger, 1977) is
not excluded. In this speculative view, release would not be related to nerve impulses, but rather to some local variations in
the extra cellular space ; this pool of glial GABA might be implicated as a neuromodulator in some type of homeostatic function.
Endogenous GABA levels represent a marker of this large pool.

Since it is not feasible with available techniques to visualize GAD and GABA-containing cells simultaneously by histochemistry, this heuristic model remains highly speculative. At least it
takes into account the unusual topographical distribution of the
transmitter and its biosynthetic enzyme.

## ORIGIN OF GAD-CONTAINING CELLS

Assuming that GAD is a satisfactory marker of the GABAergic
neurons, we then investigated possible GABAergic afferents to the
hypothalamus by looking at the origin of hypothalamic GAD-containing cells. Major afferents well described in previous neuroanatomical studies were lesioned and GAD was measured in the nuclei
which were reported to receive projections from the lesioned pathway as summarized in figure 5. Consequently nuclei that are
sparsely innervated by the major afferents as well as diffuse, ill
-defined or controversial projections, may not have been investigated in this study. None of these lesions was followed by a marked decrease in GAD activity in most of the nuclei we studied
(figure 6). A significant but still unimpressive 30-40 % decrease
was observed in two cases : in both mammillary nuclei following
midbrain hemisection, and in the periventricular nucleus after
medio-dorsal thalamus lesioning. Thus, some GAD-containing fibers
might make up a component of the mammillary peduncles and periventricular fiber network respectively. However, due to proximity
of the cut in both cases, possible nonspecific damage cannot be
entirely ruled out.

As shown in the substantia nigra where degeneration of the descending strionigral afferents was already complete four days after
the lesion, the survival time was long enough to allow a massive
decrease should a GAD-containing pathway be severed. This never
occured. Accordingly GAD is likely to be contained in cellular elements which are intrinsic to the hypothalamus. Most hypothalamic
GABAergic nerve cells are probably short interneurons providing

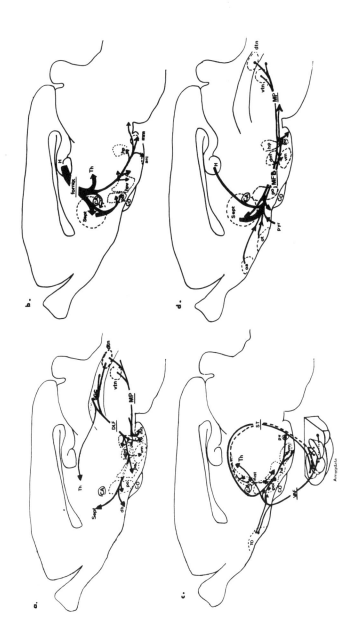

Figure 5. Schematic drawings of the major afferent projections to the various hypothalamic nuclei a) From the mesencephalic reticular formation arises the mammillary peduncle (MP) and the dorsal longitudinal fasciculus (DLF). b) The hippocampus projects through the fornix which divides in a pre- and a post-commissural component. c) The amygdala is connected by two major ipsilateral fiber systems : the stria terminalis (ST) also divided in a pre- and a post-commissural component and the ventral amygdalofugal pathway (VAF). d) The medial forebrain bundle (MFB) is a bidirectional link with medial basal teleencephalic region and the mesencephalic region.

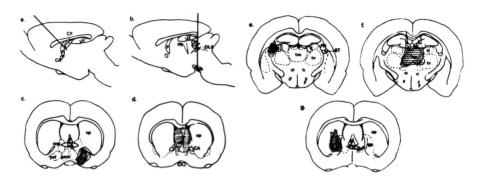

| | Midbrain | Stria terminalis | Fornix | Lateral preoptic area | Globus pallidus | Thalamus | Septum |
|---|---|---|---|---|---|---|---|
| N. Preopticus medialis | | | n.s. | | | | n.s. |
| N. Preopticus lateralis | | | | | | n.s. | n.s. |
| N. Suprachiasmatis | n.s. | | n.s. | | | | |
| N. Anterior | n.s. | n.s. | | | | | |
| N. Paraventricularis | n.s. | | | | | | |
| N. Periventricularis | n.s. | | | | | -40% | |
| N. Ventromedialis | n.s. | n.s. | n.s. | n.s. | n.s. | n.s. | n.s. |
| N. Dorsomedialis | n.s. | n.s. | n.s. | n.s. | n.s. | n.s. | |
| N. Arcuatus | n.s. | n.s. | n.s. | n.s. | n.s. | n.s. | |
| Media forebrain bundle | n.s. | n.s. | n.s. | n.s. | n.s. | n.s. | n.s. |
| N. Premammillaris | n.s. | n.s. | | | | | n.s. |
| N. Posterior | n.s. | | | | | | |
| N. Mammillaris medialis | -35% | n.s. | n.s. | | | | |
| N. Mammillaris lateralis | -40% | | n.s. | | | | |

Figure 6. Effects of the lesioning the major afferents on GAD
activity in discrete hypothalamic nuclei.
Typical lesions are schematically drawn. a) Fornix cut, b) Midbrain hemisection, c) Lateral preoptic area, d) Septum, e) Stria
terminalis, f) Dorso-medial thalamus, g) Globus pallidus.
GAD was assayed in nuclei where projections of the pathway were
described in previous anatomical studies 8-12 days after the
lesion. When significant ($p < 0.01$) GAD fall is expressed as percentage of the control. n.s. not significant; blank, not studied.
From Tappaz and Brownstein 1977.

intrahypothalamic connexions between the various nuclei. Similar
conclusions have been reported in the neostriatum (Mc Geer and
Mc Geer, 1975 and this volume) as well as in the hippocampus
(Storm-Mathisen, 1972 and this volume).


## STUDIES ON THE MEDIO BASAL HYPOTHALAMUS

The mediobasal hypothalamus is part of the hypophysiotropic
area, where hypophysiotropic hormones (releasing or inhibiting
factors) are synthetized and released and submitted to a neural
control. Since GABA has been suggested to be involved in the regulation of ACTH (Makara and Stark, 1974 ; Jones et al., 1976), LH-RH
(Ondo, 1974) and prolactin (Mioduszewski et al., 1976 ; Ondo and
Pass, 1976 ; Schally et al., 1977) understanding the organization
of the GABAergic network in this tiny region of the brain is of
paramount importance if one is to seek morphological support for
this putative regulation.

a) Deafferentiation of the mediobasal hypothalamus. In the
totally deafferented islands ventro-medial and arcuate nuclei displayed a marked decrease in GAD-activity (figure 7). This fall
seems unlikely to be due to unspecific necrotic damage. We ascertained that dopamine and its biosynthetic enzyme, tyrosine hydroxylase remained unchanged inside the island (Brownstein et al.,
1976) in agreement with the anatomy of the short tubero-infundibular dopaminergic pathway. Our results suggest that part of GAD
activity (about 60 %) in the arcuate and ventro-medial nuclei might
be localized in terminals the cell  bodies of which be outside the
mediobasal hypothalamus.

Partial deafferentation from lateral or posterior hypothalamus
still produced a moderate decrease but the rostral deafferentation
was without effect (figure 7). Therefore, the intrahypothalamic
connexions from the anterior and preoptic area to the hypothalamus
which was severed by the rostral cut, did not appear to contain
GABAergic fibers. On the other hand, there might exist some GABA-
ergic projection into the ventro-medial and arcuate nuclei originating from the lateral and posterior hypothalamus. However, as no
partial lesion led to the same decrease in GAD level as total deafferentation, it can be speculated that the GAD-containing cells
probably comprise a rather diffuse projecting system.

Complete deafferentation of the medio-basal hypothalamus did
not alter GAD levels in the median eminence. Ultrastructurally,
the median eminence is made up of intrinsic glial and ependymal
cells, fibers and processes from the tubero-infundibular parvi-
cellular neurons, and axons of passage from hypothalamo-hypophysial
tract originating outside the island. It is virtually devoid of
perikarya (Kobayashi et al., 1970). Since GAD in the median eminence appears to originate in cells intrinsic to the island, there

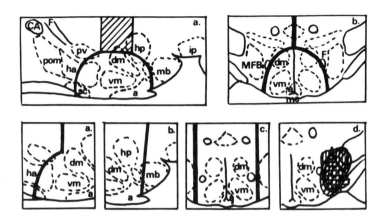

| | Total Deafferentation | Rostral cut | Bilateral parasagittal cut | MFB lesion | Posterior cut |
|---|---|---|---|---|---|
| N. Ventromedialis | - 65% | n.s | - 25% | - 20% | n.s |
| N. Arcuatus | - 60% | n.s | n.s | n.s | -30% |
| Median Eminence | n.s | n.s | | | |

Figure 7. Effect of total or partial deafferentation on GAD activity in medial-basal nuclei.
Upper drawing : Complete deafferentation (hypothalamic island) : Parasagittal (a) and coronal (b) view. Lower drawing : Partial deafferentation : Rostral cut (a), posterior cut (b), bilateral parasagittal cut (c), and medial forebrain bundle electrolytic lesion (d).
Lesions were made 8-12 days before biochemical analysis. When significant (p < 0.01) GAD is expressed as percentage of the control : n.s not significant blank : not studied.
From Tappaz and Brownstein, 1977.

exists two possible locations for GAD at this level : glial cells
or neuronal processes of the tubero-infundibular pathways.
    This alternative is being investigated using chemical lesion-
ing with kainic acid ; this excitotoxic analog of glutamate has
been reported to destroy cell bodies near the injection site while
sparing axons passing through or terminals (Olney et al., 1974 ;
Schwarcz and Coyle 1977). Preliminary results showed that there
was a decrease in GAD in the arcuate nucleus accompanied by a
parallel yet small decrease in the median eminence following injection of kainate into the third ventricle (Belin and Tappaz unpublished data). This indicates the possible existence of some GAD-
containing cell bodies lying in the arcuate nucleus and sending
short projections to the median eminence as a component of the
tubero-infundibular pathway. However only limited decreases (about
20 %) have been observed so far ; further investigations are
obviously needed to confirm these preliminary data.
    b) Distribution of GAD within the bovine median eminence. The
distribution of GAD and LHRH and TRH was studied in subdivisions
of the bovine median eminence. It was reasoned that a parallel distribution would give a topographic support for a GABAergic regulation.
GAD activity varied about 1 to 4 times with the highest values in
the caudal part. However only moderate activity was measured in the
external layers where the highest levels of LHRH and TRH were precisely found (table 2). This lack of correlation militates against
a GABAergic control of the release of LHRH and TRH, but by no means
rules it out. It is still possible that interregulations exist at
the cellular level which could be visualized only by histochemical
techniques and which are not reflected at the macroscopical level
in the biochemical mapping studies.

TABLE 2.  DISTRIBUTION OF RELEASING FACTORS[a] AND GAD[b] IN EIGHT
SUBDIVISIONS OF THE BOVINE MEDIAN EMINENCE

| Substance assayed* | Rostral | Anterior external | Anterior external | Middle external medial | Middle external lateral | Middle internal medial | Middle internal lateral | Caudal |
|---|---|---|---|---|---|---|---|---|
| TRH | 3.5 ±1.1 | 7.1 ±4.2 | 5.2 ±2.7 | 25.3 ±3.0 | 22.8 ±3.4 | 11.2 ±2.0 | 4.2 ±.4 | 1.9 ±1.1 |
| LHRH | 2.2 ±.6 | 2.6 ±.6 | 4.0 ±1.0 | 1.8 ±.3 | 4.1 ±.8 | 2.5 ±.6 | 3.3 ±.5 | 2.1 ±.2 |
| Glutamic acid decarboxylate | 4.5 ±.7 | 2.9 ±.7 | 5.0 ±.7 | 3.8 ±.6 | 5.1 ±.9 | 3.0 ±.3 | 5. ±.5 | 11.0 ±1.2 |

[a]Expressed as the concentration in ng/mg protein + SEM
[b]Expressed as nmoles product/mg protein/h + SEM.
*n = 6 for all determinations.
From Kizer et al., 1976.

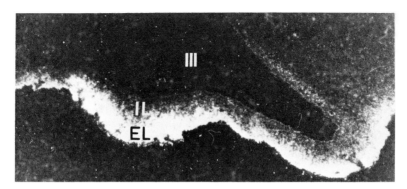

Figure 8. Dark-field autoradiography of the median eminence in the
kitten. Newborn kittens (two days old) pretreated with amino-oxyacetic acid (AOAA) were injected with tritiated GABA into the heart.
EL : External layer.    IL : Internal layer (from Aguera and Tappaz,
unpublished results).

    c) Autoradiography studies. In order to overcome these inherent
limitations of the biochemical mapping, autoradiography is being
developed in our laboratory to visualize cells which take up GABA
or GABA analogs according to methods previously described (Kelly
and Dick, 1976 and this volume) Tritiated GABA with high specific
activity was injected, either systemically into the heart in the
newborn kitten, or into the third ventricle with an excess of cold
β-alanine in the adult rat. In the kitten accumulation of silver
grains was observed in the external layer of the median eminence,
while some labelling appeared in the subependymal layer (figure 8).
In the rat heavy labelling was found all over the hypothalamus (figure 9a). Accumulation of silver grains was observed on the ependymal cells, but also on cell bodies and the neuropil. Cells which
did not take up labelled GABA were frequently seen. Non specific
labelling in glial cells must have been minimized by the simultaneous injection of an excess of cold β-alanine which is preferentially taken up by glial cells. Furthermore radio-labelled β-alanine did not provide the same pattern of labelling which, in
contrast to GABA seemed to follow the gradient of concentration
along the third ventricle. A striking feature of the labelling of
GABA was the conspicuous streaks of silver grains in the area late-
ro-basal to the third ventricle (figure 9b). This pattern did not
appear in the dorsal or lateral borders. In addition they were seen
only at the posterior level of the hypothalamus. In some cases the
streak of labelling seemed to emerge from a cell body. Thus these
streaks are likely to represent neural processes from the tubero-
infundibular tracts according to their general orientation. However
glial origin, for instance ependymal processes from the tanycytes
is possible since in a few instances β-alanine led to an analogous
yet much less conspicuous pattern. Electromicroscopy will be
needed to answer this question.

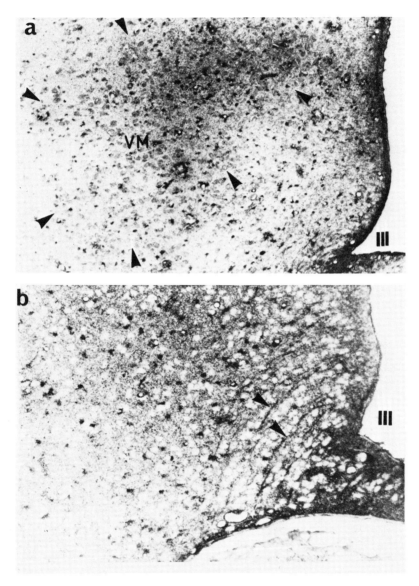

Figure 9. Autoradiography of the mediobasal hypothalamus in the rat.
Tritiated GABA was injected into the third ventricle in presence of
an excess of cold β-alanine in AOAA pretreated adult rats. (a)
Heavier accumulation is observed over the cells and neuropil in
the ventro-medial nucleus (VM). (b) Conspicuous streaks of labelling (arrows) are seen in the region basolateral to the third ventricle at the level of the posterior hypothalamus (from Aguera and
Tappaz, unpublished results).

SUMMARY

GAD activity showed an uneven pattern of distribution within
the various hypothalamic nuclei. On the other hand, endogenous GABA
levels showed a uniform distribution. These results suggest that
while GABA synthesis is likely to occur in unevenly distributed
nerve cells, most GABA may be stored in surrounding cells. As a
working hypothesis a dual localization is postulated : a small pool
of GABA is contained in nerve cells ; these cells are likely to be
GABAergic neurons involved in a well-defined neuronal circuitry.
GAD appeared to be the best marker for these cells. However the
main bulk of GABA is localized in evenly distributed cells, presumably glial cells, where it might play a neuromodulator role.

GAD activity in discrete hypothalamic nuclei was not affected
by lesions of the major afferents to the hypothalamus from the midbrain, hippocampus, amygdala, septum, thalamus and globus pallidus.
Consequently most GAD containing cells have their origin inside the
hypothalamus. In this region, GABAergic neurons are likely to be
short interneurons providing intrahypothalamic connexions. Total or
partial deafferentiations of the medial basal region provided results which suggest that such connexions exist from the lateral and
/or posterior hypothalamus into the ventro-medial and arcuate nuclei. In the median eminence GAD appeared to be contained in cells
intrinsic to the medio-basal hypothalamic island, which may be
either glial elements or neuronal processes from the tubero-infundibular pathway. Our preliminary studies do not yet allow us to
distinguish between these two possibilities.

LIST OF ABBREVIATIONS

CO:chiasma opticum. CA:commissura anterior. CF:columna fornicis.
cp:caudate putanem. db:tractus diagonalis (Broca). dtn:n. dorsalis
tegmentis. F:fornix. FH:fimbria hippocampi. FR:fasciculus retro-
flexus. Gp:globus pallidus. H:hippocampus. ip:n.interpeduncularis.
nist:n. interstitialis striae terminali. oa:n. olfactorius. ot:n. trac
tus olfactorii. Pyr: pyriform cortes. Pit:pituitary. SGC:substantia
grisea centralis. sl:n. septi lateralis. SM:stria medullaris. Th:
thalamus. TO:tuberculum olfactorium. tm:n. medialis thalami. tl:
n. lateralis thalami. tv:n. ventralis thalami. vtn:n.ventralis
tegmentis.
For the abbreviations of the hypothalamic nuclei see Table 1.

ACKNOWLEDGEMENTS

Most results reported here were obtained during the tenure of
a postdoctoral fellowship at the "National Institute of Mental
Health, N.I.H., Bethesda, USA". The work was carried out in collaboration with Dr M.J. Brownstein. I wish to thank Dr. I.J. Kopin
for his generous help and encouragement throughout this work.

REFERENCES

Albers, R.W., and Brady, R., 1959, The distribution of glutamic decarboxylase in the nervous system of the Rhesus monkey, J. Biol.
Chem. 234:926-928.

Baxter, C.F., 1969, The nature of γ-aminobutyric acid, in "Handbook of Neurochemistry (A. Lajtha, ed.), pp. 289-353, vol. 3,
Plenum Press, New York.

Bowery, N.G., Brown, D.A., Collins, G.S., Galvan, M., Marsh, S.,
and Yamini, G., 1976, Indirect effects of amino-acids on sympathetic ganglion cells mediated through the release of γ-aminobutyric acid from glial cells, Br. J. Pharmacol., 57:73-91.

Brownstein M.J., Palkovitz, M., Tappaz, M.L., Saavedra, J.M., and
Kizer, J.S., 1976, Effect of surgical isolation of the hypothalamus on its neurotransmitter content, Brain Res., 117:287-295.

Dreifuss, J.J., and Matthews, E.K., 1972, Antagonism between
strychnine and glycine and bicuculline and GABA in the ventro-
medial hypothalamus. Brain Res., 45:599-603.

Edwardson, J.A., Bennet, G.W., and Bradford, H.F., 1972, Release
of amino-acids and neurosecretory substances after stimulation
of nerve endings (synaptosomes) isolated from the hypothalamus,
Nature 240:554-556.

Fahn, S., and Cote, L.J., 1968, Regional distribution of sodium-
potassium activated adenosine triphophatase in the brain of the
rhesus monkey, J. Neurochem., 15:433-436.

Fahn, S., and Cote, L.J., 1968, Regional distribution of γ-aminobutyric acid (GABA) in brain of the Rhesus monkey, Brain Res.,
15:209-213.

Fonnum, F., 1968, The distribution of glutamate decarboxylase and
aspartate transaminase in subcellular fractions of rat and guinea
pig brain, Biochem. J., 106:401-411.

Fonnum, F. Grofova, I., Rinvik, E., Storm-Mathisen, J., and
F. Walberg, 1974, Origin and distribution of glutamate decarboxylase in substantia nigra of the cat, Brain Res., 71:77-92.

Fonnum, F., Storm-Mathisen, J., and Walberg, F., 1970, Glutamate
decarboxylase inhibitory neurones. A study of the enzyme in
Purkinje cell axons and boutons in the cat, Brain Res., 20:259-
275.

Fonnum, F., and Walberg, F., 1973, The concentration of GABA within
inhibitory nerve terminals, Brain Res., 62:577-579.

Fuxe, K., and Hökfelt, T., 1969, Catecholamines in the hypothalamus
and the pituitary gland, in "Frontiers in neuroendocrinology"
(W.F. Ganong and L. Martini, eds.) pp. 47-96, Oxford university
Press, New York.

Graham, L.T., Jr., 1973, Distribution of glutamic acid decarboxylase activity and GABA content in the olfactory bulb, Life Sci.,
12:443-447.

Hattori, T., McGeer, P.L., Fibiger, H.C., and McGeer, E.G., 1973, On the source of GABA containing terminals in the substantia nigra. Electron microscopic autoradiographic and biochemical studies, Brain Res., 54:103-114.

Iversen, L.L., and Kelly, J.S., 1975, Uptake and metabolism of $\gamma$-aminobutyric acid by neurones and glial cells, Biochem. Pharmacol., 24:933-938.

Jones, M.T., Hillhouse, E., and Burden, J., 1976, Secretion of corticotropin releasing hormone in vitro, in "Frontiers in Neuroendocrinology" (L. Martini and W.F. Ganong, eds.), pp. 195-223, vol. 4.

Kataoka, K., Bak, I.J., Hassler, R., Kim, J.S., and Wagner, A., 1974, L-glutamate decarboxylase and choline acetyltransferase activity in substantia nigra and the striatum after surgical interruption of the strio-nigral fibers in the baboon. Exp. Brain Res., 19:217-227.

Kelly, J.S., and F. Dick, 1976, Differential labeling of glial cells and GABA-inhibitory interneurons and nerve terminals following the microinjection of $\beta$ ($^3$H) Alanine, (3H) DABA and ($^3$H) GABA into single folia of the cerebellum. Cold spring harbor Symposia on quantitative biology. Vol. XL, The synapse, 93-106.

Kim, J.S., Bak, I.J., Hassler, R., and Okada, Y., 1971, Role of $\gamma$-amino-butyric acid (GABA) in the extrapyramidal motor system. 2. Some evidence for the existence of a type of GABA-rich strionigral neurones. Exp. Brain Res. 14:95-104.

Kimura, H., and Kuriyama, K., 1975, Distribution of gamma-amino butyric acid (GABA) in the rat hypothalamus : Functional correlates of GABA with activities of appetite controlling mechanisms. J. Neurochem., 24:903-907.

Kizer, J.S., Palkovits, M., Tappaz, M., Kebabian, J., and Brownstein M.J., 1976, Distribution of releasing factors, biogenic amines, and related enzymes in the bovine median eminence, Endocrinology, 98:685.

Kobayashi, H., Matsui, T., and Ishii, S., 1970, Functional election microscopy of the hypothalamic median eminence, Int. Rev. Cytol., 29:281-381.

Makara, G.B., Rappay, G., and Stark, E., 1975, Autoradiographic localization of $^3$H-Gamma-aminobutyric acid in the medial hypothalamus, Exp. Brain Res., 22:449-455.

Makara, G.B., and Stark, E., 1974, Effect of gamma-aminobutyric acid (GABA) and GABA antagonist drugs on ACTH release. Neuroendocrinology, 16:178-190.

Mangan, J.L., and Whittaker, V.P., 1966, The distribution of free aminoacids in subcellular fractions of guinea-pig brain. Biochem. J. 98:128-137.

Mc Geer, P.L., and Mc Geer, E.G., 1975, Evidence for glutamic acid decarboxylase-containing interneurons in the neostriatum, Brain Res., 9:331-335.

Mc Laughlin, B.J., Wood, J.G., Saito, K., Barber, R., Vaughn, J.E., Roberts, E., and Wu, J.Y., 1974, The fine structural localization of glutamate decarboxylase in synaptic terminals of rodent cerebellum, Brain Res., 76:377-391.

Mioduszewski, R., Grandison, L., and Meites, J., 1976, Stimulation of prolactin release in rats by GABA, Proc. Soc. Exp. Biol. Med. 151:44-46.

Okada, Y., and Shimada, C., 1975, Distribution of gamma-amino-butyric acid (GABA) and glutamate decarboxylase (GAD) activity in the guinea pig hippocampus. Brain Res., 98:202-206.

Olney, J.W., Rhee, V., and Ho, O.L., 1974, Kainic acid : a power-ful neurotoxic analogue of glutamate, Brain Res., 77:1777-1782.

Ondo, J.G., 1974, Gamma-aminobutyric acid effects on pituitary gonadotropin secretion. Science, 186:738-739.

Ondo, J.G., and Pass, K.A., 1976, The effects of neurally active amino acids on prolactin secretion, Endocrinology, 98, 1248.

Otsuka, M., Obata, K., Miyata, Y., and Tanaka, Y., 1971, Measure-ment of $\gamma$-aminobutyric acid in isolated nerve cells of cat central nervous system. J. Neurochem., 18:287-295.

Palkovits, M., Brownstein, M., Saavedra, J., and Axelrod, J., 1974, Norepinephrine and dopamine content of hypothalamic nuclei of the rat, Brain Res., 77:137-149.

Rassin, D.K., 1972, Amino acids as putative transmitters : Failure to bind to synaptic vesicles of guinea pig cerebral cortex. J. Neurochem. 19:139-148.

Ribak, C.E., Vaughn, J.E., Saito, K., Barber, R., and Roberts, E., 1976, Immunocytochemical localization of glutamate decarboxylase in rat substantia nigra, Brain Res., 116:287-298.

Ryall, R.W., 1964, The subcellular distribution of acetylcholine, substance P, 5-hydroxy tryptamine, gamma-aminobutyric acid and glutamic acid in brain homogenates. J. Neurochem. 11:131-145.

Saavedra, J.M., Brownstein, M., Palkovits, M., Kizer, J.S., and Axelrod, J., 1974, Tyrosine hydroxylase and dopamine-$\beta$-hydroxy-lase distribution in the individual rat hypothalamic nuclei. J. Neurochem. 23:869-871.

Salganicoff, L., and De Robertis, E., 1965, Subcellular distribu-tion of the enzyme of the glutamic acid, glutamine, and gamma-aminobutyric acid cycle in rat brain. J. Neurochem. 12:287-309.

Schally, A.V., Redding, T.W., Arimura A., Dupont, A., and Linthicum G.L., 1977, Isolation of gamma-amino butyric acid from pig hypo-thalami and demonstration of its prolactin release-inhibiting (PIF) activity in vivo and in vitro, Endocrinology, 100:681.

Schrier B.K., and Thompson, E.J., 1974, On the role of glial cells in the mammalian nervous system. Uptake, excretion, and meta-bolism of putative neurotransmitters by cultured glial tumor cells, J. Biol. Chem. 249:1769-1780.

Schwarcz, R., and Coyle, J.T., 1977, Striatal lesions with kainic acid : neurochemical characteristics, Brain Res., 122:235-249.

Sellström, A., and Hamberger, A., 1977, Potassium-stimulated gamma aminobutyric acid release from neurons and glia, Brain Res., 119:189-198.

Storm-Mathisen, J., 1972, Glutamate decarboxylase in the rat hippocampal region after lesions of the afferent fiber systems. Evidence that the enzyme is localized in intrinsic neurones. Brain Res., 40:215-235.

Storm-Mathisen, J., and Fonnum, F., 1971, Quantitative histochemistry of glutamate decarboxylase in the rat hippocampal region, J. Neurochem., 18:1105-1111.

Tappaz, M., and Brownstein, M., 1977, Origin of GAD-containing cells in discrete hypothalamic nuclei, Brain Res., (in press).

Tappaz, M., Brownstein, M.J., and Palkovits, M., 1976, Distribution of glutamate decarboxylase in discrete brain nuclei. Brain Res., 108:371-379.

Tappaz, M.L., Brownstein, M.J., and Kopin, I.J., 1977, Glutamate decarboxylase (GAD) and $\gamma$-aminobutyric acid (GABA) in discrete nuclei of hypothalamus and substantia nigra. Brain Res., 125: 109-121.

Weinstein, H., Roberts, E., and Kakefuda, T., 1963, Studies of subcellular distribution of gamma-aminobutyric acid and glutamic decarboxylase in mouse brain, Biochem. Pharmacol., 12:503-509.

Yagi, K., and Sawaki, Y., 1975, Recurrent inhibition and facilitation : demonstration in the tubero-infundebular system and effects of strychnine and picrotoxin, Brain Res., 84:155-159.

# IDENTIFIED <u>APLYSIA</u> NEURONS WITH RAPID AND SPECIFIC

# GLYCINE UPTAKE

C.H. Price, D.J. McAdoo, R.E. Coggeshall, and
T.M. Iliffe
Marine Biomedical Institute, Department of Human
Biochemistry and Genetics, and Department of Anatomy
University of Texas Medical Branch
Galveston, Texas 77550  USA

Glycine concentrations in individual cell bodies of the identified giant neurons R3-R14 in the parietovisceral ganglion of the mollusc <u>Aplysia californica</u> are up to 20 times higher than in neighboring neurons (Iliffe <u>et al</u>., 1977).  High concentrations of putative neurotransmitters are present in invertebrate neurons thought to use those compounds as transmitters (Otsuka <u>et al</u>., 1967; Rude <u>et al</u>., 1969; McCaman <u>et al</u>.; Weinreich <u>et al</u>., 1973). In vertebrates, relatively high concentrations of glycine are present in the ventral grey matter of the spinal cord (Aprison <u>et al</u>., 1975), where glycine is probably used as an inhibitory neurotransmitter by interneurons (Davidson, 1976; Johnston, 1976). Glycine may, therefore, be in high concentrations in R3-R14 for use as a neurotransmitter, particularly since other putative transmitters have not been found in these neurons (Cottrell, 1974; McCaman <u>et al</u>., 1976).

Because specific uptake systems for probable neurotransmitters frequently exist (Kuhar, 1973; Hökfelt and Ljungdahl, 1975; Iversen, 1975), we undertook a biochemical and autoradiographic study of glycine uptake into cell bodies of R3-R14 and other <u>Aplysia</u> neurons.

## MATERIALS AND METHODS

Ganglia were dissected from <u>Aplysia californica</u> (30 - 80 g) and incubated in artificial seawater solutions (room temp) containing labelled amino acids (8 - 20 $\mu$M; 0.1 Ci/mmol.).  Chemical agents were added to some incubation media.

For autoradiographic studies, ganglia were fixed in isotonic 3% glutaraldehyde, postfixed in 1% OsO₄, and dehydrated in a graded ethanol series. Ganglia were embedded in wax for 10 μm sections, or in plastic for thin (0.75 μm) and ultrathin sections. All sections were coated with Ilford L-4 emulsion and stored in the dark for 10 - 15 da at 4°C. Autoradiographs were developed at 17°C in Dektol and fixed in 25% hypo. Light microscope autoradiographs of unstained thin sections were photographed at 1000X mag for counting grains. Other sections were stained with methylene blue-azure A. EM autoradiographs were stained in lead citrate and examined in a Phillips 300 EM.

For biochemical analyses, ganglia incubated in ³H-glycine were fixed for 0.5 h and then immersed in chilled ethylene glycol-seawater. Individual cell bodies were identified on the basis of size, color, and location (Frazier et al., 1967) and dissected out intact. The major and minor axes of each cell were measured and cell volumes determined using the formula for an oblate spheroid. Individual cell bodies were placed in scintillation vials and dissolved in tissue solubilizer. Liquid phosphor and 0.5 ml glacial acetic acid were added and samples counted in a scintillation spectrometer.

## RESULTS AND DISCUSSION

Neurons R3-R14 were more intensely labelled than their neighbors in autoradiographs of ganglia incubated in ³H-glycine for several hours (Figure 1A). Grain counts were 3 - 4 times greater over R3-R14 than over other neurons in ganglia incubated for 1 h (Table I). No differences in uptake between R3-R14 and adjacent cells occurred in ³H-alanine, -serine, and -leucine incubations. Thus, R3-R14 take up glycine specifically and rapidly. Glia cells around R3-R14 did not preferentially take up any of the labelled amino acids.

Chemically determined ³H-glycine concentrations resulting from uptake were twice as high in R3-R14 as in other neurons (Table II). Tissue: medium ratios of radioactivity after a 1 h incubation reached 8:1 in R3-R14 and 4:1 in neighboring cells; after a 3 h incubation, these ratios increased to 17:1 and 8:1 respectively. We calculated from these results that glycine concentrations in the intact animal should reach 540 μM in R3-R14 and 250 μM in other neurons after 3 h, based on uptake from the hemolymph (32 μM in glycine). These concentrations represent 11% of the endogenous glycine found in R3-R14 and 25% of that found in other neurons (determined by gas chromatography-mass spectrometry; Iliffe et al., 1977). Extrapolation of the uptake curves from 3 h to 24 h indicates that the uptake systems of both R3-R14 and other neurons would supply the endogenous levels of glycine within 24 h.

TABLE I.   GRAIN COUNTS FROM LM AUTORADIOGRAPHS OF GANGLIA INCUBATED
IN $^3$H-GLYCINE AND OTHER $^3$H-AMINO ACIDS[a]

| Conditions | Grains/100 $\mu m^2$ cytoplasm area | | Ratio R3-R14 neighbors |
| --- | --- | --- | --- |
| | R3-R14 | neighboring cells | |
| $^3$H-Glycine | 128.4 ± 6.8[b] | 39.3 ± 4.1 | 3.3 |
| + formaldehyde fix | 63.9 ± 3.8 | 20.3 ± 2.6 | 3.2 |
| + Na$^+$ free media[c] | 44.1 ± 1.0 | 28.9 ± 1.9 | 1.5 |
| + HgCl$_2$(0.1 mM) | 12.5 ± 1.6 | 8.1 ± 2.0 | 1.6 |
| + reserpine(1.0 µg/ml) | 127.5 ± 4.2 | 40.1 ± 4.1 | 3.2 |
| + anisomycin(40 µg/ml) | 111.3 ± 6.0 | 37.8 ± 2.7 | 2.9 |
| $^3$H-Alanine | 14.9 ± 3.1 | 13.5 ± 1.1 | 1.1 |
| $^3$H-Serine | 31.7 ± 3.8 | 33.5 ± 4.5 | 0.9 |
| $^3$H-Leucine | 35.3 ± 8.1 | 42.7 ± 10.9 | 0.8 |

[a] standardized conditions: 8-20 µM $^3$H-amino acid (0.1 Ci/mmol), 1 h, 22°C, glutaraldehyde fix; [b] N ≥ 3 cells counted per condition, 5 counts per cell averaged, error limits ± SEM; [c] NaCl replaced by choline chloride.

TABLE II.   BIOCHEMICAL ANALYSES OF $^3$H-GLYCINE UPTAKE BY R3-R14 AND OTHER NEURONS

| Treatment | Cell body $^3$H-glycine concentrations (µM) | |
| --- | --- | --- |
| | R3-R14 | Other Neurons |
| Standard conditions[a] | 32 ± 5[b] | 16 ± 2 |
| Removal of Na$^+$ (5 min)[c] | 7 ± 2 | 11 ± 2 |
| HgCl$_2$ (0.1 mM; 5 min) | 14 ± 2 | 11 ± 2 |
| Ouabain (0.1 mM; 30 min) | 26 ± 4 | 13 ± 1 |
| 2,4-Dinitrophenol (1.0 mM; 30 min) | 32 ± 4 | 17 ± 3 |
| Low temp (4°C; 5 min) | 21 ± 6 | 10 ± 1 |

[a] 8.8 µM $^3$H-glycine, 1 h, 25°C; [b] each determination based on at least 10 cells of each type from at least 2 ganglia so treated, error limits ± SEM; [c] NaCl replaced by choline chloride.

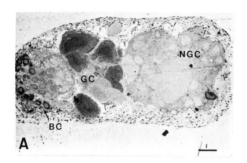 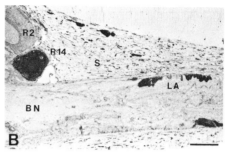

FIGURE 1.   Autoradiographs of ganglia in $^3$H-glycine (8.8 μM, 1 h).
Plastic sections (0.75 μm thick) exposed to emulsion
2 wk; dark areas are concentrations of developed silver
grains.  (A) Cross-section (lightly stained) showing 5
cell bodies of R3-R14 ("glycine cells", GC) and several
non-glycine cells (NGC).  Bag cells (BC) are also heavily
labelled.  (B) Unstained longitudinal section of caudal
portion of ganglia and branchial nerve (BN).  Glycine
cell R14 is heavily labelled as are 3 - 4 axons of
R3-R14 (LA).  Smaller neuronal processes (probably from
R3-R14) in the sheath (S) are also labelled.  Scale bars
300 μM.

Thin layer chromatographs demonstrated that less than 10% of
the radioactivity in R3-R14 from ganglia incubated in $^{14}$C-glycine
was in macromolecules after 1 h.  Thus, glycine does not appear to
undergo any special metabolic transformation, although some 25% of
the radioactivity in R3-R14 and most other neurons comigrated with
serine in TLC.  By contrast, the distribution of label in the neurosecretory "bag cells" of the ganglion was 50% macromolecular, 35%
glycine, and 15% serine.  This probably reflects the incorporation
of label into the polypeptide neurohormones synthesized by these
cells (Arch, 1972; Gainer and Wollberg, 1974).

In autoradiographs of ganglia incubated in $^3$H-glycine and fixed
in formaldehyde (a poor fixative for free amino acids; Peters and
Ashley, 1967), much of the label over R3-R14 was washed out when
compared with glutaraldehyde-fixed tissue (Table I).  The majority
of the label in the bag cells, however, remained in the cytoplasms
of those cells in both fixes.  Anisomycin, a potent protein synthesis inhibitor in Aplysia (Schwartz et al., 1971), eliminated the
numerous clusters of grains in the bag cell cytoplasms but did not
affect the high numbers of grains throughout R3-R14.  Thus, we are
confident that the major role for glycine in R3-R14 is not as a precursor for metabolic purposes.

Ratios of grain counts in the cytoplasm to those in the nucleus were near unity in the R3-R14 and neighboring neurons. Furthermore, grains were evenly distributed within the nuclear and cypoplasmic compartments. In electron microscope autoradiographs, we found no association of grains with any cellular component, including the dense-core granules that are characteristic of R3-R14 (Coggeshall, 1967). This may be due to the diffusion of free glycine during fixation; however, this lack of apparent localization parallels findings in studies of amino acid neurotransmitters in vertebrates (De Belleroche and Bradford, 1973; Hall et al., 1974).

The major processes of R3-R14, which travel down the branchial nerve, become intensely labelled when left attached to ganglia incubated in $^3$H-glycine (Figure 1B). If the branchial nerve is severed from the ganglia and incubated in $^3$H-glycine, the axons still label strongly, suggesting rapid transport across axonal membranes. Significant amounts of labelled glycine are also transported from the cell bodies of R3-R14 and down their axons, as demonstrated in autoradiographs of branchial nerves attached to, but isolated from, ganglia incubated in $^3$H-glycine.

Since tissue: media concentration ratios well above 1 for $^3$H-glycine are reached quickly in all Aplysia neurons, glycine must be taken up by active processes by all neurons. Replacement of the Na$^+$ in incubation media with choline had a relatively slight effect on neurons other than R3-R14; uptake of glycine in R3-R14, however, was reduced to approximately the level of all other neurons (Tables I and II). The presence of Hg$^{++}$ also eliminated the difference between R3-R14 and other neurons (Tables I and II). Ouabain, a sodium pump inhibitor, had little effect on uptake into any neurons, even after preincubations in the agent for 1 h. We conclude from these results that there is a glycine uptake system common to all Aplysia neurons and a special system unique to R3-R14. This R3-R14 system depends on the presence of a sodium gradient, but not directly on the activity of the Na$^+$ pump.

The rapid and selective uptake of glycine by neurons R3-R14 and their usually high endogenous glycine concentrations suggest that glycine may be used as a neurotransmitter substance by these cells. The advantage of working with single, identifiable cells mitigates many of the problems associated with vertebrate preparations (e.g., the heterogeneity of tissues in brain slices and the difficulty of achieving intact and clean synaptosome fractions). We are now searching for the terminals of R3-R14 to develop a single cell-effector tissue system that may help satisfy the criteria (e.g., Werman, 1966) needed to fully establish glycine as a neurotransmitter.

This work was supported by USPHS grants NS 12567 to DJM and NS 11255 and NS 10161 to REC.

## REFERENCES

Aprison, M.H., Daly, E.C., Shank, R.P., and McBride, W.J., 1975, Neurochemical evidence for glycine as a transmitter and a model for its intrasynaptosomal compartmentation, in "Metabolic Compartmentation and Neurotransmission" (S. Berl, D.D. Clark, and D. Schneider, eds.), pp. 37-64, Plenum, New York.

Arch, S., 1972, Polypeptide secretion from the isolated parieto-visceral ganglion of Aplysia californica, J. Gen. Physiol., 59:47-59.

Coggeshall, R.E., 1967, A light and electron microscope study of the abdominal ganglion of Aplysia californica, J. Neurochem., 22:557-559.

Cottrell, G.A., 1974, Serotonin and free amino acid analysis of ganglia and isolated neurones of Aplysia dactylomella, J. Neurochem., 22:557-559.

Davidson, N., 1976, "Neurotransmitter Amino Acids," Academic, pp. 39-56, New York.

De Belleroche, J.S. and Bradford, H.F., 1973, Amino acids in synaptic vesicles from mammalian cerebral cortex: A reappraisal, J. Neurochem., 21:441-451.

Frazier, W.T., Kandel, E.R., Kupferman, I., Waziri, R., and Coggeshall, R.E., 1967, Morphological and functional properties of identified neurons in the abdominal ganglion of Aplysia californica, J. Neurophysiol., 30:1288-1351.

Gainer, H. and Wollberg, Z., 1974, Specific protein metabolism in identifiable neurons of Aplysia californica, J. Neurobiol., 5:243-261.

Hall, Z.W., Hildebrand, J.G., and Kravitz, E.A., 1974, "Chemistry of Synaptic Transmission," p.168, Chiron Press, Newton, Masachusetts.

Hökfelt, T. and Ljungdahl, Å., 1975, Uptake mechanisms as a basis for the histochemical identification and tracing of transmitter specific neuron populations, in "The Use of Axonal Transport for Studies of Neuronal Connectivity," (W.M. Cowan and M. Cuénod, eds.), pp. 249-306, Elsevier, New York.

Iliffe, T.M., McAdoo, D.J., Beyer, C.B., and Haber, B., 1977, Amino acid concentrations in Aplysia nervous system: neurons with high glycine concentrations, J. Neurochem. 28: 1037-1042.

Iversen, L.L., Dick, R.F., Kelly, J.S., and Schon, F., 1975, Uptake and localization of transmitter amino acids in the nervous system, in "Metabolic Compartmentation and Neurotransmission," (S. Berl, D.D. Clarke, and D. Schneider, eds.), pp. 65-90, Plenum, New York.

Johnston, G.A.R., 1976, Amino acid inhibitory transmitters in the mammalian nervous system, in "Chemical Transmission in the Mammalian Central Nervous System," (C.H. Hockman and D. Bieger, eds.), pp. 31-81, University Park Press, Baltimore.

Kuhar, M.J., 1973, Neurotransmitter uptake: A tool in identifying
    neurotransmitter-specific pathways, Life Sciences, 13:
    1623-1634.

McCaman, R.E. and McCaman, M.W., 1976, Biology of individual
    cholinergic neurons in the invertebrate CNS, in "Biology of
    Cholinergic Function," (A.M. Goldberg and I. Hanin, eds.),
    pp. 485-513, Raven Press, New York.

Otsuka, M., Kravitz, E.A., and Potter, D.D., 1974, Physiological
    and chemical architecture of a lobster ganglion with part-
    icular reference to gamma-aminobutyrate and glutamate, in
    "Chemistry of Synaptic Transmission", (Z.W. Hall, J.G.
    Hildebrand, and E.A. Kravitz, eds.), pp. 183-210, Chiron
    Press, Newton, Massachusetts.

Peters, T., Jr. and Ashley, C.A., 1967, An artefact in radioauto-
    graphy due to binding of free amino acids to tissues by
    fixatives, J. Cell Biol., 33:53-60.

Rude, S., Coggeshall, R.E., and Van Orden, L.S. III, 1969,
    Chemical and ultrastructural identification of 5-hydroxy-
    tryptamine in an identified neuron, J. Cell Biol., 41:832-854.

Schwartz, H.J., Castellucci, V.F., and Kandel, E.R., 1971,
    Functioning of identified neurons and synapses in abdominal
    ganglion of Aplysia in absence of protein synthesis, J.
    Neurophysiol., 34:939-953.

Werman, R., 1966, A review - criteria for identification of a
    central nervous system transmitter, Comp. Biochem. Physiol.,
    18:745-766.

Weinreich, D., McCaman, M.W., McCaman, R.E., and Vaughn, J.E.,
    1973, Chemical, enzymatic and ultrastructural character-
    ization of 5-hydroxytryptamine-containing neurons from the
    ganglia of Aplysia californica and Tritonia diomedia,
    J. Neurochem., 20:969-976.

# NEUROTRANSMITTERS IN THE AVIAN VISUAL SYSTEM

M. Cuénod and H. Henke

Institute for Brain Research
University of Zurich
CH-8029 Zurich / Switzerland

Increasing evidence that amino acids are involved in
chemical synaptic transmission has been obtained by
subjecting them to the criteria established for neurotransmitters like acetylcholine and the catecholamines.
Their concentration relative to other regions of the
nervous system should be high, their synthetizing
enzyme(s) must show a high activity and the nerve endings
should possess a selective high affinity uptake mechanism.
All those presynaptic characteristics would then diminish
or disappear when the terminals degenerate following a
lesion of the afferent neuron or axon. Further, the transmitter candidate should be released from the nerve terminals, either through the effect of high $K^+$ concentration
or drugs like veratridine, or through electrical stimulation, diffuse or, better, applied to the corresponding
afferent pathway. Microiontophoretic application of the
amino acid should mimic the effect of the physiological
synaptic action of the transmitter on the postsynaptic
element and specific antagonists should prevent this
action. This implies the presence of specific postsynaptic receptors, and transmitters and antagonists should
bind to the receptors. Ideally these characteristics
should allow a localization of specific pre- or postsynaptic elements at the light and electron microscopic
levels using either autoradiography or immunohistochemistry. The amino acids are limited in this respect, by
some difficulties not present with the more classical

221

transmitters. They and their synthetizing enzymes usually
are present not only as a 'transmitter' pool but also as
a 'metabolic' pool. Neither the pools nor their respective enzymes can be isolated separately at the moment.
An exception is GABA where only a transmitter pool is
present so that GAD can be used as a marker enzyme.
While some postsynaptic receptors can be blocked by
rather specific antagonists, like bicuculline for the
GABA-receptor or strychnine for the glycine-receptor,
others must still be studied without this very useful
tool.

     This paper reviews evidence for some amino acids
possibly involved in synaptic transmission in the pigeon
optic tectum. The visual system of the bird is highly
developed and occupies a large part of a relatively small
central nervous system. The retinal ganglion cells project almost exclusively to the contralateral meso-dience-
phalon so that lesion or injection can be made on one
side leaving the other as control. The tectum, which is
a laminated structure, lends itself easely to anatomical
separation as well as to subcellular fractionation in
order to obtain synaptosomes. (For morphological details,
see Cajal, 1891; Karten, 1969; Nauta and Karten, 1970;
Repérant, 1973; Meier et al., 1974; Webster, 1974; Hunt
and Webster, 1975; Hunt and Künzle, 1976 a+b; Streit and
Reubi, 1977;  Cuénod and Streit, 1978.)

## HIGH AFFINITY UPTAKE OF PUTATIVE TRANSMITTERS
## IN THE AVIAN OPTIC TECTUM

     The presence of a sodium dependent high affinity
uptake mechanism in subcellular fractions enriched in
synaptosomes for a given substance has been shown to
correlate with a transmitter function of this substance,
as established by electrophysiological, pharmacological
and histochemical methods (Iversen, 1971; Logan and
Snyder, 1971; Snyder et al., 1973). It was then suggested
that such a selective mechanism is responsible for the
termination of transmitter action and the restauration
of the presynaptic pool. Henke et al. (1976a) and Henke
and Cuénod (1978) have investigated the uptake of various
putative transmitters in synaptosome containing fractions
of the pigeon optic tectum. Both high and low affinity
uptake have been observed for L-alanine, L-aspartate,

TABLE I. High affinity uptake in pigeon optic tectum

| Substrate | $K_T$ µM | $V_{max}$ nmol/mg prot /3 min |
|---|---|---|
| Alanine | 18.6 ± 9.3 | 0.3 |
| Aspartate | 6.4 ± 1.2 | 17.8 |
| Choline | 36.4 ± 4.8 | 2.0 |
| GABA | 19.1 ± 7.9 | 26.5 |
| Glutamate | 9.7 ± 1.3 | 18.9 |
| Glycine | 32.7 ± 10.0 | 4.5 |
| Proline | 41.0 ± 11.0 | 4.9 |
| Serine | 14.2 ± 7.4 | 0.5 |
| Serotonine | 39.0 ± 12.0 | 0.7 |
| Dopamine | - | - |
| Leucine | - | - |
| Taurine | - | - |

(from Henke et al., 1976a; Henke and Cuénod, 1978)

choline, GABA, L-glutamate, L-glycine, L-proline, L-serine and serotonine. In contrast, dopamine, a well established neurotransmitter, and L-leucine, an amino acid for which no indication of a transmitter function is available, were taken up by low affinity systems only (Table I). The high affinity uptake was strictly sodium and temperature dependent. That the substances taken up were trapped in organelles and not bound to membranes is indicated by the fact that 95% of the label was released by osmotic shock. In sucrose gradients, the organelles loaded by the uptake systems migrated to the density characteristic of synaptosomes, so that they might be the site of uptake, although contribution of other compartments cannot be excluded. The organelles loaded at one concentration always equilibrated at the same density irrespective of the substrate used, but the density equilibrium was systematically higher after incubation in higher concentration of any substrate. Beart (1976) observed high affinity uptake of glutamate and noradrenaline in synaptosomal fractions of pigeon optic tectum, and Bondy and Purdy (1977a), using the chick optic lobe, obtained results essentially similar to the one reported above.

In conclusion, acetylcholine, aspartate, GABA, glutamate, glycine, noradrenaline and serotonine could be involved in synaptic transmission in the avian optic tectum. For proline, Felix and Künzle (1976) have suggested an inhibitory transmitter function based on evidence obtained in the cerebellar cortex.

## L-GLUTAMATE AND THE RETINO-TECTAL PATHWAY

For their survival, the nerve terminals are entirely dependent on material provided by the cell body and migrating by axoplasmic transport. When they are severed from their cell body, they degenerate with a time course which varies from system to system. Therefore, when a pathway degenerates, the transmitter pool, its metabolic enzymes and the high affinity uptake mechanisms located in the terminals should finally disappear. This approach has been used with success in many systems, for instance in the hippocampus (Storm-Mathisen and Guldberg, 1974; Storm-Mathisen, 1977) and in the cortico-caudate pathway (Divac et al., 1977). After removal of the retina in the pigeon, the optic nerve terminals degenerate within 4 to 8 weeks (Cuénod et al., 1970). Henke et al. (1976b) observed that at the same time the high affinity uptake in the whole tectum when compared to the undegenerated control side, was decreased by 60% for glutamate, 21% for GABA, and 14% for proline, while it was increased by 18% for glycine and 25% for choline (Fig. 1). The decrease of glutamate uptake was due to a reduction of the $V_{max}$ and not to an alteration of the $K_T$. This indicates a decrease in the capacity of the uptake compartment rather than a modification of the uptake system. These observations were confirmed by Bondy and Purdy (1977b) in the chick, 3 weeks after enucleation. However, Beart (1976) failed to detect any change in the glutamate level and high affinity uptake in the pigeon optic tectum 7 days after retinal ablation. It seems thus that in the pigeon retino-tectal pathway the change in glutamate high affinity uptake appears only after degeneration times longer than those required in other systems. This variability is consistent with the known variability in survival time needed for the appearance of morphological degenerative changes.

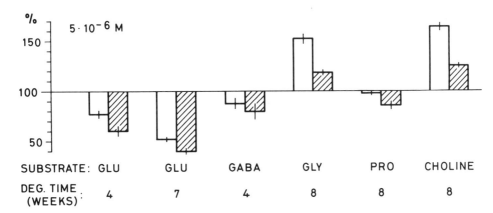

FIGURE 1. Effect of optic nerve degeneration on high
affinity uptake in tectal $P_2$ fractions. Incubation at
$5.10^{-6}$ M substrate concentration. Results expressed in
percent of control values referred to mg protein (white
columns) or to total tectum (hatched columns).
(from Henke et al., 1976b)

After retinal ablation, Henke and Fonnum (unpublished observations) observed a 20% decrease in the
glutamate pool of the tectal layers containing the optic
nerve terminal but no change in the deeper layers (Fig.2).
The concentration of aspartate was not significantly
affected by optic nerve degeneration. In the frog optic
tectum, enucleation induces within 14 to 24 days a 30%
decrease in the concentration of glutamate and a 20 to
40% decrease in that of GABA (Yates and Roberts, 1974).
In the pigeon optic lobe, cholineacetyltransferase
(ChAT) and glutamic acid decarboxylase (GAD) have different activities in the individual tectal layers (Fig.3).
Whereas Henke and Fonnum (1976) did not observe any
significant changes in these activities after retinal
ablation, a decrease of 5 - 20% for ChAT and 12% for GAD
was reported by others (Chakrabarti et al., 1974; Chakrabarti and Daginawala, 1976).

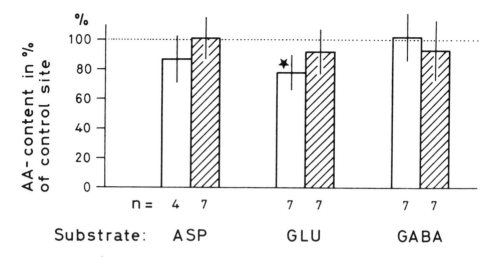

FIGURE 2. Effect of optic nerve degeneration (1-3 months)
on amino acid content in tectal layers. Layers 4-7 (white
columns) contain optic nerve terminals, while layers
8-12 (hatched columns) do not.
* $0.01<P<0.05$. (Henke and Fonnum, unpublished)

Thus in submammalian vertebrates, degeneration of
the optic nerve fibers and terminals is accompanied by
a marked decrease in the high affinity uptake and level
of glutamate as well as, to a lesser extent, of GABA.
Because the time course of degeneration is slower in the
pigeon retino-tectal neurons than in other vertebrate
systems, it is difficult to decide if the biochemical
changes are related to this primary degeneration or to
secondary, transneuronal consequences of it. Both interpretations are possible. It is tempting to speculate that
glutamate is or mimics the physiological excitatory transmitter of at least part of the avian optic nerve fibers.
While it cannot be excluded that a population of these
fibers are using GABA as transmitter, transneuronal
effects of optic nerve degeneration could explain most
of the GABA uptake decrease. Histochemically, at least
three types of neurons seem to have a selective affinity
for GABA (Hunt and Künzle, 1976b).

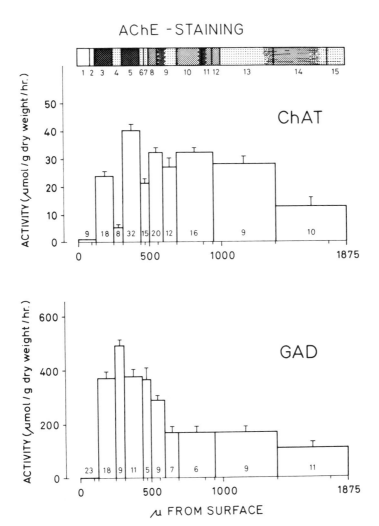

FIGURE 3. Distribution of ChAT and GAD in the tectal layers, as indicated at the top (1-15) of the pigeon optic tectum.
(from Henke and Fonnum, 1976)

Further clues on the exact localization of the glutamate uptake compartment which disappears after optic nerve degeneration could be obtained by double labelling experiment. The optic nerve terminals can be labelled by axoplasmic transport of proteins following intraocular injection of radioactive amino acids (Schonbach et al., 1971; Cuénod and Schonbach, 1971). When tectal crude mitochondrial fractions containing $^{14}C$ labelled optic nerve synaptosomes are incubated at $10^{-6}$ M concentration of $^3H$-glutamate, the two isotopes overlap perfectly in that region of sucrose density gradients which is richest in synaptosomes (Henke et al., 1976b). This indicates that glutamate is taken up with high affinity by organelles having the same sedimentation characteristics as the optic nerve synaptosomes. Beart (1976) obtained EM autoradiographic evidence that synaptosomes accumulating glutamate might belong to a retino-tectal population.

Felix and Frangi (1977) showed that microiontophoretic application of glutamate and aspartate activates a large number of tectal neurons, an effect which was antagonized by L-nuciferine. Furthermore, Felix (personal communication) observed that unit activity evoked in the optic tectum by electrical stimulation of the optic nerve is abolished by microiontophoretic application of L-nuciferine, but not of atropine or dihydro-β-erythroidine. As L-nuciferine blocks the excitatory effects of glutamate, and to a lesser degree of aspartate (Felix and Frangi, 1977), these observations support the hypothesis that glutamate is or mimics an excitatory transmitter in at least some of the retino-tectal fibers. An indication of their localisation comes from the observation that incubating tectal slices in $^3H$-glutamate leads to labelling of sublayers 4/IIc and 7/IIf, but less to 5/IId all of them containing optic nerve terminals (Hunt, personal communication; Streit, unpublished results).

In conclusion biochemical, physiological, pharmacological and histochemical evidence favors glutamate, or a substance acting like it, as an excitatory transmitter in the avian retino-tectal pathway. It is, however, most likely that different transmitters are used by various fiber types.

## GLYCINE, SERINE, ALANINE AND THE NUCLEUS ISTHMI

As mentioned above, glycine, L-serine and L-alanine are taken up by sodium dependent high affinity systems in tectal synaptosomal fractions (Henke et al., 1976a; Henke and Cuénod, 1978). Thirty minutes after injection of either tritiated glycine, serine or alanine into the lateral part of the optic tectum, autoradiographs of the optic lobe reveal an intense labelling of the perikarya in the nucleus isthmi, pars parvocellularis (Ipc) (Hunt et al., 1977) (Fig. 4). This nucleus has a reciprocal connection with the optic tectum from which it is about 4 mm apart (Cajal, 1899; Hunt and Künzle, 1976a; Hunt et al., 1977). In contrast, injection of many other amino acids labels only the Ipc neuropile, but not the cell bodies, as would be expected from an anterograde transport in the tecto-Ipc neurons. The perikaryal labelling of the nucleus Ipc after intratectal injection of [3]H-glycine, [3]H-serine or [3]H-alanine seems to be due to a retrograde, somatopetal migration of the radioactivity taken up in the zone of termination of the Ipc-tectal neurons. This interpretation is supported by the observation that the injection area must include this zone of termination in order to obtain a labelling of the Ipc perikarya (Hunt et al., 1977). The grain density over axons, perikarya and neuropile is much higher when the brains are perfused with glutaraldehyde than with formaldehyde, suggesting that the majority of the radioactivity is present in a soluble form (Fig. 4). In addition, retrograde migration of [3]H-GABA has been observed in two different types of tectal neurons (Hunt et al., 1977; Hunt and Künzle, 1976b; Cuénod and Streit, 1978).

Could these observations indicate that glycine, serine and alanine function as synaptic transmitters in some Ipc-tectal neurons, that they are taken up into specific nerve terminals and migrate towards the cell bodies? For glycine, there is evidence that specific receptors exist in the optic tectum: first, microiontophoretic application of glycine induces a strychnine sensitive inhibition of tectal neurons (Barth and Felix, 1974) and second, strychnine binding receptors have been observed in tectal membranes (Zukin et al., 1976; Le Fort et al., 1978). Exogenous glycine is released in the tectum by electrical stimulation of Ipc (Reubi and

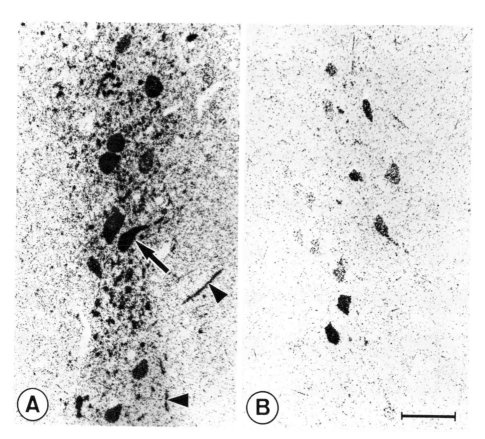

FIGURE 4. Lightfield autoradiographs of part of the
nucleus isthmi, pars parvocellularis (Ipc) following
injections of $^3$H-glycine (50 µCi in 0.2 µl during
10 min.) into the lateral tectum. A: Some heavily
labelled perikarya, one with fibrous processes (arrow),
are situated in a limited field of labelled neuropile.
Note labelled fibers (arrow-heads) in the space between
tectum and Ipc. 5% glutaraldehyde perfusion 20 min.
after injection. 1 µm Epon section. B: After perfusion
with 4% formaldehyde only the perikarya but no fibrous
elements are slightly outlined by silver grains (arrows).
Same amount of $^3$H-glycine injected and same survival and
injection time as in A. 1 µm Epon section. Scale 50 µm.
(Courtesy of P. Streit)

Cuénod, 1976). Thus glycine could be or mimics a transmitter within the Ipc-tectal pathway.

What is then the role of serine and alanine? Are
they part of a system having affinity for all three
amino acids, or are they independent of each other?
It is known that the low affinity uptake system is unspecific and takes up all small aliphatic neutral amino
acids (Blasberg, 1968), and it should also be remembered
that serine is the precursor of glycine (Aprison et al.,
1975). The distribution of the three amino acids high
affinity uptake, their interaction and the effects of
various inhibitors have been investigated (Henke and
Cuénod, 1978). (1) As can be seen in Table II, the $K_T$
for each amino acid is practically the same in the spinal
cord, the tectum and the telencephalon, suggesting a
single mechanism. However, the capacities of the systems,
as expressed by the $V_{max}$, are quite different. For glycine, the uptake capacity in spinal cord is approximately
3-4 times higher than in the tectum while no high affinity uptake was found in the telencephalon. This has
already been described for the rat (Logan and Snyder,
1971). The capacities for alanine and serine were lower
than for glycine and their $V_{max}$ distribution opposite:
highest in the telencephalon, lower in the tectum and
lowest in the spinal cord (Table II). (2) The mutual inhibition of uptake for all three amino acids was typically competitive, with one exception: Glycine uptake
was inhibited by serine and alanine in a complex and incomplete way (Fig. 5). (3) L-alanine, L-cysteine,
D-serine and L-serine inhibited the uptake of alanine
and serine equally and much stronger than that of glycine,
in contrast to betaine, glycine, imipramine and sarcosine
which affected glycine uptake more than the serine or
alanine ones (Table III). These observations could be
explained by assuming the existence of two different
compartments, a 'classical' one for glycine only and
another one, which has affinity for serine, alanine and
possibly glycine. In the spinal cord, only the glycine
specific compartment can be detected, in the telencephalon
the serine-alanine-glycine compartment is present and
both are found in the tectum.

TABLE II. KINETIC PARAMETERS OF L-ALANINE, GLYCINE AND L-SERINE UPTAKE BY P$_2$-FRACTIONS FROM PIGEON TELENCEPHALON, TECTUM AND SPINAL CORD

Kinetic parameters of L-alanine, glycine and L-serine uptake by P$_2$-fractions from the pigeon telencephalon, tectum and spinal cord. The uptake of the amino acids was measured as described in Methods. The kinetic constants were calculated according to the formulas given in the legend of Fig. 1, the number in parenthesis indicates the number of points used for calculation in the high (5-50 μM) and low (100-1000 μM) range respectively.

| | $K_T$ (μM) | | | $V_{max}$ (nmols/mg prot./3 min) | | |
| | Telencephalon | Tectum | Spinal cord | Telencephalon | Tectum | Spinal cord |
|---|---|---|---|---|---|---|
| L-alanine | 44.7 ± 21.7 (8) | 18.6 ± 9.3 (8) | 14.6 ± 4.7 (8) | 1.12 ± 0.9 | 0.26 ± 0.22 | 0.18 ± 0.20 |
| | 2210 ± 923 (8) | 1398 ± 701 (8) | 2099 ± 682 (8) | 30.2 ± 8.1 | 25.4 ± 4.2 | 5.28 ± 2.3 |
| Glycine | --- | 32.7 ± 10.2 (36) | 32.4 ± 7.9 (12) | --- | 4.49 ± 1.5 | 6.82 ± 2.7 |
| | 351 ± 70 (8) | 446 ± 220 (8) | 479 ± 189 (8) | 15.3 ± 1.5 | 13.0 ± 1.2 | 12.6 ± 3.2 |
| L-serine | 11.0 ± 2.3 (16) | 14.2 ± 7.4 (66) | 14.2 ± 6.5 (16) | 0.64 ± 0.08 | 0.48 ± 0.18 | 0.065 ± 0.04 |
| | 2224 ± 889 (8) | 2785 ± 637 (8) | 2700 ± 844 (8) | 16.8 ± 4.9 | 28.9 ± 17.1 | 3.9 ± 2.1 |

(from Henke and Cuénod, 1978)

TABLE III. EFFECT OF VARIOUS CHEMICALS ON THE UPTAKE OF L-ALANINE,
GLYCINE AND L-SERINE

The substances were added simultaneously with the amino acid, the substrate
concentration was $10^{-5}$M. Results are means $\pm$ S.E.M. for four determinations
of uptake under standard conditions. Values are listed only if different
from controls at $P < 0.05$. N.S. means not significantly different from
control.

| Substance | concentration | uptake in % of control ($10^{-5}$M) | | |
|---|---|---|---|---|
| | | alanine | glycine | serine |
| L-alanine | $10^{-3}$ | 30 $\pm$ 4 | 68 $\pm$ 7 | 17 $\pm$ 0 |
| L-cysteine | $10^{-3}$ | 17 $\pm$ 8 | 59 $\pm$ 5 | 13 $\pm$ 2 |
| L-serine | $10^{-3}$ | 30 $\pm$ 2 | N.S. | 31 $\pm$ 6 |
| D-serine | $10^{-3}$ | 42 $\pm$ 7 | 75 $\pm$ 10 | 27 $\pm$ 3 |
| Glycine | $10^{-3}$ | 58 $\pm$ 8 | 17 $\pm$ 4 | 50 $\pm$ 2 |
| Betaine | $10^{-3}$ | N.S. | 68 $\pm$ 4 | N.S. |
| Sarcosine | $10^{-3}$ | N.S. | 15 $\pm$ 4 | N.S. |
| Imipramine | $10^{-4}$ | N.S. | 60 $\pm$ 2 | N.S. |
| β-alanine | $10^{-3}$ | N.S. | 63 $\pm$ 15 | 79 $\pm$ 2 |
| D-alanine | $10^{-3}$ | 70 $\pm$ 3 | 61 $\pm$ 6 | 65 $\pm$ 10 |
| Apamine | $10^{-4}$ | 63 $\pm$ 2 | 37 $\pm$ 4 | 40 $\pm$ 2 |
| p-chloromercuri-<br>sulfonic acid | $10^{-4}$ | 18 $\pm$ 6 | 0 | 0 |
| L-cysteic acid | $10^{-3}$ | 68 $\pm$ 12 | 74 $\pm$ 1 | 76 $\pm$ 3 |
| Juglone | $10^{-4}$ | 6 $\pm$ 11 | 7 $\pm$ 2 | 8 $\pm$ 6 |
| Ouabain | $10^{-4}$ | 33 $\pm$ 7 | 66 $\pm$ 5 | 65 $\pm$ 5 |

No significant effect had:  GABA, taurine, cholinbromide, ethanolamine,
lactate, pyrurate, hydroxypyrurate, 3-P-hydroxypyrurate, D-phospho-L-serine,
sodium acetate, glycylglycine hydrochloride, glycyl-L-serine, glycyl-L-ala-
nine, L-seryl-L-alanine, L-seryl-L-alanine, L-seryl-glycine, strychnine
and tetanus toxine.

(from Henke and Cuénod, 1978)

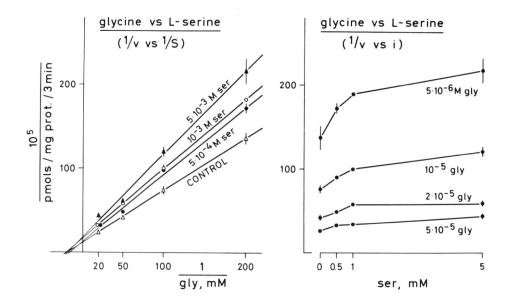

FIGURE 5. Inhibition of glycine uptake by L-serine
(similar pattern for L-alanine, not shown).
(from Henke and Cuénod, 1978)


Le Fort et al. (1978) have shown the presence of
glycine specific strychnine binding to tectal membranes,
using the technique described by Young and Snyder (1973)
(Table IV). This indicates the existence of glycine
receptors in the tectum, having the same $K_D$ than in
the spinal cord. The demonstration of glycine sensitive
strychnine binding in the telencephalon and even in the
cerebellum suggests that these areas contain some glycinergic terminals too. Their number, however, must be small
since no high affinity uptake was measured in the telencephalon (Table II). The superimposed ubiquitous low
affinity uptake prevents measurements of high affinity
uptake systems with small capacities. That the glycine
sensitive strychnine binding in the telencephalon is not
connected to the serine, alanine, glycine system is indicated by the finding that serine is not more potent
here in displacing bound strychnine than it is in the
spinal cord.

TABLE IV. Affinity constants ($K_D$) and maximal binding values ($B_{max}$) of glycine sensitive [3]H-strychnine binding in the pigeon CNS (Le Fort et al., 1978)

| CNS-region | $K_D$ (nM) | $B_{max}$ (fmols/mg prot.) |
|---|---|---|
| Telencephalon | 2.3 ± 0.9 | 92 ± 34 |
| Tectum | 5.0 ± 3.2 | 275 ± 42 |
| Cerebellum | 6.0 ± 4.0 | 20 ± 11 |
| Spinal cord | 5.0 ± 1.4 | 1000 ± 180 |

As previously mentioned, optic nerve degeneration results in a 18% increase of glycine high affinity uptake (Fig. 1). In contrast, a 20% decrease in the glycine specific strychnine binding was observed after retinal ablation (Le Fort et al., 1978). These observations are difficult to interprete at the moment. However, they could be explained by assuming a degeneration of glycinoceptive neurons followed by a sprouting of glycinergic terminals.

SUMMARY

This review presents an attempt to study the relevance of some amino acids as transmitters in the avian visual system. Emphasis has been given, whenever possible, to obtain quantitative estimates of pre- and postsynaptic elements as well as information on their histochemical localization (Cuénod and Streit, 1978). Evidence has been given that glutamate may be the excitatory transmitter in some retino-tectal fibers and that glycine and GABA are involved in tectal inhibition. The existence of an uptake system with high affinity for serine, alanine and possibly glycine has been demonstrated in telencephalon, tectum and spinal cord.

ACKNOWLEDGEMENT

The authors are grateful to Dr. P. Streit for valuable advice and to J. Gubler, M. Jäckli, D. Savini and E. Schneider for excellent technical assistance.

This work was supported by Grants 3.744.76 and 3.636.75 from the Swiss National Science Foundation, the Dr. Eric Slack-Gyr Foundation, the Emil Barrel Foundation and 'Stiftung für wissenschaftliche Forschung der Universität Zürich'.

REFERENCES

Aprison, M.H., Daly, E.C., Shank, R.P., and McBride, W.J., 1976, Neurochemical evidence for glycine as a transmitter and a model for its intrasynaptosomal compartmentation, in "Metabolic Compartmentation and Neurotransmission", (S. Berl, D.D. Clarke and D. Schneider, eds.), pp. 37-63, Plenum Press, New York.

Barth, R., and Felix, D., 1974, Influence of GABA and glycine and their antagonists on inhibitory mechanisms of pigeon's optic tectum, Brain Res. 80: 532-537.

Beart, P.M., 1976, An evaluation of L-glutamate as the transmitter released from optic nerve terminals of the pigeon, Brain Res. 110:99-114.

Blasberg, R.G., 1968, Specificity of cerebral amino acid transport: a kinetic analysis, in "Brain Barrier Systems", Progress in Brain Research, Vol. 29 (A. Lajtha and D.H. Ford, eds.), pp. 245-256, Elsevier, Amsterdam.

Bondy, S.C., and Purdy, J.L., 1977a, Development of neurotransmitter uptake in regions of the chick brain, Brain Res. 119:403-416.

Bondy, S.C., and Purdy, J.L., 1977b, Putative neurotransmitters of the avian visual pathway. Brain Res. 119:417-426.

Cajal, S.R., 1891, Sur la fine structure du lobe optique des oiseaux et sur l'origine réelle des nerfs optiques, Int.Mschr.Anat.Physiol. 8:337-366.

Cajal, S.R., 1899, Adiciones a nuestros trabajos sobre los centros ópticos de las aves, Rev.trimest. Microgr. 4:77-86.

Chakrabarti, T., and Daginawala, H.F., 1976, Effect of
    unilateral visual deprivation and visual stimulation
    on the activities of glutamate decarboxylase,
    GABA-α ketoglutarate transaminase, aspartate
    aminotransferase and hexokinase of the optic lobe
    of the adult pigeon, J.Neurochem. 27:273-276.
Chakrabarti, T., Dias, P.D., Roychowdhury, D., and
    Daginawala, H.F., 1974, Effect of unilateral
    visual deprivation on the activities of acetyl-
    cholinesterase, cholinesterase and carbonic
    anhydrase of the optic lobe of pigeon. J.Neurochem.
    22:865-867.
Cuénod, M., Sandri, C., and Akert, K., 1970, Enlarged
    synaptic vesicles as an early sign of secondary
    degeneration in the optic nerve terminals of the
    pigeon, J.Cell Sci. 6:605-613.
Cuénod, M., and Schonbach, J., 1971, Synaptic proteins
    and axonal flow in the pigeon visual pathway,
    J.Neurochem. 18:809-816.
Cuénod, M., and Streit, P., 1978, Amino acid transmitters
    and local circuitry in optic tectum, in "The Neuro-
    sciences: Fourth Study Program" (F.O. Schmitt and
    F.G. Worden, eds.), MIT Press, Cambridge, Mass.
    and London.
Divac, I., Fonnum, F., and Storm-Mathisen, J., 1977,
    High affinity uptake of glutamate in terminals of
    corticostriatal axons, Nature 266:377-378.
Felix, D., and Frangi, U., 1977, Dimethoxyaporphine as
    an antagonist of chemical excitation in the pigeon
    optic tectum. Neuroscience Letters 4:347-350.
Felix, D., and Künzle, H., 1976, The role of proline in
    nervous transmission, Adv.Biochem.Psychopharm.
    15:165-173.
Henke, H., and Cuénod, M., 1978, Uptake of L-alanine,
    glycine and L-serine in the pigeon central nervous
    system, submitted.
Henke, H., and Fonnum, F., 1976, Topographical and sub-
    cellular distribution of choline acetyltransferase
    and glutamate decarboxylase in pigeon optic tectum,
    J.Neurochem. 27:387-391.
Henke, H., Schenker, T.M., and Cuénod, M., 1976a,
    Uptake of neurotransmitter candidates by pigeon
    optic tectum, J.Neurochem. 26:125-130.

Henke, H., Schenker, T.M., and Cuénod, M., 1976b,
    Effects of retinal ablation on uptake of gluta-
    mate, glycine, GABA, proline and choline in pigeon
    tectum, J.Neurochem. 26:131-134.

Hunt, S.P., and Künzle, H., 1976a, Observations on the
    projections and intrinsic organization of the
    pigeon optic tectum: An autoradiographic study
    based on anterograde and retrograde, axonal and
    dendritic flow, J.Comp.Neur. 17:153-172.

Hunt, S.P., and Künzle, H., 1976b, Selective uptake and
    transport of label within three identified neuronal
    systems after injection of $^3$H-GABA into the pigeon
    optic tectum: An autoradiographic and Golgi study,
    J.Comp.Neur. 170:173-190.

Hunt, S.P., Streit, P., Künzle, H., and Cuénod, M., 1977,
    Characterization of the pigeon isthmo-tectal path-
    way by selective uptake and retrograde movement of
    radioactive compounds and by Golgi-like horseradish
    peroxidase labeling, Brain Res. 129:197-212.

Hunt, S.P., and Webster, K.E., 1975, The projection of
    the retina upon the optic tectum of the pigeon,
    J.Comp.Neur. 162:433-446.

Iversen, L.L., 1971, Role of transmitter uptake mecha-
    nisms in synaptic neurotransmission, Brit.J.Pharmacol
    41:571-591.

Karten, H.J., 1969, The organisation of the avian telen-
    cephalon and some speculations on the phylogeny of
    the amniote telencephalon, Ann.N.Y.Acad.Sci. 167:
    164-179.

Le Fort, D., Henke, H., and Cuénod, M., 1978, Glycine
    specific $^3$H-strychine binding in the pigeon CNS,
    in preparation.

Logan, W.J., and Snyder, S.H., 1971, Unique high affinity
    uptake systems for glycine, glutamic and aspartic
    acids in central nervous tissue of the rat, Nature
    234:297-299.

Meier, R.E., Mihailovic, J., and Cuénod, M., 1974,
    Thalamic organization of the retino-thalamo-hyper-
    striatal pathway in the pigeon (Columba livia),
    Exp.Brain Res. 19:351-364.

Nauta, W.J.H., and Karten, H.J., 1970. A general profile
    of the vertebrate brain with sidelights on the
    ancestry of cerebral cortex, in "The Neurosciences:
    2nd Study Programme", (F.O. Schmitt, ed.), pp. 7-26,
    Rockefeller University Press, New York.

Repérant, J., 1973, Nouvelles données sur les projections visuelles chez le pigeon (Columba livia), J.Hirn-forschung. 14:151-187.

Reubi, J.C., and Cuénod, M., 1976, Release of exogenous glycine in the pigeon optic tectum during stimulation of a midbrain nucleus, Brain Res. 112:347-361.

Schonbach, J., Schonbach, C., and Cuénod, M., 1971, Rapid phase of axoplasmic flow and synaptic proteins: An electron microscopical autoradiographic study, J.Comp.Neur. 141:485-498.

Snyder, S.H., Yamamura, H.I., Pert, C.B., Logan, W.J., and Bennett, J.P., 1973, Neuronal uptake of neurotransmitters and their precursors in studies with 'transmitter' amino acids and choline, in "New Concepts in Neurotransmitter Regulation", (A.J. Mandell, ed.), pp. 195-222, Plenum Press, New York.

Storm-Mathisen, J., 1977, Glutamic acid and excitatory nerve endings: reduction of glutamic acid uptake after axotomy, Brain Res. 120:379-386.

Storm-Mathisen, J., and Guldberg, H.C., 1974, 5-Hydrosytryptamine and noradrenaline in the hippocampal region: Effect of transection of afferent pathways on endogenous levels, high affinity uptake and some transmitter-related enzymes, J.Neurochem. 22:793-803.

Streit, P., and Reubi, J.C., 1977, A new and sensitive staining method for axonally transported horseradish peroxidase (HRP) in the pigeon visual system, Brain Res. 126:530-537.

Webster, K.E., 1974. Changing concepts of the organization of the central visual pathways in birds, in "Essays on the nervous system", (R. Bellairs, and E.G. Gray, eds.), pp. 258-298, Clarendon Press, Oxford.

Yates, R.A., and Roberts, P.J., 1974, Effects of enucleation and intra-ocular colchicine on the amino acids of frog optic tectum, J.Neurochem. 23:891-893.

Young, A.B., and Snyder, S.H., 1973, Strychnine binding associated with glycine receptors of the central nervous system, Proc.Nat.Acad.Sci. Vol.70, 10:2832-2836.

Zukin, S.R., Young, A.B., and Snyder, S.H., 1975, Development of the synaptic glycine receptor in chick embryo spinal cord, Brain Res. 83:525-530.

# NEUROTRANSMITTERS OF THE MAMMALIAN VISUAL SYSTEM

R. Lund Karlsen

Norwegian Defence Research Establishment
Division for Toxicology
P O Box 25, N-2007 Kjeller, Norway

## RETINA

The retina is a layered structure, easy to obtain, and well described anatomically (Stell, 1972; Dowling, 1970) and is therefore a structure suitable for neurochemical investigations. Up till now a huge amount of information has been gained on the localization of putative neurotransmitters in the retina by microdissection techniques and autoradiography, for review (Graham, 1974; Bonting, 1976; Voaden, this volume).

In the present report I will mainly deal with the effects of toxic lesions on retina to describe the localization of neurotransmitter candidates in the rat retina (Lund-Karlsen & Fonnum, 1976; Lund-Karlsen, 1978). Subcutaneous injection of high doses of sodium glutamate to new born rats has been used to destroy retinal neurons, (Olney, 1967; Olney, 1974). In light microscopy the ganglion cells, amacrine cells and horizontal cells have disappeared (Lucas & Newhouse, 1957). The photoreceptors and Müllerian cells are intact, whereas the bipolar cells degenerate after 3 months (Potts et al., 1969). This finding has further been confirmed on the electron microscopic level (Hansson, 1970). Thus the treatment leaves a retina dominated by photoreceptors and glia (Figure 1.). The glial part of the retina, the Müllerian cells, may be destroyed by intravitreal injection of the gliotoxic compound DL-α-aminoadipic acid. (Olney et al., 1971). Four h. after the injection of this compound, the heavy staining of the Müllerian cells normally found, had completely disappeared (Figure 2.). The lesion was not permanent, however, as the Müllerian cells had regained their staining abilities after 24 h. Microscopically the photoreceptors and the retinal neurons look normal after this treatment.

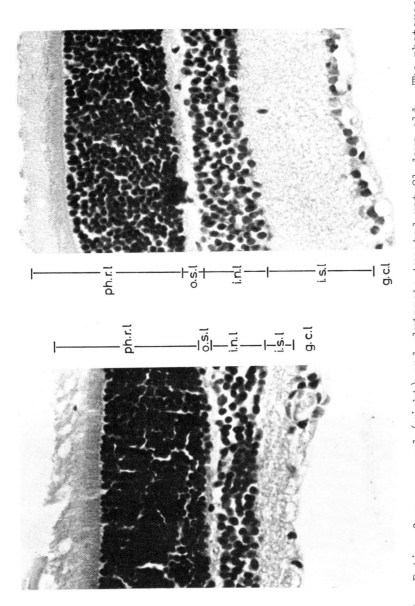

Figure 1.   Retina from a normal (right) and glutamate treated rat 21 days old.  The photoreceptor layer (ph.r.l.) and the outer synaptic layer (o.s.l.) are unaffected by the treatment. The inner nuclear layer (i.n.l.) is reduced in thickness and the inner synaptic layer (i.s.l.) and ganglion cell layer (g.c.l.) are heavily reduced (haematoxylin & eosin, ×400).

From:   Lund Karlsen & Fonnum, 1971.

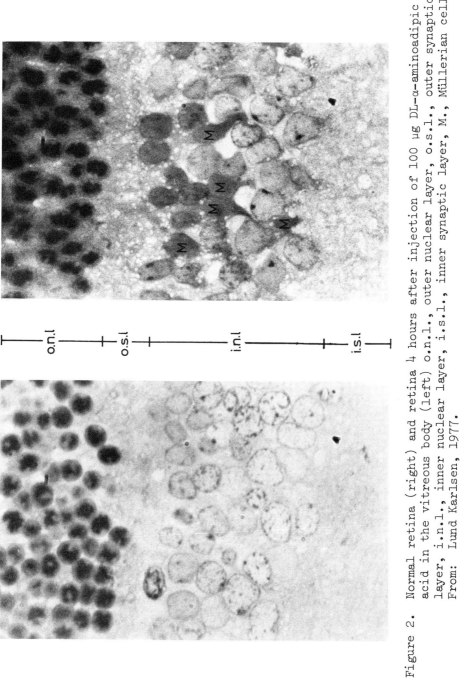

Figure 2.  Normal retina (right) and retina 4 hours after injection of 100 μg DL-α-aminoadipic acid in the vitreous body (left) o.n.l., outer nuclear layer, o.s.l., outer synaptic layer, i.n.l., inner nuclear layer, i.s.l., inner synaptic layer, M., Müllerian cells. From:  Lund Karlsen, 1977.

Following the glutamate lesion the cholinergic parametres
ChAT, AChE and high affinity uptake  of choline were severely reduced (Lund-Karlsen & Fonnum, 1976; Lund-Karlsen, 1978) (Table 1).
These observations are in agreement with results obtained by dissecting the retina into individual layers where the cholinergic
marker enzyme, ChAT, is mainly found in the inner synaptic layer
(Graham, 1974; Ross & MacDougal, 1976). In this layer a population
of amacrine cells is most probably responsible for the enzyme
activity  (Nichols & Koelle, 1968; Ross & MacDougal, 1976). Of
special interest was the finding that the high affinity uptake of
choline was reduced almost to the same extent as ChAT activity,
indicating in line with previous work that choline is mainly taken
up by cholinergic nerve terminals (Simon et al., 1976). Injection
of DL-α-aminoadipic acid on the other hand did not affect the
cholinergic parametres (Table 2).

Dopamine is mainly responsible for the catecholamine fluorescence found in retina (Häggendal & Malmfors, 1965; Ehinger & Falck;
1971) and is localized to the amacrine cells. In some species
(goldfish, Cebus monkey) this population of amacrine cells, named
interplexiform neurons, are found to project from the inner to the
outher synaptic layer (Dowling & Ehinger, 1975). As expected after
destruction of amacrine cells by glutamate, AAD activity was reduced by 70% (Table 1). This reduction in AAD activity was much
less pronounced than the reductions observed for ChAT and GAD.
Studies from other regions of the brain, however, suggest that
catecholaminergic neurons might be more resistant to the toxic
effect of glutamate than  cholinergic and GABAergic neurons
(Schwarz & Coyle, 1977; Walaas & Fonnum, 1978).

By immunocytochemical techniques GAD is mainly found localized
to a proportion of the amacrine cells (Wood et al., 1975) and by
microdissection the highest level of GABA and GAD is found in the
inner synaptic layer (Graham, 1972). In agreement to these
observations the glutamate lesion was accompanied by 90% reduction
in GAD activity, whereas the GABA level was reduced by 60% (Table
1). Destruction of the Müllerian cells did not affect GAD activity
(Table 2). Glutamate treatment also reduced the high affinity uptake of GABA in retinal homogenates by 60% (Table 1) suggesting
mainly uptake into GABAergic nerve terminals, probably derived
from the amacrine cells. However, when the high affinity uptake of
GABA was measured on intact retina after glutamate treatment, no
reduction was observed (Table 1). By autoradiographic techniques
the neuronal uptake of GABA is difficult to demonstrate. After
in vitro incubation of the rat retina with labelled GABA only the
Müllerian cells were labelled (Marshall & Voaden, 1974). However,
4 hours after injection of GABA into the vitreous body amacrine
cells are labelled as well (Bruun & Ehinger, 1974). The glial uptake of GABA on intact retina thus seems to mask the neuronal uptake which is best demonstrated on retinal homogenates. In agree-

TABLE 1. ENZYME ACTIVITIES, AMINO ACID CONCENTRATION AND HIGH AFFINITY UPTAKE IN THE NORMAL RAT RETINA. IN PARENTHESIS ARE GIVEN THE ACTIVITY (OR LEVEL) IN PERCENT OF NORMAL VALUES AFTER THE GLUTAMATE LESION

| Enzyme activities μ mole/h/g protein | Amino acid conc. μ mole/g protein | High affinity uptake homogenate p mole/3 min/mg protein | High affinity uptake intact retina p mole/3 min/mg protein |
|---|---|---|---|
| | aspartate 40 (52%) | aspartate 20 (67%) | |
| | glutamate 71 (63%) | glutamate 19 (61%) | glutamate 1.6 (106%) |
| | glycine 49 (46%) | glycine 6 (40%) | |
| | alanine 23 (43%) | | |
| GAD 107 (9%) | GABA 31 (32%) | GABA 53 (36%) | GABA 30.2 (104%) |
| | | DABA 5.8 (36%) | DABA 0.7 (57%) |
| | | β-alanine 4.9 (100%) | β-alanine 4.1 (170%) |
| | glutamine 55 (60%) | | |
| | taurine 158 (87%) | taurine 1.2 (100%) | |
| AChE 7900 (26%) | | | |
| ChAT 126 (0.5%) | | choline 1.1 (18%) | |
| AAD 1.6 (27%) | | | |

From: Lund Karlsen & Fonnum, 1976
Lund Karlsen, 1978.

TABLE 2.   ENZYME ACTIVITIES AND HIGH AFFINITY UPTAKE IN NORMAL RAT
           RETINA.   IN PARENTHESIS ARE GIVEN THE VALUES IN PERCENT
           OF NORMAL ACTIVITIES FOUR HOURS AFTER INTRAVITRAL INJEC-
           TION OF DL-α-AMINOADIPIC ACID

| Enzyme activities | High affinity uptake Intact retina | | |
|---|---|---|---|
| p mole/h/mg protein | p mole/3 min/mg protein | | |
| GAD    153 (95%) | GABA | 33 | (72%) |
| | β-alanine | 4.5 | (44%) |
| | DABA | 0.6 | (116%) |
| | glutamate | 1.6 | (75%) |
| ChAT    96 (88%) | choline | 1.3 | (85%)[*] |

[*]homogenate.

From Lund Karlsen, R., 1978.

ment the injection of DL-α-aminoadipic acid reduced GABA uptake on
intact retina (Table 2) thus demonstrating the glial component of
the uptake.   When the GABA analogue diamino-n-butyric acid (DABA)
was used no discrepancies between the uptakes on homogenates and
intact retinae were observed after the glutamate lesion (Table 1),
and DL-α-aminoadipic acid injection was without any effect (Table
2) in agreement with the concept that DABA labels neuronal structures and not glia (Dick & Kelly, 1975).   Four hours after injection of DL-α-aminoadipic acid the high affinity uptake of β-alanine
which mainly labels glia (Schon & Kelly, 1975) was reduced by 55%.
on intact retinae.   However, 24 hours after the injection, at a
time when the Müllerian cells had regained their staining abilities, the β-alanine uptake had returned to normal (Table 2).
These observations are in agreement with autoradiographic studies
demonstrating β-alanine uptake into the Müllerian cells (Iversen,
1975).   Glutamate treatment did not affect β-alanine uptake on
retinal homogenates, but on intact retinae the uptake was increased
by 70%, indicating that the glutamate lesion is accompanied by
glioses.   The differences observed between the uptake studies of
GABA, DABA and β-alanine on retinal homogenates and intact retinae
can best be explained on the basis that glial uptake mechanisms are
destroyed by homogenization, whereas nerve terminals form synaptosomes with intact uptake mechanisms.   GABA is taken up into both
glial and neuronal elements whereas β-alanine is mainly taken up
into glial cells and DABA into neuronal cells.

Due to the central position of aspartate and glutamate in brain metabolism, nerve terminals suspected of using these amino acids as their transmitter are difficult to trace biochemically. In the rat retina aspartate and glutamate are by microdissection found to be evenly distributed among the retinal layers, although differencies among species occur (Graham et al., 1968; Voaden, this volume). The retinal concentrations of these amino acids were reduced by 40% after glutamate treatment (Table 1), suggesting a higher concentration of these amino acids in retinal neurons than in the Müllerian cells. This lesion reduced the high affinity uptake of aspartate and glutamate retinal homogenates by 30% (Table 1), indicating the presence of neuronal high affinity uptake mechanisms. On intact retina DL-α-aminoadipic acid reduced the glutamate uptake by 25% (Table 2) whereas the uptake in glutamate lesioned intact retinae was unaffected (Table 1). These observations indicate glial as well as neuronal uptake mechanisms for these amino acids. As autoradiographic studies only demonstrate glial uptake of aspartate and glutamate in the rat retina (White & Neal, 1976), the cellular localization of the neuronal high affinity uptakes of these amino acids is difficult to explain.

The role of glycine as a neurotransmitter in CNS is reviewed by Aprison & Nadi (this volume). In several species glycine is consistently demonstrated by autoradiography to be taken up by amacrine cells (Ehinger & Falck, 1971; Bruun & Ehinger, 1974; Voaden et al., 1974). In agreement with the probable localization of glycine to the amacrine cells the glutamate lesion reduced the glycine level and high affinity uptake by 50% (Table 1). The release of preloaded glycine from the rabbit retina by stimulation with flickering light strengthens the case for glycine as a retinal neurotransmitter (Lindberg Bauer, 1975; Ehinger & Lindberg Bauer, this volume).

The retinal concentration of taurine is extremely high (Pasantes-Morales et al., 1972) (Table 1) and taurine is mainly localized to the photoreceptors (Orr et al., 1976). By stimulation with flickering light preloaded taurine is slowly released from the retina (Pasantes-Morales et al., 1973), and chickens raised in the dark have a higher retinal concentration of taurine than controls (Pasantes-Morales et al., 1973). These and other experiments suggest that taurine is a retinal neurotransmitter or modulator of neuronal activity (review, Mandel et al., 1976). In the glutamate treated retinae the level and high affinity uptake of taurine was unchanged (Table 1) in agreement with intact photoreceptor layer.

In contrast to other regions of the CNS where the high affinity uptakes of GABA, glutamate and aspartate have been suggested as useful tools in tracing transmitter specific nerve terminals (Snyder et al, 1973) the rat retina is dominated by the glial uptakes into the Müllerian cells. For studies of the neuronal GABA uptake this problem can partly be overcome by using DABA. To study the neuronal

uptake of aspartate or glutamate no such compounds exist. Fortunately the glial uptake mechanisms seem to be more vulnerable to
homogenization than neuronal uptake mechanisms.


## VISUAL PATHWAYS

The anatomy and especially the neurophysiology of the central
part of the visual system is well described, establishing a sound
foundation for neurochemical studies (Polyak, 1957; Kuffler &
Nichols, 1976).

The optic tract, originating in the retinal ganglion cells,
terminates in the superior colliculus (S.C) and dorsal lateral
geniculate body (DLG). In common laboratory animals such as rat,
guinea pig and rabbit the crossing of fibres in chiasma is nearly
complete (more than 90%) (Polyak, 1957), making these animals suitable for denervation studies. Following enucleation degenerating
nerve terminals are found in stratum griseum superficiale in the
S.C. (rat, Langer & Lund, 1974) and in the DLG, (rat, Montero and
Guillery, 1968). The DLG projects uncrossed fibres to the primary
visual cortex (area 17) (Valverde, 1968). After destruction of
the DLG or enucleation of new born animals a reduced number of
spines is observed on the dendrites of the pyramidal cells in area
17 (mouse) (Valverde, 1968). This lesion is in addition accompanied
by a reduction in the number of dendritic spines of the pyramidal
cells in the contralateral peristriatal cortex (mouse, Valverde &
Estéban, 1968). The S.C. projects further to thalamic structures
mainly outside the DLG, forming the socalled extrageniculate visual
system (tree shrew, Casagrande et al., 1972).

The DLG and S.C. are also under cortical control. After visual
cortex ablation degenerating nerve terminals are found within a week
in the deeper part of the stratum griseum superficiale of the S.C.
(rat), and in the DLG (rat, cat) ipsilateral to the lesion (Lund,
1966; Gosavi & Dubey, 1972; Guillery, 1967). After weeks the lesion
is accompanied by degeneration of neuronal cells in the DLG, but
not in the S.C. (rat, Montero & Guillery, 1968; Lund, 1966). The
corticofugal fibre projections to the DLG and S.C. are uncrossed,
but if visual cortex ablation is performed during the first week
of life a crossed fibre projection to these structures from the
cortex can be demonstrated (rat, Mustari & Lund, 1976), illustrating
the plasticity of the visual system.


## BIOCHEMICAL STUDIES

The activity of the cholinergic marker enzyme ChAT in low in
the optic nerve (Graham, 1974) and roughly of the same magnitude
in the SC, DLG, area 17 and 18 (Tables 3, 4). In the rabbit the

ACh concentration in the DLG is reduced by 20% 3 weeks after enucleation, whereas no changes were found in the S.C. AChE activity was unchanged in both structures (Miller et al., 1969). ChAT activity was also unaffected in the S.C. of the rabbit after enucleation (Siou & Israel, 1969). In the rat ChAT activity is unchanged from control values both in S.C. and DLG 1 - 6 weeks after enucleation of adult animals and similar results are observed if enucleation is performed at birth (Table 4). Likewise ChAT activity is unaffected in area 17 and 18 following this operation (Table 4). In the rabbit visual cortex ablation was accompanied by 20 reduction in ACh concentration in the DLG, but not in the S.C. (Miller et al., 1969), whereas visual cortex ablation of the rat had no effects on ChAT activity in DLG and S.C. (Table 3). These results exclude the possibility that the connections between the S.C., DLG and the visual areas of the cortex are cholinergic. The small changes in ACh concentration found weeks after surgery is probably due to secondary changes.

In the rat GAD activity, GABA concentration and high affinity uptake of GABA is much higher in the S.C. than in the DLG and the visual cortical areas (Table 3, 4). In the rat these GABAergic parametres were unaffected both by enucleation (at birth, adults) and by ablation of the visual cortex in all the structures studied (Table 3, 4) indicating that these connections are not GABAergic. These observations are in agreement with the work of Okada (1974) who found that the GABA concentration in the S.C. of the rabbit was unaffected by enucleation, visual cortex ablation and cutting of the commissural fibres of the S.C. By dissection of the layers of the S.C. Okada found that the GABA concentration was highest in the most superficial layer. In the visual cortex of the rat GAD positive neurons, (probably stellate neurons), are demonstrated in all cortical layers by the immunocytochemical technique (Ribak, 1977) and by autoradiography (Chronwall & Wolf this volume).

Whereas the aspartate and glutamate concentrations are euqal in the S.C. and DLG the high affinity uptake of these amino acids are three times higher in the latter structure and even higher in the visual cortex (Table 3). In the optic nerve (cat), however, the concentration of aspartate and glutamate are very low (Johnson & Aprison, 1971). Enucleation of new born rats did not change the high affinity uptake of L-glutamate or D-aspartate in the S.C., DLG, area 17 and area 18 when the animals were examined at 6 weeks of age (Table 4). This indicates that neither glutamate nor aspartate is the transmitter of the optic nerve, of the fibres from the DLG to area 17 nor of the commissural fibres from area 17 to area 18. Similar results were observed when adult rats were enucleated and examined 1 - 6 weeks after surgery. In other species, however, the situation may be different. In the frog the level of glutamate was reduced in the optic lobe 1 - 2 weeks after enucleation (Yates & Roberts, 1974). Similar results were observed in the optic lobe

TABLE 3. EFFECT OF ABLATION OF RIGHT VISUAL CORTEX ON BIOCHEMICAL PARAMETRES IN THE SUPERIOR
COLLICULUS, DORSAL LATERAL GENIFULATE BODY AND VISUAL CORTEX

| | superior colliculus | | dorsal lateral geniculate body | | visual cortex | |
|---|---|---|---|---|---|---|
| | right | left | right | left | control | left |
| L-glutamate uptake | 49 ± 6 | 91 ± 7 | 80 ± 16 | 315 ± 36 | 447 ± 49 | 435 ± 40 |
| D-aspartate uptake | 21 ± 3 | 37 ± 5 | 111 ± 26 | 242 ± 59 | | |
| glutamate concentration | 93 ± 12 | 112 ± 13 | 82 ± 11 | 120 ± 2 | | |
| GABA uptake | 78 ± 14 | 78 ± 14 | 28 ± 6 | 31 ± 8 | | |
| GABA concentration | 69 ± 10 | 61 ± 10 | 26 ± 4 | 26 ± 5 | | |
| glutamate decarboxylase | 635 ± 24 | 610 ± 19 | 227 ± 17 | 219 ± 17 | | |
| choline acetyltransferase | 61 ± 10 | 61 ± 8 | 47 ± 8 | 50 ± 11 | | |
| carnitine acetyltransferase | 100 | 100 | 100 | 100 | | |

The primary visual cortex was removed by suction on adult rats. 7 days before the animals were killed. The values represent: high affinity uptake p mole/3 min/mg protein; GABA and glutamate concentration: μ mole/g protein; glutamate decarboxylase and choline acetyltransferase: n mole/h/mg protein; carnitine acetyltransferase, arbitrary units (mean ± SD from 6 experiments). The values on the left side were unchanged from controls.

(From: Lund Karlsen & Fonnum, 1978)

TABLE 4. THE EFFECT OF UNILATERAL ENUCLEATION (RIGHT SIDE) ON NEW BORN ANIMALS IN THE PRIMARY VISUAL CORTEX (AREA 17), ACCESSORY VISUAL CORTEX (AREA 18), SUPERIOR COLLICULUS AND DORSAL LATERAL GENICULATE BODY

| | area 17 | | | area 18 | | |
|---|---|---|---|---|---|---|
| | left | right | control | left | right | control |
| D-aspartate uptake | 350 ± 42 | 383 ± 42 | 350 ± 40 | 355 ± 38 | 313 ± 41 | 369 ± 30 |
| choline acetyltransferase | 54 ± 10 | 49 ± 8 | 55 ± 10 | 58 ± 8 | 51 ± 10 | 56 ± 11 |
| glutamate decarboxylase | 182 ± 18 | 183 ± 16 | 180 ± 10 | 179 ± 20 | 173 ± 20 | 170 ± 15 |

| | superior colliculus | | | dorsal lateral geniculate | | |
|---|---|---|---|---|---|---|
| | left | right | control | left | right | control |
| D-asparate uptake | 37 ± 5 | 41 ± 9 | 36 ± 5 | 242 ± 59 | 255 ± 43 | 245 ± 30 |
| choline acetyltransferase | 60 ± 5 | 61 ± 5 | 62 ± 5 | 53 ± 6 | 50 ± 11 | 47 ± 8 |
| glutamate decarboxylase | 635 ± 29 | 610 ± 19 | 620 ± 20 | 227 ± 17 | 219 ± 17 | 220 ± 20 |

The animals were examined at 40 days of age. The values are mean ± SD from 5 separate experiments and represent the same units as in Table 3.

of the pigeon where both the high affinity uptake of L-glutamate
and glutamate concentration was severely reduced 4 - 7 weeks after
enucleation (Henke et al., 1976; Cuenod et al, this volume). However, this reduction might be due to secondary changes as degeneration of the optic nerve terminals is fairly advanced within a week
after enucleation in the pigeon (Repérant & Angaut, 1977).

The concentration of 5-hydroxytryptamine, noradrenaline and
dopamine are very low in the optic nerve (Bogdanski et al., 1957;
Cobbin et al., 1965) making these substances less credible as transmitter candidates for this nerve. The activity of AAD in the S.C.
and DLG was unaffected by enucleation 7 days after sugery.
The optic nerve has a fairly high concentration of ergothioneine
(Crossland et al., 1966), this compound has, however, no electrophysiological effect in the DLG (Tebécis, 1973). From these studies
it seems that the chemical nature of the neurotransmitter of the
optic nerve remains unknown. However, the possibility exists, as
there are different populations of ganglion cells (Dowling, 1970),
that several unknown substances might be involved in carrying information from the retina to the DLG and S.C.

As for the decending pathway from the visual cortex to the DLG
and S.C., however, recent experiments in our laboratory suggest that
glutamate is the neurotransmitter of this pathway (Lund Karlsen &
Fonnum, 1978). The reductions in high affinity uptake of D-aspartate and L-glutamate occurred in parallel to degeneration of nerve
terminals in the DLG and S.C. after visual cortex ablation (Guillery,
1967). The reduction, which was ipsilateral to the lesion, was
first detected after 3 days and was maximally developed after 7
days (Table 3). At this time the reductions in high affinity uptake
of D-aspartate and L-glutamate were 75 and 50% in the DLG and S.C.
respectively. In separate experiments the uptake was found to be
most active in the synaptosomal fraction where also the most pronounced reduction after lesion occurred. Other parametres included
GAD, ChAT, carnitine acetyltransferase and high affinity GABA uptake were unaffected (Table 3), indicating that the reduction in
L-glutamate uptake cannot be due to secondary changes. As L-glutamate and L-aspartate are taken up by the same mechanism. (Balcar
& Johnston, 1973) they can only be differentiated by amino acid
analysis. This showed 34 and 17% reductions in the level of glutamate in the DLG and S.C. respectively without any changes of the
other amino acids (Table 3). These observations indicate that nerve
terminals from the visual cortex to the DLG and S.C. contain high
concentrations of glutamate and have a high affinity uptake mechanism for this amino acid and suggest that glutamate is the transmitter of this pathway.

REFERENCES

Balcar, V.J. & Johnston, G.A.R., 1973, High affinity uptake of transmitters: studies on the uptake of L-aspartate, GABA, L-glutamate and glycine in cat spinal cord, J. Neurochem., 20:529-539.

Bogdanski, D.F., Weissbach, H. & Udenfriend, S., 1957, The distribution of serotonin, 5-hydroxytryptophan decarboxylase and monoamine oxidase in brain, J. Neurochem., 1:272-278.

Bonting, S.L., 1976, Transmitters in the visual process (Bonting, S.L. ed.), Pergamon Press.

Bruun, A. & Ehinger, B., 1974, Uptake of certain possible neurotransmitters into retinal neurons of some mammals., Exp. Eye. Res., 19:435-437.

Casagrande, V.A., Harting, J.K., Hall, W.C. & Diamond, J.T., 1972, Superior colliculus of the tree shrew: A structural and functional subdivision into superficial and deep layers, Science, 177:444-447.

Cobbin, L.B., Leeder, S. & Pollard, J., 1965, Smooth muscle stimulants in extracts of optic nerve, optic tracts and lateral geniculate bodies of sheep, Brit. J. Pharmacol., 25:295-306.

Crossland, J., Mitchell, J.F. & Woodruff, G.N., 1966, The presence of ergothioneine in the central nervous system and its probable identity with the cerebellar factor, J. Physiol. (London), 182:427-438.

Dick, F. & Kelly, J.S., 1975, L-2,4-Diaminobutyric acid (L-DABA) as a selective marker for inhibitory nerve terminals in rat brain, Bit. J. Pharmacol., 53:439 P.

Dowling, J.E., 1970, Organization of vertebrate retinas, Invest. Ophthalmol., 9:655-680.

Dowling, J.E. & Ehinger, B., 1975, Synaptic organization of the aminecontaining interplexiform cells of the goldfish and Cebus monkey retinas, Science, 188:270-273.

Ehinger, B. & Falck, B., 1971, Autoradiography of some suspected neurotransmitter substances: GABA, glycine, glutamic acid, histamine, dopamine and L-DOPA, Brain Res., 33:157-172.

Gosavi, V.S. & Dubey, P.N., 1972, Projection of striate cortex to the dorsal lateral geniculate body in the rat, J. Anat. (London), 113:75-82.

Graham, L.T., 1972, Intraretinal distribution of GABA content and GAD activity, Brain Res., 36:476-479.

Graham, L.T., 1974, Comparative aspects of neurotransmitters in the retina. In: The Eye. Volume 6. Comparative Physiology. (Davson, H. & Graham, L.T., eds.), pp 283-342, Academic Press, N.Y., London.

Graham, L.T., Lolley, R.N. & Baxter, C.F., 1968, Effect of illumination upon levels of γ-aminobutyric acid and glutamic acid in frog retina in vivo, Fed. Proc., 27:463.

Guillery, R.W., 1967, Patterns of fibre degeneration in the dorsal lateral geniculate nucleus of the cat following lesions in the visual cortex, J. comp. Neurol., 130:197-222.

Hansson, H.A., 1970, Utrastructure studies on long-term effects
of MSG on rat retina, Virchows Arch. B.Z. (Cell Pathol.),
6:1-19.

Häggendal, J. & Malmfors, T., 1965, Identification and cellular
localization of the catecholamines in the retina and choroid
of the rabbit, Acta Physiol. scand., 64:58-66.

Iversen, L.L., Dick, F., Kelly, J.S. & Schon, F., 1975, Uptake and
localization of transmitter amino acids in the nervous system. In: Metabolic compartmentation and neurotransmission.
NATO advanced study institute series. (Berl, S., Clarke, D.D.
& Schneider, D., Eds.), Vol 6, pp. 65-89.

Johnson, J.L. & Aprison, M.H., 1971, The distribution of glutamate
and total free amino acids in thirteen specific regions of
the cat central nervous system, Brain Res., 26:141-148.

Kuffler, S.W. & Nichols, J.S., 1976, The visual world cellular
organization and its analysis. In: From Neuron to Brain,
(Kuffler, S.W. & Nichols, J.S., Eds.), Sunderland, Massachusetts.

Langer, T.P. & Lund, R.D., 1974, The upper layers of the superior
colliculus of the rat: A Golgi study, J. comp. Neur., 158:
405-436.

Lindberg-Bauer, A., 1975, Light evoked release of glycine from
rabbit retina, Acta Ophthal., 125:30-31.

Lucas, D.R. & Newhouse, J.P., 1957, The toxic effect of sodium L-
glutamate on the inner layers of the retina, Arch. Ophthal.
58:193-201.

Lund, R.D., 1966, The occipitotectal pathway of the rat, J. Anat.,
100.1:51-62.

Lund Karlsen, R., 1978, The toxic effect of sodium glutamate and
DL-α-aminoadipic acid on rat retina: Changes in high affinity
uptake of putative transmitter, J. Neurochem., Submitted for
publication.

Lund Karlsen, R. & Fonnum, F., 1976, The toxic effect of sodium
glutamate on rat retina: Changes in putative transmitters and
their corresponding enzymes, L. Neurochem., 27:1437-1441.

Lund Karlsen, R. & Fonnum, F., 1978, Evidence for glutamate as a
neurotransmitter in the corticofugal fibres to the dorsal
lateral geniculate body and the superior colluculus in rats,
Brain Res., Submitted for publication.

Mandel, P., Pasantes-Morales, H. & Urban, P.F., 1976, Taurine, a
putative transmitter in retina. In: Transmitters in the
visual process. (Bonting, S.L., ed.), pp. 89-105, Pergamon
Press.

Marshal, J. & Voaden, M., 1974, An investigation of the cells in-
corporating ($^3$H) GABA and ($^3$H) glycine in the isolated retina
of the rat, Exp. Eye. Res., 18:367-370.

Miller, E., Heller, A. & Moore, R.E., 1969, Acetylcholine in rabbit
visual system nuclei after enucleation and visual cortex ablation, Pharm. Exp. Ther., 165:117-125.

Montero, V.M. & Guillery, R.W., 1968, Degeneration in the dorsal
    lateral geniculate nucleus of the rat following interruption
    of the retinal or cortical connections, J. Comp. Neur.,
    134:211-292.
Mustari, M.J. & Lund, R.D., 1976, An aberrant crossed visual cor-
    ticotectal pathway in albino rat, Brain Res., 112:37-44.
Neal, M.J., 1976, Amino acid transmitter substances in the verte-
    brate retina, Gen. Pharmac., 7:321-332.
Nichols, C.W. & Koelle, G.B., 1968, Comparison of the localiza-
    tion of acetylcholinesterase and non-specific cholinesterase
    activities in mammalian and avian  retinas, J. Comp. Neurol.,
    133:1-15.
Okada, I., 1974, Distribution of γ-aminobutyric acid (GABA) in the
    layers of superior colliculus of rabbit, Brain Res., 75:363-
    365.
Olney, J.W., 1969, Glutamate - induced retinal degereration in
    neonatal mice.  Electron microscopy of the evolving lesion,
    J. Neuropath. exp. Neurol., 28:455-474.
Olney, J.W., 1974, Toxic effects of glutamate and related amino
    acids on the developing central nervos system.  In:  Heritable
    disorders of amino acid metabolism.  (Nyhan, W.H., Ed.),
    pp. 501-512, John Wiley, New York.
Olney, J.W., Ho, O.L. & Rhee, V., 1971, Cytotoxic effects of acidic
    and sulphur  containing amino acids on the infant mouse cen-
    tral nervous system, Exp. Brain. Res., 14:61-76.
Orr, H.T., Cohen, A.I. & Carter, J.A., 1976, The levels of free
    taurine, glutamate, glycine and γ-amino butyric acid during
    the postnatal development of the normal and dystrophic retina
    of the mouse, Exp. Eye. Res., 23:377-384.
Pasantes-Morales, H., Klethi, J., Leidig, M. & Mandel, P., 1972,
    Free amino acids of chicken and rat retina, Brain Res.,
    41:494-497.
Pasantes-Morales, H., Urban, P.F., Klethi, J. & Mandel, P., 1973,
    Light stimulated release of $^{35}$S-taurine from chicken retina,
    Brain Res., 51:375-378.
Polyak, S., 1957, The vertebrate visual system.  (Klüver, H., Ed.),
    University of Chicago Press, Chicago.
Potts, A.M., Modrell, R.W. & Kingsbury, C., 1960, Permanent frac-
    tionation of the electroretinogram by sodium glutamate, Am.
    J. Ophthal., 50:900-907.
Repérant, J. & Angaut, P., 1977, The retinotectal projections in
    the pigeon.  An experimental optical and electron microscope
    study, Neuroscience, 2:119-140.
Ribak, C.E., 1977, The immunocytochemical localization of GAD
    within stellate neurons of rat visual cortex, Anatomical
    Record, 187:692-693.
Ross, C.D. & MacDougal, D.B., 1976, The distribution of choline
    acetyltransferase in vertebrate retina, J. Neurochem.,
    26:521-526.

Schon, F. & Kelly, J.S., 1975, Selective uptake of ($^3$H) β-alanine by glia: association with the glial uptake system for GABA, Brain Res., 86:243-247.

Schwarcz, R. & Coyle, J.T., 1977, Kainic acid: neurotoxic effects after intraocular injection, Invest. Optithal., 16:141-148.

Simon, J.R., Atweh, S. & Kuhar, M.I., 1976, Sodium-dependent high affinity choline uptake: a regulatory step in the synthesis of acetylcholine, J. Neurochem., 26:909-922.

Siou, G. & Israel, M., 1969, Recherches experimentales sur la distribution de la choline-acetyltransferase dans le tectum opticum du Lapin, C.R. Soc. Biol., 3:594-598.

Snyder, S.H., Young, A.B., Bennett, J.P. & Mulder, A.H., 1973, Synaptic biochemistry of amino acids, Fed. Proc., 32:2039-2047.

Stell, W.K., 1972, The morphological organization of the vertebrate retina. In: Handbook of sensory physiology. (Fuortes, M.G.F., Ed.), 7:112-213, Springer-Verlag, Berlin.

Tebécis, A.K., 1973, Studies on the identity of the optic nerve transmitter, Brain Res., 63:31-42.

Valverde, F., 1968, Structural changes in the area striata of the mouse after enucleation, Exp. Brain. Res., 5:274-292.

Valverde, F. & Esteban, M.E., 1968, Peristriate cortex of mouse: location and the effects of enucleation on the number of dendritic spines, Brain Res., 9:145-148.

Voaden, M., Marshall, J. & Murani, N., 1974, The uptake of $^3$H-γ-aminobutyric acid and $^3$H glycine by the isolated retina of the frog, Brain Res., 67:115-132.

Wallaas, I. & Fonnum, F., 1978, The effect of parenteral glutamate treatment on the localization of neurotransmitters in the mediobasal hypothalamus, Brain Res., Submitted for publication.

Wood, J.S., MacLaughlin, B.J. & Vaughn, I.E., 1976, Immunocytochemical localization of GAD in electron microscopic preparations of rodent CNS. In: GABA in nervous system function, (Roberts, E., Chase, T.N. & Tower, D.B., Eds.), pp. 133-148, Raven Press, New York.

Yates, R.A. & Roberts, P.J., 1974, Effects of enucleation and intraocular colchicine on the amino acids of frog optic tectum, J. Neurochem., 23:891-893.

THE LOCALIZATION AND METABOLISM OF NEUROACTIVE AMINO ACIDS

IN THE RETINA

M. J. Voaden

Department of Visual Science
Institute of Ophthalmology
London WC1H 9QS

The retina is an integral part of the central nervous system and has
an overall metabolic organization resembling that in the brain.  In
line with this neurotransmission is, in general, chemically mediated
and, of the neuroactive amino acids, there is evidence showing that
glutamate, aspartate, glycine, ४ -aminobutyrate (GABA) and taurine
are potential retinal neurotransmitters (Graham, 1974; Mandel et
al., 1976; Neal, 1976; Voaden, 1976).

The amino acid concentrations in the retina are similar to those
in the brain except that taurine levels are higher (Table 1).  There
is considerable variation in the reported values for retinal taurine
but how this relates to the estimation techniques is not clear as
dansylation has yielded values for the rat retina of about 14 - 90
µmoles /gm wet wt. (Lund Karlsen and Fonnum, 1976; Yates and Keen,
1975), whereas results from amino acid analyzers range between 10 -
40 µmoles /gm wet wt. (Pasantes-Morales et al., 1972; Macaione et
al., 1974).  There is therefore no immediate explanation.  However,
even in the lower ranges taurine can be considered concentrated as
compared to other amino acids.

## 1. LOCALIZATION OF ENDOGENOUS AMINO ACIDS

The distribution of neuroactive amino acids in the retina has
been studied in detail in three species, the monkey, rat and frog,
and the results are summarized in Figs. 1 & 2.  This data has been
obtained by analysing horizontal, sometimes microdissected, retinal
slices.  These will be enriched in specific neuronal cell types
because of the ordered arrangement of the cells of the retina (cf.
Fig.3).  However most fractions will also contain glial cytoplasm

TABLE I.   AMINO ACID CONCENTRATIONS IN THE RETINA

| | Amino acid | Concentration range* (μmoles / gm wet wt.) | |
|---|---|---|---|
| | | Retina | Brain |
| Excitatory | Glutamate | 2.7-14.8 | 7.8-12.5 |
| | Aspartate | 0.4- 5.3 | 1.5- 2.7 |
| Inhibitory | Glycine | 1.0- 7.4 | 0.6- 1.5 |
| | GABA | 1.6- 5.3 | 0.8- 2.3 |
| | Taurine | 9.6-90.0 | 1.3- 5.4 |
| | Glutamine | 0.8-10.5 | 2.2- 5.6 |

*Recalculations have been based on a retinal water content of 85%, and protein of 10%.
Brain values are from McIlwain and Bachelard (1971), and retina from Pasantes-Morales et al. (1972); Cohen et al. (1973); Macaione et al. (1974); Starr (1975); Yates and Keen (1975); Lund Karlsen and Fonnum (1976); Kennedy et al. (1977) and Voaden et al. (1977a).

contributed by the Müller cells that run radially through the tissue, their extremities forming the outer and inner limiting membranes.

The morphometry of the glial cytoplasm has been studied in detail in the rat retina, where it is estimated to contribute 43% of the total volume of the ganglion cell / nerve fibre layer but only 5% of the photoreceptor nuclei sections (Rasmussen, 1972). The full distribution is shown in Fig. 4.

The levels of amino acids in retinal glia are not known but data is available that does allow the formulation of an estimate. The parenteral administration of sodium glutamate to weanling rats will degenerate inner neurones of the retina, leading eventually to tissue composed mainly of photoreceptors and collapsed glial cells. The free amino acid content of both normal and glutamate treated retinas, as measured by Lund Karlsen and Fonnum (1976) is shown in Table II.   The percentage contribution that each amino acid makes to the photoreceptor and inner retinal layers of the rat retina is also known (Voaden et al., 1977a) and it is possible, therefore, to obtain an estimate of the amino acid levels in the glial enriched inner retina of the glutamate treated animals (Tables II and III).

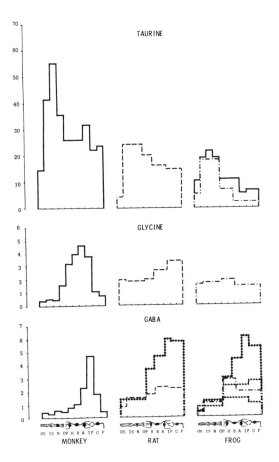

FIGURE 1. The distribution of amino acids in the retina : taurine, glycine and GABA (μmoles / gm wet wt. retina).

Data for the monkey retina (━━━━) are from Orr et al. (1976) (taurine) and Berger et al. (1977). Values for rat and frog are from Kennedy et al. (1977) (━ ━ ━), Graham (1974) (▸♦♦♦♦♦ ; dark-adapted retina) and Graham et al. (1970) (▰▰▰▰▰▰ ; top value light-adapted, lower dark-adapted). The amino acid distribution in the frog (━•━•━) is based on data obtained by Kennedy & Voaden (1974) and on the amino acid levels in shaken off frog photoreceptor outer segments (unpublished observations). Recalculations have been based on 10% protein, 85% water contents for monkey and rat retinas and 89% water content for the frog retina.

The retinal layers are OS - photoreceptor outer segments; IS - photoreceptor inner segments; N - photoreceptor nuclei; OP - outer plexiform layer; H - horizontal cells; B - bipolar cells; A - amacrine cells; IP - inner plexiform layer; G - ganglion cells; F - nerve fibre layer.

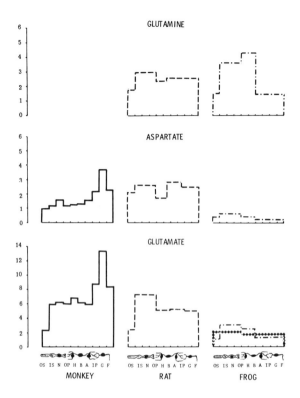

FIGURE 2. The distribution of amino acids in the retina : glutamine, aspartate and glutamate (μmoles / gm wet wt. retina).
    Notations and retinal layers are as designated in Fig. 1.

It must be emphasized that the tissue is only glial-enriched since, at the age the amino acids were measured (21 days) some neurones would still be present. In addition gliosis may have occurred. The estimates for the amino acid concentrations in the retinal glia are based on many approximations, however when they are compared with values found for glial fractions obtained from brain homogenates or with amino acid levels in cerebral gliomas, similarities are apparent (Table III).

From the data in Table II, it is possible also to estimate the tissue pools of each amino acid present in photoreceptor cells, neurones of the inner retina and glial cells. The results from these calculations (Table II) suggest that, in the rat retina, the glutamate, aspartate and glutamine pools are predominantly neuronal and are distributed evenly between photoreceptors and the inner retina

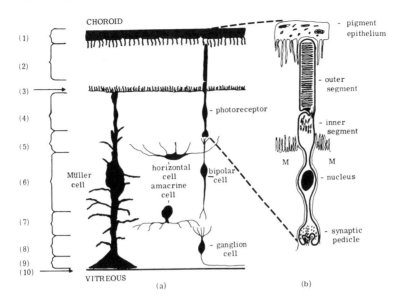

FIGURE 3. Schematic diagram of a) the major constituents of the vertebrate retina and b) a rod photoreceptor. The layers are : (1) pigment epithelium; (2) photoreceptor outer limbs; (3) outer limiting membrane; (4) outer nuclear layer; (5) outer plexiform layer; (6) inner nuclear layer; (7) inner plexiform layer; (8) ganglion cell layer; (9) nerve fibre layer; (10) inner limiting membrane. The arrangement shown does not signify a 1:1 numerical relationship between photoreceptor, bipolar and ganglion cells. M = Müller cell cytoplasm.

Glycine and GABA may also be largely neuronal but differ from glutamate and aspartate in that they are concentrated in the inner retinal neurones. Finally the sulphonic amino acid taurine shows a particular concentration in photoreceptor cells but is present also as the major amino acid in glia and in the inner neuronal pool. The lower percentage of the tissue amino acids in the glial pool does not mean that they are necessarily less concentrated in these cells as the Müller fibres form only 10% of the total tissue volume (Rasmussen 1972, 1973). Assuming that 32% of the tissue volume is extracellular space (as estimated with $^3$H-inulin) the glia, therefore, may form about 14% of the cell space.

Derivation of the above pools has, in part, been based on amino acid distributions obtained from retinal slicing. Some measure of agreement with the data shown in Figs. 1 & 2 might therefore be expected. However, we can also ask how far finer sectioning of the inner retina supports the evidence for neuronal pools obtained from

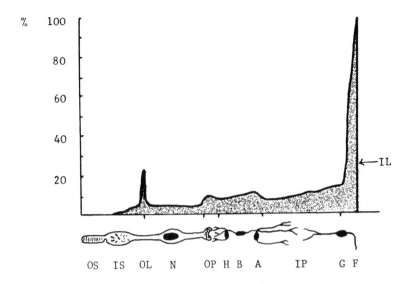

FIGURE 4. The distribution of glial cytoplasm through the rat
retina (% total retinal volume). Redrawn from Rasmussen (1972).
The retinal layers are as designated in Fig. 1. OL - outer
limiting membrane; IL - inner limiting membrane.

glutamate degeneration and how far there is agreement between
laboratories.

As regards the distribution of retinal taurine (Fig. 1), it is
clear from all the studies that the major pool is present in the
photoreceptor cells. This is supported by additional observations
of Orr et al. (1976) and Voaden et al. (1977a) and by amino acid
levels in retinas with degenerate photoreceptors (Cohen et al.,
1973). In addition, the presence of an inner neuronal pool is also
suggested. Mention was made earlier of the disparity in taurine
levels reported in the literature. There is the possibility,
however, of a genuine species difference between the frog (where
the estimates for taurine are consistently low) and the mammalian
retinas; it may be that there is not a glial pool of taurine in the
frog retina (cf. Voaden et al., 1977a).

Glycine and GABA, in contrast to taurine, appear to have their
major location in inner retinal neurones (Fig. 1). This is most
evident in the monkey retina where the distributions strongly support
the conclusions from glutamate degeneration (cf. also Cohen et al.,
1973) and where peaks are seen in the amacrine and inner plexiform
layers of the tissue. There is some discrepancy as to the finer
location of GABA in the frog retina, but this may, in part, be due
to changes in pool sizes according to the adaptational state of the

TABLE II.  PUTATIVE AMINO ACID POOLS IN NEURONES AND GLIA OF THE RAT RETINA

| Amino acid | 21 day normal retina (a) | % in photoreceptor layer * | Photoreceptor layer of 'a' (b) | Inner retina of 'a' (c) | Glutamate treated retina (d) | Glia-enriched inner retina = d-b (e) |
|---|---|---|---|---|---|---|
| Glutamate | 31.2 | 42 | 13.1 | 18.1 | 16.5 | 3.4 |
| Aspartate | 17.6 | 42 | 7.4 | 10.2 | 7.7 | 0.3 |
| Glycine | 21.6 | 25 | 5.4 | 16.2 | 8.4 | 3.0 |
| GABA | 13.6 | 17 | 2.3 | 11.3 | 3.7 | 1.4 |
| Taurine | 60.7 | 55 | 33.4 | 27.3 | 44.0 | 10.6 |
| Glutamine | 24.2 | 40 | 9.7 | 14.5 | 12.1 | 2.4 |

| | 'Glial' contribution** to photoreceptor layer (f) | Photoreceptors | | Inner neurones | | 'glia' | |
|---|---|---|---|---|---|---|---|
| | | (b-f) | %total | (c-e) | %total | (e+f) | %total |
| Glutamate | 0.9 | 12.4 | 40 | 14.7 | 47 | 4.1 | 13 |
| Aspartate | 0.1 | 7.3 | 42 | 9.9 | 56 | 0.4 | 2 |
| Glycine | 0.8 | 4.8 | 22 | 13.1 | 61 | 3.6 | 17 |
| GABA | 0.4 | 2.0 | 15 | 10.0 | 73 | 1.7 | 13 |
| Taurine | 2.8 | 31.2 | 51 | 16.7 | 28 | 12.8 | 21 |
| Glutamine | 0.6 | 9.2 | 38 | 12.1 | 50 | 2.9 | 12 |

Values are expressed as n.moles / retina or equivalent.  Data from Lund Karlsen and Fonnum (1976).
The protein content of the normal retina was 440 µg and the glutamate treated retina 367 µg.
* Voaden et al.(1977a);  ** 21% of total glial pool, Rasmussen (1972)

TABLE III. AMINO ACID CONCENTRATIONS IN BRAIN AND RETINAL GLIA
(μ MOLES / GM WET WEIGHT)

| Amino acid | Source of glial tissue | | | |
|---|---|---|---|---|
| | Rabbit[1] brain | Rat[2] cortex | Human[3] glioblastoma | Rat[4] retina |
| Glutamate | 3.3 | 2.1 | 4.2 | 2.9 |
| Aspartate | 1.0 | 0.6 | 0.8 | 0.3 |
| Glycine | 0.5 | 0.3 | 3.1 | 2.5 |
| GABA | 0.7 | 0.5 | 0.5 | 1.2 |
| Taurine | 0.6 | - | 1.2 | 8.9 |
| Glutamine | 0.6 | - | 3.8 | 2.0 |

Recalculations based on a tissue protein content 10% of wet weight.
1. Subcellular fraction; Sellström et al. (1975), 2. Subcellular
fraction; Nagata et al. (1974), 3. Lefauconnier et al. (1976),
4. Derived from column 'e' Table II by assuming a uniform distribution of tissue protein and thence that 32.3% was present in the
glial-enriched portion (as assessed from the relative areas of
photoreceptor and inner retina in a glutamate treated animal; Lund
Karlsen and Fonnum, 1976).

tissue (Graham, 1974; Voaden, 1976). Similar changes have not been
found in the rat.

Photoreceptor pools of glutamate, aspartate and glutamine appear to
be present in all three species (Fig. 2), and, with the finer slicing
of the monkey retina, inner neuronal pools of glutamine and aspartic
acids are evident, with striking peaks in the ganglion cell layer
of the tissue. The significance of this localization is not known.
There is a possibility that glutamic acid may be a neurotransmitter
released by ganglion cell axons in the optic tectum of pigeons
(Henke et al., 1976) but no information is available on primate
retinas.

In all of the above studies the glial pools are not readily
assessed since, in general, slicing has not been fine enough to
allow discrimination. Nevertheless, supporting the evidence from
glutamate degeneration (Table II), the amino acid levels in the
nerve fibre layer of the monkey show that all the neuroactive amino
acids are potentially present in the Müller cells.

## II. SOURCES OF ENDOGENOUS AMINO ACIDS

There are two ways in which endogenous pools of a compound may be built up. One is by direct uptake, the exogenous source being other cells or the blood stream, and the other is by in situ synthesis from precursors.

### Taurine

There is evidence that the blood stream is a major and, in some species, an essential source of retinal taurine. Cats, maintained on a taurine-free diet, loose their photoreceptor cells, and dietary methionine or cysteine will not halt the progression of the lesion (Berson et al., 1976). There is species variation, however, as there was no evidence of photoreceptor degeneration in rabbits maintained for 16 weeks on essentially the same diet (Lake, Marshall, Morjaria and Voaden, unpublished observations).

The entry of taurine into the retina is restricted by the blood-retinal barrier (cf. Miller and Steinberg, 1976). However, from the blood stream, it is actively taken up by the pigment epithelium (Lake et al., 1977; Voaden et al., 1977a) and then, over several hours, passes into the neural retina, where it enters photoreceptors and more proximal cells. Once there it appears to be remarkably stable with very little turnover or metabolism under normal environmental conditions.

In vitro, exogenously-applied taurine is taken up by photoreceptors and, with species variation, by Müller cells and inner neurones. Glial uptake of taurine is not seen in the frog (Lake et al., 1977) although it is readily apparent in, for example, rat, cat and rabbit retinas (Ehinger, 1973; Voaden et al., 1977a).

Autoradiography and uptake studies suggest that it might be possible to build up the endogenous pools of taurine in retina from exogenous sources of the amino acid. However, it is probable also that there is in situ synthesis, as cysteine oxidase and cysteine sulphinate decarboxylase activities have been demonstrated in rat and ox retinas (Macaione and Di Giorgio, 1977; Pasantes-Morales et al., 1976). In the rat retina, Pasantes-Morales and colleagues found that the level of cysteine sulphinate decarboxylase increased when the photoreceptor cells developed. Slicing or autoradiography are needed to see if this is because of a direct association of the enzyme with photoreceptors or if it is a reflection of increased functional activity.

## Glycine

The observation of peak levels of glycine in the amacrine cell layer of the monkey retina (Fig. 1) correlates well with the uptake of exogenously-applied glycine into subpopulations of amacrine cells (Bruun and Ehinger, 1974; Voaden, 1976). The glycine, once accumulated, is tightly held and not extensively metabolised. However endogenous localization is not as precise as suggested by the autoradiography and precursors must be sought. At present these are not known. A preliminary autoradiographical study with [3]H-serine has failed to reveal labelling of specific cells (Bauer and Ehinger, 1977).

## Glutamate, Aspartate and GABA

Although there may be as much as 85% of the retinal content of glutamate, aspartate and GABA localized in neurones (Table II), nevertheless when their sites of uptake are identified by autoradiography, the major initial influx in mammalian retinas is found to occur into glial cells (Fig. 5; Bruun and Ehinger, 1974; White and Neal, 1976; Voaden, 1976): all three amino acids are then actively metabolised. Correlating with this succinic-semialdehyde dehydrogenase and GABA-$\alpha$-oxoglutarate transaminase are present in Müller cells (Moore and Gruberg, 1974; Hyde and Robinson, 1974).

There is doubt as to the extent of neuronal uptake of the above amino acids in mammalian retinas, but it is clear that uptake will not explain fully the large neuronal stores. They must be formed from endogenous precursors. A potential precursor of neuroactive amino acids in the CNS is glutamine (see eg. Van den Berg, 1973).

Glutamine is a metabolic product of glutamate, aspartate and GABA in the retina and in vitro readily passes out from its sites of formation and accumulates in the incubation medium (Starr, 1975). In vivo, high concentrations (>500µM) are present in vitreous humour (Altman and Dittmer, 1974), implying that endogenous retinal pools could be maintained. In addition, it is formed within the tissue from eg. glucose and acetate (Starr, 1975). It is, therefore, available continuously as a substrate. In line with this, when retinas are pulse-labelled with [3]H-glutamine (4µM) and then incubated in the presence of unlabelled glutamine (400µM) for various times a conversion of the amino acid into glutamate, aspartate and GABA can be detected (Table IV; see also Starr, 1975). [3]H-glutamine can enter all the cells of the retina (Marshall and Voaden, 1976) but, following further incubation with unlabelled glutamine, autoradiography suggests that the main sites of neuroactive amino acid formation are amacrine and ganglion cells (Fig. 6).

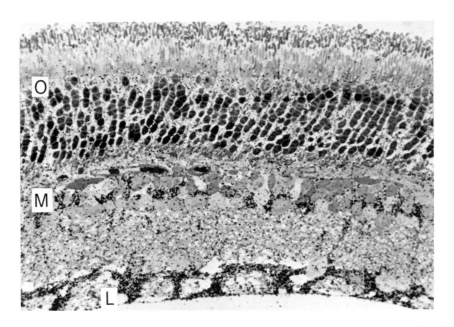

FIGURE 5. Cat retina incubated for 30 min, at 37°C, with L-$\left[\text{G-}^3\text{H}\right]$ aspartic acid (100 μCi/ml; 178 mCi/mmol). Fixation was with glutaraldehyde followed by osmium tetroxide, and Ilford L4 photographic emulsion was used for the autoradiography.

Exposed grains are present throughout Müller cells; over their terminal expansions at the inner limiting membrane (L), over cell bodies (M) and over the outer limiting membrane (O).  ( X 400 ). (Marshall and Voaden, unpublished observations.)


In the longer incubations, it is only the label in GABA that stabilizes or increases (Table IV), suggesting that this may be the main end product. Glutamic decarboxylase activity is also greatest in the amacrine cell, inner plexiform amd ganglion cell layers of the rat retina (Graham, 1974; Voaden, 1976) and EM immunohistochemistry has localised the enzyme to amacrine synaptic terminals (Wood et al., 1976). There is, therefore, very good biochemical evidence supporting the premise that, in the rat, GABA is a transmitter of some amacrine cells.

Many studies suggest that this is true also in the frog retina. In addition, there is evidence that, in eg. the goldfish, frog and pigeon, GABA may also be a transmitter for horizontal cells. A major species difference between these retinas and the mammals so far investigated, is that GABA does not appear, from autoradiography, to enter the glia in frog, goldfish or pigeon, the main uptake

TABLE IV.   GLUTAMINE METABOLISM IN THE RETINA

| Animal | Amino acid | Time of Incubation | | | % of total soluble counts at 60 min |
| --- | --- | --- | --- | --- | --- |
| | | 5 | 5+25 | 5+55 | |
| RAT | aspartate | 2.8± 0.4 | 1.8±0.4 | 1.1±0.2 | 2.6±0.7 |
| | glutamate | 51.9± 9.0 | 21.3±3.1 | 9.6±1.2 | 18.5±1.2 |
| | glutamine | 239.6±30.7 | 27.1±6.2 | 7.3±1.3 | 14.0±1.8 |
| | GABA | 10.3± 2.1 | 26.0±2.5 | 26.6±2.7 | 58.2±2.1 |
| CAT | aspartate | 1.6 | 1.1 | 0.5 | 1.8 |
| | glutamate | 43.0 | 22.0 | 7.1 | 28.2 |
| | glutamine | 200.0 | 28.0 | 8.4 | 33.6 |
| | GABA | 3.1 | 5.0 | 7.3 | 29.3 |

Retinas were incubated for 5 min with 4.35 X $10^{-6}$ M $^3$H-glutamine and then 'chased' with 4.35 X $10^{-4}$ M unlabelled glutamine for the times indicated.  Radioactive counts are expressed as dpm X $10^{-3}$ / mg. wet wt. retina ± SEM.  Data for the rat are based on 3-5 estimations and are given as mean ± SEM.  Values for the cat are from single experiments.
(Lake, Marshall, Morjaria and Voaden, unpublished observation.)

occurring with variation into horizontal, amacrine and ganglion cells.  This has been discussed by Voaden (1976) and will not be considered in detail here.  However it should be noted that GABA synthesis from glutamate has been demonstrated directly in the horizontal cells of the goldfish (Lam, 1975).

GABA is also present at a relatively high level in the horizontal cell layer of the rat retina (Fig. 1).  Its source and function(s) are not known.  However glucose and acetate are readily converted to glutamate, aspartate and GABA (Starr, 1975), and autoradiography following incubation of the rat retina with $^3$H-glucose has shown labelling of photoreceptor and horizontal cells (Marshall and Voaden, 1976).  Preliminary quantitative studies indicate that glucose is converted to all three amino acids in both photoreceptor cells and in the inner retina, but that more GABA synthesis occurs proximal to the photoreceptors (Table V).

III.  GLUTAMINE, GLUTAMATE AND METABOLIC COMPARTMENTATION

When radioactive glutamate, aspartate or GABA are metabolised by eg. the rat retina the specific activity of the total tissue glutamine, a metabolite, is higher than that of its immediate precursor, glutamate (Starr, 1974; Voaden et al., 1977b).  A

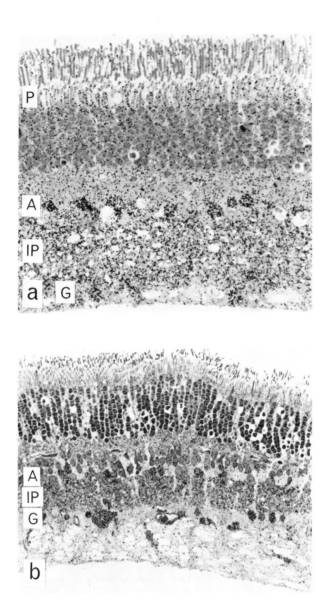

FIGURE 6. Light microscope autoradiographs of a) rat and b) cat retinas incubated for 5 min with 4.35 X $10^{-6}$ M L-[G-$^3$H] glutamine (26 Ci/mmol), and then 'chased' for 55 min with 4.35 X $10^{-4}$ M unlabelled glutamine. Activity can be seen principally in the position of amacrine (A) and ganglion cells (G) and over the inner plexiform layer (IP). Label is also present in photoreceptors (P). (Lake, Marshall, Morjaria and Voaden, unpublished observations.)

TABLE V.  GLUCOSE CONVERSION TO AMINO ACIDS IN THE RAT RETINA

| Amino acid | % of total radioactivity | | |
|---|---|---|---|
| | Photoreceptor layer (80μ) | inner retina | whole retina |
| Aspartate | $3.1 \pm 0.3$ | $3.4 \pm 0.2$ | 6.5 |
| Glutamate | $14.7 \pm 1.5$ | $18.5 \pm 2.3$ | 33.2 |
| Glutamine | $1.8 \pm 0.2$ | $4.7 \pm 0.8$ | 7.6 |
| GABA | $1.9 \pm 0.4$ | $5.5 \pm 0.5$ | 7.4 |
| Total in amino acids | 21.4 | 33.2 | 54.6 |

Retinas were incubated in the presence of 5mM D-$[U-^{14}C]$glucose (327mCi/mmol) for 30 min at 37°C, and sliced as described by Voaden et al., (1977a) using 3mm. diameter trephines (three were combined for each analysis).  Results are the mean of 4 incubations ± SEM.  The mean dpm / 3mm trephine of retina was $2.6 \times 10^4$. (Morjaria and Voaden, unpublished observations).

possible explanation for this anomalous labelling might be that metabolism is occurring via a minor tissue pool of glutamate of high specific activity, thus producing glutamine of high activity. Autoradiography suggests that these pools are in glial cells.  In theory the glutamine is then able to leave the glia and to mix, perhaps freely, with the remaining tissue pools (see above), thus tending to raise the specific activity of the total tissue glutamine. Glutamate cannot do this, since glial cells are its principal site of uptake.  Released glutamate taken up again into the glia, would change not only the specific activity of the glial pool of glutamate but also that of the glutamine formed.  When the total tissue specific activities are measured, the glial pool of glutamate would be diluted by the unlabelled neuronal pools of the amino acid.  To some extent this would also occur for glutamine but the effect might perhaps be lessened by the lower overall concentrations of glutamine as compared to glutamate in mammalian retinas (cf. Fig. 2; see also individual authors Table I).  Against this explanation is the fact that, even after 30-45 mins of incubation with the radioactive substrate, it is still only the glial cells that are principally labelled (Fig. 5; White and Neal, 1976; Voaden, 1976). However, it is recognised that there is a considerable loss of label from CNS tissues when they are fixed in glutaraldehyde, followed by osmium tetroxide,and then processed for autoradiography. It may be that insufficient label is present in the neurones to withstand this method of processing.  Alternatively, there may be a differential loss from a specific location or of a specific amino acid. Present evidence suggests that this does not occur.

In the frog retina radioactive glutamate is taken up by glial cells and again the anomalous specific activity ratios for glutamate and glutamine are found (Kennedy et al., 1974). However, when GABA is metabolised, the reverse is seen (Voaden et al., 1977b; but cf. Starr, 1975). This is also true of the pigeon retina and, in both species, GABA enters extensively into, and is metabolised by, neurones (see Voaden, 1976). As in the rat retina, glutamine is produced, is readily lost from both retinas (Starr, 1975), and is also potentially able to re-enter all cells. In contrast, however, any glutamate produced from the GABA and released from the tissue would not be taken up by the cells that produced it but would enter the glia, labelling more of the tissue pools. In theory these movements would tend to eliminate the 'compartmentation' effect, although, again, the results from autoradiography imply that they might not occur to any great extent.

The data in Fig. 2 suggest that the glutamate concentration is lower in the frog retina than in the mammalian retinas. This results in approximately equal concentrations of glutamate and glutamine (see also Kennedy et al., 1974; Starr, 1975). Moreover the glutamine may be concentrated more in inner neurones. Both of these factors might help to equalise or reverse the relative tissue specific activities of the glutamine and glutamate. A higher concentration of glutamine than glutamate has been found by Voaden et al. (1977a) for the pigeon retina, but Starr (1975) reports glutamine at a level 6% that of glutamate. Further studies are needed, therefore, to investigate this, and also the overall basis for the observations implying a compartmentation of amino acid metabolism in mammalian retinas.

## ACKNOWLEDGEMENT

I am grateful to my colleagues Dr. J. Marshall, Dr. N. Lake and Miss B. Morjaria for allowing me to quote unpublished work in this review. And I thank the Medical Research Council for financial support of our research.

## REFERENCES

Altman, P. L., and Dittmer, D. S., 1974, in "Biology Data Book, 2nd Edition, Volume III", Federation of American Societies for Experimental Biology, Bethesda, Maryland.
Bauer, B., and Ehinger, B., 1976, Failure of [3]H-serine to induce radioactivity in presumed glycinergic retinal neurones, Experientia 32:1460-1461.

Berger, S. J., McDaniel, M. L., Carter, J. G., and Lowry, O. H., 1977, Distribution of four potential transmitter amino acids in monkey retina, J. Neurochem. 28:159-163.

Berson, E. L., Hayes, K. C., Rabin, A. R., Schmidt, S. Y., and Watson, G., 1976, Retinal degeneration in cats fed casein. II Supplementation with methionine, cysteine, or taurine, Invest. Ophthalmol. 15:53-58.

Bruun, A., and Ehinger, B., 1974, Uptake of certain possible neurotransmitters into retinal neurones of some mammals, Exp. Eye Res. 19:435-447.

Cohen, A. I., McDaniel, M., and Orr, H., 1973, Absolute levels of some free amino acids in normal and biologically fractionated retinas, Invest. Ophthalmol. 12:686-693.

Ehinger, B., 1973, Glial uptake of taurine in the rabbit retina, Brain Research 60:512-516.

Graham, L. T. Jr., 1974, Comparative aspects of neurotransmitters in the retina, in "The Eye Volume 6, Comparative Physiology" (H. Davson and L. T. Graham, Jr., eds), pp. 283-342, Academic Press, New York.

Graham, L. T., Baxter, C.F., and Lolley, R. N., 1970, In vivo influence of light or darkness on the GABA system in the retina of the frog (Rana pipiens), Brain Research 20:379-388.

Henke, T. E., Schenker, T. M., and Cuénod, M., 1976, Effects of retinal ablation on uptake of glutamate, glycine, GABA, proline and choline in pigeon tectum, J. Neurochem. 26:131-134.

Hyde, J. C., and Robinson, N., 1974, Localisation of sites of GABA catabolism in the rat retina, Nature 248:432-433.

Kennedy, A. J., Voaden, M. J., and Marshall, J., 1974, Glutamate metabolism in the frog retina, Nature London 252:50-52.

Kennedy, A. J., Neal, M. J., and Lolley, R. N., 1977, The distribution of amino acids within the rat retina, J. Neurochem. 29: 157-159.

Lake, N., Marshall, J., and Voaden, M. J., 1977, The entry of taurine into the neural retina and pigment epithelium of the frog, Brain Research 128:497-503.

Lam, D. M. K., 1975, Biosynthesis of ɣ-aminobutyric acid by isolated axons of cone horizontal cells in the goldfish retina, Nature 254:345-347.

Lefauconnier, J., Portemer, C., and Chatagner, F., 1976, Free amino acids and related substances in human glial tumours and in fetal brain : comparison with normal adult brain, Brain Research 117:105-113.

Lund Karlsen, R., and Fonnum, F., 1976, The toxic effect of sodium glutamate on rat retina : changes in putative transmitters and their corresponding enzymes, J. Neurochem. 27:1437-1441.

Macaione, S., and Di Giorgio, R. M., 1977, Subcellular distribution of cysteine oxidase activity in ox retina, Life Sciences 20: 617-622.

Macaione, S., Ruggeri, P., De Luca, F., and Tucci, G., 1974, Free amino acids in developing rat retina, J. Neurochem. 22:887-891.

Mandel, P., Pasantes-Morales, H., and Urban, P. F., 1976, Taurine,
    a putative transmitter in retina, in "Transmitters in the
    Visual Process" (S. L. Bonting, ed.), pp. 89-105, Pergamon
    Press, London.
Marshall, J., and Voaden, M. J., 1976, unpublished observation
    cited by Voaden (1976).
McIlwain, H., and Bachelard, H. S., 1971,"Biochemistry of the
    central nervous system, 4th Edition", Churchill Livingstone,
    London.
Miller, S., and Steinberg, R. H., 1976, Transport of taurine, L-
    methionine and 3-o-methyl-D-glucose across frog retinal pigment
    epithelium, Exp. Eye Research 23:177-190.
Moore, C. L., and Gruberg, E. R., 1974, The distribution of succinic
    semialdehyde dehydrogenase in the brain and retina of the tiger
    salamander (Ambystoma tigrinum), Brain Research 67:479-488.
Nagata, Y., Mikoshiba, K., and Tsukada, Y., (1974), Neuronal cell
    body enriched and glial cell enriched fractions from young and
    adult rat brains : preparation and morphological and biochemical
    properties, J. Neurochem. 22:493-503.
Neal, M. J., 1976, Amino acid transmitter substances in the verte-
    brate retina, Gen. Pharmacol. 7:321-332.
Orr, H. T., Cohen, A. I. and Lowry, O. H., 1976, The distribution
    of taurine in the vertebrate retina, J. Neurochem. 26:609-611.
Pasantes-Morales, H., Klethi, J., Ledig, M., and Mandel, P., 1972,
    Free amino acids of chicken and rat retina, Brain Research 41:
    494-497.
Pasantes-Morales, H., Lopez-Colome, A. M., Salceda, R., and Mandel,
    P., 1976, Cysteine sulphinate decarboxylase in chick and rat
    retina during development, J. Neurochem. 27:1103-1106.
Rasmussen, K-E., 1972, A morphometric study of the Müller cell
    cytoplasm in the rat retina, J. Ultrastructure Res. 39:413-429.
Rasmussen, K-E., 1973, A morphometric study of the Müller cells,
    their nuclei and mitochondria, in the rat retina, J. Ultra-
    structure Res. 44:96-112.
Sellström, A., Sjöberg, L-B., and Hamberger, A., 1975, Neuronal and
    glial systems for ɣ-aminobutyric acid metabolism, J. Neurochem.
    25:393-398.
Starr, M. S., 1974, Evidence for the compartmentation of glutamate
    metabolism in isolated rat retina, J. Neurochem. 23:337-344.
Starr, M. S., 1975, A comparative study of the utilization of glucose,
    acetate, glutamine and GABA as precursors of amino acids by
    retinae of the rat, frog, rabbit and pigeon, Biochem. Pharmacol.
    24:1193-1197.
Van den Berg, C. J., 1973, A model of compartmentation in mouse
    brain based on glucose and acetate metabolism, in "Metabolic
    compartmentation in the brain" (R. Balázs and J. E. Cremer,
    eds.), pp. 137-166, Macmillan, London.
Voaden, M. J., 1976, ɣ-Aminobutyric acid and glycine as retinal
    neurotransmitters in "Transmitters in the Visual Process" (S. L.
    Bonting, ed.), pp. 107-125, Pergamon Press, London.

Voaden, M. J., Lake, N., Marshall, J., and Morjaria, B., 1977a,
     Studies on the distribution of taurine and other neuroactive
     amino acids in the retina, Exp. Eye Research 25:249-257.
Voaden, M. J., Lake, N., and Nathwani, B., 1977b, A comparison
     of ɣ-aminobutyric acid metabolism in neurones versus glial
     cells using intact isolated retinae, J. Neurochem. 28:457-459.
White, R. D., and Neal, M. J., 1976, The uptake of L-glutamate by
     the retina, Brain Research 111:79-93.
Wood, J. G., McLaughlin, B. J., and Vaughn, J. E., 1976, Immunocyto-
     chemical localization of GAD in electron microscopic prepara-
     tions of rodent CNS, in "GABA in Nervous System Function"
     (E. Roberts, T. Chase, and D. B. Tower, eds.), pp. 133-148,
     Raven Press, New York.
Yates, R. A., and Keen, P., 1975, The effect of optic stalk section
     on the amino acid content of rat retina, Brain Research 99:
     166-169.

# LIGHT-INDUCED RELEASE OF AMINO ACIDS FROM THE RETINA

B. Bauer and B. Ehinger

Departments of Ophthalmology and Histology

University of Lund, Lund, Sweden

## INTRODUCTION

The ultrastructural morphology of the retina strongly suggests that most of the signal transmission between its neurons is by means of chemical synapses. It is important to determine the substances that can serve as transmitters in these synapses, and to identify precisely the ones that operate with a given substance. With such knowledge it becomes possible to influence the synapses in a pre-dictable way in normal or pathological conditions. This is of more than purely academic importance as more and more selective and po-tent psychoactive drugs are coming in use. Most if not all these drugs are likely to exert their effects at chemical synapses. In-deed, knowledge about which synapses that use a defined transmitter is of prime importance also outside the clinical wards: contrast sensitivity or sensitivity to small moving objects in the periphery are examples of functions likely to be mediated through chemical synapses in the retina and which are very important for traffic safety. Several other examples could be listed. However, if a drug selectively impairs either (or a similar function) this is not likely to be detected by traditional clinical trials. Knowledge of the un-derlying  synaptic mechanisms can then aid in deciding on specia-lized tests for selected drugs, and which tests to perform.

The retina is a part of the CNS providing several experimental advantages for neurochemical and neuropharmacological studies. It can be isolated without much injury and kept for hours in a viable condition, responding to light (Ames and Gurian 1960, Gouras and Hoff 1970). The responses of the tissue can be monitored by recording the ERG or by intracellular recording, and the well defined, layered

structure of the retina facilitates the correlation of neurochemical
and neurophysiological findings with anatomical structure. Furthermore the retina is very thin, with very short diffusion pathways
(Ames and Nesbett 1966), and the extracellular fluid therefore
equilibrates rapidly with the bathing fluid. This is a clear advantage in release studies, for example. Moreover, the absence of a
barrier in the diffusion pathways makes retinal preparations very
suitable for pharmacological studies, since compounds can be applied
to the cellular elements under study in known concentrations.
Finally, it is reasonable to assume that the retina utilizes transmitter substances which also occur in the rest of the CNS. Therefore
the study of retinal transmitters, in addition to providing information on visual physiology, may also provide clues to understanding
central synaptic mechanisms in general.

Three criteria are usually recognized as being the most important for identifying a substance as a neurotransmitter:
1. The substance must be synthesized and/or stored presynaptically
   in the nerve endings from which it is released
2. The substance must be released upon presynaptic stimulation and
   appear in the extracellular fluid in the vicinity
3. Postsynaptic applications of the substance must mimic the action
   seen when the presynaptic system is stimulated

In addition, other criteria have been recognized, the most important being that there must be a mechanism for the removal of the
transmitter from the postsynaptic region and that specific antagonists should be able to block both natural transmission and the
action of exogenously applied transmitter. Several of these criteria
have been established for glycine and GABA in the retina (see Neal
1976 b, or Voaden 1976) and for some time they have therefore been
suspected to be retinal neurotransmitters. However, the second criterion has not been demonstrated; that is, it has not been shown
that either glycine or GABA can be released by normal presynaptic
nerve stimulation. The aim of the present work was therefore to
study the possibility of releasing amino acids from the retina with
both light flashes and other types of stimulation. In particular,
the work was concentrated on glycine, GABA and a few similar amino
acids.

It has been shown that certain retinal amacrine neurons will
accumulate and retain exogenously applied glycine (Fig 1), GABA
(Fig 2) and a few more related $\Omega$-amino acids (Ehinger 1976, Bauer
and Ehinger 1977 a). Glycine or GABA accumulated this way mixes in-
distinguishably with the endogenous glycine or GABA (Snyder et al
1973, Neal and Iversen 1969). Thus both morphological autoradiographic experiments as well as biochemical tests suggest that en-
dogenously applied [$^3$H]-amino acid could be used as tracer for the
endogenous neurotransmitter amino acid and this is a fundamental

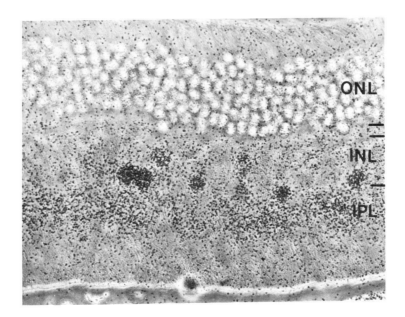

Fig 1. Autoradiograph of rabbit retina 2 hours after the intravitreal injection of 25 µCi [³H] -glycine. There is radioactivity throughout the inner plexiform layer and in certain cell bodies in the inner nuclear layer. ONL, outer nuclear layer; INL, inner nuclear layer; IPL, inner plexiform layer. Phase contrast micrograph, X 480.

prerequisite for the work summarized here.

## METHODS

The concentration of free amino acids in the retina is about ten times higher on a molar ratio than for instance the biogenic amines, which are also presumed neurotransmitters. Thus, it seems likely that only a small fraction of the total tissue content is actually the mobile neurotransmitter, and our work was therefore aimed at using systems capable of detecting small and fairly rapid changes in the release. The initial experiments were done with pre-retinal perfusion in living cats (Ehinger and Lindberg 1974, Ehinger and Lindberg-Bauer 1976) with a technique similar to that used by Kramer (1971). After removal of the anterior segment of the eye and the vitreous, a preretinal stream of fluid is maintained between two cannulas placed 10 mm apart in close proximity with the retina. In later experiments we superfused the rabbit retina in vitro in a specially designed apparatus (Bauer 1977 a). This was found less troublesome than the in vivo experiments and also offered better

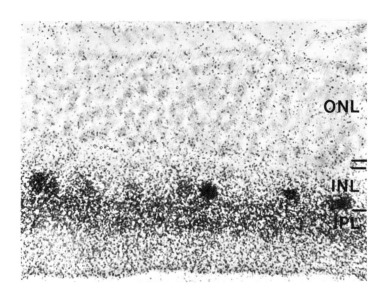

Fig 2. Autoradiograph of rabbit retina 4 hours after the intravitreal injection of 25 μCi [3H] -GABA. There is radioactivity in
the inner plexiform layer and in cell bodies in the innermost part
of the inner nuclear layer. Designation of layers like in Fig 1.
Phase contrast micrograph, X 480.

control of e.g. concentration of applied drugs.

In all cases the retina was labelled by intraocular application
of the tritiated amino acid in vivo. The advantage is that long
application times can be used without running the risk that the
retina deteriorates. This is important because with [3H] -GABA one
has to wait several hours to get rid of the initial heavy glial
labelling (cf Ehinger, 1977). On the other hand, the in vivo labelling results in rather varying absolute radioactivities in different retinas, resulting in the need for an efficient normalization
procedure of the radioactivity efflux curves to make them comparable.
Of several possible procedures, the simplest and most efficient for
the present purposes was found to be to let a computer scale the
efflux curve so that during the five minutes preceding the stimulation it would always attain the same position on the plot. Also,
the experiments were run in a standardized fashion so that the
start of the stimulation was at a fixed time after the start of the
superfusion (with some deliberate exceptions).

The superfusion speed was in all cases 1 ml/min and the effluent
was collected in 1 ml fractions and usually analysed for radioactivity without further fractionation. In order to inhibit reuptake,

the amino acid being tested was usually continuously present (1mM) in non-radioactive form in the superfusate. In the case of GABA it was found that this decreased the amount of tritiated GABA metobolites from 80 to 30 per cent in the superfusate (Bauer 1977 b).

Up to the start of superfusion the experiments were run in ambient laboratory light (190 lux) and thereafter in darkness. Light stimulation was with 2 flashes/sec from a xenon flash tube. The average illumination then was 1.75 lux, but the peak of the flash rapidly reached 2175 lux and then decreased exponentially with a time constant of 0.4 msec.

Changes in the release rate were assessed by comparing with Student s two-tailed t-test the slope of a least squares regression line during stimulation with the slope of a similar line from the control curve.

## RESULTS AND COMMENTS

### Light evoked release of glycine from cat and rabbit retina

Release of radioactive glycine has been demonstrated by electrical stimulation and high $K^+$ concentration in the CNS (Hammerstad et al 1971, Hopkin and Neal 1971, Roberts and Mitchell 1972) and the results have been taken as evidence that glycine is a synaptic transmitter. The validity of these model systems for studying the release of a neurotransmitter rests on the assumption that exogenously administered glycine mixes with endogenous pools and that electrical stimulation or high $K^+$ concentration cause a depolarization of neuronal membranes, similar to physiological stimulation. As discussed above, $[^3H]$ -glycine appears to mix with the endogenous glycine, so that the release of $[^3H]$ -glycine can be taken as a measure of release of endogenous glycine. However, the assumption that electrical stimulation or high $K^+$ concentration replicates physiological nerve activity is questionable. Electrical stimulation has been shown to be able to release non-transmitter amino acids (Orrego and Miranda 1976) and high $K^+$ concentration to release, for example, GABA from tissue where it is unlikely to act as a neurotransmitter (Bowery and Brown 1972). We therefore studied the effect of flashing light on the release of $[^3H]$ -glycine, first in vivo in anaesthetized cats. Intermittent light stimulation evoked an increased release of radioactivity (p<0.001) from cat retina preloaded with $[^3H]$ -glycine (Ehinger and Lindberg 1974, Ehinger and Lindberg-Bauer 1976). Because of technical difficulties, the in vivo experiments were changed to in vitro studies. However, the demonstration of a light evoked release in vivo is of importance since in vivo experiments reflect more closely the normal situation than in vitro experiments. On the other

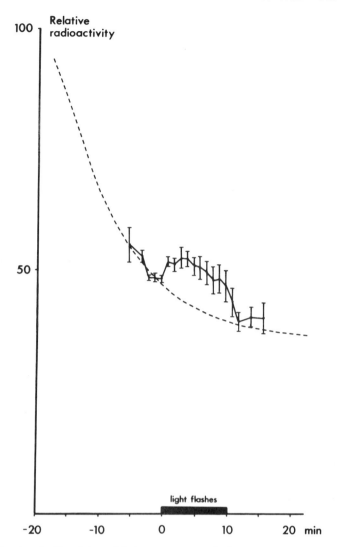

Fig 3. Effect of flashing light on the efflux of radioactivity in vitro from rabbit retinas preloaded in vivo (2 hours) with $[^3H]$-glycine. The broken line is the spontaneous efflux of radioactivity when retinas are kept in the dark. (The time for start of stimulation is marked 0 which was 17-25 min. from the start of superfusion). S.e.m. are indicated by vertical bars; 10 experiments. (From Ehinger and Lindberg-Bauer 1976).

hand, in vitro experiments have the advantages that the experimental procedure is easier. In addition the effect of different stimuli are more easily studied, the release is not subject to any dilution by the blood stream, and the results are therefore more consistently reproducible.

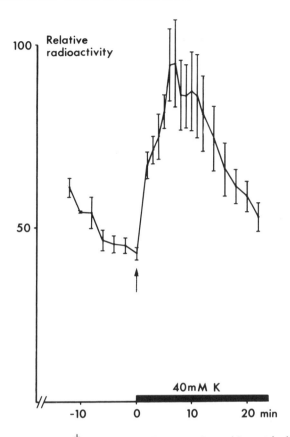

Fig 4. Effect of 40 mil $K^+$ on the release of radioactivity from rabbit retinas preloaded _in vivo_ (2 hours) with $[^3H]$-glycine. The increase is much more pronounced than with light stimulation. Y axis: relative radioactivity of the superfusate. $K^+$ was added 30 min after the start of the superfusion, at time 0 on the X axis. Average of four experiments. The vertical bars indicate the standard errors of the means.


When rabbit retina preloaded with $[^3H]$-glycine was stimulated _in vitro_ by light flashes the release of radioactivity increased significantly ($p < 0.001$, Fig 3). The increase is much less marked than that induced by depolarization with 40 mM $K^+$ (Fig 4, Bauer 1977 a), demonstrating the importance of a sensitive analysis system. If the flashing light was exchanged for continuous light there was no change in the spontaneous efflux of radioactivity.

The site of uptake was checked by autoradiography and found after both preretinal perfusion in cats and intravitreal injection in rabbits to be in amacrine cells and not, or only insignificantly,

present in the glia. This is in good agreement with previous results
(Ehinger and Falck 1971, Bruun and Ehinger 1972, Voaden et al 1974).
It therefore seems likely that these neurons are the source of the
light-evoked increase in radioactivity. This is further supported
by the observation that flashing light is necessary to release the
radioactivity because amacrine cells are known to respond readily
to changes in illumination (see Rodieck 1973). There was also good
correlation between the start of light stimulation and the change
in the efflux of radioactivity when the time between the start of
the experiment and the start of stimulation was varied. This clearly
demonstrated the relationship between stimulation and increased release.

The light-evoked release of $[^3H]$-glycine was inhibited by omitting
Ca $^{2+}$ from the perfusion medium and adding 2 mM-EDTA. It was not
sufficient to only omit Ca$^{2+}$, possible because the depletion from
tissue stores was then not complete enough, as suggested by Hammerstad et al (1971).

It was not possible to detect any light-induced release of
radioactivity from retinas preloaded with $[^3H]$-valine. This amino
acid is not selectively taken up by neurons (Ehinger 1972) and is
not suspected to be a neurotransmitter. The negative results with
$[^3H]$-valine shows that the light-induced release of glycine is not
a nonspecific reaction that can be obtained with any amino acid,
and thus supports the postulation that glycine is a retinal neurotransmitter.

Chromatographic experiments showed that in the experiments
with $[^3H]$-glycine the main part of released radioactivity was in
glycine and it can therefore be concluded from our results that
intermittent light stimulation releases $[^3H]$-glycine from rabbit
retinal neurons preloaded with it. These experiments (Ehinger and
Lindberg-Bauer 1976) thus for the first time demonstrated that
physiological stimulation, in this case light flashes, will release glycine from neurons both in vivo and in vitro, which is one
of the three main criteria needed to establish it as a neurotransmitter. Glycine may be a neurotransmitter in the amacrine cells not
only in rabbit and cat retina but presumably also in all other species with neuronal uptake in the retina.

Adding unlabelled glycine to the superfusion medium in experiments with $[^3H]$-glycine labelled retinas resulted in an increased
efflux of $[^3H]$-glycine, presumably by exchange diffusion or by reuptake competition (Bauer 1977 a). A number of other neutral ⍺-amino
acids were also found to elicit a release of glycine and this raises
the possibility that such amino acids when applied, for example,
iontophoretically can have indirect effects by releasing glycine
from nearby neurons. Caution must therefore be advised in interpreting the results of such experiments so as not to misinterpret
them as a direct inhibitory effect of the applied amino acid.

Glutamic acid, an acidic amino acid, also evoked an increased efflux of [3H]-glycine as promptly as unlabelled glycine did. An increased release was not expected, judging from the results by Crnic et al 1973. They tested the effect of different amino acids on the efflux of [3H]-glycine and [3H]-GABA, and found group specificity for amino acid exchange diffusion and no increased efflux of [3H]-glycine when exposing a [3H]-glycine preloaded rat brain to glutamic acid. However, it is known that glutamic acid may have a neuroactive role in the CNS (see Krnjević 1974). Therefore it was of interest to test if the evoked release of [3H]-glycine by glutamic acid could be inhibited by suppressing synaptic transmission. Lowering the $Ca^{2+}$ level or elevating the $Mg^{2+}$ level blocks retinal synapses (Masland and Ames 1976), and the effect of unlabelled glutamic acid on the efflux of [3H]-glycine was significantly reduced ($p < 0.05$) when the retina was superfused in a medium containing a low $Ca^{2+}$ and high $Mg^{2+}$ concentration. Thus the effect of glutamic acid on the efflux or [3H]-glycine from rabbit retina seems to be more than heteroexchange, possibly an effect on the synaptic membrane. It is unlikely to be caused by spreading depression since the concentration of glutamic acid is too low (Van Harreveld and Fifkowa 1971).

## Photic release of radioactivity from rabbit retina preloaded with 3H-GABA

In rabbits autoradiography demonstrated a predominately neuronal localization of radioactivity 4 hours after intravitreal injection of [3H]-GABA (Fig 2.)(Ehinger and Falck 1971, Marshall and Voaden 1975). Ehinger (1977) has also shown that at short times (2 hours or less) after intravitreal injection of [3H]-GABA or after short incubations the radioactivity has a mainly glial distribution. The radioactivity appears to be well retained in neurons but more rapidly lost from the glia (Ehinger 1977). This difference between glial and neuronal retention of radioactivity makes it possible to study either a mainly glial or a mainly neuronal release of radioactivity by starting the superfusion of the preloaded retina at a time when the radioactivity is localized either mainly in glia or mainly in neurons.

As shown in Fig 5 there was a significantly ($p < 0.005$) increased release of radioactivity when a retina preloaded with [3H]-GABA was stimulated by light flashes four hours later (Bauer 1977 b). Chromatographic analysis of the superfusate showed that at least 40% of the radioactivity was released as [3H]-GABA. The efflux curve of [3H]-GABA closely matched the efflux curve of crude radioactivity. Thus light flashes will evoke an increased release of [3H]-GABA from rabbit retina (Bauer 1977 b).

If continuous light was exchanged for flashing light no increased release was seen. It is known that amacrine cells readily

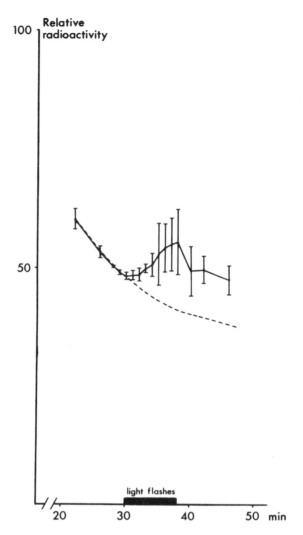

Fig 5. Effect of flashing light stimulation on the efflux of radioactivity in vitro from rabbit retinas preloaded in vivo  (4 hours)
with [³H]-GABA. The broken line is the spontaneous efflux of radioactivity when retina is kept in the dark. S.e.m. are indicated by
vertical bars; 5 experiments. From Bauer 1977 b.


respond to changes in illumination and consequently it seems likely
that the amacrine cells, which autoradiography shows contain much
[³H]-GABA (4 hours after the injection), are the source of the light-
induced increase in radioactivity of the superfusate. Can the photically evoked release of radioactivity originate from glia? If so,
it should be possible to demonstrate an increased release of radio-

activity also when the release of radioactivity originates mainly
from glia. This is the case 2 hours after the intravitreal injection
of [$^3$H]-GABA. However, no photic release of radioactivity was then
demonstrable, and flashing light will thus not release any significant portion of the glial stores which readily accumulate large
amounts of [$^3$H]-GABA (Bauer 1977 b). There should be a small neuronal release in these experiments but presumably it is concealed by
the dominating spontaneous glial efflux.

Calcium ions are thought to play an important role in the release of various neurotransmitters. In studies with GABA the $Ca^{2+}$-
dependence is also an important criterion in interpreting the nature
of the GABA release. The neuronal release seems to be $Ca^{2+}$-dependent
in CNS tissue whereas the nonspecific form of GABA release, such as
that observed by Bowery and Brown (1972) seems to be less $Ca^{2+}$-depen-
dent (Minchin 1975, Sellström and Hamberger 1977). Lowering $Ca^{2+}$ levels or elevating $Mg^{2+}$ levels in the superfusion medium blocks synaptic transmission (Masland and Ames 1976) but does not interfere
with the ability of photoreceptors to respond to light (Dowling and
Ripps 1973, Cervetto and Piccolino 1974, Kaneko and Shimazaki 1975).
No increased release of [$^3$H]-GABA from neurons could be induced by
light flashes under such conditions. Thus the light induced release
of [$^3$H]-GABA is $Ca^{2+}$-dependent which supports the assumption that
is is a neuronal release. In conjunction with the other available
pieces of evidence (see above and Voaden 1976) the present demonstration of a light-induced release of radioactivity from retinas
preloaded with [$^3$H]-GABA strongly suggests that GABA is the transmitter of certain amacrine cells of the rabbit retina.

GABA is rapidly metabolized. AOAA blocks the GABA degrading
enzyme, GABA-T, and is therefore used to depress the metabolism of
GABA. However, in experiments where AOAA ($10^{-4}$M) was added, only
a weak and insignificant light evoked release was observed (Bauer
1977 b). The action of AOAA is known to be rather nonspecific and
it has been shown that under certain conditions it inhibits the
GABA uptake (Snodgrass and Iversen 1973). It would seem that AOAA
also interferes with GABA release although our experiments do not
show how. Consequently AOAA does not seem to be a suitable additive
when light induced neuronal release of GABA is studied, especially
at the concentrations used here.

When the animals were anaesthetized with pentobarbitone no
light-evoked release of [$^3$H]-GABA could be demonstrated (Bauer and
Ehinger 1977 c). The spontaneous efflux of [$^3$H]-GABA was also re-

duced when pentobarbitone ($10^{-3}$M) was added to the superfusion
fluid (Bauer 1977 b). A similar effect has been noted in rat brain
slices where pentobarbitone competitively inhibits GABA uptake and
reduces both the spontaneous efflux and the accelerated efflux produced by elevated $K^+$ or ouabain (Cutler et al 1974). The mechanism
underlying this effect is not clear. Cutler et al (1974) suggest
that pentobarbitone may interfere with membrane transport and our
experiments are compatible with such a hypothesis.

In contrast to the results with [$^3$H]-GABA the efflux of [$^3$H]-
glycine is not affected by pentobarbitone up to $10^{-3}$M concentration
(Bauer, unpublished results). Furthermore, in a previous study a
light-evoked release of [$^3$H]-glycine from retina was demonstrable
in pentobarbitone anaesthetized rabbits and cats (Ehinger and Lindberg 1974, Ehinger and Lindberg-Bauer 1976). Thus the neuronal release of glycine does not seem to be affected by pentobarbitone,
neither in vitro nor in vivo, in contrast to the effect on the neuronal release of GABA. This is important to note because it demonstrates that the effect of pentobarbitone is not a nonspecific, general, membrane-blocking action. Furthermore, it demonstrates that
not only is the uptake mechanism for GABA and glycine different in
the rabbit retina (Bruun and Ehinger 1972), but that there also are
fundamental differences in the release mechanisms, making them
differently sensitive to different drugs.

Retinal uptake and release of [$^3$H]-DABA

Considerable species variation has been noted in the [$^3$H]-GABA
uptake into the retina. Four hours after an intravitreal injection
the localization was predominately glial in such species as rats and
cynomolgus monkeys, whereas it was mainly neuronal in, for example,
rabbits, guinea-pigs and cats (Bruun and Ehinger 1974, Marshall and
Voaden 1974, Voaden 1976). [$^3$H]-GABA therefore offers little assistance  in identifying putative GABA-ergic retinal neurons with autoradiography in some species. It was therefore desirable to study analogues of GABA not entering, e.g., the so-called GABA shunt in the
cellular metabolism, but which simulate the neurotransmitter function of GABA.

In the CNS DABA has been considered as a substrate for the
neuronal uptake mechanism for GABA (see Iversen et al.1975). The
high affinity neuronal uptake of GABA is inhibited by DABA but the
glial uptake is affected to a much smaller extent (Iversen and
Johnston 1971, Schon and Kelly 1974). The DABA uptake is also inhibited by the same compounds which are effective inhibitors of the
[$^3$H]-GABA uptake, and the kinetic parameters for the DABA uptake
closely match those found for GABA (see Iversen et al. 1975).
Furthermore, DABA has been demonstrated to be taken up by cerebral
cortex and cerebellum into nerve terminals with a distribution
closely comparable to that previously obtained with [$^3$H]-GABA,
whereas no uptake was found over satellite glial cells (see Iversen

et al. 1975). Therefore DABA has been suggested to be a suitable marker for neurons operating with GABA as a transmitter.

Four hours after the intravitreal injection of $[^3H]$-DABA radio-activity appeared in the rabbit retina mainly in the inner plexi-form layer and in cell bodies with the location which corresponds to that of amacrines (Bauer and Ehinger 1977 a). It was very simi-lar to that seen with $[^3H]$-GABA. It was not possible from the auto-radiograms to assert unequivocally that the neurons which take up and retain DABA were also the same as those that take up GABA. However, the distribution of radioactivity after intravitreal in-jection of $[^3H]$-DABA fits best with the one seen after intravitre-al injection of $[^3H]$-GABA. Therefore it is reasonable to assume that $[^3H]$-DABA labels GABA-ergic neurons in the retina. On the other hand autoradiograms shortly after intravitreal injection of $[^3H]$-DABA (30 min.) or after brief (15 min.) incubation in $[^3H]$-DABA showed that there was not only a neuronal uptake of $[^3H]$-DABA but also a glial one (Bauer and Ehinger 1977 a). Biochemical uptake studies with short incubation times thus show the glial up-take and not the neuronal one. The uptake was found to be tempera-ture dependent as expected by an active energy dependent mechanism and was there a high affinity component in it ($K_m$ 2.11 x $10^{-5}$M and V max 2.38 x $10^{-5}$ moles/mg/min.), which also has been reported for the glial uptake of GABA (Starr and Voaden 1972, Goodchild and Neal 1973, Schon and Kelly 1974). The DABA uptake in our experiments in rabbit retina was significantly inhibited by GABA but not by gly-cine, $\beta$-alanine or $\epsilon$-aminocaproic acid (Bauer and Ehinger 1977 a). The results suggest that DABA and GABA may have a common glial up-take system.

A glial uptake system for DABA may explain the observation by Goodchild and Neal (1973) and by Neal (1976 a) that the GABA uptake was inhibited by DABA in rat retina, where GABA is mainly taken up by glia (Neal and Iversen 1972, Bruun and Ehinger 1974, Marshall and Voaden 1974).

After intravitreal injections of $[^3H]$-DABA in rats there was marked radioactivity in some cells with the localization consistent with that of amacrines and in the inner plexiform layer (at 1/2, 2 and 4 hours after the injection). In cats the radioactivity had the same localization as in rats but was weaker. In guinea-pigs, the distribution of radioactivity was the same at 1/2 and 4 hours as in rats. However, in addition to a neuronal labelling in the inner layers of the inner nuclear layer there was a significant glial labelling (Bauer and Ehinger 1977 a). The study thus shows that $[^3H]$-DABA gives less variability in the neuron marking than $[^3H]$-GABA and from this point of view $[^3H]$-DABA is therefore the preferable sub-stance of the two for labelling neurons. The improvement when using $[^3H]$-DABA is most marked in rats. The distribution of labelled neurons

and the uptake characteristics are very similar between [3H] -DABA
and [3H] -GABA, both in this work and in previous studies on rat and
cat brain (see Iversen et al. 1975, Kelly and Dick 1976) so that
it would seem that [3H] -DABA is a good marker for GABA neurons.

In the retina [3H] -DABA is strongly retained in neurons as is
illustrated by the observation that neuronal radioactivity is readily demonstrable as much as 24 hours after the intravitreal injection.
This may be one reason why DABA is a good neuronal marker despite
the presence of a high affinity glial uptake.

When [3H] -DABA preloaded (4 hours) rabbit retinas were stimulated by flashing light it was not possible to demonstrate any significantly increased release of radioactivity, which seems to indicate that DABA is more strongly bound to the neurons than GABA. The
general experimental conditions do not seem to be a restricting
factor of the light-induced release of [3H] -DABA since [3H] -GABA,
[3H] -glycine and [3H] - $\beta$ -alanine under identical conditions can be
released by flashing light from neuronal stores in rabbit retina
(Ehinger and Lindberg-Bauer 1976, Bauer 1977 b, Bauer and Ehinger
1977 b). [3H] -DABA is on the other hand released by depolarizing
the tissue with K+ (40 mM), which indicates that it is not alto-
gether impossible to release it (Bauer and Ehinger 1977 a).

In a retina with neurons containing [3H] -DABA the effect of
an applied amino acid on the efflux of radioactivity is a measure
of the degree to which the amino acid will interfere with the neuronal transport system of [3H] -DABA. In such experiments GABA and
$\beta$ -alanine increased the release of [3H] -DABA, whereas glycine did
not (Bauer and Ehinger 1977 a). It would thus seem that DABA, GABA
and $\beta$ -alanine may have a common neuronal release mechanism in contrast to that of glycine.

DABA has previously been suggested to be a selective inhibitor
or neuronal GABA uptake since it affects uptake in cortical slices
but not sensory (see Iversen et al. 1975) or sympathetic ganglia
(Bowery and Brown 1972). However, Leach et al. (1976) have reported
both a neuronal and a glial labelling in rat cerebral cortex by
[3H] -DABA, and in bulk isolated fractions of glia and synaptosomes
DABA inhibited the GABA uptake equally well (Sellström and Hamberger 1975). Similarly, our experiments also show that in the retina [3H] -DABA is labelling not only neurons but glia as well. However, DABA is not as well retained by glia as by neurons and therefore the net effect is that DABA labels neurons better than GABA,
particularly in rats. Nevertheless, the observation indicate that
[3H] -DABA labelling should not be used indiscriminately.

Stimulated release of [3H] - $\beta$ -alanine from rabbit retina

$\beta$ -alanine has been suggested to act as a selective inhibitor

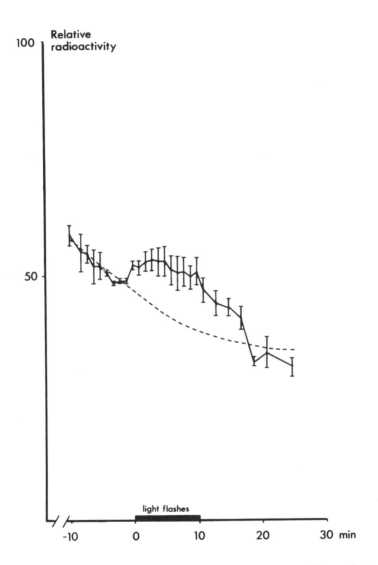

Fig 6. Effect of flashing light on the efflux of radioactivity in vitro from rabbit retinas preloaded in vivo with $[^3H]$-$\beta$-alanine. The broken line is the spontaneous efflux of radioactivity in the dark. The time for the start of stimulation is marked 0 (which was 20-25 min. from the start of superfusion). S.e.m. are indicated by vertical bars; 8 experiments. From Bauer and Ehinger 1977 b.

for the high-affinity GABA-uptake in glial cells (Schon and Kelly
1974) and an exclusive glial localization of $[^3H]$-$\beta$-alanine has
been reported by Schon and Kelly (1975) in rat cerebral cortex and
sensory ganglia. However, in rabbit retina autoradiography has shown
that the site of uptake is mainly in inner plexiform layer, in cells
with a localization corresponding to that of amacrines as well as
in some ganglion cells (Ehinger 1972, Bruun and Ehinger 1974, Bruun
et al. 1974). In our study the site of uptake was checked by autoradiography two hours after the intravitreal injection of $[^3H]$-$\beta$-
alanine and was the same as that described above in rabbit retina.
A significantly (p < 0.001) increased efflux of radioactivity was
seen when rabbit retina preloaded with $[^3H]$-$\beta$-alanine was stimulated with light flashes (Bauer and Ehinger 1977 b, Fig 6). Chromatographic experiments showed that it was mainly $\beta$-alanine that was
released and previous studies have shown that only very little $\beta$-
alanine appears as metabolites (Bruun et al. 1974, Johnston 1977).
Thus the increased efflux of radioactivity means that $\beta$-alanine
can be released by physiological, light-induced nerve activity in
the retina. It seems most likely that the amacrines, which autoradiography shows contain the highest concentration of radioactivity,
are the source of the light-induced increase of radioactivity in
the superfusate in these experiments.

To get more information about the transport system of $\beta$-ala-
nine, the influence of an added amino acid on the efflux of $[^3H]$-
$\beta$-alanine was studied. In these experiments $\beta$-alanine (0.5 and
5 mM) evoked an increased efflux of $[^3H]$-$\beta$-alanine, presumably
by exchange diffusion or by competition for its reuptake. Similar effects have been demonstrated for glycine on the efflux of
$[^3H]$-glycine from rabbit retina (Bauer 1977 a) and for GABA on the
efflux of $[^3H]$-GABA from frog retina (Kennedy and Voaden 1974).
When GABA (0.5 or 5 mM) was added to the superfusion medium there
was also an immediate increased efflux of $[^3H]$-$\beta$-alanine. 5 mM
GABA had nearly the same effect as 5 mM $\beta$-alanine. Glycine, on the
other hand, was much less effective (Bauer 1977 a). 5 mM glycine
evoked a slight increase on the efflux of radioactivity but the
effect of 0.5 mM glycine was insignificant. Uptake studies on rabbit
retina have also shown that the uptake of $\beta$-alanine is competitively
inhibited by GABA but is unaffected by glycine (Bruun et al 1974).
Thus it seems that $\beta$-alanine may use the same transport system as
GABA in the retina.

40 mM $K^+$ evoked a strongly increased efflux of $[^3H]$-$\beta$-alanine.
Similarly, a potassium stimulated release of $[^3H]$-$\beta$-alanine has recently been demonstrated by Johnston (1977) from rat spinal cord and
from rat cerebral cortex. A difference was found between the two
sites. In the spinal cord the $K^+$ evoked release was $Ca^{2+}$-dependent,
suggesting a neuronal origin of the $[^3H]$-$\beta$-alanine. On the other
hand the $K^+$ induced release of $[^3H]$-$\beta$-alanine in cerebral cortex

was $Ca^{2+}$ independent indicating a release from other cells than
neurons, presumably glia, which in rat cerebral cortex accumulate
[$^3$H] - $\beta$-alanine. The localization of radioactive $\beta$-alanine in the
spinal cord has not yet been reported but it seems that $\beta$-alanine
may share the same transport system as GABA in the spinal cord and
be transported into a compartment which most likely is associated
with nerve terminals (Johnston 1977). The results indicate that
$\beta$-alanine both in rabbit retina and in rat spinal cord  is transported in a different manner than in the cerebral cortex, and that
it is not as exclusively a glial marker as was first proposed. Also,
uptake studies confirm that the retina differs from CNS in handling
$\beta$-alanine. In the brain, DABA is supposed to be a selective inhibitor of neuronal uptake of GABA, and should not affect the glial
uptake. Conversely, $\beta$-alanine is supposed to affect the glial uptake, and should therefore inhibit glial uptake of GABA better
than DABA does. However, the reverse was found to be true in rat
retina (Neal 1976 a).

It has thus been shown that in rabbit retina [$^3$H] - $\beta$-alanine
is taken up mainly by amacrine cells (Bruun and Ehinger 1972,
Bruun et al. 1974) from which it is released by physiological stimulation with light flashes (Bauer and Ehinger 1977 b). $\beta$-alanine
seems to use a neuronal transport system in common with GABA. The
results support the suggestion that $\beta$-alanine may act as a "false
transmitter" mimicking GABA in the retina (Bruun et al. 1974) but
may also indicate that it may have a neuroactive role of its own
in the rabbit retina. However, further main criteria have to be
fulfilled before $\beta$-alanine can be considered as a neurotransmitter.
It remains to be shown that it is stored and/or synthesized presynaptically in the retina and that the application of $\beta$-alanine
mimics the action seen when the presynaptic system is stimulated.

## ACKNOWLEDGEMENTS

This work was supported by grants from the Swedish Medical Research
council (project 04X-2321), the Faculty of Medicine at the University of Lund, the C-B Nathhorsts Stiftelse, and the H Järnhardts Stiftelse.

REFERENCES

Ames, A., and Gurian, B., 1960, Measurement of function in an
    in vitro preparation of mammalian central nervous tissue,
    J. Neurophysiol. 23:676-691.
Ames, A., and Nesbett, B., 1966, Intracellular and extracellular
    compartments of mammalian central nervous tissue, J. Physiol.
    184:215-238.
Bauer, B., 1977 a, Factors affecting the spontaneous release of
    [3H]-glycine from rabbit retina, Acta Ophthal. 55: in press.
Bauer, B., 1977 b, Photic release of radioactivity from rabbit re-
    tina preloaded with [3H]-GABA, Exp. Brain Res. in press.
Bauer, B., and Ehinger, B., 1977 a, Retinal uptake and release
    of [3H]-DABA, Exp. Eye Res. in press.
Bauer, B., and Ehinger, B., 1977 b, Stimulated release of [3H]-$\beta$-
    alanine from rabbit retina, Brain Res. 120:447-457.
Bauer, B., and Ehinger, B., 1977 c, Light evoked release of radio-
    activity from rabbit retinas preloaded with [3H]-GABA, Experi-
    mentia 33:470-471.
Bowery, N.G., and Brown, D.P., 1972, $\gamma$-aminobutyric acid uptake
    by sympathetic ganglia, Nature New Biol. 238:89-91.
Bruun, A., and Ehinger, B., 1972, Uptake of the putative neurotrans-
    mitter, glycine into rabbit retina, Invest. Ophthal. 11:191-
    198.
Bruun, A., and Ehinger, B., 1974, Uptake of certain possible neuro-
    transmitters into retinal neurons of some mammals, Exp. Eye
    Res. 19:435-447.
Bruun, A., Ehinger, B., and Forsberg, A., 1974, In vitro uptake of
    $\beta$-alanine into rabbit retinal neurons, Exp. Brain Res. 19:
    239-247.
Cervetto, L., and Piccolino, M., 1974, Synaptic transmission between
    photoreceptors and horizontal cells in the turtle retina,
    Science 183:417-419.
Crnic, D.M., Hammerstad, J.P., and Cutler, R.W.P., 1973, Accelerated
    efflux of [14C] and [3H] amino acids from superfused slices of
    rat brain, J. Neurochem. 20:203-209.
Cutler, R.W.P., Markowitz, D., and Dudzinsky, D.S., 1974, The effect
    of barbiturates on [3H]-GABA transport in rat cerebral cortex
    slices, Brain Res. 81:189-197.
Dowling, J., and Ripps, H., 1973, Effects of magnesium on horizontal
    cell activity in the skate retina, Nature 242:101-103.
Ehinger, B., 1970, Autoradiographic identification of rabbit retinal
    neurons that take up GABA, Experientia 26:1063.
Ehinger, B., 1972, Cellular location of the uptake of some amino
    acids into the rabbit retina, Brain Res. 46:297-311.
Ehinger, B., 1976, Selective neuronal accumulation of $\Omega$-amino acids
    in the rabbit retina, Brain Res. 107:541-554.
Ehinger, B., 1977, Glial and neuronal uptake of GABA, glutamic acid
    glutamine and glutathione in rabbit retina, Exp. Eye Res. in

press.

Ehinger, B., and Falck, B., 1971, Autoradiography of some suspected neurotransmitter substances: GABA, glycine, glutamic acid, aspartatic acid, histamine, dopamine and L-DOPA, Brain Res. 33:157-172.

Ehinger, B., and Lindberg, B., 1974, Light-evoked release of glycine from the retina, Nature 251:727-728.

Ehinger, B and Lindberg-Bauer, B., 1976, Light-evoked release from cat and rabbit retina, Brain Res. 113:535-549.

Gouras, P., and Hoff, M., 1970, Retinal function in an isolated, perfused mammalian eye, Invest. Ophthal. 9:388-399.

Goodchild, M., and Neal, M.J., 1973, The uptake of $[3H]$-$\gamma$-aminobutyric acid by the retina, Br. J. Pharmac. 47:529-542.

Hammerstad, J.P., Murray. J.E., and Cutler, R.W.P. , 1971, Efflux of amino acid neurotransmitters from rat spinal cord slices. II. Factors influencing the electrically induced efflux of $[14C]$-glycine and $[3H]$-GABA. Brain Res. 35:357-367.

Hopkin, J., and Neal, M.J., 1971, Effect of electrical stimulation and high potassium concentrations on the efflux of $[14C]$-glycine from slices of spinal cord. Br. J. Pharmac. 42:215-223.

Iversen, L.L., Dick, F., Kelly, J.S., and Schon, F., 1975, Uptake and localization of transmitter amino acids in the nervous system, In Berl, S., Clarke, D. and Schneider, D. (eds.), Metabolic compartmentation and neurotransmission, Plenum Press, pp 65-90.

Iversen, L.L., and Johnston, G.A.R., 1971, GABA uptake in rat central nervous system: comparison of uptake in slices and homogenates and the effects of some inhibitors, J. Neurochem. 18:1939-1950.

Johnston, G.A.R., 1970, Effects of calcium on the potassium-stimulated release of radioactive $\beta$-alanine and $\gamma$-aminobutyric acid from slices of rat cerebral cortex and spinal cord, Brain Res. 121:179-181.

Kaneko, A., and Shimazaki, H., 1975, Effects of external ions on the synaptic transmission from photoreceptors to horizontal cells in the carp retina, J. Physiol. 252:509-522.

Kelly, J.S., and Dick, F., 1976, Differential labelling of glial cells and GABA-inhibitory interneurons and nerve terminals following the microinjection of $\beta$-$[3H]$alanine, $[3H]$-DABA and $[3H]$-GABA into single folia of cerebellum. In Cold Spring Harbor Symposia on quantitative biology, Vol. 60, The Synapse, Cold Spring Harbor Laboratory, pp. 93-106.

Kennedy, A.J., and Voaden, M.J., 1974, Factors affecting the spontaneous release of $[3H]$-$\gamma$-aminobutyric acid from the frog retina in vitro, J. Neurochem. 22:63-71.

Kramer, S.G., 1971, Dopamine: a retinal neurotransmitter. I. Retinal uptake, storage and light-stimulated release of $[3H]$-dopamine in vivo. Invest. Ophthal. 10:438-452.

Krnjević, K., 1974, Chemical nature of synaptic transmission in
    vertebrates, Physiological Reviews 54:418-540.
Leach, M.J., Riddel, D.R., and Winkley, C.M., 1976, Uptake of
    L-2,-4 diamino 4-$^3$H butyric acid into slices of rat cere-
    bral cortex, J. Neurochem. 27:1281-1282.
Marshall, J., and Voaden, M., 1974, An investigation of the cells
    incorporating [$^3$H]-GABA and [$^3$H]-glycine in isolated retina
    of the rat, Exp. Eye Res. 18:367-370.
Marshall, J., and Voaden, M., 1975, Autoradiographic identification
    of the cells accumulating [$^3$H]-$\gamma$-aminobutyric acid in
    mammalian retinae: a species comparison, Vision Res. 15: 459-
    461.
Masland, R., and Ames, A., 1976, Responses to acetylcholine of
    ganglion cells in isolated mammalian retina, J. Neurophysiol.
    39:1220-1235.
Minchin, M.C.W., 1975, Factors influencing the efflux of [$^3$H]-
    gamma-aminobutyric acid from satellite glial cells in rat
    sensory ganglia, J. Neurochem. 24:571-577.
Neal, M.J., 1976 a, The uptake and release of $\gamma$-aminobutyric
    acid (GABA) by the retina. In Levi, Battistin, Lajtha (eds.):
    "Transport phenomena in the nervous system", Plenum Press,
    N.Y. London, pp. 211-220.
Neal, M.J., 1976 b, Amino acid transmitter substances in the verte-
    brate retina, Gen. Pharmac. 7:321-332.
Neal, M.J., and Iversen, L.L., 1969, Subcellular distribution of
    endogenous and [$^3$H] aminobutyric acid in rat cerebral cortex,
    Journal of Neurochemistry 16:1245-1252.
Neal, M.J., and Iversen, L.L., 1972, Autoradiographic localization
    of [$^3$H]-GABA in rat retina, Nature New Biol. 235:217-218.
Orrego, F., and Miranda, R., 1976, Electrically induced release of
    [$^3$H]-GABA from neocortical thin slices. Effects of stimulus
    waveform and of amino-oxyacetic acid. J. Neurochem. 26:1033-
    1038.
Roberts, P.J., and Mitchell, J.F., 1972, The release of amino acids
    from the hemisected spinal cord during stimulation, J. Neuro-
    chem. 19:2473-2481.
Rodieck, R.W., 1973, In:"The Vertebrate Retina", Freeman and Co.,
    San Francisco, Calif., pp. 506-509.
Schon, F., and Kelly, J.S., 1974, The characterization of [$^3$H]-GABA
    uptake into satellite glial cells of rat sensory ganglia, Brain
    Res. 66:289-300.
Schon, F., and Kelly, J.S., 1975, Selective uptake of [$^3$H]-$\beta$-ala-
    nine by glia: association with the glial uptake system for
    GABA. Brain Res. 86:243-257.
Sellström, A., and Hamberger, A., 1975, Neuronal and glial systems
    for  -aminobutyric acid transport, J. Neurochem. 24:847-852.
Sellström, A., and Hamberger, A., 1977, Potassium-Stimulated $\gamma$-
    amino-butyric acid release from neurons and glia. Brain Res.
    119:189-198.

Snodgrass, S.R., and Iversen, L.L., 1973, Effects of amino-oxyacetic acid on [$^3$H] -GABA uptake by rat brain slices, J. Neurochem. 20:431-439.

Snyder, S., Yamamura, H., Pert, C., Logan, W., and Bennet, J., 1973, Neuronal uptake of neurotransmitters and their precursors: studies with "transmitter" amino acids and choline. In Mandel, A. (ed.):"New concepts in neurotransmitter regulation", Plenum Press N.Y. London, pp. 195-222.

Starr, M., and Voaden, M., 1972, The uptake of [$^{14}$C] -aminobutyric acid by the isolated retina of the rat, Vision Res. 12:549-557.

Van Harreveld, A., and Fifkowa, E., 1971, Effects of glutamate and other amino acids on the retina, J. Neurochem. 18:2145-2154.

Voaden, M., 1976, Gamma aminobutyric acid and glycine as retinal neurotransmitters, In Bonting, S.L. (ed.):"Transmitters in the Visual Process", Pergamon Press, pp. 107-126.

Voaden, M., Marshall, J., and Murani, N., 1974, The uptake of [$^3$H] - $\gamma$-aminobutyric acid and [$^3$H]glycine by the isolated retina of the frog, Brain Res. 67:115-132.

# CLASSIFICATION AND LOCATION OF NEURONS TAKING UP $^3$H-GABA IN THE VISUAL CORTEX OF RATS

B.M. Chronwall and J.R. Wolff

Dept. Neurobiology, Neuroanatomy, Max-Planck-Institute

for Biophysical Chemistry, P.B. 968, D-3400 Göttingen

## INTRODUCTION

There is converging evidence from biochemical and electro-physiological work suggesting that GABA acts as an inhibitory transmitter in the neocortex (Baxter, 1970; Krnjević, 1976). However, except for the reports of Hökfelt and Ljungdahl (1971, 1972), suggesting that neurons in lamina I (LI) to LIII take up $^3$H-GABA, little is known of the type and position of neurons which might take up, produce and utilize GABA. This preliminary report presents an autoradiographic study of the distribution of neurons taking up $^3$H-GABA and their location in various layers of the adult rat neocortex.

## MATERIALS AND METHODS

Trepanations were made over area 17 on adult Sprague-Dawley rats one week before the experiment to minimize edema. Under urethane anesthesia 2 μl, containing 50-150 μCi of 4-amino-n-G-$^3$H butyric acid ($^3$H-GABA) were injected under pressure into various depths. For comparison a mixture of aminooxyacetic acid (AOAA) and $^3$H-GABA was injected into animals pretreated with AOAA (80 mg/kg body weight) for 30 minutes. Preparation of autoradiographs: 0-45 minutes after the injection animals were perfused intracardially with 2.5% glutaraldehyde in cacodylat buffer. Tissue was embedded in Epon 812. Semithin sections were cut at 3-4 μm, dipped in Ilford L4 or K2 emulsion, exposed 8-12 days at 4°C and developed in Kodak D19b.

RESULTS

## General Features of the Labelling

Silver grains were found over cells of the pia mater, some endothelial cells and pericytes of pial and intracerebral vessels, astrocytic and neuronal somata and elements of the neuropil. In edematous areas labelled axonterminal-like structures became more prominent (comparable to results from uptake in slices (Neal and Iversen, 1969; Hökfelt and Ljungdahl, 1970; Iversen and Bloom, 1972 and own unpublished results)), whereas the labelling of neuronal somata was diminished.

The intensity of the labelling varied greatly between different neurons of the same section; heavily labelled neurons were often found adjacent to moderately or very lightly labelled neurons (fig. 1a). These findings were consistent for the neurons concerned through serial sections. The variability in labelling was observed in all cortical layers and in all types of labelled neurons.

Main dendrites, identifiable as relatively thick, straight and smooth processes may be labelled along much of their length (fig. 2c and 3), especially those which are vertically oriented and penetrate LII to LV and the upper LVI. Thinner, branched, tortuous and beaded labelled structures appear to be axons.

## Distribution and Types of Labelled Neurons

Labelled neurons have been found in all layers of the neocortex as well as in the subcortical white matter. LI is the only cortical layer where almost all cells are labelled in the zone into which $^3$H-GABA has diffused (fig. 1a). Labelled cells are found in all levels of LI. In the superficial half the perikarya of the neurons are larger and the longer axis horizontally oriented (fig. 1a and e). These neurons might be Cajal-Retzius cells (fig. 1c). On the other hand, smaller neurons showing multipolar or vertically oriented, elongated perikarya are situated in the deep half of LI (fig. 1a, b and f). These neurons are probably identical with small spiny stellates (fig. 1d). Upper LII contains small labelled neurons (fig. 1b). These neurons are sometimes surrounded by a labelled axonal network resembling that of the small basket cell.

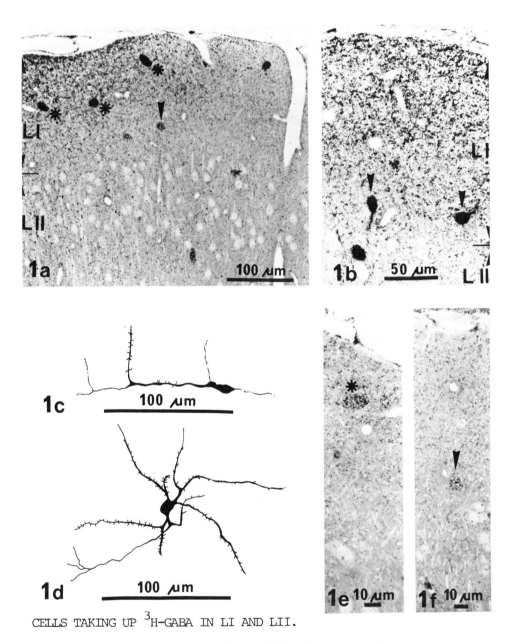

CELLS TAKING UP ³H-GABA IN LI AND LII.

Neurons in the upper part of LI ( ✱ ): fig. 1a and 1e.
Fig. 1c Drawing of a Golgi preparation of a Cajal-Retzius cell.

Neurons in the lower part of LI ( ▼ ): fig. 1a, 1b and 1f.
Fig. 1d Drawing of a Golgi preparation of a small spiny stellate.

Lower LII, LIII and LIV contain a relatively higher number of labelled neurons, most of which are fusiform in shape with vertically arranged main dendrites (fig. 2b-e). In several cases it was possible to follow at least the first branching of the upper or lower main dendrite (fig. 2e) indicating that they may branch dichotomously near the perikarya. These neurons might not represent a uniform population, but may have at least some characteristic features in common with the "cellule à double bouquet dendritique" of Cajal (fig. 2a) (cf. Colonnier, 1966; fig. 11, Szentágothai, 1973). The unipolar cells could also belong to other types such as the star pyramids (Szentágothai, 1976). Neurons of various size with more angular somata are also found in these laminae. The large ones in LIV sometimes show dendrites extending in all directions (fig. 3). These could belong to the group of stellate cells described by Kelly and Van Essen (1974) as exerting inhibitory effects on other cortical cells.

In LV only a few labelled neurons have been found. Numerous neurons of a great variety of types and sizes are labelled in LVI: horizontally oriented cells with fusiform, rounded or multiangular somata can be recognized (fig. 5). The glial elements of the white matter  showing a massive uptake can be discriminated from the few isolated labelled neurons by their smaller size (fig. 4). According to recent observations in our laboratory, these scattered subcortical neurons as well as the Cajal-Retzius cells belong to the pallial anlage in which the first neurons appear before the formation of the cortical plate (Rickmann et al., in press).

Although a few seemingly unipolar neurons have been observed with a vertically oriented ascending dendrite thus resembling to some extent pyramidal neurons, none of these cells could be identified as unipolar or producing basal dendrites.


DISCUSSION

The number of neurons labelled in the different preparations can be modified by many factors (i.e., amount of $^3$H-GABA injected, distance to the injection site, degree of edema and other reasons discussed by Hökfelt and Ljungdahl (1971)). However, even in those preparations which showed the highest number of labelled cells only a small fraction of all cortical neurons were labelled with $^3$H-GABA.

The degree of labelling is probably governed not only by the surrounding concentration of $^3$H-GABA or type of neuron, but also by some temporal function and/or metabolic condition of the neuron concerned.

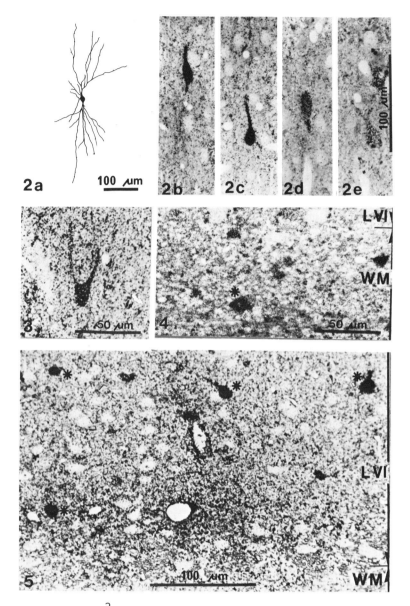

CELLS TAKING UP [3]H-GABA IN LIII – LVI AND THE SUBCORTICAL
WHITE MATTER.

Fig. 2a Drawing of a Golgi preparation of a "cellule à double
bouquet".
Fig. 2b-e Vertically oriented neurons in LIII –LV.
Fig. 3 Multipolar neuron in LV.
Fig. 4 One horizontal neuron ( ✱ ) in the white matter (WM).
Fig. 5 Labelled neurons ( ✱ ) in LVI.

From the great variations of the intensity of labelling and the number of neurons labelled in each preparation, it is clear that negative results cannot be evaluated and that the number of neurons capable of $^3$H-GABA uptake probably is underestimated with the present method.

From the orientation of the main dendrites and the long axis of the perikarya of labelled cells, three main systems of neurons seem to be labelled by $^3$H-GABA in the rat's visual cortex: (1) horizontally oriented neurons in upper LI, deep LVI and the subcortical white matter, (2) vertically oriented dendrites originating in LII to LIV and (3) neurons in all layers with dendrites extending in all directions. Each of these groups contains large and small neurons.

Careful experimentation combining a variety of methods must be done, before specific morphological types of neurons can be identified as capable of rapid $^3$H-GABA uptake. In this study, the most positive identifications can be made on LI neurons.

## REFERENCES

Baxter, C.F., 1970, The nature of γ-aminobutyric acid, in "Handbook of Neurochemistry," Vol. 3 (A. Lajtha, ed.), pp. 289-253, Plenum Press, New York - London.

Colonnier, M.L., 1966, The structural design of the neocortex, in "Brain and Conscious Experience," (J.C. Eccles, ed.), pp. 1-23, Springer-Verlag, Berlin-Heidelberg-New York.

Hökfelt, T., and Ljungdahl, Å., 1971, Uptake of [$^3$H]noradrenalin and γ-[$^3$H] aminobutyric acid in isolated tissue of rat: An autoradiographic and fluorescent microscopic study, Prog. Brain Res. 34: 87-102.

Hökfelt, T., and Ljungdahl, Å., 1972, Autoradiographic identification of cerebral and cerebellar cortical neurons accumulating labeled gamma-aminobutyric acid ($^3$H-GABA), Exp. Brain Res. 14: 354-362.

Iversen, L.L., and Bloom, F.E., 1972, Studies of the uptake of $^3$H-GABA and $^3$H glycine in slices and homogenates of rat brain and spinal cord by electron microscopic autoradiography, Brain Res. 41: 131-143.

Kelly, J.P., and Van Essen, D.C., 1974, Cell structure and function in the visual cortex of the cat, J. Physiol. 238: 515-547.

Krnjević, K., 1976, Inhibitory action of GABA and GABA-mimetics on vertebrate neurons, in "GABA in Nervous System Function" (E. Roberts, T.N. Chase, and D.B. Tower, eds.), pp. 269-281, Raven Press, New York.

Neal, M.J., and Iversen, L.L., 1969, Subcellular distribution of
    endogenous and [3H] γ-aminobutyric acid in rat cerebral cortex,
    J. Neurochem. 16: 1245-1252.
Rickmann, M., Chronwall, B.M., and Wolff, J.R., in press,
    On the development of non-pyramidal neurons and axons outside
    the cortical plate: The early marginal zone as a pallial
    anlage.
Szentágothai, J., 1973, Synaptology of the visual cortex, in
    "Handbook of Sensory Physiology," Vol. VII/3 (R. Jung, ed.),
    pp. 270-321, Springer-Verlag, Berlin-Heidelberg-New York.
Szentágothai, J., 1976, Basic circuitry of the neocortex, Exp.
    Brain Res. Suppl. 1: 282-287.

# GABA AGONISTS AND UPTAKE INHIBITORS OF RESTRICTED CONFORMATIONS: STRUCTURE-ACTIVITY RELATIONS

Povl Krogsgaard-Larsen

Department of Chemistry, The Royal Danish School of

Pharmacy, DK-2100 Copenhagen, Denmark

The central γ-aminobutyric acid (GABA) system seems to be involved in the development of certain neurological and psychiatric disorders like Huntington's chorea (McGeer and McGeer, 1976; Enna *et al.*, 1977), Parkinson's disease (Hornykiewicz *et al.*, 1976), and possibly schizophrenia (Van Kammen, 1977). These diseases may be treated by pharmacologic manipulation of the GABA mediated synaptic mechanisms by using agents which specifically interact with and increase neurotransmitter function. A prerequisite of the development of such compounds on a rational basis is information about the mechanism of action of GABA at the molecular level and elucidation of the "active conformations" of GABA. Due to the considerable flexibility of the molecule of GABA (Ham, 1974; Pullman, 1976; Pullman and Berthod, 1975) these aspects have to be studied indirectly by investigations of relationships between structure and biological activity of model compounds, the molecular structure and flexibility of which are systematically changed.

The mechanism with which GABA interacts with its post synaptic receptors has been the subject of considerable interest. Based on the theory that the interaction of the GABA antagonist bicuculline with the GABA receptors is the consequence of structural similarities between GABA and certain parts of the molecule of bicuculline, the preferred conformations of this alkaloid under different conditions have been studied (Gilardi, 1973; Kier and George, 1973; Andrews and Johnston, 1973). These investigations, however, have not shed light on the conformational basis of GABA-receptor interactions, mainly because the molecule of GABA is not unequivocally reflected by any structural elements of bicuculline (Curtis *et al.*, 1970 ; Steward *et al.*, 1971; Gilardi, 1973; Steward *et al.*, 1975). This approach is further complicated by the recent finding that bicucul-

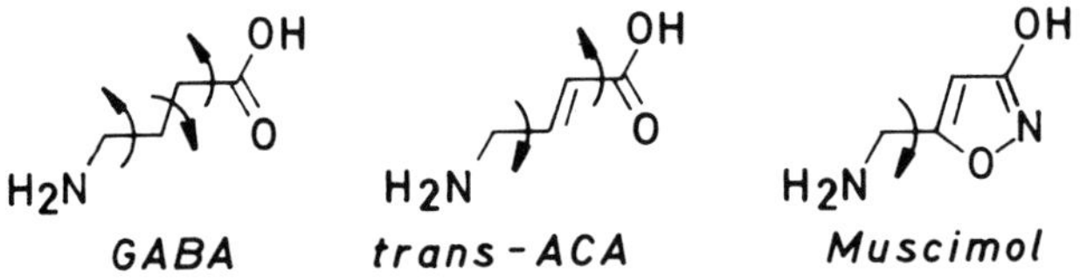

FIGURE 1. The conformational mobility of the molecules of GABA and the GABA agonists *trans*-ACA and muscimol as illustrated by the rotational freedon round carbon-carbon single bonds.

line and GABA agonists may interact with different receptor sites or even with different types of GABA receptors (Möhler and Okada, 1977).


                              GABA AGONISTS

    The "active conformations" of GABA with respect to its pre and post synaptic receptors may be elucidated *via* structure-activity studies on compounds of semirigid structure which mimic the activity of GABA on its receptors. Such compounds are of pharmacological interest *per se* and may be model compounds for the development of therapeutically useful GABA agonists. Muscimol (5-aminomethyl-3-isoxazolol) (Curtis *et al.*, 1971; Johnston *et al.*, 1968) and *trans*-4-aminocrotonic acid (*trans*-ACA) (Johnston *et al.*, 1975a) are powerful GABA agonists with respect to bicuculline-sensitive GABA receptors. Furthermore the conformational mobility of these compounds is reduced as compared with that of GABA, as depicted in Figure 1.

    Contrary to *trans*-ACA, which is also a potent inhibitor of GABA uptake (Beart *et al.*, 1972) and a substrate for GABA:2-oxoglutarate aminotransferase (GABA T) (Beart and Johnston, 1973), muscimol is an almost specific GABA agonist, being only a weak inhibitor of GABA uptake (Johnston, 1971). A series of isoxazole derivatives related to muscimol have been tested as GABA agonists on single neurones by using microelectrophoretic techniques (Krogsgaard-Larsen *et al.*, 1975). The results of these studies compared with those of affinity binding experiments using [3]H GABA as a ligand (Krogsgaard-Larsen *et al.*, unpublished) according to the general procedure of Enna and Snyder (1975) are summarized in Table I. With the exception of the isoxazoles *7* and *8*, which are inactive with respect to displacement of [3]H GABA from GABA receptor sites but moderately potent as depressants of neuronal firing *in vivo* (Krogsgaard-Larsen *et al.*, 1975) there is a reasonable agreement between the results of the two series of experiments. The inhibitory effects on the firing of single

TABLE I.   MUSCIMOL ANALOGUES AS GABA AGONISTS

| Isoxazole No | Formula | % Inhibition | $IC_{50}$ ($\mu M$) | Rel. Potency | pK Values |
|---|---|---|---|---|---|
| | GABA | | $0.34 \pm 0.007$ | − − − [+] | 4.0;10.7 |
| 1 (Muscimol) | | $103 \pm 4$ | $0.024 \pm 0.003$ | − − − − [+] | 4.8;8.4 |
| 2 | | $91 \pm 1$ | $10 \pm 2$ | − − − [+] | 5.1;9.5 |
| 3 | | $35 \pm 3$ | $140 \pm 37$ | n.t. | 5.1;9.3 |
| 4 | | n.s. | | n.t. | — |
| 5 | | $22 \pm 5$ | — | (−) | 5.4;10.4 |
| 6 | | $89 \pm 1$ | $7 \pm 1$ | − − − [+] | 4.7;8.5 |
| 7 | | n.s. | | − − [0] | 4.7;8.4 |
| 8 | | n.s. | | − − [0] | 4.7;8.5 |
| 9 | | $13 \pm 4$ | — | − [0] | 4.8;8.8 |
| 10 | | n.s. | | 0 | — |
| 11 | | n.s. | | n.t. | 4.6;8.6 |
| 12 | | n.s. | | 0 | 5.3;9.7 |
| 13 | | n.s. | | 0 | 4.7;10.0 |
| 14 | | n.s. | | 0 | 5.1;10.4 |
| 15 | | n.s. | | n.t. | 5.3;10.6 |

The potency of muscimol analogues as inhibitors of $^3H$ GABA binding, stated as % inhibition when tested at $10^{-4}$ M and as $IC_{50}$ values, and as depressants of neuronal firing compared to that of GABA − − −. Zero indicates no activity, n.s. not significant, and n.t. not tested. Effects of doubtful significance are cited in brackets and antagonism by BMC is indicated in square brackets.

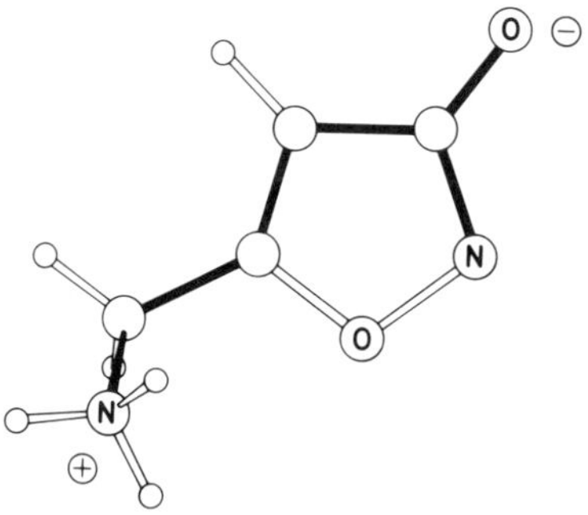

FIGURE 2.   The conformation of muscimol in the crystalline state as established by X-ray analysis.

neurones of the isoxazoles 7 and 8, however, are bicuculline methochloride (BMC)-insensitive (Krogsgaard-Larsen et al., 1975).

Of the compounds listed in Table I muscimol is the most powerful GABA agonist.  The isoxazoles 2 and 6, obtained by introduction of an additional carbon atom into the side chain of muscimol, are still potent GABA agonists equipotent with GABA but weaker than muscimol.  More extensive molecular manipulations of muscimol by further elongation of the side chain, by introduction of alkyl groups into the 4-position of the 3-isoxazolol nucleus, or by removal of the aminoalkyl groups from the 5- to the 4-position of the ring result in compounds with drastically reduced affinity for the GABA receptors.

Although muscimol and its analogues are depicted in the unionized forms they have zwitterionic structures.  It is evident from Table I that the differences in potency of the compounds as GABA agonists are not simply explained by their slightly different protolytic properties (pK values).  Furthermore there is no conspicuous relationship between the biological activity and the number of carbon atoms separating the charged centres of the compounds.  The affinity for the GABA receptors apparently depends on the ability of the compound to attain a definite conformation, the "active conformation" during interaction with the receptor macromolecule.  Based on a comparison of the semirigid structure and the remarkable potency of muscimol as a GABA agonist the "active conformation" of muscimol might be assumed to be identical with its preferred conformations (Kier and Truitt, 1970; Krogsgaard-Larsen et al., 1975).  In agreement with this hypothesis the low-energy conformations of muscimol have been studied.  Molecular orbital (MO) calculations predict an extended conformation of muscimol (Kier and Truitt, 1970), and in two different crystal forms extended but slightly twisted conformations are

observed (Brehm *et al.*, 1972; Brehm, unpublished) as shown in Figure 2.  Consequently muscimol and GABA might be expected to bind
to the GABA receptors in a more or less extended conformation.

Low-energy conformations of flexible and even semirigid GABA
analogues, however, do not necessarily reflect "active conformations" of GABA.  Muscimol may interact with the receptor macromolecule in a conformation, in which the angle between the side chain
and the plane of the ring is different from that of the low-energy
conformations.  If that is the case the rotational energy barrier
of the side chains of muscimol and related compounds may be the factor of decisive importance for their potency as GABA agonists.
Based on MO calculations the rotational energy barrier of the aminomethyl side chain of muscimol is relatively low (Kier and Truitt,
1970; Borthwick, unpublished communications).  Structural modifications of the molecule of muscimol may increase this energy barrier
or even prevent some muscimol analogues from adopting a conformation recognizable by the GABA receptors.  Such effects, probably
combined with direct steric hindrance to interaction with the GABA
receptors, may explain the considerable reduction or complete loss
of activity as GABA agonists of the muscimol analogues listed in
Table I.

As part of the conformation-activity studies on GABA and GABA
agonists a series of bicyclic muscimol analogues has been developed.
In these compounds the aminoalkyl side chains are built into an additional ring structure and locked in different conformations
(Table II).

The accessible conformations of that part of the molecule of
isoxazole *23*, which is related to muscimol, are within a narrow
range and similar to the low-energy conformations of muscimol.  In
the isoxazoles *16* (THIP) and *20* the side chain of muscimol is twisted *ca*. 180° and locked in slightly different conformations.  Of the
bicyclic isoxazoles listed in Table II only THIP was found to be a
potent inhibitor of GABA binding (Krogsgaard-Larsen *et al.*, unpublished).  In microelectrophoretic experiments THIP was shown to be
a potent GABA agonist with respect to bicuculline-sensitive GABA
receptors on feline spinal interneurones *in vivo* (Krogsgaard-Larsen
*et al.*, 1977).  The above findings compared with the inactivity of
THIP with respect to GABA uptake and as an inhibitor of GABA T and
L-glutamate 1-carboxylase (Krogsgaard-Larsen *et al.*, unpublished)
indicate that THIP is a specific GABA agonist.  Isoxazole *20* is
closely related to but much weaker than THIP as an inhibitor of GABA
binding, and isoxazole *23* is inactive.  As a result of its bicyclic
structure THIP has an extra alkyl substituent on the amino group and
in the 4-position of the isoxazole ring as compared with muscimol.
As shown in Tables I and II methylations of the 4-position or the
amino group of muscimol result in pronounced reductions of the po-

TABLE II. SOME BICYCLIC MUSCIMOL ANALOGUES AS GABA AGONISTS

| Isoxazole No | Formula | % Inhibition | $IC_{50}$ ($\mu M$) | Rel. Potency | pK Values |
|---|---|---|---|---|---|
| N-Methyl muscimol | | $59\pm1$ | $63\pm7$ | n.t | — |
| 16 | | $97\pm1$ | $2.6\pm0.5$ | --- (−) [+] | 4.4;8.5 |
| 17 | | $39\pm4$ | $88\pm22$ | 0 | 4.8;9.2 |
| 18 | | $31\pm2$ | — | (−) | 4.3;9.1 |
| 19 | | $27\pm3$ | — | n.t. | 3.3;9.6 |
| 20 | | $21\pm3$ | — | n.t. | 4.6;8.6 |
| 21 | | n.s. | | n.t. | 4.5;9.8 |
| 22 | | n.s. | | n.t. | 4.6;9.9 |
| 23 | | n.s. | | n.t. | 4.5;8.3 |

The potency of some bicyclic muscimol analogues as inhibitors of [3]H GABA binding, stated as % inhibition when tested at $10^{-4}$ M and as $IC_{50}$ values, and as depressants of neuronal firing compared to that of GABA - - -. Zero indicates no activity, n.s. not significant, and n.t. not tested. Effects of doubtful significance are cited in brackets and antagonism by BMC is indicated in square brackets.

tency with respect to displacement of [3]H GABA from its receptor sites. In the light of these findings THIP is remarkably potent as a GABA agonist, and THIP may be locked in an energetically unfavourable conformation which represents the conformation, in which muscimol interacts with the GABA receptors. The inactivity of isoxazole 23 as a GABA agonist further supports the proposal that the "active conformation" of muscimol is different from its low-energy conformations (see Figure 3).

Since the 3-isoxazolol nucleus of muscimol and muscimol analogues can be regarded as a masked carboxyl group the above findings

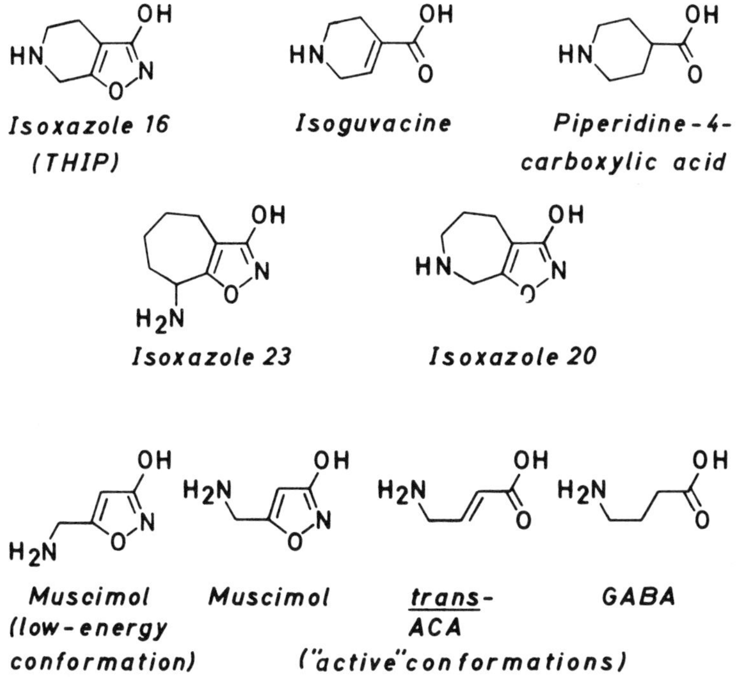

Isoxazole 16
(THIP)

Isoguvacine

Piperidine-4-
carboxylic acid

Isoxazole 23

Isoxazole 20

Muscimol
(low-energy
conformation)

Muscimol

trans-
ACA
("active"conformations)

GABA

FIGURE 3. A depiction of the proposed "active conformations" of muscimol, *trans*-ACA, and GABA and the structures of some key model compounds.

prompted the preparation and biological investigations of isoguvacine (1,2,3,6-tetrahydropyridine-4-carboxylic acid), the monocyclic amino acid related to THIP (Figure 3). Like THIP isoguvacine was shown to be a specific GABA agonist equipotent with muscimol as determined on feline spinal interneurones *in vivo* (Krogsgaard-Larsen *et al.*, 1977).

A series of cyclic amino acids related to isoguvacine has been tested as GABA agonists (Table III). The saturated analogue of isoguvacine, piperidine-4-carboxylic acid, was weaker than isoguvacine as a GABA agonist but almost equipotent with GABA as established in microelectrophoretic experiments on spinal neurones of cats (Krogsgaard-Larsen *et al.*, 1977). Isoguvacine and in particular piperidine-4-carboxylic acid, however, are weaker than GABA with respect to displacement of [3]H GABA from receptor sites on membrane fractions isolated from rat brains (Krogsgaard-Larsen *et al.*, unpublished). The structure-activity studies summarized in Table III

TABLE III.   ISOGUVACINE AND RELATED AMINO ACIDS AS GABA AGONISTS

| Compound | Formula | % Inhibition | $IC_{50}$ ($\mu M$) | Rel. Potency |
|---|---|---|---|---|
| THIP (Isoxazole16) | | $97 \pm 1$ | $2.6 \pm 0.5$ | − − − (−) [+] |
| Isoguvacine | | $91 \pm 6$ | $1.4 \pm 0.1$ | − − − − [+] |
| Piperidine-4-carboxylic acid | | $87 \pm 3$ | $15 \pm 2$ | − − − [+] |
| N-Methyl GABA | | $18 \pm 1$ | − | 0 * |
| N-Methyl isoguvacine | | n.s | | n.t |
| N-Methyl piperidine-4-carboxylic acid | | n.s | | n.t |
| Guvacine | | n.s | | 0 ** |
| Nipecotic acid | | n.s | | (−) + |
| Gabaculine | | n.s ++ | | 0 ++ |

The potency of some amino acids as inhibitors of $^3$H GABA binding, stated as % inhibition when tested at $10^{-4}$ M and as $IC_{50}$ values, and as depressants of neuronal firing compared to that of GABA − − −. Zero indicates no activity, n.s. not significant, and n.t. not tested.  Effects of doubtful significance are sited in brackets and antagonism by BMC is indicated in square brackets.  * From Curtis and Watkins, 1960, ** from Lodge et al., 1977, † from Krogsgaard-Larsen et al., 1975, and †† from Allan et al., 1977.

emphasize the remarkable structural specificity of the GABA receptors.  Thus the N-methyl derivatives of isoguvacine and piperidine-4-carboxylic acid are inactive as inhibitors of GABA binding.  Similarly an open-chain analogue of piperidine-4-carboxylic acid, N-methyl GABA, is almost inactive as a GABA agonist in vivo (Curtis and Watkins, 1960) and in vitro (Krogsgaard-Larsen et al., unpublished).  The substrate-competitive inhibitors of GABA uptake guvacine (Johnston et al., 1975b) and nipecotic acid (Krogsgaard-Larsen and Johnston, 1975; Johnston et al., 1976a, 1976b) have very little

or no affinity for the GABA receptors *in vitro* (Krogsgaard-Larsen
*et al.*, unpublished) and *in vivo* (Lodge *et al.*, 1977; Krogsgaard-
Larsen *et al.*, 1975). Furthermore gabaculine, a potent inhibitor
of GABA T (Rando and Bangerter, 1976; Allan *et al.*, 1977) has no
affinity for the GABA receptors *in vivo* and *in vitro* (Allan *et al.*,
1977). Isoguvacine and piperidine-4-carboxylic acid are conformationally restricted amino acids which represent partially folded
conformations of *trans*-ACA and GABA, respectively. The results
summarized in Table III compared with the rigid and flattened
structure of THIP indicate that muscimol, *trans*-ACA, and GABA may
interact with the GABA receptors in partially folded and almost
planar conformations (Figure 3).

The muscimol analogues so far discussed have been obtained by
replacing the aminomethyl side chain of muscimol by various aminoalkyl groups and keeping the 3-isoxazolol ring intact. Other possible structural changes of muscimol are alterations of the heterocyclic ring, and a series of muscimol analogues has been developed
in which only the structure of the ring has been systematically

TABLE IV.  SOME HETEROCYCLIC MUSCIMOL ANALOGUES AS GABA AGONISTS

| Compound | Formula | % Inhibition | $IC_{50}$ ($\mu M$) | Rel. Potency | pK Values |
|---|---|---|---|---|---|
| Muscimol | | 103±4 | 0.024±0.003 | − − − − [+] | 4.8 ; 8.4 |
| Thio-muscimol | | 114±2 | 0.12±0.01 | − − − − [+] | 6.1 ; 8.9 |
| Iso-muscimol | | 42±1 | 377±55 | −   [0] | 2.6 ; 9.0 |
| Aza-muscimol | | 16±3 | — | − −  [0] | 6.2 ; 9.8 |
| 1-Methylaza-muscimol | | 26±1 | — | n.t. | 8.0 ; 10 |
| 2-Methylaza-muscimol | | 17±2 | — | n.t. | 5.5 ; 9.8 |

The potency of some heterocyclic muscimol analogues as inhibitors of
$^3$H GABA binding stated as % inhibition when tested at $10^{-4}$ M and as
$IC_{50}$ values, and as depressants of neuronal firing compared to that
of GABA − − −. Zero indicates no activity, n.s. not significant,
and n.t. not tested. Effects of doubtful significance are cited in
brackets and antagonism by BMC is indicated in square brackets.

changed. This series of muscimol analogues has been tested as GABA
agonists in affinity binding and microelectrophoretic experiments.
The relationships between potencies as GABA agonists, molecular
structures, and protolytic properties are summarized in Table IV.
It is evident that the affinity for the GABA receptors and the protolytic properties of the compounds are strictly dependent on the
structure of the heterocyclic rings. There is, however, no simple
relationship between the potencies of these muscimol analogues as
GABA agonists and their pK values. Isomuscimol, azamuscimol, and
derivatives of it are almost inactive as inhibitors of GABA binding.
Although depicted in the unionized forms the compounds listed in
Table IV are zwitterions, and despite an immediate structural similarity with muscimol isomuscimol, azamuscimol, and derivatives of
it may not be recognized by the GABA receptors because the charge
distributions of their molecules are different from those of GABA,
muscimol, and thiomuscimol. Alternatively the differences between
the structures of e.g. muscimol and isomuscimol may result in different rotational energy barriers of the side chains. Further
structure-activity studies on pertinent model compounds may shed
light on these aspects. The moderate depression of neuronal firing
recorded for azamuscimol (Krogsgaard-Larsen et al., 1975) is not
antagonized by BMC and may be unrelated to the GABA receptors.


INHIBITORS OF GABA UPTAKE


     With respect to inhibition of GABA uptake the closely related
bicyclic isoxazoles 18 ($IC_{50}$ 624 ± 55 µM)(Krogsgaard-Larsen and
Johnston, 1975) and 21 ($IC_{50}$ 402 ± 27 µM)(Krogsgaard-Larsen et al.,
unpublished) proved to be more potent than muscimol. Based on the
structural relationship between the 3-isoxazolol nucleus and the
carboxyl group nipecotic acid, the cyclic amino acid analogue of isoxazole 18, was tested and shown to be a potent inhibitor of GABA
uptake (Krogsgaard-Larsen and Johnston, 1975). Nipecotic acid was
later shown to be a substrate-competitive inhibitor of GABA uptake
which combines with the transport carrier and penetrates the tissue
(Johnston et al., 1976a, 1976b). These findings compared with the
semirigid structure of nipecotic acid make it a possible model compound for studies of the mechanism of action and the physiological
role of the GABA transport system (Curtis et al., 1976).

     The above findings for nipecotic acid prompted the development
and investigations of structurally related compounds (Figure 4).
Guvacine (1,2,5,6-tetrahydropyridine-3-carboxylic acid), an unsaturated analogue of nipecotic acid isolated from the betel nut, is
almost equipotent with R(-)-nipecotic acid as an inhibitor of GABA
uptake (Johnston et al., 1975b). Kinetic studies suggest that the
mechanism of interaction of guvacine with the GABA transport carrier

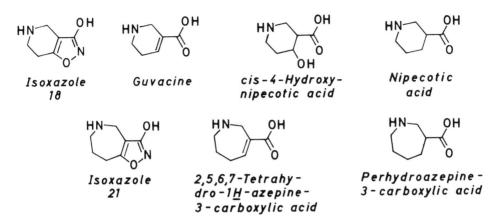

FIGURE 4.  The structures of isoxazole 18 (4,5,6,7-tetrahydroisoxa-
zolo|4,5-c|pyridin-3-ol) and isoxazole 21 (5,6,7,8-tetrahydro-4H-
isoxazolo|4,5-c|azepin-3-ol) and related cyclic amino acids.

is similar to that described above for nipecotic acid (Johnston *et
al.*, 1975b).  More recently (±)-*cis*-4-hydroxynipecotic acid has been
synthesized (Krogsgaard-Larsen, unpublished) and shown to be a potent
and probably a substrate-competitive inhibitor of GABA uptake (Johnston *et al.*, unpublished).  The structural specificity of the GABA
uptake system with respect to this class of inhibitors has been elucidated *via* structure-activity studies on a number of related compounds (Table V).  The observation that the isoxazole 21 is equipotent with the isoxazole 18 as an inhibitor of GABA uptake prompted
the syntheses of 2,5,6,7-tetrahydro-1H-azepine-3-carboxylic acid and
perhydroazepine-3-carboxylic acid, the seven-membered ring analogues
of guvacine and nipecotic acid, respectively (Figure 4) (Krogsgaard-
Larsen and Thyssen, unpublished).  Surprisingly these cyclic amino
acids proved to be two orders of magnitude weaker than guvacine and
nipecotic acid with respect to inhibition of GABA uptake.  Furthermore 5-methyl guvacine, isoguvacine, and β-proline are very weak of
inactive as GABA uptake inhibitors.  The structural specificity of
the GABA uptake system is further supported by the recent studies on
some nipecotic analogues by Johnston *et al.*, 1977.  Ecgonine, the
amino acid skeleton of cocain, is structurally related to *cis*-4-hy-
droxynipecotic acid but it is inactive with respect to GABA uptake.
Similarly the compounds obtained by removal of the N-methyl group
and the hydroxy group of ecgonine, nor-ecgonine and nortropane-2-
carboxylic acid, respectively, are inactive.  Based on these results
it may be concluded that nipecotic acid, guvacine, and *cis*-4-hydroxy-
nipecotic acid reflect the conformation of GABA in which it is transported by its carrier.  The cyclic structure of these amino acids

TABLE V.   CYCLIC AMINO ACIDS AS INHIBITORS OF GABA UPTAKE

| Compound | Formula | % Inhibition | $IC_{50}$ (µM) | Potentiation of GABA |
|---|---|---|---|---|
| Guvacine | | $98 \pm 1$[†] | $8 \pm 1$[†] | +[*] |
| (±)-5-Methyl guvacine | | $46 \pm 1$ | $547 \pm 22$ | n.t |
| 2,5,6,7-Tetrahydro-1H-azepine-3-carboxylic acid | | $23 \pm 2$ | — | n.t |
| Isoguvacine | | n.s | | |
| (-)-Nipecotic acid | | — | $5 \pm 1$[††] | +[**] |
| (+)-Nipecotic acid | | — | $30 \pm 2$[††] | +[**] |
| (±)-perhydro-azepine-3-carboxylic acid | | $52 \pm 2$ | $502 \pm 49$ | n.t |
| (±)-β-Proline | | n.s | | |
| (+)-Nortropane-2-carboxylic acid | | n.s | | |
| (±)-cis-4-hydroxy-nipecotic acid | | $95 \pm 1$ | $12 \pm 2$ | n.t |
| Ecgonine | | n.s | | |
| Nor-ecgonine | | n.s | | |

The inhibitory effects of some cyclic amino acids on the uptake of GABA into rat brain slices stated as % inhibition when tested at $5 \times 10^{-4}$ M and as $IC_{50}$ values.  The potentiation of the depressant action of GABA on spinal neurones in cats by the amino acids was determined in microelectrophoretic experiments.  * From Lodge et al., 1977, ** from Curtis et al., 1976, † from Johnston et al., 1975b, and †† from Johnston et al., 1976a.

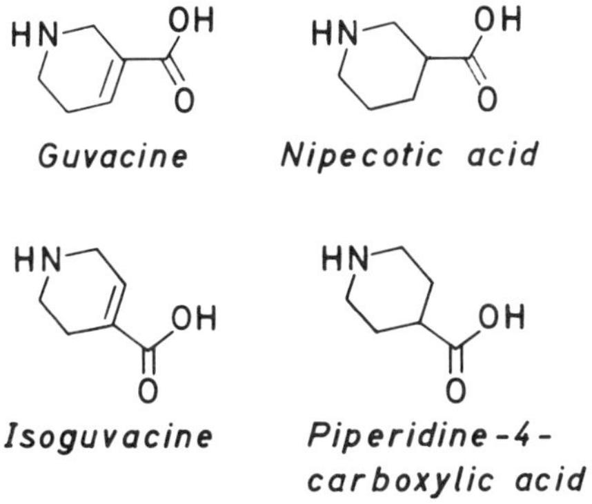

*FIGURE 5.* A comparison of the structures of the potent inhibitors of GABA uptake guvacine and nipecotic acid, and the potent GABA agonists isoguvacine and piperidine-4-carboxylic acid.

indicate that GABA is transported in a partially folded conformation. However, since no part of the molecules of nipecotic acid, guvacine, or *cis*-4-hydroxynipecotic acid unequivocally reflects the structure of GABA conclusive evidence concerning the interaction of GABA with its transport carrier at the molecular level can not be derived from these studies.

The present structure-activity studies support previous findings that different conformational modes of GABA interact with its receptors and uptake system (Krogsgaard-Larsen *et al.*, 1975). Thus the potent GABA agonists, as for example isoguvacine and piperidine-4-carboxylic acid (Beart *et al.*, 1972) are inactive or very weak, respectively, as inhibitors of GABA uptake. The potent GABA uptake inhibitors guvacine (Johnston *et al.*, 1975b) and nipecotic acid (Krogsgaard-Larsen and Johnston, 1975) on the other hand are inactive as inhibitors of GABA binding, and guvacine (Lodge *et al.*, 1977) and nipecotic acid (Krogsgaard-Larsen *et al.*, 1975) are very weak or inactive as depressants of firing of central neurones (Figure 5). GABA seems to be transported in a folded conformation different from that, in which it interacts with its receptors. Since gabaculine, a conformationally restricted inhibitor at the active site of GABA T (Rando and Bangerter, 1976; Allan *et al.*, 1977), is inactive as a GABA agonist and a relatively weak inhibitor of GABA uptake (Allan *et al.*, 1977) GABA may interact with GABA T in a conformation different from those recognized by its receptors and transport system.

In this structure-activity analysis the biological activities of the model compounds have been determined *in vitro* on tissue, membrane, and enzyme preparations from rat brains and by electrophoretic application of the substances on single spinal neurones of cats. Consequently the interpretations of the biological results are not complicated by factors like differences in metabolism, ability to penetrate biological membranes, and distribution in brain tissue. The attempts to correlate the observed effects with affinities for receptors, transport carriers, and active sites of enzymes, however, still involve fundamental problems, and such aspects may be further elucidated in future studies on the interactions of model compounds with purified enzymes and macromolecules responsible for binding of GABA to its receptors and transport carriers.


PHARMACOLOGICAL CONSIDERATIONS


The next steps in the development of the pharmacology of the GABA system include studies of compounds with potent and specific actions on the GABA system in pertinent animal behavioural models. Extremely powerful behavioural effects have been observed on rats after injections of muscimol into substantia nigra (Scheel-Krüger *et al.*, 1977; Waddington, 1977). It has been concluded that muscimol can be characterized as a powerful and selective GABA agonist after systemic administration to rats (Naik *et al.*, 1976). Muscimol is metabolized in mice (Ott *et al.*, 1975) and the possibility that metabolites of muscimol contribute to the effects observed after systemic administration of muscimol can not be excluded (Naik *et al.*, 1976). The relative potencies of a number of muscimol analogues after injections into substantia nigra have been determined, and the results are in agreement with the biological results summarized in Tables I, II, and IV (Arnt *et al.*, unpublished).

The ubiquity of the GABA system in the mammalian central nervous system may limit the possibilities of treatment of the above mentioned mental diseases *via* pharmacologic manipulations of the GABA synaptic mechanisms. Stimulation of GABA receptors by administration of GABA agonists or by inhibition of GABA uptake or GABA T may activate the entire system and provoke a variety of undesirable effects. However, future investigations may disclose the existence of several GABA systems in the mammalian central nervous system characterized in different structural specificities of pre and post synaptic receptors (Johnston, 1976), uptake systems, and metabolizing enzymes. In any case pharmacochemists are faced with the important and urgent task of developing compounds with which the function of GABA synapses in different brain areas can be selectively manipulated.

*Acknowledgements* – This work was supported by grants from The Danish Medical Research Council. It is a pleasure to acknowledge the close collaboration of Professor D. R. Curtis and Drs. G. A. R. Johnston and D. Lodge, The Australian National University, Canberra, Australia, and my colleagues Drs. L. Brehm and H. Hjeds, Mrs. K. Thyssen and Mr. T. Honoré, and the skilful assistance of Mrs. B. Hare and Mr. S. Stilling.

## REFERENCES

Allan, R.D., Johnston, G.A.R., and Twitchin, B., 1977, Effects of gabaculine on the uptake, binding and metabolism of GABA, *Neuroscience Letters* 4:51-54.

Andrews, P.R. and Johnston, G.A.R., 1973, Molecular orbital and proton magnetic resonance studies of bicuculline, *Nature New Biol.* 243:29-30.

Beart, P.M. and Johnston, G.A.R., 1973, Transamination of analogues of γ-aminobutyric acid by extracts of rat brain mitochondria, *Brain Res.* 49:459-462.

Beart, P.M., Johnston, G.A.R., and Uhr, M.L., 1972, Competitive inhibition of GABA uptake in rat brain slices by some GABA analogues of restricted conformation, *J. Neurochem.* 19:1855-1861.

Brehm, L., Hjeds, H., and Krogsgaard-Larsen, P., 1972, The structure of muscimol a GABA analogue of restricted conformation, *Acta Chem. Scand.* 26:1298-1299.

Curtis, D.R., Duggan, A.W., Felix, D., and Johnston, G.A.R., 1970, GABA, bicuculline and central inhibition, *Nature* 226:1222-1224.

Curtis, D.R., Duggan, A.W., Felix, D., and Johnston, G.A.R., 1971, Bicuculline, an antagonist of GABA and synaptic inhibition in the spinal cord of the cat, *Brain Res.* 32:69-96.

Curtis, D.R., Game, C.J.A., and Lodge, D., 1976, The *in vivo* inactivation of GABA and other inhibitory amino acids in the cat nervous system, *Exp. Brain Res.* 25:413-428.

Curtis, D.R. and Watkins, J.C., 1960, The excitation and depression of spinal neurones by structurally related amino acids, *J. Neurochem.* 6:117-141.

Enna, S.J. and Snyder, S.H., Properties of γ-aminobutyric acid (GABA) receptor binding in rat brain synaptic membrane fractions, *Brain Res.* 100:81-97.

Enna, S.J., Stern, L.Z., Wastek, G.J., and Yamamura, H.I., 1977, Neurobiology and pharmacology of Huntington's disease, *Life Sciences* 20:205-211.

Gilardi, R.D., 1973, The configuration and conformation of bicuculline, a GABA antagonist, *Nature New Biol.* 245:86-88.

Ham, N.S., 1974, NMR studies of solution conformations of physiologically active amino acids, *in* "Molecular and Quantum Pharmacology" (E. Bergmann and B. Pullman, eds.), pp.256-263, D. Reidel Publ. Comp., Dordrecht-Holland.

Hornykiewicz, O., LLoyd, K.G., and Davidson, L., 1976, The GABA system, function of the basal ganglia, and Parkinson's disease, *in* "GABA in Nervous System Function" (E. Roberts, T.N. Chase, and D.B. Tower, eds.), pp.479-485, Raven Press, New York.

Johnston, G.A.R., 1971, Muscimol and the uptake of γ-aminobutyric acid by rat brain slices, *Psychopharmacologia* 22:230-233.

Johnston, G.A.R., 1976, Physiologic pharmacology of GABA and its antagonists in the vertebrate nervous system, *in* "GABA in Nervous System Function" (E. Roberts, T.N. Chase, and D.B. Tower, eds.), pp.395-411, Raven Press, New York.

Johnston, G.A.R., Curtis, D.R., Beart, P.M., Game, C.J.A., McCulloch, R.M., and Twitchin, B., 1975a, *cis-* and *trans-*4-aminocrotonic acid as GABA analogues of restricted conformation, *J. Neurochem.* 24:157-160.

Johnston, G.A.R., Curtis, D.R., DeGroat, W.C., and Duggan, A.W., 1968, Central actions of ibotenic acid and muscimol, *Biochem. Pharmac.* 17:2488-2489.

Johnston, G.A.R., Krogsgaard-Larsen, P., and Stephanson, A., 1975b, Betel nut constituents as inhibitors of γ-aminobutyric acid uptake, *Nature* 258:627-628.

Johnston, G.A.R., Krogsgaard-Larsen, P., Stephanson, A.L., and Twitchin, B., 1976a, Inhibition of the uptake of GABA and related amino acids in rat brain slices by the optical isomers of nipecotic acid, *J. Neurochem.* 26:1029-1032.

Johnston, G.A.R., Stephanson, A.L., and Twitchin, B., 1976b, Uptake and release of nipecotic acid by rat brain slices, *J. Neurochem.* 26:83-87.

Johnston, G.A.R., Stephanson, A.L., and Twitchin, B., 1977, Piperazic acid and related compounds as inhibitors of GABA uptake in rat brain slices, *J. Pharm. Pharmac.* 29:240-241.

Kier, L.B. and George, J.M., 1973, Molecular orbital studies on the conformation of bicuculline and β-hydroxy GABA, *Experientia* 29:501-502.

Kier, L.B. and Truitt, E.B.Jr., 1970, Molecular orbital studies on the conformation of γ-aminobutyric acid and muscimol, *Experientia* 26:988-989.

Krogsgaard-Larsen, P. and Johnston, G.A.R., 1975, Inhibition of GABA uptake in rat brain slices by nipecotic acid, various isoxazoles and related compounds, *J. Neurochem.* 25:797-802.

Krogsgaard-Larsen, P., Johnston, G.A.R., Curtis, D.R., Game, C.J.A., and McCulloch, R.M., 1975, Structure and biological activity of a series of conformationally restricted analogues of GABA, *J. Neurochem.* 25:803-809.

Krogsgaard-Larsen, P., Johnston, G.A.R., Lodge, D., and Curtis, D.R., 1977, A new class of GABA agonists, *Nature* 268:53-55.

Lodge, D., Johnston, G.A.R., Curtis, D.R., and Brand, S.J., 1977, Effects of the areca nut constituents arecaidine and guvacine on the action of GABA in the cat central nervous system, *Brain*

*Res.*, in the press.

McGeer, P.L. and McGeer, E.G., 1976, The GABA system and function of the basal ganglia: Huntington's disease, *in* "GABA in Nervous System Function" (E. Roberts, T.N. Chase., and D.B. Tower, eds.), pp.487-495, Raven Press, New York.

Möhler, H. and Okada, T., 1977, GABA receptor binding with $^3$H(+)bicuculline methiodide in rat CNS, *Nature* 267:65-67.

Naik, S.R., Guidotti, A., and Costa, E., 1976, Central GABA receptor agonists: Comparison of muscimol and baclofen, *Neuropharmacology* 15:479-484.

Ott, J., Wheaton, P.S., and Chilton, W.S., 1975, Fate of muscimol in the mouse, *Physiol. Chem. & Physics* 7:381-384.

Pullman, B., 1976, Quantum-mechanical studies on the effect of water on the conformation of two biologically important zwitterionic systems: Polar head of phospholipids and GABA, *in* "Environmental Effects on Molecular Structure and Properties" (B. Pullman, ed.), pp.55-80, D. Reidel Publ. Comp., Dordrecht-Holland.

Pullman, B. and Berthod, H., 1975, Molecular orbital studies on the conformation of GABA (γ-aminobutyric acid), *Theoret. Chim. Acta (Berl.)* 36:317-328.

Rando, R.R. and Bangerter, F.W., 1976, The irreversible inhibition of mouse brain γ-aminobutyric acid (GABA)-α-ketoglutaric acid transaminase by gabaculine, *J. Am. Chem. Soc.* 98:6762-6764.

Scheel-Krüger, J., Arnt, J., and Magelund, G., 1977, Behavioural stimulation induced by muscimol and other GABA agonists injected into the substantia nigra, *Neuroscience Letters* 4:351-356.

Steward, E.G., Borthwick, P.W., Clarke, G.R., and Warner, D., 1975, Agonism and antagonism of γ-aminobutyric acid, *Nature* 256:600-601.

Steward, E.G., Player, R.B., Quilliam, J.P., Brown, D.A., and Pringle, M.J., 1971, Molecular conformation of GABA, *Nature New Biol.* 233:87-88.

Van Kammen, D.P., 1977, γ-Aminobutyric acid (GABA) and the dopamine hypothesis of schizophrenia, *Am. J. Psychiat.* 134:138-143.

Waddington, J.L., 1977, GABA-like properties of flurazepam and baclofen suggested by rotational behaviour following unilateral intranigral injection: A comparison with the GABA agonist muscimol, *Br. J. Pharmac.* 60:263P-264P.

MUSCIMOL ANALOGUES INJECTED INTO SUBSTANTIA NIGRA:

A VALUABLE NEW IN VIVO MODEL FOR GABA-ERGIC DRUGS

J. Arnt[1], J. Scheel-Krüger[2], G. Magelund[2], P. Krogsgaard-Larsen[3] and H. Hjeds[3]

1)Department of Pharmacology, Royal Danish School of Pharmacy, DK-2100 Copenhagen, Denmark
2)Psychopharmacological Research Laboratory, Sct. Hans
Mental Hospital, Roskilde, Denmark, and
3)Department of Chemistry, Royal Danish School of Pharmacy, DK-2100 Copenhagen, Denmark

We have recently shown that unilateral injection of GABA into
the caudal part of substantia nigra, zona reticulata induced contralateral turning in rats. This effect was mimicked by small amounts
of three GABA-ergic drugs, muscimol, baclofen and imidazole acetic
acid (Scheel-Krüger et al, 1977). The GABA-antagonists bicuculline
methiodide and picrotoxin in contrast induced ipsilateral turning.
These results have now been extended to a series of semirigid structural analogues of GABA related to muscimol in the purpose to evaluate the sensitivity of this in vivo model in comparison to micro-
electrophoretic and membrane receptor studies.

Male Wistar rats were stereotaxically implanted with stainless
steel guide cannulas vertically above substantia nigra at the co-
ordinates A 1,6 L 2,1 (König and Klippel, 1963) under pentobarbital
anaesthesia as described previously. Four days after operation
saline or test substances dissolved in water or saline (dependent
on drug concentration) were injected in a volume of 1 microliter
into handheld unanaesthetized animals. Immediately after the injection the rats were placed on a large open field for continuous
behavioral observation. After the experiments all needle tracks
were histologically verified after cresylviolet staining.

All compounds were injected at usually three to four dose levels. The lowest dose which gave a significant turning response
is shown in table 1. Generally the rats reached their maximum turn-

TABLE 1.   Turning behavior after GABA agonists into substantia nigra.

| Compound | Formula | Dose | | Turning response | |
|----------|---------|------|------|------|------|
| | | μg | nM | Max. frequency (t/min) | Duration (min) |
| GABA | | 100 | 970 | 4-28 | 4-30 |
| Muscimol | | 0.03 | 0.26 | 12-30 | 60-120 |
| Baclofen | | 0.1 | 0.47 | 12-31 | > 150 |
| THIP | | 0.3 | 2.1 | 8-18 | 30-85 |
| Homo-muscimol | | 0.6 | 4.7 | 12-18 | 20-25 |
| 5'-Methyl-muscimol | | 1.0 | 7.8 | 5-30 | 30-90 |
| Thio-muscimol | | 3.0 | 23 | 6-15 | 6-7 |
| 4-Methyl-muscimol | | 15 | 117 | 15-40 | 40-80 |
| Iso-muscimol | | 85 | 746 | 0 | 0 |

The potency of GABA agonists injected unilaterally into substantia nigra, stated as the minimum dose, (in micrograms and nanomoles) inducing a strong contralateral turning behavior, expressed as turns/minute and duration of action.  0 indicates no effect.

ing rate short after the injection.  The longlasting drugs maintained usually this rate for a relatively long period and then slowly decreased.  The shortlasting drugs homomuscimol and thiomuscimol
reached their maximal turning rate immediately and then quickly declined in activity.  In contrast, saline did not give a significant
behavioral response on any occasion.

   These preliminary data show a clear distinction in activity
of the different drugs.  Muscimol is by far the most active GABA
agonist available but also baclofen shows considerable activity.
When other analogues of muscimol were tested there were a remarkable decrease or complete loss in activity.  Generally, there is
fairly good correlation between the potency in this behavioral model compared to ability to displace [3]H-GABA binding or depress feline spinal neurones (Krogsgaard-Larsen, this meeting; Krogsgaard-
Larsen et al, 1975).  However, our in vivo model provide a better
quantitative evaluation of the potency of these compounds than
possible with electrophysiological methods.  There are some discrepancies between the turning activity and receptor affinities
in vitro.  First, GABA itself is very weak in our model probably
because GABA in vivo is very rapidly removed from the receptor
sites by neuronal and glial high-affinity uptake and metabolized.
Secondly, baclofen has an unclear mechanism of action.  It shows
strong activity in the substantia nigra, but is recently reported
as inactive in displacing [3]H-Bicuculline methiodide binding (Möhler
and Okada, 1977), but no data seem available of its ability to displace [3]H-GABA binding.  Pharmacological data suggest also some unspecific effects of baclofen (Naik et al, 1976).  The sulphur analogue of muscimol, thiomuscimol, is very strong in both receptor
binding assay and in microelectrophoresis but is much weaker and
shortlasting after injection into substantia nigra.  The reason for
this difference is unclear but could be due to differences in diffusion rate or alternatively a rapid metabolism in the brain tissue.  The close similarity of homomuscimol and muscimol makes it
unlikely that diffusion differences are responsible for the short-
lasting effect of homomuscimol.  It may be suggested that this drug
is more easily metabolized because of its longer aminogroup containing side chain.

   On condition that the compounds under study have been found
active and specific in receptor affinity binding assays or electrophysiologically, our in vivo model represents a most useful quantitative approach for evaluation of comparative potency in vivo of
GABA agonists.  Contralateral turning is not specific for GABA-ergic drugs since we recently have found other neurotransmitters including glycine, noradrenaline, substance P and the glutamic acid
analogue kainic acid able to induce this behavioral response (results in preparation).

Acknowledgement.  This work was supported by grant number 512-7182 from Danish Medical Research Council.

REFERENCES

Krogsgaard-Larsen, P., Johnston, G.A.R., Curtis, D.R., Game, C.J.A., and McCulloch, R.M., 1975, Structure and biological activity of a series of conformationally restricted analogues of GABA, J. Neurochem 25:803-809.

König, J.F.R., and Klippel, R.A., 1963, The rat brain.  A stereotoxic atlas of the forebrain and lower parts of the brain stem, R.E. Krieger Publishing Co.

Möhler, H., and Okada, T., 1977, GABA receptor binding with $^3$H(+) bicuculline-methiodide in rat CNS, Nature 267:65-67.

Naik, S.R., Guidotti, A. and Costa, E., 1976, Central GABA receptor agonists: Comparison of muscimol and baclofen, Neuropharmacology 15:479-484.

Scheel-Krüger, J., Arnt, J., and Magelund, G., 1977, Behavioural stimulation induced by muscimol and other GABA agonists into the substantia nigra, Neuroscience Letters 4:351-356.

# UPTAKE, EXCHANGE AND RELEASE OF GABA IN ISOLATED NERVE ENDINGS

G. Levi[+], M. Banay-Schwartz[o] and M. Raiteri[^]

[+]Laboratory of Cell Biology, Via Romagnosi 18/A, Rome

[o]N.Y.State Research Institute for Neurochemistry, New York

[^]Institute of Pharmacology, Catholic University, Rome, Italy

## I. INTRODUCTION

In the last three years there has been considerable controversy on the GABA transport system of nerve endings, and, in particular, on the role of high affinity uptake in the termination of the action of synaptically released GABA (Iversen, 1975; Iversen and Kelly, 1975; Lake and Voaden, 1976; Levi and Raiteri, 1974; Levi and Raiteri, 1975a and 1975b; Levi et al., 1976a; Martin, 1976; Raiteri et al., 1975; Ryan and Roskoski, 1977; Sellström et al., 1976; Simon et al., 1974; Storm-Mathisen et al., 1976).

The aim of the present article is to interpret the data on synaptosomal GABA transport in a more unitary fashion than it has generally been done. In other words, we shall try to abandon the probably arbitrary distinction among different transport systems (such as high and low affinity uptake, homoexchange, carrier-mediated release) and to consider synaptosomal GABA transport as a single complex function, capable of being finely modulated by cationic and substrate concentrations.

For this purpose, we shall briefly summarize our first data on GABA exchange, and present more recent results, both published and unpublished, on which our present views on GABA transport are based. We shall then analyze some criticisms and different interpretations given to the exchange phenomenon, and see how these fit into our unitary view.

## II. GABA HOMOEXCHANGE

In 1974 and 1975 we and other authors reported that a large
part of the accumulation of radioactive GABA by synaptosomes observed
in high affinity uptake studies could be accounted for by a homoexchange process, rather than by a net uptake mechanism (Levi and Raiteri, 1974; Raiteri et al., 1975; Simon et al.,1974). In other
words, we noted that the entry of exogenous GABA into synaptosomes
was coupled with the exit, from synaptosomes, of comparable amounts
of endogenous GABA, at least in the concentration range of the high
affinity uptake system. The characteristics of the exchange process
were practically identical to those of the high affinity uptake.
Homoexchange was concentration dependent and saturable, and the apparent Vmax and Km values were similar to those of the high affinity uptake. Other common features were: substrate specificity, $Na^+$-
dependence and temperature-dependence (Levi and Raiteri, 1974; Raiteri et al., 1975; Simon et al., 1974). We concluded that the kinetic parameters of the GABA transport system performing net uptake
should be re-evaluated, and we tentatively suggested that, in case
a high affinity net uptake system did not exist, the inactivation
of the synaptically released GABA might be performed by an uptake
system with high capacity and low affinity (Levi and Raiteri, 1975a;
Raiteri et al., 1975).

The lack of a significant net uptake of GABA in synaptosomes
incubated in media containing low concentrations of the amino acid
has been subsequently confirmed in several other laboratories (Ryan
and Roskoski, 1977; Sellström et al., 1976; Storm-Mathisen et al.,
1976). We were aware of the fact that these observations raised,
rather than solved, a number of problems. In particular, what seemed
to us difficult to rationalize was the possible functional role of
a transport system apparently uncapable of performing any useful
work, namely net transport in one or the other direction.

In other terms, the problem could be set as follows: if an exchange process similar to that described in synaptosomes were present also in nerve terminals of the living brain, this process would
tend to maintain certain (subliminal?) concentrations of GABA in the
synapse. What function could this GABA have?

## III. NET RELEASE OF GABA INDUCED BY EXTRACELLULAR GABA. MECHANISMS OF GABA RELEASE

### A. Conditions in Which Extracellular GABA Promotes Its Own Release

It seemed logical to approach this problem by studying the stimulated release of GABA from synaptosomes in the presence of small
concentrations of extracellular GABA. In a number of experimental

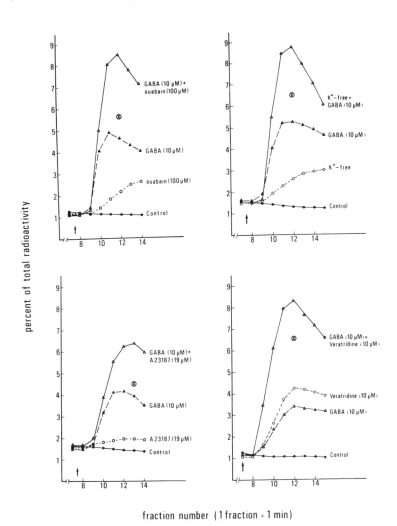

fraction number (1 fraction ≈ 1 min)

Fig. 1 - Supra-additive release of GABA from synaptosomes. Purified rat brain synaptosomes were prelabeled with 0.5 μM $^3$H-GABA in a Krebs-Ringer medium at pH 7.35, and then superfused on Millipore filters with standard medium (Raiteri et al., 1975). After some minutes (see arrows), the superfusion media were changed as indicated in the various panels. The radioactivity released in each fraction was expressed as percentage of the total radioactivity recovered (total fractions plus radioactivity remaining in the superfused filters). Amino-oxyacetic acid (10 μM) was present in all the media used. Each curve is the average of 2-6 duplicate experiments. The circled cross shows the calculated peak point of a purely additive release. The experiments with A23187 and ouabain are from Levi et al., 1976b.

conditions which depolarize synaptosomal membranes and inhibit the influx of GABA in uptake experiments, the net release of $^3$H-GABA was greately potentiated by the presence of a small concentration of GABA in the extracellular fluid. Fig. 1 shows these experiments. Each panel of the figure presents a curve of spontaneous release of $^3$H-GABA and a curve of release of $^3$H-GABA induced by 10 $\mu$M unlabeled GABA. A third curve refers to the release of $^3$H-GABA induced by one of the following drugs or conditions: 1) the calcium ionophore A23187 (19 $\mu$M); 2) veratridine (10 $\mu$M); 3) ouabain (100 $\mu$M); 4) K$^+$-free medium. In all cases the stimulated release of $^3$H-GABA was relatively modest. The fourth curve of each panel shows that the addition of 10 $\mu$M GABA to the superfusion media in the various conditions mentioned above caused a release of $^3$H-GABA which was greater than the sum of the release induced by unlabeled GABA alone plus that induced by each of the other stimulating conditions alone. Since in all four conditions the influx of GABA into synaptosomes was more or less markedly inhibited, this "supra-additive" release cannot be accounted for by an acceleration of a 1:1 homoexchange, but represents a net release of $^3$H-GABA, superimposed to the release caused by the drug alone (Levi et al., 1976b). In order to understand the mechanisms by which these supra-additive releasing effects were obtained, it was necessary to investigate how each of the various releasing agents tested elicited GABA release.

### B. Carrier-Mediated and Non-Carrier-Mediated Release.

The observation that the supra-additive releasing effect was still present when saturating concentrations of GABA were used to stimulate $^3$H-GABA release in the presence of maximal doses of ouabain or A23187, or in the absence of extracellular K$^+$ (unpublished observations) suggested that the release evoked by GABA or by the other agents had a different mechanism. Further support to this concept came from studies in which we attempted a discrimination between carrier-mediated and non-carrier-mediated release of GABA. For this purpose we exploited some interesting observations of Simon and Martin,(1973) on the inhibitory effect of L-2,4-diaminobutyric acid (DAB) on GABA transport. We studied the release of GABA in DAB pretreated synaptosomes, which exhibited only a minimal residual transport of GABA, thinking that, if GABA exited from synaptosomes utilizing the membrane transport system, efflux should be inhibited (Levi et al., 1976c). Fig. 2 shows that pretreatment of synaptosomes with 100 $\mu$M DAB did not affect the spontaneous release of $^3$H-GABA, but inhibited about 70% the GABA-stimulated $^3$H-GABA release, confirming the involvement of the membrane carrier in this type of release. On the other hand, Fig. 3 shows that the release of GABA caused by any of the other conditions tested (including 56 mM KCl, veratridine, A23187, ouabain, lack of K$^+$ and a purified toxin from black widow venom) was not inhibited in DAB pretreated synaptosomes. Al-

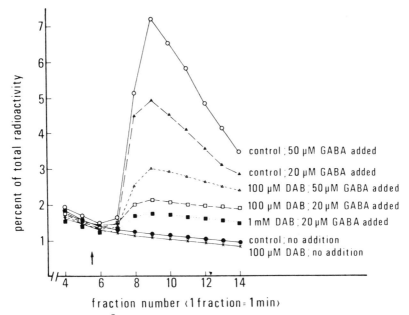

Fig. 2 - Release of [3]H-GABA from synaptosomes pretreated with L-dia-
minobutyric acid (DAB). Purified synaptosomes were incubated for 10
min with 0.2 μM [3]H-GABA (controls) or with 0.5 μM [3]H-GABA and 0.1
or 1 mM DAB, and then superfused with standard medium. After 5.5
min (see arrow) the medium of some of the superfusion chambers was
replaced with new medium containing 20 or 50 μM unlabeled GABA. For
other details, see Fig. 1. Each curve is the average of 2-4 duplicate experiments. Data from Levi et al., 1976c.


though these data leave open the problem of the mechanism by which
GABA is released under these conditions, it appears that the mechanism does not involve the DAB-inhibited GABA carrier (Levi et al.,
1976c). Incidentally, it may be worth mentioning that we have successfully utilized a similar procedure of blocking the membrane carrier for discriminating between carrier-mediated and "exocytotic-
like" release of biogenic amines from nerve endings (Raiteri et al.,
1977a; Raiteri et al., 1977b).

    Fig. 4 shows that the supra-additive release of [3]H-GABA, that
is the excess of release observed when synaptosomes were treated
with exogenous GABA plus one of the conditions depicted in Fig. 2,
was greatly reduced in DAB-treated synaptosomes, and thus appears
to be mediated by the DAB-inhibited carrier.

    In conclusion, the findings described above indicate that the
supra-additive release is due to an increased outward transport of

GABA triggered by the presence of extracellular GABA. Since the inward transport of GABA is partly inhibited in the conditions in which
the supra-additive release is observed, one can conclude that the
stoichiometry of the GABA homoexchange process is changed in the

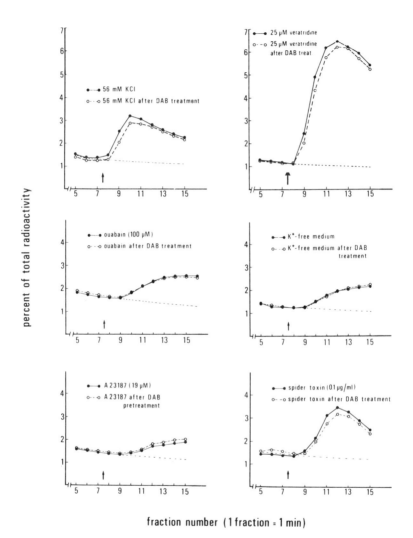

fraction number (1 fraction = 1 min)

Fig. 3 - Effect of pretreatment with 100 μM DAB on the synaptosomal
release of ³H-GABA elicited by various agents. Experimental conditions as described in the Fig. 2 caption. The releasing agents were
added when indicated by the arrows. Each curve is the average of 2-
6 experiments run in duplicate or triplicate. All the data, except
those obtained with veratridine, are from Levi et al., 1976c.

direction of net outward transport (Levi et al., 1976b)

What are the factors allowing this change in the stoichiometry of GABA homoexchange?

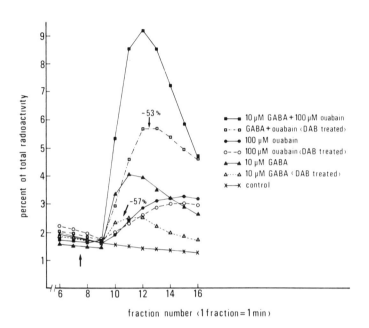

fraction number (1 fraction = 1 min)

Fig. 4 - Effect of pretreatment with 100 μM DAB on the supra-additive release of $^3$H-GABA elicited by unlabeled GABA and ouabain. Experimental conditions as described in the Fig. 2 caption, except that crude synaptosomal fractions (P$_2$ fractions) were used. The percentages of release inhibition given in the figure were calculated from the difference in the peak points of the curves, after subtracting the spontaneous release, and, in the experiments with GABA + ouabain, the release due to ouabain alone. Averages of 2 experiments are given.

C. Prominent Role of Changes Induced in Cationic Fluxes.

All the conditions studied in the experiments reported in Fig. 1 (namely: ouabain, lack of K$^+$, veratridine and the ionophore A23187) have the common effect of producing profound changes in cationic fluxes across the synaptosomal membrane. We shall briefly examine these changes, in order to assess their possible role in effecting

GABA release. Ouabain and lack of extracellular K$^+$ are known to inhibit the Na$^+$-K$^+$-ATPase (Schwartz et al., 1972). The most important consequence is an increase of the concentration of intrasynaptosomal Na$^+$ (Abdel-Latif, 1973; Archibald and White, 1974). However other cations are also affected. The level of intrasynaptosomal K$^+$ decreases (Goddard and Robinson, 1976; Blaustein and Goldring, 1975) and, according to several, but not all (Kamino et al., 1974), authors (Goddard and Robinson, 1976; Stahl and Swanson, 1969; Swanson et al., 1974), the influx of Ca$^{2+}$ increases. The effects of ouabain (alone or with added exogenous GABA) on $^3$H-GABA release were maintained unchanged in the absence of extracellular Ca$^{2+}$ (Fig. 5),

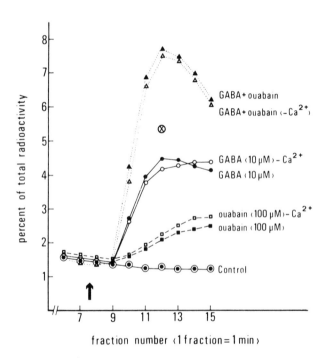

Fig. 5 - Effect of Ca$^{2+}$-deprivation on the synaptosomal release of $^3$H-GABA induced by ouabain and unlabeled GABA. In the experiments without Ca$^{2+}$, incubation and superfusion were performed with Ca$^{2+}$-free media. Other experimental details as described in the Fig. 1 caption. Each curve is the average of 2 duplicate experiments.

which seems to exclude the likelihood of a major role of $Ca^{2+}$ in the phenomena observed.

Thus, a probable reason for the GABA releasing effect of ouabain and $K^+$-free media is the increase of intracellular $Na^+$ concentration. As previously discussed, however, the membrane carrier does not seem to mediate the release induced by these conditions. This finding, together with the observation that synaptosomes prelabeled with $^3H$-GABA in a $Na^+$-rich medium do not lose $^3H$-GABA upon incubation or superfusion in a $Na^+$-free medium (Raiteri et al., 1975; Simon et al., 1974), support the concept that a favorable $Na^+$ gradient alone is not sufficient to drive carrier-mediated outward transport of GABA (Levi and Raiteri, 1976). The situation is quite different when the carrier-mediated transport of GABA is activated by exogenous GABA. In this case, the increased influx of $Na^+$ induced by ouabain and, possibly (as we shall discuss later) the decreased level of intracellular $K^+$, determine a potentiation of carrier-mediated release and therefore a predominance of outward versus inward GABA transport: in other words, the stoichiometry of GABA homoexchange is in favor of net outward transport.

Let's now consider the effects of veratridine. This drug depolarizes synaptosomes by increasing the permeability of the $Na^+$ channels (Blaustein and Goldring, 1975); the increased influx of $Na^+$ is accompanied by an increased influx of $Ca^{2+}$ and both are abolished by tetrodotoxin (Blaustein, 1975; Li and White, 1977). The neurotransmitter release induced by veratridine is generally considered to be $Ca^{2+}$-dependent, similar to the release induced by high $K^+$ depolarization (Blaustein, 1975; Redburn et al., 1976). Our experiments are in contrast with this generalization, since we could show that extracellular $Ca^{2+}$, at a concentration of 2.7 mM, consistently depressed, rather than stimulated, the veratridine-induced, tetrodotoxin-sensitive GABA release (Fig. 6). At a lower concentration (0.9 mM) $Ca^{2+}$ was no longer inhibitory: in fact, veratridine induced the same release of GABA in the presence of 0.9 mM $Ca^{2+}$, in the absence of $Ca^{2+}$, and in the absence of $Ca^{2+}$ with 0.2 mM EDTA (data not shown). It should be noted that in the same experimental conditions, 2.7 mM $Ca^{2+}$ strongly potentiated the veratridine-induced release of norepinephrine and dopamine, and the high $K^+$ -induced release of GABA and of biogenic amines (Raiteri et al., 1975; Raiteri et al., 1977 and unpublished observations), so that the data of Fig. 6 can be hardly attributed to our technical procedure. In conclusion, the release of GABA induced by veratridine, either alone or in combination with exogenous GABA, seems related to the influx of $Na^+$, but not to that of $Ca^{2+}$. As discussed above for ouabain, only the release triggered by exogenous GABA in the presence of the drug appears to be carrier-mediated, whereas that caused by veratridine alone does not seem to be mediated by the DAB-inhibited carrier.

The experiments presented so far suggest that when $Na^+$ influx

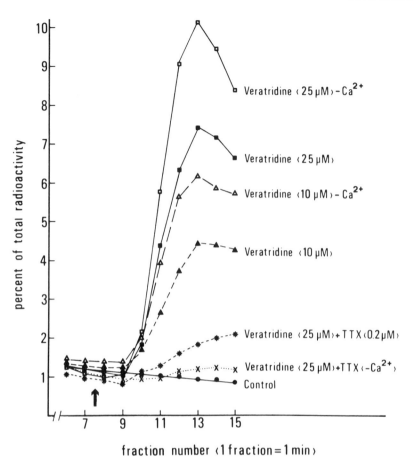

Fig. 6 - Inhibitory effect of $Ca^{2+}$ on the synaptosomal release of $^3H$-GABA induced by veratridine. Experimental conditions as described in the Fig. 1 caption. The arrow indicates the time of addition of veratridine (10 or 25 μM) to the superfusion medium. Tetrodotoxin (0.2 μM), when present, was added together with veratridine. Each curve is the average of 2 duplicate experiments.

is increased, $Na^+$ has a predominant role in promoting the outward transport of GABA triggered by extracellular GABA. The data obtained with the $Ca^{2+}$ ionophore A23187, (Levi et al., 1976b) which are similar to those obtained with ouabain, lack of $K^+$ and veratridine, indicate that also $Ca^{2+}$ can promote the outward transport of GABA triggered by exogenous GABA. The effects of A23187 were entirely $Ca^{2+}$-dependent. It is interesting that in studies of GABA uptake, $Ca^{2+}$ was shown to stimulate GABA transport at low, but not at high, $Na^+$ concentrations (Martin and Smith III, 1972). The situation may be similar in the case of GABA efflux.

The effects of inhibitors of the $Na^+$ $-K^+$ $-ATPase$ and of veratridine, which are all conditions leading to an increased concentration of intrasynaptosomal $Na^+$ (Goddard and Robinson, 1976; Li and
White, 1977), on the stoichiometry of GABA homoexchange may generate the idea that the lack of net uptake and the presence of a 1:1
homoexchange observed in synaptosomes could be due to the abnormally
high internal $Na^+$ concentration reported in synaptosomes incubated
in standard media (Goddard and Robinson, 1976; Li and White, 1977;
Marchbanks, 1975). An interpretation of this type has been given to
our first results on GABA exchange by Lake and Voaden (1976). However, the possibility that the GABA release elicited by exogenous GABA
is artificially high in synaptosomes because of their higher than normal
$Na^+$ content seems disproved by the experiments shown in Fig. 7. In
the first set of experiments synaptosomes were prelabeled with

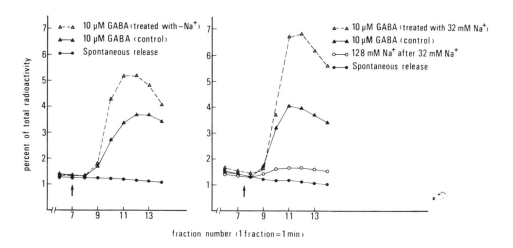

Fig. 7 - Effect of $Na^+$ -depletion on the synaptosomal release of $^3H$-
GABA elicited by exogenous GABA. Left panel: synaptosomes were incubated in a standard medium (with 130 mM $Na^+$) for 20 min at 37° (10
min of equilibration and 10 other minutes in the presence of 0.5 μM
$^3H$-GABA); then they were superfused for 7.5 min with standard medium
(controls) or with a $Na^+$ -free medium ($Na^+$ replaced by sucrose).
The superfusion was then continued (see arrow) with standard medium
containing 10 μM GABA. The lower curve shows the spontaneous release
of $^3H$-GABA from synaptosomes not treated with $Na^+$-free medium. Right
panel: the control synaptosomes were treated as described above.
Other synaptosomes from the same preparation were incubated and superfused in a medium containing 32 mM $Na^+$ (the missing $Na^+$ was replaced with sucrose). At the time indicated by the arrow, the superfusion was continued with standard medium, with or without 10 μM
GABA. Other experimental details were as in the Fig. 1 caption.
Each curve is the average of 3 experiments run in triplicate.

$^3$H-GABA in a standard medium, and then superfused for 7.5 min either
with standard medium (controls) or with a Na$^+$ -free medium. The latter treatment should rapidly deplete intracellular Na$^+$ (Banay-Schwartz
et al., 1976; Blaustein, 1975; Li and White, 1977). The superfusion
was then continued with a standard medium containing 10 µM GABA
(which in some experiments was $^{14}$C-labeled). The GABA induced $^3$H-
GABA release, rather than being depressed in Na$^+$-depleted synaptosomes, was stimulated more than in controls. The simultaneous uptake
of $^{14}$C-GABA did not differ significantly in control and Na$^+$-depleted
synaptosomes.One might argue that the treatment with Na$^+$-free media
was not enough effective. Therefore, in order to prevent any accumulation of Na$^+$, we ran an other set of experiments in which synaptosomes were never allowed to stay in Na$^+$-rich media before the beginning of the exchange period (Fig. 7). In these experiments, the synaptosomes were exposed to a medium containing only 32 mM Na$^+$ during
the labeling period with $^3$H-GABA and during the first minutes of superfusion. Then they were exposed to standard medium containing 10
µM GABA. Also in this case, the GABA induced $^3$H-GABA release was
stimulated rather than decreased. It should be noted that the mere
restoration of the normal concentration of extracellular Na$^+$ caused
only a modest release of GABA.

The significance of these experiments seems to go beyond just
showing that the GABA-stimulated GABA release is not a consequence
of the Na$^+$ enrichment taking place during incubations in normal media. In fact, the result obtained with Na$^+$ depleted synaptosomes is
paradoxically similar to the supra-additive release observed in conditions leading to an increased intrasynaptosomal concentration of
Na$^+$ (see Fig. 1). The effect could not be attributed to the accumulation of Ca$^{2+}$ that may occur during the incubation or superfusion
with media containing low or no Na$^+$ (Blaustein and Oborn, 1975). In
fact, it was observed also when the whole experiment was run in
Ca$^{2+}$ -free media. If we look more carefully at the experiments with
ouabain or with K$^+$ -free media (Fig. 1), we may have the clue to
this paradox. It can be noted that the supra-additive release is
immediate, and reaches its peak when the effect of ouabain or of
K$^+$ deprivation is still quite below its maximum. Thus, it seems
plausible that the influx of Na$^+$, rather than the establishment of
a high intracellular Na$^+$ concentration, determines the conditions
in which the homoexchange of GABA is characterized by a high efflux/
influx ratio. This interpretation would fit very well to the experiments in which the supra-additive release was observed in Na$^+$-de-
pleted synaptosomes (Fig. 7). In fact, when these are exposed to a
Na$^+$ -rich medium, a rapid, tetrodotoxin-insensitive influx of Na$^+$
takes place (Li and White, 1977). This Na$^+$ influx, by itself, has
only a little effect on GABA release. However, the presence of extracellular GABA triggers a homoexchange process, characterized by
an efflux/influx ratio greater than 1, similarly to what observed
with ouabain, veratridine etc.

To summarize this section, we have shown that a number of conditions which have the common feature of increasing the influx of $Na^+$ or $Ca^{2+}$, or both, and which, under some aspects, mimic events occurring during physiological stimulation, are capable of altering the stoichiometry of the basal GABA homoexchange. The result of this altered stoichiometry is a substantial net carrier-mediated release of GABA.

It may be interesting to mention that a supra-additive releasing effect was not observed when synaptosomes were superfused in a medium containing a depolarizing concentration of KCl and GABA. Although this finding was somewhat disappointing, it may have several explanations: high potassium media are either deficient in $Na^+$ or hypertonic, and both these factors might affect GABA transport; more important, high $K^+$ media determine not only an increased influx of $Ca^{2+}$, which is responsible for a large part of the evoked release of GABA (Blaustein, 1975; Raiteri et al., 1975; Redburn et al., 1976) (and this release does not appear to be carrier-mediated (Levi et al., 1976c; Fig. 3)), but also       a large increase in the intrasynaptosomal concentration of $K^+$ (Goddard and Robinson, 1976) which may inhibit the outward carrier-mediated transport of GABA (see Section V), and thus prevent the occurrence of a supra-additive release when extracellular GABA is present.

## IV. INTRASYNAPTOSOMAL POOLS SUSCEPTIBLE OF BEING RELEASED OR EXCHANGED

The validity of the conclusions drawn from the data discussed so far could be seriously hampered if the radioactive GABA taken up by synaptosomes during the pre-labeling step of our release studies were released more easily than the bulk of the endogenous GABA pool, under some of the experimental conditions employed: for example, if exogenous GABA exchanged with a pool of intrasynaptosomal GABA having a specific radioactivity much higher than that of the total GABA contained in the synaptosomes, exchange rates would have been overestimated. Similarly, the supra-additive releasing effects described in the previous paragraphs could be only apparent, and result from an increase in the specific radioactivity of the GABA released, rather than from an increase in the actual amount of GABA released.

In previous experiments we had compared, in the same synaptosomes, the release of the $^{14}C$-GABA metabolically derived from $^{14}C$-glutamate  to that of the $^3H$-GABA taken up (Levi et al., 1976a). The results obtained showed that $^{14}C$- and $^3H$-GABA were released in a similar way, both spontaneously and under homoexchange conditions. This experiment, although suggesting a similar behavior of two GABA pools of different origin, (recent synthesis and uptake), does not say anything about the bulk of the endogenous GABA pool, which is

probably neither recently synthesized, nor recently taken up. Therefore, we designed another experiment which allowed us to compare
the behavior of the GABA recently taken up to that of the endogenous
GABA. Synaptosomes were prelabeled with radioactive GABA and then
superfused under various of the conditions discussed in the previous paragraphs. The specific radioactivity of GABA was measured

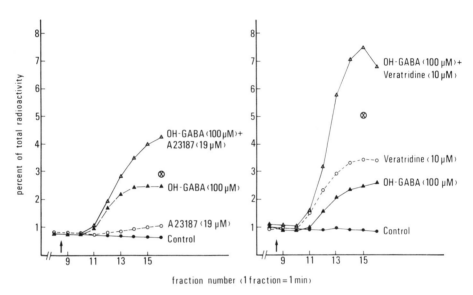

fraction number (1 fraction = 1 min)

Fig. 8 - Supra additive release of synaptosomal ³H-GABA elicited by
gamma-amino-beta-hydroxybutyric acid (OH-GABA) in the presence of
veratridine or ouabain. Experimental conditions as described in the
Fig. 1 caption. Each curve is the average of 2-3 duplicate experiments.

in synaptosomes at zero time (at the beginning of superfusion) and
at the end of the superfusion period, and in pooled fractions of
the superfused medium before and during the stimulation period. For
obvious reasons, we could not use exogenous GABA to promote homoexchange; we overcame this difficulty by using gamma-amino-beta-hydroxybutyric acid (OH-GABA), a GABA analog utilizing the same transport  system as GABA (Iversen and Johnston, 1971; Levi, 1972; Raiteri et al., 1975) and causing, as GABA, a supra-additive release of
GABA in the appropriate conditions (Fig. 8).

TABLE I. EFFECT OF VARIOUS AGENTS ON THE SPECIFIC RADIOACTIVITY OF THE GABA RELEASED FROM SYNAPTOSOMES

| Releasing agent | Relative specific radioactivity of GABA | | | | | |
|---|---|---|---|---|---|---|
| | OH–GABA 100 $\mu$M | KCl 56 mM | Veratr. 10 $\mu$M | OH–GABA +veratr. | A23187 19 $\mu$M | OH–GABA +A23187 |
| Synaptosomes (zero time) | 100 | 100 | 100 | 100 | 100 | 100 |
| Medium (pre-stimulation) | 103 | 106 | 106 | 94 | 96 | 104 |
| Medium (stimulation) | 113 | 96 | 126 | 123 | 96 | 132 |
| Synaptosomes (superfused) | 97 | 105 | 89 | 78 | 103 | 94 |

released over control during stimulation (nmoles/mg protein)

| 0.89 | 2.11 | 1.43 | 4.56 | 0.02 | 1.36 |
|---|---|---|---|---|---|

Purified rat brain synaptosomes were incubated for 10 min in a medium containing 0.5 $\mu$M radioactive GABA. Aliquots of the suspension were superfused with standard medium for 10 min, and then with new medium containing the releasing agents, shown in the Table, up to the 16th min. GABA was measured on perchloric acid extracts of the synaptosomes at the beginning (zero time) and at the end of superfusion, and on pooled fractions (pools of 5 fractions of 1 min) of the superfused media, by ion exchange chromatography followed by reaction with o-phtalaldehyde. The effuent of the chromatographic column was split, in order to measure the radioactivity present in the GABA peak. The GABA specific radioactivities (cpm/nmole) are expressed as relative values, taking the specific radioactivity in synaptosomes at zero time as 100. The relative specific radioactivity of GABA in the uptake medium was 3000 at the beginning of the incubation, and approximately 800 at the end of the incubation. Averages of 2-5 separate experiments, and of 2-10 determinations are presented.

The results concerning the specific radioactivity of GABA in
the various experimental phases are presented in the upper part of
Table I. For convenience, the specific radioactivity of GABA in syn-
naptosomes at zero time was taken as 100. Values above 100 in the
superfused medium indicate a preferential release of the radioactive GABA taken up. Looking at these results, several points can be
made: 1) the GABA taken up by synaptosomes over a short period of
incubation does not distribute homogeneously within the endogenous
pool. 2) Under some of the conditions tested, the GABA recently taken up is released preferentially, with respect to the endogenous
GABA. Among these conditions is the depolarization induced by veratridine, but not that caused by media containing high $K^+$. The different behavior observed in these two conditions is noteworthy. 3)
OH-GABA exchanges with a GABA pool having a specific radioactivity
just above average. The result is at the border-line of significance. 4) The compartmentation of the radioactive GABA taken up by synaptosomes  is probably less pronounced than it appears at first
sight. In fact, the highest specific radioactivities observed in the
superfused media were only 20-30% higher than those measured in synaptosomes  at zero time, but were several folds lower than the specific radioactivity of the GABA present in the medium during the
incubation preceeding the superfusion. 5) The compartmentation of
the radioactive GABA taken up is not such to influence the interpretation of our exchange and release studies. Judging from the experiments with OH-GABA alone (Table I), our basal exchange rates might
have been overestimated of about 15% and a correction of this magnitude would not change the results in a significant way. As to the
supra-additive releasing effects previously described, the lower
part of Table I shows that they are clearly detectable also when the
results are expressed in terms of actual nmoles of GABA released,
rather than in terms of radioactivity.

## V. IS HOMOEXCHANGE OF GABA AN IN VITRO ARTIFACT?

The concept of GABA homoexchange did not appear as appealing
as that of high affinity uptake, and in several recent reports it
has been argued that the homoexchange present in incubated synaptosomes could result from artifactual situations. In the living brain,
net, high affinity uptake would instead be operating. We shall briefly analyze the arguments for or against this concept. Whatever conclusion may be reached on this point, it has to be remembered that
the high affinity uptake theory was based on results obtained in the
supposedly artifactual situation present in in vitro experiments.

### A. Abnormal Ionic Gradients of Incubated Synaptosomes

Sellström et al. (1976) confirmed that, in incubated synaptosomes, no net uptake of GABA is detectable at concentrations below

100 µM, but reached the conclusion that, in vivo, in resting conditions, the balance point at which net uptake of GABA begins could
be at a concentration of extracellular GABA of about 1 µM (that is
in the range of high affinity uptake systems). This conclusion was
based on several assumptions: 1) that the energy for GABA transport
resides entirely in the ionic gradient. 2) That three $Na^+$ and one
$K^+$ are co-transported with one molecule of GABA. 3) That the membrane potential of isolated nerve endings is much lower than that of
nerve endings in vivo. These assumptions do not seem to us fully
justified. From the first assumption it would be expected that the
outward transport of GABA is facilitated when the extracellular concentration of $Na^+$ is decreased or nullified, to create a favorable
$Na^+_{in}$ - $Na^+_{out}$ gradient. However, in these conditions, the efflux
of GABA does not increase (Raiteri et al., 1975; Simon et al., 1974).
Moreover, it would be also expected that decreasing the intracellular concentration of $Na^+$ to create a more favorable $Na^+_{out}$ - $Na^+_{in}$
gradient, should facilitate GABA influx. To test this, we superfused synaptosomes with standard (128 mM $Na^+$) or with a $Na^+$ -free medium for 10 min to deplete intracellular $Na^+$ (Banay-Schwartz et al.,
1976; Li and White, 1977), and then we continued the superfusion
for 5 min with standard medium containing 10 µM $^3H$-GABA. No increase in the uptake of GABA could be observed in these conditions. Taking the uptake of GABA in controls as 100, the uptake in $Na^+$ -de-
pleted synaptosomes was 93+4 (average of 6 experiments +S.D.). As
to the second assumption, the literature contains no direct evidence that $K^+$ is co-transported with GABA, but only the suggestion that
it might be, and that, if it were, concentrative uptake of GABA would
be facilitated (Martin, 1976). Finally, we are not aware of data in
the literature supporting the statement that the membrane potential
of incubated synaptosomes is substantially lower than that of nerve
endings in vivo. In contrast, in the only study in which, to our
knowledge, this problem was analyzed, Blaustein and Goldring (1975)
calculated a membrane potential of -55 to -60 mV for synaptosomes
incubated in 132 mM $Na^+$, 5 mM $K^+$ and 1.2 mM $Ca^{2+}$. This value is remarkably close to the resting potentials measured directly with microelectrodes in mammalian central neurons (Li, 1959; Phillips,
1956).

     To conclude, the statement that the point at which net uptake
of GABA begins in vivo could correspond to an extracellular GABA
concentration of 1 µM (Sellström et al., 1976) appears premature.
It may not even be crucial to determine exactly this point, until
more is known about the concentration of GABA in the synaptic cleft,
at rest or after stimulation. It should be noted that, in more general terms, Sellström et al. (1976) agree with us in considering
cationic concentrations of primary importance for determining the
ratio between GABA influx and efflux, and therefore the direction
of net transport.

     Lake and Voaden, in a paper on GABA transport in retina (Lake

and Voaden, 1976) suggested that homoexchange of GABA in synaptosomes may be an artifact deriving from an increased (spontaneous and
GABA-stimulated) efflux consequent to the higher than normal level
of $Na^+$ present in incubated synaptosomes. We have already commented
upon this point in Section III, C.


B. Abnormally High Concentration of GABA in Isolated Nerve Endings

In a very recent, stimulating paper, Ryan and Roskowski (1977)
noted that synaptosomes partially depleted of their endogenous content of GABA by a preincubation in a medium containing 56 mM KCl, and
then incubated in a medium with 1-4 mM KCl, exhibited a net uptake
of 10 $\mu$M GABA. In contrast, net uptake was very limited, as compared to the accumulation of radioactivity, in synaptosomes not previously treated with high $K^+$. The authors attributed the net uptake
of GABA observed after treatment with high $K^+$ to the partial depletion of the endogenous GABA and suggested that normal synaptosomes
may be in a condition in which their uptake capacity is virtually
saturated, due to the high GABA content. They also inferred that
GABA-depleted synaptosomes may simulate a post-release situation of
nerve endings in vivo.

We have repeated the experiments of Ryan and Roskowski, and
confirmed their results; however, our interpretation of the data
differs considerably. It has been shown that the synaptosomal content of $K^+$ is increased 2.5 times after only 3 min incubation in a
medium containing 50 mM KCl (Goddard and Robinson, 1976). Since high
concentrations of $K^+$ inhibit GABA transport (Blaustein and King,
1976; Martin, 1976), we thought that a more than doubled concentration of $K^+$ in synaptosomes might decrease the carrier-mediated efflux of GABA stimulated by exogenous GABA. If this were true, the
increased influx/efflux ratio observed by Ryan and Roskowski would
be explained. In order to test this possibility, we designed an experiment in which synaptosomes were preloaded with $K^+$ in conditions
preventing any GABA depletion. Synaptosomes resuspended in 0.32 M
sucrose were diluted 1:4 in a solution of 160 mM KCl or NaCl and
left for 90 min at 0°. After centrifugation, the GABA content of
the synaptosomes was identical in the two preparations (Table II).
The synaptosomes were then resuspended in a Krebs-Ringer solution
containing 2 mM KCl. After 5 min equilibration, 10 $\mu$M radioactive
GABA was added, and uptake over a 10 min period was determined by
measuring the accumulation of radioactivity in the tissue and the
decrease of radioactivity and of actual GABA concentration in the
medium. The KCl-treated synaptosomes exhibited a substantial increase in net GABA uptake, and only a modest increase in radiochemical
uptake, as compared to the NaCl-treated controls, which suggests that
the carrier-mediated efflux of GABA is decreased when the intrasynaptosomal $K^+$ content is raised above that of controls.
These preliminary findings confirm and extend a previous observation

of Martin (1976) who reported a higher uptake of radioactive (?)
GABA in $K^+$-loaded synaptosomes.

TABLE II. UPTAKE OF GABA BY SYNAPTOSOMES SUBJECTED TO HIGH KCl
CONCENTRATIONS

| Treatment before uptake | GABA concentr. (nmoles/mg protein) | GABA uptake after KCl (% of control) | |
|---|---|---|---|
| | | Chemical | Radiochem. |
| None (zero time) | 15.9 | | |
| Experiment A: 90 min at 0° in 120 mM $K^+$ | 11.5 | 135 | 120 |
| 90 min at 0° in 120 mM $Na^+$ (controls) | 11.3 | | |
| Experiment B: 10 min at 37° in 56 mM $K^+$ | 7.4 | 140 | 114 |
| 10 min at 37° in normal medium (controls) | 15.4 | | |

Experiment A: Purified rat brain synaptosomes were resuspended in
0.32 M sucrose at a protein concentration of about 10 mg/ml. An
aliquot was taken for GABA determination (zero time); other aliquots
were diluted 1:4 in a solution of 160 mM NaCl (controls) or 160 mM
KCl, kept at 0° for 90 min, and then centrifuged. The concentration
of GABA was measured in perchloric acid extracts of some of the pellets. Other pellets were resuspended in a glucose-containing Krebs-
Ringer medium (with 2 mM KCl) buffered at pH 7.35 with HEPES-Tris.
The suspensions (1-2 mg of synaptosomal protein) were equilibrated
for 5 min at 37°, and then incubated for 10 min in the presence of
10 μM $^3$H-GABA. Uptake was stopped by centrifugation. Chemical uptake was determined by measuring the decrease in the concentration of
GABA in the medium after incubation, radiochemical uptake by measuring the loss of radioactivity from the medium and the accumulation
of radioactivity into synaptosomes. GABA was measured by ion exchange chromatography (Levi et al., 1972). Averages of 4 experiments
run in duplicate are presented.
Experiment B: Synaptosomes were resuspended in 0.32 M glucose and
diluted 1:10 either in standard Krebs-Ringer medium (controls), or
in a medium containing 56 mM KCl (replacing an equivalent amount of
NaCl). After a 10 min incubation at 37°, the suspensions were centrifuged, and then treated as described above for experiment A. The
data presented refer to one experiment run in duplicate.

It seems therefore plausible that the increased net uptake of GABA observed by Ryan and Roskowski (1977) after treatment with high $K^+$ has to be attributed to the elevated intrasynaptosomal content of $K^+$, rather than to the diminished GABA concentration. Since the $K^+$ concentration of nerve endings in vivo is not expected to increase above the values present in resting conditions, during or after depolarization, their finding may have little bearing to the problem of GABA high affinity uptake in vivo. At any rate, their and our own data seem to confirm the importance of $K^+$ as one of the cations involved in the modulation of GABA fluxes.

## VI. UNITARY INTERPRETATION OF GABA TRANSPORT IN SYNAPTOSOMES CENTERED ON A BASAL HOMOEXCHANGE PROCESS

All the data discussed so far fit into an interpretation of GABA transport which aims at unifying the multiple GABA transport systems currently described (high and low affinity uptake, exchange, carrier-mediated efflux). This interpretation is tentatively proposed for central nerve endings, and may not be valid for other preparations exhibiting GABA transport, such as glia or retina; moreover, it may have to be readjusted as long as new data will appear. In synthesis, the in vitro results available can be summarized as follows:

1) In normal conditions of incubation or superfusion (high $Na^+$, low $K^+$) synaptosomes do not perform a net uptake of GABA, when the amino acid is present at low concentrations ($< 20$ $\mu$M) in the medium. In these conditions, a homoexchange process, with an apparent ratio of GABA influx/efflux approximating unity is observed. Data obtained on the inwardly directed component indicate that the process is highly $Na^+$-dependent (Iversen and Neal, 1968; Kuriyama et al., 1969; Levi and Raiteri, 1975a; Simon et al., 1974), shows $Ca^{2+}$-dependence only at low $Na^+$ concentrations (Martin and Smith III, 1972) and is inhibited by high concentrations of $K^+$ (Martin, 1976).

2) The stoichiometry of the basal 1:1 homoexchange of GABA can be changed in the direction of net outward transport (i.e. carrier-mediated **efflux > carrier-**mediated influx) by conditions causing an increased influx of $Na^+$ and/or of $Ca^{2+}$ into synaptosomes. Some of these conditions (ouabain, veratridine) also cause a rapid fall in the concentration of intracellular $K^+$ (Li and White, 1977), which may contribute to determine a higher efflux/influx ratio.

3) The stoichiometry of basal 1:1 homoexchange of GABA is shifted in the direction of net inward transport (**i.e. influx>efflux**) when the extracellular concentration of GABA is relatively high (100 $\mu$M or more (Iversen and Neal, 1968; Levi and Raiteri, 1974; Raiteri et al., 1975; Sellström et al., 1976; Simon et al., 1974) in normal ionic conditions. Alterations of the concentrations of some ionic

species may also favor this shift. For example, an increase of intracellular $K^+$ is likely to depress the efflux component of the homoexchange process.

4) Carrier-mediated transport of GABA seems to require $Na^+$ and
GABA at both sides of the membrane. In fact, a favorable $Na^+$ gradient
alone (lack of extracellular $Na^+$) is not sufficient to promote a carrier-mediated outward transport of GABA. In this respect, the behavior of GABA differs markedly from that of catecholamines (Raiteri
et al., 1977a; Raiteri et al., 1977b).

One can certainly find in the literature arguments for or against an extrapolation of the results obtained in vitro with synaptosomes to phenomena occurring in nerve endings in vivo. We like to
believe that the arguments in favor outbalance slightly the arguments against this extrapolation. Therefore, we tentatively suggest
that, in the case of "GABA-ergic" nerve endings, the following situations may exist:

1) A resting phase, in which small extracellular concentrations
of GABA are maintained in the synapse by a basal 1:1 homoexchange
process.

2) A release phase, in which the ionic alterations accompanying depolarization (influx of $Na^+$ and of $Ca^{2+}$, possibly efflux of
$K^+$), besides causing some non-carrier-mediated release of GABA by
themselves, cause a modification of the stoichiometry of GABA homoexchange, in the sense of an increased outward/inward flux ratio.
The net release of GABA would thus be potentiated by the very presence of GABA out of the nerve ending membrane.

3) A reuptake phase, in which an inversion of the flux ratio
would be facilitated by the increased concentration of extracellular GABA consequent to the release phase, and possibly by the inversion of the ionic fluxes characteristic of the restoration phase
following depolarization.

We intentionally avoided speaking of the affinity of the transport system, first because the knowledge on this point is somewhat
confused, second because the problem may not be as crucial as it
appeared some time ago. Simon et al. (1974) found a high affinity Km
for the exchange process., but the Km for net uptake has not been
measured. It cannot be excluded that, under the circumstances in
which net uptake is possible, a high affinity interaction occurs
between extracellular GABA and the membrane carrier. We do not think
that our interpretation of the GABA transport system would suffer
if such high affinity interactions did exist.

Acknowledgment. We thank Mr. Alberto Coletti for excellent technical assistance, and Eli Lilly and Co. for a gift of the ionophore A23187. Part of the studies reported were supported by Research Grant n. 922 of the North Atlantic Treaty Organization and by Grant n. CT 76.01555.04 of the Italian National Research Council.


## VII. REFERENCES

Abdel-Latif, A.A., 1973, Ion transport in the synaptosome and Na$^+$ -K$^+$ -ATPase, in "Methods of Neurochemistry", Vol. 5 (R. Fried, ed.) pp. 147-188, M. Dekker, New York.

Archibald, J.T., and White, T.D., 1974, Rapid reversal of internal Na$^+$ and K$^+$ of synaptosomes by ouabain, Nature 252:595-596.

Banay-Schwartz, M., Teller, D.N. and Lajtha A., 1976, Energetics of low affinity amino acid transport into brain slices, in "Transport Phenomena in the Nervous System" Vol. 69 of Adv. Exp. Med. Biol. (G. Levi, L. Battistin and A. Lajtha, eds.) pp. 349-370, Plenum Press, New York.

Blaustein, M.P., 1975, Effects of potassium, veratridine and scorpion venom on calcium accumulation and transmitter release by nerve terminals in vitro, J. Physiol. 247:617-655.

Blaustein, M.P.,and Goldring, J.M., 1975, Membrane potentials in pinched-off presynaptic terminals monitored with a fluorescent probe: evidence that synaptosomes have potassium diffusion potentials, J. Physiol. 247:589-615.

Blaustein, M.P., and King, A.C., 1976, Influence of membrane potential on the sodium-dependent uptake of gamma-amino-butyric acid by presynaptic nerve terminals: experimental observations and theoretical considerations, J. Membrane Biol. 30:153-173.

Blaustein, M.P., and Oborn, C.J., 1975, The influence of sodium on calcium fluxes in pinched-off nerve terminals in vitro, J. Physiol. 247:657-686.

Goddard, G.A., and Robinson, J.D., 1976, Uptake and release of calcium by rat brain synaptosomes, Brain Res. 110:331-350.

Iversen, L.L., 1975, High affinity uptake of neurotransmitter amino acids, Nature 253:481.

Iversen, L.L., and Johnston, G.A.R., 1971, GABA uptake in rat CNS: comparison of uptake in slices and in homogenates and the effect of some inhibitors, J. Neurochem. 18:1939-1950.

Iversen, L.L., and Kelly, J.S., 1975, Uptake and metabolism of $\gamma$-aminobutyric acid by neurons and glial cells, Biochem. Pharmacol. 24:933-938.

Iversen, L.L., and Neal, M.J., 1968, The uptake of ($^3$H)GABA by slices of rat cerebral cortex, J. Neurochem. 15:1141-1149.

Kamino, K., Uyesaka, N., and Inouye, A., 1974, Calcium-binding of synaptosomes isolated from rat brain cortex. I. Effects of high external potassium ions, J. Membr. Biol. 17:13-26.

Kuriyama, K., Weinstein, H., and Roberts, E., 1969, Uptake of $\gamma$-aminobutyric acid by mitochondrial and synaptosomal fractions from rat brain, Brain Res. 16:479-492.

Lake, N., and Voaden, M.J., 1976, Exchange versus net uptake of exo-
    genously-applied ɣ-aminobutyric acid in retina, J. Neurochem.
    27:1571-1574.
Levi, G., 1972, Transport systems for GABA and for other amino acids
    in incubated chick brain tissue during development, Arch. Bio-
    chem. Biophys. 151:8-21.
Levi, G., Amaldi, P., and Morisi, G., 1972, Gamma-aminobutyric acid
    (GABA) uptake by the developing mouse brain in vivo, Brain Res.
    41:435-451.
Levi, G., and Raiteri, M., 1974, Exchange of neurotransmitter amino
    acid at nerve endings can simulate high affinity uptake, Nature
    253:735-737.
Levi, G., and Raiteri, M., 1975a, Transport of GABA in nervous tis-
    sues, in "Biological Membranes, Neurochemistry", FEBS Meeting,
    Vol. 41 (J. Montreuil and P. Mandel eds.), pp. 81-93, North-
    Holland, Amsterdam.
Levi, G., and Raiteri, M., 1975b, Reply, Nature 253:481-482.
Levi, G., and Raiteri, M., 1976, Synaptosomal transport processes,
    Int. Rev. Neurobiol. 19:51-74.
Levi, G., Poce, U., and Raiteri, M., 1976a, Uptake and exchange of
    GABA and glutamate in isolated nerve endings, in "Transport
    Phenomena in the Nervous System", Vol. 69 of Adv. Exp. Med.
    Biol. (G. Levi, L. Battistin and A. Lajtha, eds) pp. 273-289,
    Plenum Press, New York.
Levi, G., Roberts, P.J., and Raiteri, M., 1976b, Release and exchan-
    ge of neurotransmitters in synaptosomes: effects of the iono-
    phore A23187 and of ouabain, Neurochem. Res. 1: 409-416.
Levi, G., Rusca, G., and Raiteri, M., 1976c, Diaminobutyric acid: a
    tool for discriminating between carrier-mediated and non-car-
    rier-mediated release of GABA from synaptosomes? Neurochem.
    Res. 1:581-590.
Li, C.L., 1959, Cortical intracellular potentials and their respon-
    ses to strychnine, J. Neurophysiol. 22:436-450.
Li, P.P., and White, T.D., 1977, Rapid effects of veratridine, tetro-
    dotoxin, gramicidin D, valinomycin and NaCN on the Na$^+$, K$^+$ and
    ATP contents of synaptosomes, J. Neurochem. 28:967-975.
Marchbanks, R.M., 1975, The chloride content, anionic deficit and
    volume of synaptosomes, J. Neurochem 25:463-470.
Martin, D.L., 1976, Carrier-mediated transport and removal of GABA
    from synaptic regions, in "GABA in Nervous System Function"
    (E. Roberts, T.N. Chase and D.B. Tower, eds) pp. 347-386, Raven
    Press, New York.
Martin, D.L., and Smith III, A.A., 1972, Ions and the transport of
    gamma-aminobutyric acid by synaptosomes, J. Neurochem. 19:841-
    855.
Phillips, C.G., 1956, Intracellular records from Betz cells in cat,
    Q.Jl.exp.Physiol. 41:58-69.
Raiteri, M., del Carmine, R., Bertollini, A., and Levi, G., 1977a,
    Effect of desmethylimipramine on the release of $^3$H-norepinephri-
    ne induced by various agents in hypothalamic synaptosomes, Mol.

    Pharmacol. 13:(in press).
Raiteri, M., Cerrito, F., Cervoni, A.M., del Carmine, R., Ribera,
    T., and Levi, G., 1977b, Studies on the uptake and release of
    dopamine in synaptosomes, Symposium on "Dopamine", Southampton
    (in press).
Raiteri, M., Federico, R., Coletti, A., and Levi, G., 1975, Release
    and exchange studies relating to the synaptosomal uptake of
    GABA, J. Neurochem. 24:1243-1250.
Redburn, D.A., Shelton, D., and Cotman, C.W., 1976, Calcium-depen-
    dent release of exogenously loaded $\gamma$-amino- U-$^{14}$C- butyrate
    from synaptosomes: time course of stimulation by potassium,
    veratridine, and the calcium ionophore A23187, J. Neurochem.
    26:297-303.
Ryan, L.D., and Roskoski, R. jr., 1977, Net uptake of $\gamma$-aminobuty-
    ric acid by a high affinity synaptosomal transport system, J.
    Pharmacol. exp. Ther. 200:285-291.
Schwartz, A., Lindenmayer, G.E., and Allen, J.C., 1972, The Na$^+$,K$^+$
    -ATPase membrane transport system: importance of cellular func-
    tion, Curr. Top. Membr. Transp. 3:1-82.
Sellström, A., Venema, R., and Henn, F., 1976, Functional assessment
    of GABA uptake or exchange by synaptosomal fractions, Nature
    264:652-653.
Simon, J.R., and Martin, D.L., 1973, The effects of L-2,4-diamino-
    butyric acid on the uptake of gamma-aminobutyric acid by a
    synaptosomal fraction from rat brain, Arch. Biochem. Biophys.
    157:348-355.
Simon, J.R., Martin, D.L., and Kroll, M., 1974, Sodium-dependent ef-
    flux and exchange of GABA in synaptosomes, J. Neurochem. 23:
    981-991.
Stahl, W.L., and Swanson, P.D., 1969, Uptake of calcium by subcellu-
    lar fractions isolated from ouabain treated cerebral tissue,
    J. Neurochem. 16:1553-1563.
Storm-Mathisen, J., Fonnum, F., and Malthe-Sørenssen, D., 1976, GABA
    uptake in nerve terminals, in "GABA in Nervous System Function"
    (E. Roberts, T. N. Chase and D.B. Tower, eds) pp. 387-394, Ra-
    ven Press, New York.
Swanson, P.D., Anderson, L., and Stahl, W.L., 1974, Uptake of cal-
    cium ions by synaptosomes from rat brain, Biochim. Biophys.
    Acta 356:174-183.

CIS 3-AMINOCYCLOHEXANE CARBOXYLIC ACID, A SELECTIVE INHIBITOR AND

SUBSTRATE FOR THE NEURONAL GABA UPTAKE PROCESS

N.G. BOWERY and M.J. NEAL

Departments of Pharmacology, St. Thomas's Hospital
Medical School, London SE1 7EH & The School of Pharmacy
29/39 Brunswick Square, London WC1N 1AX, U.K.

GABA which is now generally believed to be an important
inhibitory synaptic transmitter substance in the vertebrate central
nervous system (see Krnjević 1974) is thought to be inactivated
after its release  from nerve terminals by uptake processes which
are present in some neurones and glia (see Iversen & Kelly, 1975).
These transport processes for GABA in neurones and glia have very
similar properties but can be distinguished by their structural
requirements (Bowery  et al, 1976).  We have found that a conformationally-restricted analogue of GABA, cis 3-aminocyclohexane carboxylic acid (ACHC), which has previously been reported to competitively
inhibit GABA transport in slices of cerebral cortex (Beart et al,
1972), is a relatively selective inhibitor of neuronal GABA transport
(Bowery et al, 1976).  Studies with radiolabelled ACHC ($^3$H-ACHC)
indicate that the analogue is a selective substrate for the neuronal
GABA transport process.

The selective inhibition of neuronal GABA transport processes
was revealed by studying the uptake of $^3$H-GABA by isolated slices of
rat cerebral cortex, frog retinae, rat retinae and rat  sympathetic
ganglia.  Autoradiographic studies with $^3$H-GABA have shown a predominantly neuronal uptake in cortical slices (Iversen & Bloom,1972)
and frog retinae (Voaden et al, 1974) and a glial uptake in rat
retinae (Neal & Iversen, 1972) and ganglia (Young et al, 1973).
The effects of ACHC and some other structural analogues of GABA
on $^3$H-GABA uptake by these tissues are summarised in Table 1.  The
uptake of $^3$H-GABA (0.1 μM) by cortical slices and frog retinae was
50% inhibited (IC$_{50}$) by ACHC at a concentration of 62 μM and 960 μM
respectively but uptake in rat retinae and sympathetic ganglia (and
rat spinal ganglia; another tissue in which GABA is taken up by
glia (Schon & Kelly, 1974)) was unaffected by ACHC at concentrations

351

TABLE I.  EFFECT OF ACHC AND OTHER ANALOGUES ON GABA UPTAKE

| Analogue | Concentration of analogue that inhibits uptake of $^3$H-GABA (0.1 $\mu$M) by 50% ($IC_{50}$ $\mu$M) | | | |
| | Neuronal uptake | | Glial uptake | |
| | Cortical slices | Frog retina | Rat retina | Sympathetic ganglia |
|---|---|---|---|---|
| β-alanine | NE (20,000) | NE | 390 | 59 |
| Nipecotic acid | 12 | 1000 | 640 | 200 |
| DABA | 66 | 180 | 58 | NE |
| 4-Aminotetrolic acid | 330 | | NE | NE |
| Cis 3-aminocyclo-hexane carboxylic acid (ACHC) | 62 | 960 | NE | NE |

Cerebral cortical slices (Iversen & Neal, 1968), retinae (Good-child & Neal 1973) and sympathetic ganglia (Bowery & Brown, 1972) were incubated for 10 min (30 min for ganglia) at 25°C in 0.1 $\mu$M $^3$H-GABA in the absence or presence of analogue. The inhibition of $^3$H-GABA uptake produced by 3 or 4 concentrations of each analogue was measured and used to obtain the $IC_{50}$ value. The value at each concentration of analogue was the mean of 3 - 6 results and the s.e.m.s. were less than 10%

up to 1 mM.

The properties of ACHC which confer this specificity are of interest. In aqueous solution ACHC is likely to exist as the zwitterionic form and from pK measurements it seems that the molecule exists predominantly in the diequatorial conformation (Hewgill & Jefferies 1955). In this conformation the compound represents a partially restricted, partially folded, analogue of GABA where the separation of zwitterionic centres (mean of the two N ....O distances) is approximately 5.6 Å (Bowery et al, 1976). In contrast β-alanine, in which the corresponding distance is approximately 3.8 Å (Jose & Pant 1965) is a relatively selective inhibitor of glial GABA transport (see Iversen & Kelly, 1975). This suggests that the selectivity of inhibitors of GABA uptake is probably related to the separation of their zwitterionic centres. The upper limit of this separation for interaction at glial uptake sites is apparently lower than that at neuronal uptake sites. This is supported by the fact that 4-aminotetrolic acid, where the zwitterionic centres

have a minimum separation of 5.46 Å was also found to be a selective
inhibitor of the neuronal GABA transport system (Table 1). In
contrast, nipecotic acid has a smaller separation of charged centres
(approximately 4.5 Å) and interacts with both neuronal and glial
transport sites for GABA (Table 1). L-2,4-diamino-n-butyric acid
(DABA) in which the charged centres are separated by approximately
4.93 Å (Jones 1976) showed greater selectivity than nipecotic acid
for neuronal GABA transport sites. However, DABA is almost as
potent in inhibiting GABA uptake in rat retina and cortical slices
(Table 1). This lack of selectivity is presumably due to the
greater flexibility of this molecule. A summary of the GABA transport processes mainly inhibited by GABA analogues together with
their structures is shown in Table 2.

Further evidence that ACHC interacts mainly with neuronal
GABA transport sites was obtained in studies with $^3$H ACHC. These
indicated that ACHC is a relatively selective substrate for the
system(s) mediating the transport of GABA into neurones. This was
ascertained by measuring the uptake of $^3$H ACHC in the tissues previously mentioned, i.e. cortical slices, frog retinae, rat retinae,
sympathetic ganglia and spinal ganglia.

Tritiated ACHC (specific activity 132 mCi/mmol) was obtained
from the Radiochemical Centre, Amersham, U.K. and purified by thin

TABLE II.  SUMMARY OF SELECTIVITY AND STRUCTURES OF GABA ANALOGUES

| ANALOGUE | STRUCTURE | Distance † between charged centres(Å) | GABA transport process inhibited |
|---|---|---|---|
| β-alanine | $H_3\overset{+}{N}$ ... C | 3·83 | Glial |
| Nipecotic acid (Chair conformation -equitorial) | $H_3\overset{+}{N}$ ... C | 4·49 | Neuronal + Glial |
| 2,4-DABA | $\overset{+}{N}H_3$ $H_3\overset{+}{N}$ ... C | 4·93 ∅ | Neuronal + (Glial) |
| 4,Aminotetrolic acid | $H_3\overset{+}{N}$—≡—C | 5·46 | Neuronal |
| cis-ACHC (diequitorial) | $H_3\overset{+}{N}$ ... C | 5·6 | Neuronal |
| GABA | $H_3\overset{+}{N}$ ... C | <1·5–6·2 | Neuronal + Glial |

†for references see Bowery et al (1976) except ∅ Jones (1976)

layer chromatography (Neal & Bowery 1977). The uptake of $^3$H-ACHC determined by incubation of the tissues in 0.1 μM $^3$H-ACHC was most rapid in cortical slices incubated at 37°C. The tissue:medium ratio at 30 min was 11.5. At 25°C the ratio was 6.4. In frog retinae at 25°C the ratio after 30 min. incubation was 2.4 whereas in rat sympathetic and spinal ganglia it was only 0.7 even after 60 min. incubation. The value of 0.7 indicates accumulation only in the extracellular water. The rat retina, in which GABA uptake is predominantly glial, was found to accumulate about the same amount of $^3$H-ACHC when incubated at 37°C as the frog retina at 25°C. This is not consistent with ACHC having affinity only for the neuronal GABA transport system but it is possible that the amacrine cells of the inner nuclear layer of this tissue accumulate GABA (& ACHC) to a small extent. $^3$H-GABA uptake into the Mueller glial cells might normally mask this component. However, we have no autoradiographical evidence to substantiate this possibility, only in the frog retina do we have evidence of the localization of $^3$H ACHC. In this tissue accumulated $^3$H-ACHC is confined to the horizontal cells which take up GABA (Voaden et al 1974). The low specific activity of the $^3$H-ACHC has so far prevented us obtaining unequivocal evidence for the location in the other tissues.

We have studied the characteristics of $^3$H-ACHC uptake in cortical slices in some detail. The uptake was temperature sensitive and required the presence of sodium in the external medium. Total replacement of sodium by lithium or sucrose abolished uptake. Ouabain (10 μM), sodium cyanide (1 mM) and parachloromercuribenzene sulphonic acid (10 μM)inhibited the uptake of $^3$H-ACHC (10 min at 37°C). The uptake values expressed as per cent of control ± s.e.m.s. were 38.6 ± 1.75, 25.4 ± 1.91 and 36.6 ± 1.42 respectively (4 determinations in each case).

$^3$H-ACHC uptake followed simple Michaelis-Menten kinetics. Graphical and computer analysis of uptake data obtained at ACHC concentrations between 5 μM and 1 mM indicated that a single transport process was involved with an apparent Km of 85.1 ± 6.22 μM and Vmax of 80.2 ± 3.66 n mol/min/g.

The uptake of 0.1 μM $^3$H-ACHC by cortical slices was specific and was not inhibited by 5 mM glycine, L-glutamate, 2-amino-n-butyric acid, ornithine or taurine (Fig.1). L-Proline, L-histidine and β-alanine at 5 mM significantly inhibited the uptake of $^3$H-ACHC although 1 mM β-alanine was without effect. In contrast GABA & DABA strongly inhibited the uptake of $^3$H-ACHC. We could find no evidence of any metabolism of accumulated $^3$H-ACHC in cortical slices during 30 min incubation at 37°C (Neal & Bowery 1977) and 10 mM ACHC does not inhibit rabbit brain GABA-**T** (L.J. Fowler - personal communication). These results are in agreement with an earlier report that ACHC is not a substrate for

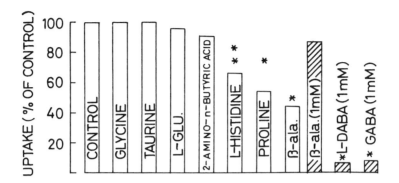

Fig. 1:  The effect of amino acids on the uptake of $^3$H-ACHC by
cortical slices.  Amino acids were tested at 1 mM or 5 mM against
the uptake of $^3$H-ACHC (0.1 μM) during 10 min. at 37°C after preincubation of the slices with the amino acid for 10 min at 37°C.
The results are the means of 4-8 determinations.  The s.e.m.s.
were less than 5%.

* p < 0.001
** p < 0.002

mitochondrial GABA-T (Beart & Johnston, 1973).

    In further experiments cortical slices and frog retinae were
incubated in 0.1 μM $^3$H-ACHC for 30 min. and then superfused with
radioactive-free medium at 0.5 ml/min.  Tritium was released into
the medium at a rate (k $\approx$ 0.001 min$^{-1}$) marginally greater than
for $^3$H-GABA (in the presence of 100 μM amino-oxyacetic acid, k
0.0007 min$^{-1}$) when compared in parallel experiments.  The addition
of potassium chloride (final K$^+$ concentration = 25 mM) to the
external medium accelerated the efflux rate of $^3$H-ACHC and $^3$H-GABA
similarly.  This increase in efflux was abolished in both cases
in the absence of Ca$^{++}$ and presence of 20 mm Mg$^{++}$ but was restored
on replacing calcium.

    It is still premature to suggest that ACHC may be a useful tool
for gaining information about neuronal as distinct from glial systems
involving GABA however, evidence obtained so far would support this
idea.

REFERENCES

Beart, P.M. and Johnston, G.A.R. 1973.  Transamination of analogues
    of γ-aminobutyric acid by extracts of rat brain mitochondria.
    Brain Res. 49, 459 - 462.

Beart, P.M., Johnston, G.A.R. and Uhr, M.L. 1972. Competitive inhi-
    bition of GABA uptake in rat brain slices by some GABA analogues of
    restricted conformation.  J. Neurochem. 19, 1855-1861.

Bowery, N.G. and Brown,D.A. 1972.  γ-aminobutyric acid uptake by
    sympathetic ganglia.  Nature, New Biol. 238, 89-91.

Bowery, N.G., Jones, G.P. and Neal, M.J. 1976. Selective inhibition
    of neuronal GABA uptake by cis-1,3-aminocyclohexane carboxylic
    acid, Nature (Lond), 264, 281 - 284.

Goodchild, M. and Neal, M.J. 1973. The uptake of $(^3H)$-γ-aminobutyric
    acid by the retina  Br.J.Pharmac. 47, 529-542.

Hewgill, F.R. and Jefferies, P.R. 1955.  The epimeric (±)-3-amino-
    cyclohexane carboxylic acids. J.chem.Soc.   2767-2772.

Iversen, L.L. and Bloom, F.E. 1972. Studies of the uptake of $(^3H)$
    GABA and $(^3H)$ glycine in slices and homogenates of rat brain
    and spinal cord by electron microscopic autoradiography.
    Brain Res. 41, 131-143.

Iversen, L.L. and Kelly, J.S. 1975. Uptake and metabolism of γ-amino
    butyric acid by neurons and glial cells, Biochem.Pharmac. 24
    933 - 938.

Jones, G.P. 1976.  Ph.D. Thesis.  University of London.

Jose, P. & Pant, L.M. 1965.  The crystal and molecular structure of
    β-alanine.  Acta Crystallogr. 18, 806 - 810.

Krnjevic, K. 1974. Chemical nature of synaptic transmission in verte-
    brates.  Physiol.Rev. 54, 418 - 540.

Neal, M.J. and Bowery, N.G. 1977.  Cis 3-aminocyclohexane carboxylic
    acid:a substrate for the neuronal GABA transport system,
    Brain Res. (in press).

Neal, M.J. and Iversen, L.L. 1968.  The uptake of $^3H$-GABA by slices
    of rat cerebral cortex.  J.Neurochem. 15, 1141 - 1149.

Neal, M.J. and Iversen, L.L. 1972.  Autoradiographic localization
    of$(^3H)$ GABA in rat retina.  Nature new Biol. 235, 217 - 218.

Schon, F. and Kelly, J.S. 1974.  Autoradiographic localization of
    $^3H$ GABA and $^3H$-glutamate over satellite glial cells. Brain
    Res. 66, 275 - 288.

Voaden, M.J., Marshall, J. and Murani, N. 1974.  The uptake of $(^3H)$
    GABA and $(^3H)$ glycine by the isolated retina of the frog.
    Brain Res. 67, 115 -132.

Young, J.A.C., Brown, D.A., Kelly, J.S. and Schon, F. 1973.  Auto-
    radiographical localization of sites of $(^3H)$-γ-aminobutyric
    acid accumulation in peripheral autonomic ganglia.  Brain Res.
    63, 479 - 486.

# PROPERTIES OF THE ACCUMULATION OF D-[$^{14}$C]ASPARTATE INTO

# RAT CEREBRAL CRUDE SYNAPTOSOMAL FRACTION

G. Takagaki

Department of Neurochemistry, Tokyo Metropolitan

Institute for Neurosciences, Fuchu-shi, Tokyo, Japan

For the cerebral accumulation of L-glutamate and L-aspartate, the existence of two processes of uptake possessing high and low affinities has been generally postulated. This is mainly based on the presence of a break in the Lineweaver-Burk plots using radio-labelled substrates. The accumulation of labelled D-glutamate was recently shown to occur only by a 'low affinity' system into rat cerebral P$_2$ fraction(Km=0.80 mM)(Takagaki, 1976) as well as into cerebral slices(Benjamin and Quastel, 1976). Davies and Johnston (1976) demonstrated that D-aspartate is accumulated in rat cereb-ral slices by a 'high affinity' uptake. The uptake of D-[$^{14}$C]-aspartate into rat cerebral P$_2$ fraction also proceeds by a 'high affinity' system, having an apparent Km of 15.1 $\mu$M(Fig. 1). The maximal velocity of D-aspartate uptake is higher than that of the 'high affinity' component of L-aspartate uptake and almost equal to that of L-glutamate under the same incubation conditions. In the P$_2$ fraction, any rapid metabolism of D-glutamate and D-aspartate is not observed in contrast to their L-isomer(Takagaki, 1976; 1977). In this connection, the D-isomers can be used to analyze the trans-port in the absence of metabolism.

## UPTAKE OF D-[$^{14}$C]ASPARTATE

The following observations were made on the uptake of D-[$^{14}$C]-aspartate into rat cerebral P$_2$ fraction. (1) The requirement of sodium is almost absolute and obligatory. (2) The affinity of the carrier for the substrate is increased by increasing sodium concent-ration in the medium, but the maximal velocity is not altered (Fig. 1). (3) Omission of potassium from the medium also inhibits the uptake competitively. (4) Whereas thallium, rubidium and ammo-

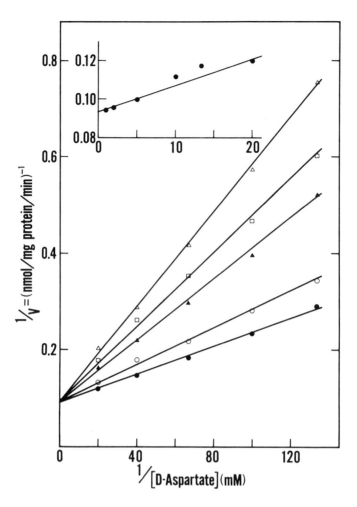

FIGURE 1. Double reciprocal plots of the uptake of D-[$^{14}$C]-
aspartate into rat cerebral P$_2$ fraction. The rat cerebral P$_2$
fraction was incubated in air at 37 °C in the standard medium containing glucose(5 mM) at a protein concentration of approximately
1 mg/ml medium. After a 10 min-preincubation, D-[$^{14}$C]aspartate
(10 µM) was added. The uptake was measured using the conventional
Millipore techniques after 1 min-incubation, and expressed as nmol
of aspartate per mg protein of the P$_2$ fraction. The sodium concentration in medium was changed by replacing sodium chloride with
equimolar choline chloride. When the effect of ouabain was examined, it was added to the medium at the beginning of the preincubation. The points are means of 6-8 independent experiments.
Key: ●, control medium, Na$^+$, 137.8 mM; ○, Na$^+$, 84.2 mM;
     □, Na$^+$, 31.0 mM; ▲, 5 x 10$^{-5}$M ouabain; △, 5 x 10$^{-4}$M ouabain

nium are the efficient substitutes for potassium in exhibiting Na-
K-ATPase activity of the P$_2$ fraction, the uptake is activated only
by rubidium in the absence of potassium. (5) Ouabain is a competitive inhibitor on the uptake(Fig. 1). (6) The uptake is strongly
inhibited by L-cysteate and L-cysteine sulfinate, but not by L-
homocysteate and D-cysteate. These observations were in common with
the uptake of L-aspartate as well as of L- and D-glutamate. With
the exception of the absolute requirement of sodium, these properties were not observed on the uptake of GABA into the P$_2$ fraction.
The uptake of L-glutamate was competitively inhibited by D-aspartate.
This was observed at low substrate concentrations('high affinity'
process) as well as at high concentrations('low affinity' process).
The uptake of D-glutamate, which is transported by a single 'low
affinity' system, was also inhibited competitively by D-aspartate.
These observations are consistent with the possibility that a common
transport carrier is involved for both the high and low affinity
uptake processes of these amino acids.

It was previously shown that the rate of uptake of L-glutamate
into the P$_2$ fraction is less markedly inhibited by ouabain than that
of D-glutamate(Takagaki, 1976). This is in accord with the present
results that ouabain inhibits the uptake of either L- or D-glutamate
in a competitive manner and that a common carrier site is involved,
the Km of which for L-glutamate is very low by comparison to that
for the D-isomer.

EXCHANGE WITH GLUTAMATE

It is often stated that only putative neurotransmitters possess
a sodium-dependent 'high affinity' uptake system, and that the presence of such an uptake system represents one of the criteria for
considering a given compound a neurotransmitter candidate. The high
affinity uptake is postulated to be important in regulating the
extracellular level of transmitters and terminating their synaptic
activity. In the experimental conditions of the uptake studies
the observed accumulation of radioactivity may not be due to an
actual net accumulation, but simply due to an exchange process
(Levi and Raiteri, 1976). The amounts of glutamate and aspartate
in the P$_2$ fraction as well as in the medium were determined using
the double isotope dansylation method(Joseph and Halliday, 1975),
after incubating the P$_2$ fraction with D-aspartate(10 $\mu$M)(Table 1).
The amount of aspartate increased in the P$_2$ fraction, and decreased
in the medium. At the same time, the amount of glutamate decreased
in the P$_2$ fraction, and increased in the medium. Mechanisms of this
apparent exchange of aspartate with glutamate should be further
studies in relation to their possible role as neurotransmitters.
By the addition of 50 mM-KCl, both aspartate and glutamate were
released from the P$_2$ fraction(Table 1).

TABLE 1. AMOUNTS OF ASPARTATE AND GLUTAMATE IN RAT CEREBRAL $P_2$ FRACTION AND MEDIUM AFTER THE INCUBATION WITH D-ASPARTATE (10 µM)

| Incubation | Medium | | $P_2$ fraction | |
|---|---|---|---|---|
| | Aspartate | Glutamate | Aspartate | Glutamate |
| | (nmol/ml) | | (nmol/mg protein) | |
| Without addition | | | | |
| 0 min | $5.88 \pm 1.88$ | $11.55 \pm 2.57$ | $23.68 \pm 2.50$ | $48.86 \pm 3.20$ |
| 5 min | $6.89 \pm 1.92$ | $12.94 \pm 2.88$ | $24.30 \pm 2.48$ | $47.87 \pm 4.07$ |
| 10 min | $6.83 \pm 1.07$ | $12.21 \pm 0.96$ | $23.97 \pm 1.80$ | $44.69 \pm 3.56$ |
| 20 min | $7.91 \pm 1.22$ | $11.99 \pm 1.62$ | $23.84 \pm 1.43$ | $39.72 \pm 2.05$ |
| With 10 µM-D-aspartate | | | | |
| 1.5 min | $12.08 \pm 2.69$ | $15.23 \pm 2.43$ | $27.14 \pm 1.60$ | $44.92 \pm 3.67$ |
| 5 min | $10.77 \pm 1.70$ | $15.31 \pm 2.12$ | $28.91 \pm 2.22$ | $42.77 \pm 4.28$ |
| 10 min | $8.60 \pm 1.07$ | $11.62 \pm 1.46$ | $31.88 \pm 1.71$ | $45.69 \pm 2.37$ |
| 20 min | $10.76 \pm 1.69$ | $13.81 \pm 2.37$ | $29.04 \pm 3.06$ | $41.70 \pm 2.81$ |
| With 10 µM-D-aspartate for 7.5 min, then 50 mM-KCl added, and incubation continued further for 12.5 min. | $33.60 \pm 2.62$ | $38.60 \pm 2.82$ | $9.76 \pm 1.21$ | $13.66 \pm 1.37$ |

The rat cerebral $P_2$ fraction was incubated as described in Fig. 1 at a protein concentration of as exactly as possible 1.0 mg/ml medium. At the end of the incubation under conditions indicated, 1 ml-aliquot of the incubating suspension was passed through a single 0.65 µm Millipore filter and the filter was washed with 0.9 %-NaCl. The combined filtrate and washings was used for measuring aspartate and glutamate in the medium. The whole Millipore filter was extracted with 5 %-TCA for 48 hrs at 0 °C. The TCA extract was used for measuring aspartate and glutamate in the $P_2$ fraction. By ion-exchange resin column-chromatography (Dowex AG-1), a fraction containing both aspartate and glutamate was obtained from the combined filtrate and washings as well as from the TCA extract of the Millipore filter. The amounts of aspartate and glutamate in the fraction from the column were measured using the double isotope dansylation method and polyamide TLC. Means ± S.D. of 6-8 independent experiments are given.

REFERENCES

Benjamin, A.M. and Quastel, J.H., 1976, Cerebral uptakes and exchange
    diffusion in vitro of L- and D-glutamates, J.Neurochem. 26: 431-
    441.
Davies, L.P. and Johnston, G.A.R., 1976, Uptake and release of D- and
    L-aspartate by rat brain slices, J.Neurochem. 26: 1007-1014.
Joseph, M.H. and Halliday, J., 1975, A dansylation microassay for
    some amino acids in brain, Analyt.Biochem. 64: 389-402.
Levi, G. and Raiteri, M., 1976, Synaptosomal transport processes,
    Int.Rev.Neurobiol. 19: 51-74.
Takagaki, G., 1976, Properties of the uptake and release of glutamic
    acid by synaptosomes from rat cerebral cortex, J.Neurochem. 27:
    1417-1425.
Takagaki, G., 1977, Sodium and potassium ions and accumulation of
    labeled D-aspartate and GABA in crude synaptosomal fraction
    from rat cerebral cortex, J.Neurochem.(accepted for publication)

# THE EFFECT OF GLUTAMATE ON THE STRUCTURE AND $K^+$-TRANSPORT OF SYNAPTOSOMES

Ferenc Hajós and András Csillag

1st Department of Anatomy, Semmelweis

University Medical School, 1450 Budapest

In earlier studies (Hajós and Csillag, 1976) it has been demonstrated that the $K^+$-loss of synaptosomes was accompanied by an increased electron-density of the presynaptic ground cytoplasm with evenly distributed synaptic vesicles and occasionally by the swelling of intrasynaptosomal mitochondria. This morphology was found consistently after incubation in iso-osmolar sucrose or in saline media where conditions favoured $K^+$-outflow from synaptosomes (ouabain, tetracain, lithium, valinomycin, gramicidin, oligomycin, rotenone, cooling). If synaptosomes were incubated in the saline medium with no inhibitors, at room temperature, an active uptake of $K^+$ took place with a concomitant morphological change as a result of which synaptosomes resembled the well preserved in situ nerve endings, i.e. they had a light ground cytoplasm synaptic vesicles, accumulated against the presynaptic membrane, and condensed mitochondria. In this work the effect of glutamate known to interfere with the ion-movements (Goddard and Robinson, 1976; McIlwain et al., 1969; Pull et al., 1970; Tan et al., 1977), and morphology (Abraham et al., 1971; Van Harreveld and Fifkova, 1971), of the brain tissue was studied in synaptomomal fractions incubated in saline media.

Synaptosomal fractions of 80 - 90% purity were prepared and processed for electron microscopy as described earlier (Hajós, 1975). Samples of 8 - 12 mg protein were added to 7.5 ml of the medium containing 64 mM NaCl, 1 or 4 mM KCl, 0.8 mM $MgCl$ , 8 mM Tris-HCl buffer (pH 7.4), 1.25 mM pyruvate, 0.75 mM malate, 0.5 mM phosphate, 0.2 mM EGTA and 160 mM sucrose. $K^+$-movements were monitored with an OP-K-7113-D type potassium-selective valinomycin membrane electrode (Radelkis, Budapest). Glutamate was added in 10

or 20 mM concentrations.  For electron microscopy synaptosomes were
fixed by the addition of a formaldehyde-glutaraldehyde mixture
(Karnovsky, 1964) at the beginning or after a 10 min. period of the
incubation with and without glutamate.  In the latter cases $K^+$-
movements were followed prior to fixation.

As shown in Figure 1. there was a 30 - 40% decrease in $K^+$-uptake
after the administration of glutamate.  Control synaptosomes showed
at the peak of their $K^+$ accumulation the "light" configuration
characteristic of intact, well-preserved nerve endings (Figure 2.).
Fractions incubated with glutamate and showing a reduced $K^+$-uptake
contained 25 - 30% "dark" synaptosomes (Figure 3.).

Our findings suggest that glutamate interferes with the $K^+$-
uptake of synaptosomes.  This is in agreement with data concerning
the effect of glutamate on the ionic composition of brain tissue
(McIlwain et al., 1969; Pull et al., 1970).  Reports concur in
observing $Na^+$-uptake into and $K^+$-release from the intracellular
compartment.  As on the basis of earlier results (Hajós and Csillag,
1976) the "dark" synaptosomal configuration is thought to be the

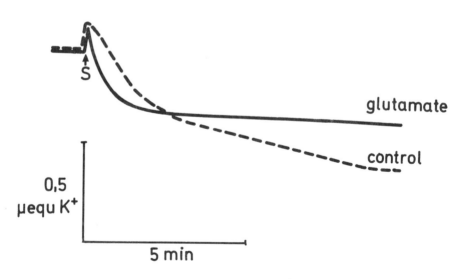

Fig. 1.  The effect of glutamate on the $K^+$ uptake of synaptosomes.

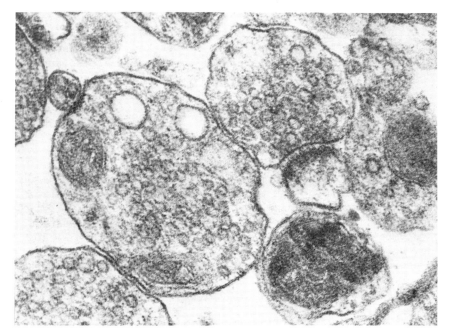

Fig. 2.  Electron micrograph of synaptosomes after accumulation
of K$^+$ ions.

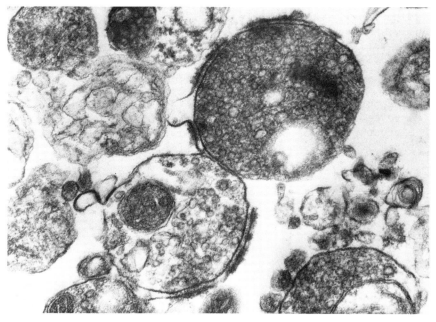

Fig. 3.  Electron micrograph of synaptosomes after incubation with
glutamate.

morphological correlate of $K^+$-outflow the present EM findings indicate that a sub-population of 25 - 30% of the total fraction can be held responsible for the decrease of net $K^+$-uptake. It is assumed that this sub-population reacts to glutamate with $K^+$-release and is regarded to be selectively depolarized. Owing to the condensation of the affected synaptosomes their separation seems to be feasible.

## REFERENCES

Abraham, R., Dougherty, W., Goldberg, L. and Coulston, F., 1971, The response of the hypothalamus to high doses of monosodium glutamate in mice and monkeys. Cytochemistry and ultrastructural study of lysosomal change, Exp. Mol. Pathol., 15:43-60.

Goddard, G.A. and Robinson, J.D., 1976, Uptake and release of calcium by rat brain synaptosomes, Brain Res., 110:331-350.

Hajós, F., 1975, An improved method for the preparation of synaptosomal fractions in high purity, Brain Res., 93:485-489.

Hajós, F., and Csillag, A., 1976, Structural changes in vitro of isolated nerve endings. I. Effect of cations, Brain Res., 112:207-213.

Karnovsky, M.J., 1964, A formaldehyde-glutaraldehyde fixative of high osmolarity in electron microscopy, J. Cell Biol., 27:137A.

McIlwain, H., Harvey, J.A., and Rodriguez, G., 1969, Tetrodotoxin on the sodium and other ions of cerebral tissues, excited electrically and with glutamate, J. Neurochem., 16:363-370.

Pull, I., McIlwain, H., and Ramsey, R.L., 1970, Glutamate, calcium ion-chelating agents and the sodium and potassium ion contents from the brain, Biochem. J., 116:181-187.

Tan, A.T., Trang, D., Renand, L.P., and Martin, J.B., 1977, Effect of somatostatin on calcium transport in guinea pig cortex synaptosomes, Brain Res., 123:193-196.

Van Harreveld, A., and Fifkova, E., 1971, Light and electron-microscopic changes in central nervous tissue after electrophoretic injection of glutamate, Exp. Mol. Pathol., 15:61-81.

ON THE METABOLIC AND INTRASYNAPTIC ORIGIN OF AMINO ACID

TRANSMITTERS

H.F. Bradford, J.S. de Belleroche and H.K. Ward

Department of Biochemistry

Imperial College, London S.W.7.

## GLUTAMINE AS PRECURSOR OF TRANSMITTER AMINO ACIDS

We have previously shown that /U$^{14}$C/-glutamine when presented as substrate to incubated mammalian synaptosome preparations labels the glutamate pool to about 50% of the specific radioactivity of the added glutamine over a 60 min. period (Table 1). The concentration of glutamine employed was that found in mammalian CSF, namely 0.5mM, and glucose was also present at CSF levels (5mM) in all experiments. Aspartate at 40% and GABA at 20% showed lower but still substantial carbon contributions from glutamine.

In view of the large contribution to transmitter amino acids which appears to be made by glutamine, as well as from glucose, it became of interest to examine whether the pools generated from these two substrates were contained in a single compartment, or whether some distinction existed between them. For instance, one might serve the purposes of energy metabolism and the other provide amino acids for synaptic release.

To pursue this idea, we incubated 'beds' of synaptosomes with /U$^{14}$C/-glucose (2.5mM) and /$^{3}$H/-glutamine, and after rinsing, transferred to fresh medium containing the depolarizing alkaloid veratrine (75µM) which released transmitter amino acids (Fig. 1). Separation and analysis of these amino acids produced specific radioactivity values which implied that released glutamate in particular was 67% derived from glutamine rather than glucose (Fig. 2a). Similar experiments employing /U$^{14}$C/-label in both glucose and glutamine but with separate tissue samples in the same experiment, allowed an equivalent analysis to be made. Specific radioactivities from these single-label experiments (Fig. 2b) showed a similar pattern of results, with released glutamate being

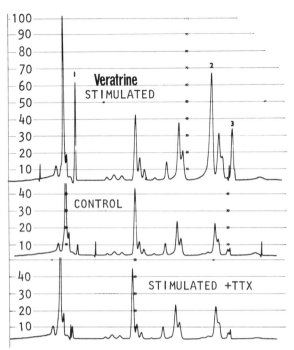

Fig. 1.   Chromatograms showing veratrine stimulation of amino acid
release from cortical synaptosomes.   Veratrine at 75μM was added
for 30 min after a 30 min preincubation period.   Tetrodotoxin at
1μM was included in the incubation fluid as shown.   1, GABA;
2, glutamate;   3, aspartate.   The glutamate peak represents 560
pmol.   (from Y.S. Luqmani;   Ph.D. Thesis, University of London).

TABLE I   INCORPORATION OF /U-$^{14}$C/ GLUTAMINE INTO AMINO ACIDS OF
               SYNAPTOSOMES

|  | Specific radioactivities of amino acids (μCi/μmol) | | |
|  | 0 min | 30 min | 60 min |
| --- | --- | --- | --- |
| Glutamine 0.50mM (0.32μCi/ml) |  |  |  |
| Aspartate | 0 | 0.140$^+$0.020(4) | 0.251$^+$0.018(4) |
| Glutamate | 0 | 0.274$\pm$0.009(4) | 0.301$\pm$0.035(4) |
| GABA | 0 | 0.087$\pm$0.006(4) | 0.131$\pm$0.016(4) |
| Glutamine 8.30mM (1.22μCi/ml) |  |  |  |
| Aspartate | 0 | 0.52(2) | 0.85(2) |
| Glutamate | 0 | 0.66(2) | 0.94(2) |
| GABA | 0 | 0.32(2) | 0.45(2) |

Legend to Table I
Synaptosome beds were incubated at 37°C in Krebs-bicarbonate
medium, containing glucose at 10mM and glutamine at 0.50mM and
8.30mM, with specific radioactivities of 0.622μCi/μmole and
0.122μCi/μmole, respectively. Values are mean ± S.E.M. for the
number of samples in parentheses. (from Bradford & Ward, 1976).

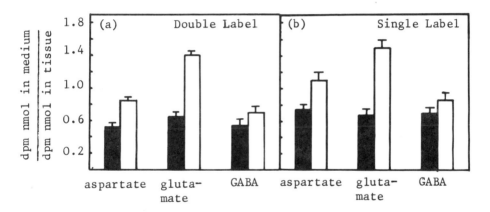

Fig. 2.    Ratios of specific radioactivities of aspartate,
glutamate and GABA in synaptosome tissue and incubation medium
after exposure to Veratrine 75μM for 10 min.   Synaptosome beds
were incubated for 45 min. in Krebs-NaHCO$_3$ containing glucose
(2.5mM) and glutamine (0.5mM).   (a) $^3$H-glutamine (white histobar),
/U$^{14}$C/-glucose (black histobar) added to same vessel, or (b)
/U$^{14}$C/-glutamine (white), /U$^{14}$C/-glucose (black) to separate
vessels.   After rinsing, beds were transferred to fresh medium
containing veratrine. Absolute specific activities in tissue:
glucose and glutamine 5000 dpm/nmol (a) $^3$H-glutamate, 1900; $^{14}$C-
glutamate, 750.   (b) $^{14}$C-glutamate (glutamine) 1400; $^{14}$C-glutamate
(glucose) 600.   Values are mean ± SD. for at least 6 values for
each histobar.

derived 80%    more from glutamine than glucose.    These results
also confirm that a high contribution is made by glutamine to the
tissue glutamate, aspartate and GABA in spite of its low concentration relative to glucose (one fifth) in the medium.

The respiratory rates, $K^+$ levels, and therefore glucose utilisation by synaptosomes are maximal at 1mM glucose (Fig. 3) thus
validating the use of 2.5mM glucose in the medium rather than the
5.0mM levels commonly found in CSF and plasma (Bradford et al,
1977).    These lower glucose concentrations were employed in the
experiments reported here to establish the optimal ratio between
$^3H$ and $^{14}C$ whilst using the smallest amounts of these isotopes
which were consistent with this ratio.    Also, since glucose utilisation was maximal at 1.0mM, this concentration should be taken
as the effective glucose level in making comparison with glutamine
uptake and metabolism, any extra glucose (e.g. 2.5mM) being present
simply as excess.

The data of Fig. 2 may be compared with that of Table 1 and
can be seen to confirm our earlier finding that glutamine makes
at least a 50% contribution to the carbon skeletons of glutamate
and GABA.    For aspartate the picture remains less clear since
using $^3H$-glutamine or $^{14}C$-glutamine as precursor gave different
answers in terms of specific radioactivity, $^{14}C$-labelling indicating glutamine to be the main source and $^3H$-glutamine showing
glucose as main precursor.    However, in terms of the proportion
of the total isotope present (i.e. tissue plus medium) which is
released to the medium, $H^3$ labelled glutamate and aspartate both
showed twice the release of their $^{14}C$-labelled counterparts
(Bradford et al, 1977 and Fig. 2).

Only low levels of amino acids and therefore of radioactivity
were recovered in the medium from unstimulated synaptosomes.    It
was not therefore possible to measure accurately the specific
radioactivities of transmitter amino acids present in the medium
before the efflux due to stimulation.

Glutaminase activity of synaptosomes.    The enzyme which allows the
use of glutamine as a substrate is glutaminase I.    It is phosphate
stimulated and found enriched in the mitochondrial (65%) and synaptosome (35%) fractions from brain (Salganicoff & de Robertis, 1965;
Bradford & Ward, 1976).    As it is a mitochondrial enzyme it is
located in nerve-ending mitochondria together with the enzyme
systems (i.e. citric acid cycle, transaminases) which produce
glutamate and aspartate from glucose.    The maximal activity of
glutaminase is high (16mM substrate conc.) and the rates measured
for incubated synaptosomes with glutamine at its CSF level (0.5mM)
was only about 8% of the maximal value without added phosphate
(Table 2).

TABLE II    GLUTAMINASE ACTIVITY IN SYNAPTOSOMES AND CEREBRAL
            HOMOGENATES

| | μmol glutamine hydrolysed/100mg protein/h | |
| --- | --- | --- |
| | No addition | Phosphate added |
| Autoanalysis | | |
| Homogenate | 58±4 (5) | 233±14 (5) |
| Synaptosomes | 102±4 (12) | 439±32 (9) |
| Incubated synaptosomes | | |
| 0.10mM glutamine | 1.48        (3) | |
| 0.50mM glutamine | 8.24±0.36 (6) | |
| 8.30mM glutamine | 42.6        (2) | |

Synaptosomes were either analysed for glutaminase activity by
ammonia release using Nessler's reagent, 16.6mM glutamine, 0.05M
potassium borate buffer in an autoanalytical system or by following the depletion of glutamine from the incubation medium of
synaptosome beds over 60 min periods of incubation at 37°C.
Krebs-bicarbonate incubation medium containing 1.2mM phosphate
and 10mM glucose.    Rates were linear over 60 min.    Values are
mean ± S.E.M. for number of samples shown in parentheses.
(from Bradford & Ward, 1976).

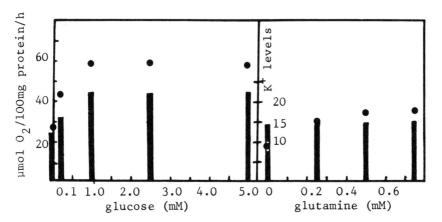

Fig. 3. Respiratory rates (black spots)and potassium content(black
histobars) of synaptosome suspensions. Cortical synaptosomes were
incubated for 60 min in Krebs-NaHCO$_3$ containing substrates as shown
(a) glucose (b) glutamine. Potassium levels in the tissue were
estimated by flame-photometry. The central y-axis gives K$^+$/100mg
protein. Data gives mean for four closely grouped values.

DIFFERENTIAL LABELLING OF INTRASYNAPTIC COMPARTMENTS

In a different series of experiments attempts were made to cause differential labelling of sub-synaptic compartments by intra-ventricular injection of /U$^{14}$C/-glucose followed by subsequent in vitro incubation of the synaptosomes from the injected brain with the same isotope. Preliminary experiments with /$^3$H/-acetate showed that in contrast to $^{14}$C-glucose, intraventricular injection did not adequately label transmitter amino acids of synaptosomes and subsequent in vitro incubation of synaptosomes with $^{14}$C-acetate also produced few counts in vesicles. For this reason /$^{14}$C/-glucose was selected as the substrate for the labelling experiments.

Depolarizing agents and transmitter release. The procedure was to prepare cerebral cortical synaptosomes from brain injected with /U$^{14}$C/-glucose and to incubated these in Krebs-bicarbonate medium containing 10mM glucose and /U$^{14}$C/-glucose at 1μC/μmol. Potassium stimulation was applied as a 50mM increase in K$^+$ concentration after 10 min. for a period of 10 min. Veratrine (75μM) was similarly applied. The synaptosome suspensions were sedimented at the end of incubation and hypo-osmotically ruptured to prepare sub-fractions essentially as described by Marchbanks (1968) and Whittaker and Sheridan (1965). Control experiments showed only a small diffusion of labelled amino acids from the soluble to other fractions deeper in the gradient during centrifugation in the absence of tissue. Morphological characterisation of the synaptic vesicle fraction showed that it consisted almost entirely of 50nm profiles with occasional extended membrane fragments (de Belleroche & Bradford, 1973).

The specific radioactivity data of Fig. 4 show that amino acid transmitters released by K$^+$ were equivalent (nCi/nmol) to those recovered in the cytoplasmic fraction. In contrast, the aspartate and GABA of the vesicle and membrane fractions were significantly different from that released. With veratrine as the stimulating agent (Fig. 5) the specific radioactivities of glutamate and GABA recovered in vesicles were significantly lower than the equivalent values for the released amino acids. As with K$^+$-stimulation, cytoplasmic glutamate and GABA were the closest to the released amino acids in specific radioactivity.

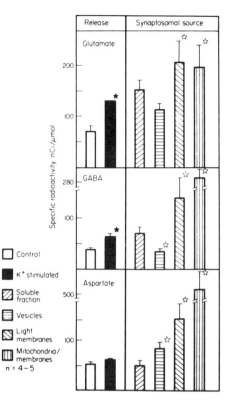

Fig. 4. The effect of potassium stimulation on the specific radioactivities of amino acids released from the synaptosome subfractions. Specific radioactivities (nCi/μmol) of amino acids released to the incubation medium (release) were measured in control and K⁺ stimulated conditions. Amino acid pool sizes (μmol) and radioactivity (nCi) in the synaptosome subfractions were measured after incubation under control or stimulated conditions and the specific radioactivities of the amino acid released by stimulation were determined (synaptosomal source) from the difference in pool size and radioactivity between control and stimulated paired samples. The values are means with the S.E.Ms shown by bars. The black asterisk indicates that the specific radioactivity of amino acid released by K⁺ stimulation was significantly greater than the control released amino acid P < 0.01. The unfilled asterisk indicates that the value is significantly different from that of the amino acid released to the medium by stimulation, P < 0.01. (from de Belleroche & Bradford, 1977).

Depolarizing agents and pool turnover. The cytoplasmic pool sizes of glutamate, GABA and aspartate showed substantial decreases following potassium or veratrine stimulation (Figs. 6 and 7). For K⁺-stimulation, the decrease in the transmitters of cytoplasmic pool was equivalent to 30-50% (80% for GABA) of the extra amount recovered in the incubation fluid, and for veratrine-stimulation, the losses from the cytoplasmic pool was almost twice the amounts released to the medium. Any decreases in the transmitter pools of vesicles, mitochondria or membranes were very small ( 5%) in comparison to those of the cytoplasm. The apparently much smaller fall in the cytoplasmic pool induced by K⁺ stimulation is probably due to the increased synthesis of transmitter amino acids induced by this agent causing partial replacement of the released pool. Certainly, the much higher specific radioactivities of the synaptosomal subfractions after exposure to high K⁺ (Fig. 4, cf. Fig.5) support this proposition, and $K^+$ is known to stimulate respiration through its effect on pyruvate kinase (McIlwain & Bachelard 1971).

Measurement of the rates of synthesis of the transmitter amino acids from /U$^{14}$C/-glucose by whole synaptosomes, and their turnover in synaptic vesicles showed the latter to be only fractions of a percent of the transmitter release occurring during 10min ( 3-15nmol /mg. whole synaptosome protein, see Figs. 6 & 7). The proportion of synaptosome protein recovered as vesicles was 4%. These calculations indicate that insufficient transmitter would be available in vesicles to allow the possibility that the vesicles take up transmitter from the cytoplasm and empty it into the synaptic cleft perhaps many times during the period of stimulation. Even if one sets the likely proportion of intact nerve-ending protein present in the vesicles at a maximum of 30% then the vesicle fraction prepared by us would still provide only a fraction of the total transmitter released. However, this hypothesis also predicts that the specific radioactivities of the cytoplasmic and vesicular pools should be identical since they would stand in a precursor-product relationship. However, Figs. 5 & 6 show that these are, in fact, mostly very different.

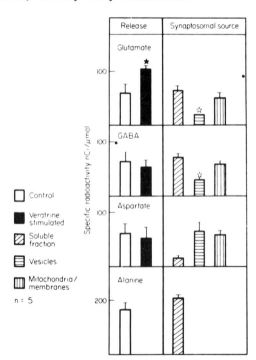

Fig. 5. The effect of veratrine stimulation on the specific radio-activities of amino acids released from the synaptosome subfractions. (From de Belleroche and Bradford, 1977).

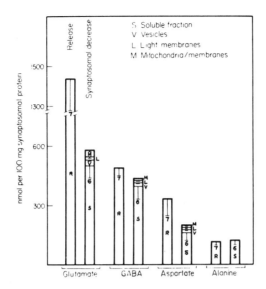

Fig. 6. The effect of potassium stimulation on amino acid release
and loss from the synaptosome subfractions. The release of amino
acid induced by K$^+$ (56mM) stimulation is shown as a histogram (r)
with the decrease in pool size of amino acid in the synaptosome subfractions (S,V,L and M) by the side. The decrease in pool size was
obtained by subtracting the value of the stimulated amino acid pool
from the control value. The values are means (nmol/100mg synaptosomal protein) with the bars indicating the S.E.Ms and the number of
experiments shown by the bars. (From de Belleroche and Bradford, 1977).

## SUMMARY AND CONCLUSIONS

The studies which are described indicate an important role
for glutamine as a precursor of certain brain amino acids since it
makes a contribution equivalent to that of glucose.  In the past
glutamine has been considered to have a passive role in the brain,
accumulating in the CSF as a result of glutamine synthetase
activity responding to increased NH$_4$$^+$ or glutamine in the plasma
or CSF.  In fact NH$_4$$^+$ appears to cause glutamine accumulation by
inhibiting glutamine breakdown via glutaminase rather than by
stimulating its synthesis (Bradford & Ward, 1976). The data we are
presenting here indicates that glutamine is probably the principle
precursor of transmitter glutamate released in response to depolarization.  The released GABA and aspartate appear to receive as much
as a 50% contribution from glutamine.  Extrapolated from synaptosomes to the in situ nerve-terminal this conclusion suggests a new
and important role for both glutamine and glutaminase in the brain.

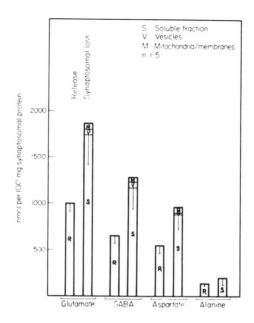

Fig. 7. The effect of veratrine stimulation on amino acid release
and loss from the synaptosome subfractions. The release of amino acid
induced by veratrine stimulation is shown as histograms (R) with the
decrease in pool size of amino acid in the synaptosome subfractions
(S,V,M) shown by the side. The values are means (nmol/100mg synaptosomal protein) with the bars indicating the S.E.Ms and the number of
experiments was 5 (from de Belleroche and Bradford, 1977).

The whole concept of a 'glutamine cycle' between neurons and glia
is well established (Balazs et al., 1973;  Benjamin and Quastel,
1974) and a central role for glutamine as principal precursor of
glutamate and other amino acid transmitters would fit in well with
such a cycle.

     The second category of experimental results described above
favoured the conclusion that the transmitter released from synaptosomes in response to treatment with depolarizing agents comes
directly from the cytoplasm.  Although no clear evidence was
obtained for the involvement of the whole vesicle fraction in the
release process, our results could not entirely rule out the possibility that a sub-population of vesicles was involved, though
their rate of 'filling and emptying' would have to be extremely
rapid to account for the volume of transmitter released.


ACKNOWLEDGEMENT

     We should like to thank the M.R.C. for funds awarded to
support this work (M.R.C. Programme Grant).

## REFERENCES

Balazs, R., Patel, A.J. and Richter, D., 1973 in 'Metabolic Compartments in the Brain' (R. Balazs and J.E. Cremer eds.) pp. 167-184, MacMillan, London.

de Belleroche, J.S. & Bradford, H.F., 1977. On the site of origin of transmitter amino acids released by depolarization of nerve terminals in vitro. J. Neurochem. 28: in press.

de Belleroche, J.S. & Bradford, H.F., 1973. Amino acids in synaptic vesicles from mammalian cerebral cortex: a reappraisal. J. Neurochem. 21: 441-445.

Benjamin, A.M. & Quastel, J.H., 1974. Fate of L-glutamate in the brain. J. Neurochem. 23: 457-464.

Bradford, H.F. & Ward, H.K., 1976. On glutaminase in mammalian synaptosomes. Brain Research 110: 115-125.

Bradford, H.F., Ward, H.K. and Thomas, A.J., 1977. Glutamine as a substrate for nerve-endings. Submitted for publication.

Marchbanks, R.M., 1968. Exchangeability of radioactive acetylcholine with the bound acetylcholine of synaptosomes and synaptic vesicles. Biochem. J. 106: 87-95.

McIlwain, H. & Bachelard, H.S., 1971, p. 162, 3rd edition, in 'Biochemistry and the CNS', Churchill Livingstone.

Salganicoff, L. & de Robertis, E., 1965. Subcellular distribution of the enzymes of the glutamic acid, glutamine and GABA cycles in rat brain. J. Neurochem. 12: 287-309.

Whitaker, V.P. & Sheridan, N.M., 1965. The morphology and acetylcholine content of isolated cerebral cortical synaptic vesicles. J. Neurochem. 12: 363-372.

GLUTAMATE AS A CNS NEUROTRANSMITTER: PROPERTIES OF RELEASE,

INACTIVATION AND BIOSYNTHESIS

Carl W. Cotman and Anders Hamberger[x]

Dept of Psychobiology, University of California, Irvine
California 92717, USA
[x]) Institute of Neurobiology, Medical Faculty
University of Göteborg, Göteborg 33, Sweden

## INTRODUCTION

At present glutamic acid is the molecule most likely to be the
major excitatory transmitter in the mammalian CNS. It has many
of the properties expected if it is to serve in such a role.
The glutamic acid concentration in brain is higher than that of
any other amino acid, and it seems to be present in sufficiently
high levels to serve as a transmitter in a variety of different
neurons. When glutamic acid is applied iontophoretically to the
various neurons throughout the CNS it most commonly has a powerful
excitatory action (Davidson, 1976). In some cases this excitatory
effect is specific: e.g., olfactory bulb neurons are relatively
unresponsive to iontophoretically applied glutamate whereas hippocampal or cerebral cortex neurons are quite sensitive (Van
Baumgarten et al., 1963). In contrast to the effect on CNS neurons,
when glutamate is applied to the muscle surface at a neuromuscular
junction, for example, it has no effect (Curtis and Watkins, 1965).
The excitatory effect of glutamate is restricted to extracellular
application in that intracellularly applied glutamate has no such
effect (Takeuchi and Takeuchi, 1963). The depolarization which
results from extracellular application of glutamate in many cases
appears to be due to an increase in the permeability to Na ions
(Curtis et al. 1972) which is not blocked by tetrodotoxin
(McIlwain et al., 1969). Glutamic acid is released from nerve
endings (Sandoval et al, 1977; de Belleroche and Bradford, 1972),
and it is concentrated by a high affinity uptake process (Logan
and Snyder, 1971).

Glutamate has been proposed to be a transmitter in a variety
of CNS systems (see Davidson, 1976). It may be a transmitter of
the lateral olfactory tract (Bradford and Richards, 1976; Yamamoto

and Matsui, 1976), cerebellar parallel fibres and perhaps mossy
fibres (Young et al, 1974; McBride et al, 1976; Sandoval and
Cotman, 1977), the entorhinal input to the dentate gyrus (Nadler et
al, 1976, 1977; White et al, in press), the CA1 field of hippocampus (Biscoe and Straughan, 1966; Dudar, 1974; Spencer et al,
1976; Segal, 1976; Storm-Mathisen, 1977), the mossy fibres of the
hippocampus (Crawford and Connors, 1973; Storm-Mathisen, 1977) as
well as a variety of other cells throughout the CNS. However, the
proof that these proposed systems are in fact glutamatergic, is
insufficient in most if not all cases. What is needed is a rigorous
study in a single system of the criteria a substance must fulfill
in order to be identified as a transmitter. In such a study it
would be anticipated that not only would som of the ambiguity
associated with the identification of glutamatergic pathways
be clarified but, in addition, much would be learned about the
properties of glutamate in brain.

In evaluating a role of glutamate as a transmitter, it is
necessary to fulfill a number of criteria: 1) Glutamate must be
released upon stimulation in a manner which is dependent on Ca and
antagonised by Mg, and the quantities released must be sufficient
to allow its action as a transmitter. 2) The effect of glutamate
on the postsynaptic cell should be identical to the action of the
natural transmitter. The time course should be the same and the
candidate should cause the same permeability changes at the postsynaptic membrane and the same metabolic responses in the postsynaptic neuron. The action of the natural transmitter should be
similarly affected by specific glutamate antagonists. 3) An
inactivation mechanism should exist. Generally inactivation in the
CNS appears to occur by way of high affinity, Na dependent uptake
so that such a transport process should be present. 4) Presynaptic
terminals should contain the machinery to manufacture and store
glutamate and to control its synthesis. Glutamate synthesis should
increase in response to stimulation so that the tissue can maintain
appreciable pools for release under a wide variety of stimulus
conditions.

We selected the dentate gyrus of the hippocampal formation to
study the properties of glutamate in relationship to a possible
transmitter function. There is now extensive interest in hippocampal function and plasticity, and this area provides a particularly well-defined anatomical substrate for the analysis of
specific fiber tracts converging on a single cell type. Also there
already exists information on a number of the transmitters in the
hippocampal formation. Aspartate is a candidate for the commissural and associational transmitter (Nadler et al, 1976), GABA is
the transmitter of interneurons (Storm-Mathisen, 1976), serotonin
is the transmitter of the Raphe input (Moore and Halaris, 1975) and
norepinephrine is the transmitter of the locus coeruleus input
(Blackstad et al, 1967; Segal and Bloom, 1974; Pickel et al, 1974).
It would be particularly valuable for mechanistic and functional
studies to complete this list and identify the perforant path

transmitter. This input is the major excitatory input from the cerebral cortex to the hippocampus and displays a number of forms of plasticity such as habituation (Mays and Best, 1965; Alger and Tyler 1976; Tyler and Alger, 1976) and long term potentiation (Alger and Tyler, 1976; Bliss and Gardner-Medwin, 1973; Bliss and Lomo, 1973; Douglas and Goddard, 1975).

The dentate gyrus provides an almost ideal system in which chemical, anatomical, and electrophysiological studies can be correlated. The dentate gyrus consists primarily of a single cell type (granule cells) which receives its major input from the entorhinal cortex (Fig. 1). The entorhinal projection accounts for approximately 60% of the total terminals on the granule cells (Matthews et al, 1976), and the projection is almost entirely unilateral. The entorhinal cortex can be ablated so that the properties specific to the entorhinal afferents can be evaluated directly in the same animal by comparison of the control and denervated sides. Moreover, hippocampal electrophysiology is reasonably well studied in vivo as well as in vitro using hippocampal slices. Hippocampal slices are particularly well suited to carry out detailed neurophysiological and pharmacological experiments under carefully controlled conditions.

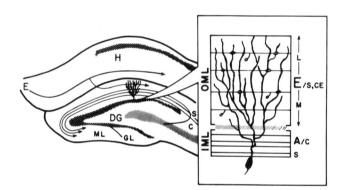

Fig. 1    Structure of the hippocampus. The granule cells in the dentate gyrus (DG) are arranged in a layer (GL) such that the dendrites and afferents are organized in a zone called the molecular layer (ML). The major projection to the molecular layer is from the entorhinal cortex (E).

In this paper we will report on our evaluation of glutamate as a transmitter of the perforant path input to the dentate gyrus. We will evaluate each criterion in turn in order to see if definitive evidence exists on whether or not glutamate is the transmitter. We will also describe some of the properties of the regulation of glutamate biosynthesis in relationship to its release.

## RELEASE OF ENDOGENOUS GLUTAMATE

In 1973 Crawford and Connor discovered that when the entorhinal input to the dentate gyrus is stimulated in vivo, glutamate can be collected from the hippocampus by perfusion techniques. Accordingly Crawford and Connor suggested that glutamate may be a transmitter in the hippocampus. However, in intact animals it is not possible to determine precisely the origin of released glutamate or to evaluate the dependency on divalent ions, which is one of the important criteria in identifying release specific to stimulus-secretion coupling processes. In order to circumvent these problems we have selected to study slices of the dentate gyrus in vitro using perfusion techniques.

We prepared slices of the dentate gyrus from the dendritic-afferent field of the granule cells (the molecular layer) by free hand dissection with the aid of a stereomicroscope. This preparation provides a nearly pure population of the dendritic and afferent field of a single cell type (see Fig. 1). The synaptic input in the molecular layer originates primarily from the entorhinal cortex but there are in addition minor projections from the septum, the contralateral hippocampal pyramidal cells (the commissural system) and the ipsilateral hippocampal pyramidal cells (the associational system). Also a few interneurons are present which are GABAnergic (Storm-Mathisen, 1976).

In a typical experiment slices are placed on a support filter and chemically stimulated with various media (low K medium consisting of 3 mM KCl in a modified Kreb's Ringer bicarbonate medium, a high K medium consisting of 56 mM KCl also in the Kreb's Ringer bicarbonate medium and a high K - Ca medium consisting of 56 mM KCl and 2 mM free $CaCl_2$ in the Kreb's Ringer bicarbonate medium). As shown in Fig. 2, in the presence of low K medium glutamate efflux is in the range of 1 nmol/mg tissue/min. When the tissue is depolarized by the introduction of the high K medium, glutamate efflux increases 2 or 3 times and than stabilizes at that level for a period of time. Introduction then of the high K-Ca medium further stimulates release so it is approximately twice that seen in the high K medium (or about 8 times that in the low K medium). Glutamate release decreases again upon returning to the high K medium and is stimulated again upon reintroduction of the high K-Ca medium. About 5% of the tissue glutamate is released per minute in a Ca-dependent manner. In other experiments using a slightly larger slice which includes portions of the hilus, Mg inhibits release and barium substitutes for Ca (Nadler et al, 1977). Veratridine, another depolarizing agent also supports release. Release is obtained in the absence of Na, and Ca has no effect in the absence of depolarization (Nadler et al, 1977). The release of GABA, a known transmitter in the dentate gyrus, exhibits properties in all respects identical to glutamate (Sandoval et al, 1977).

In order to determine whether release can also be elicited by electrical stimulation, the following experiment was done. Slices

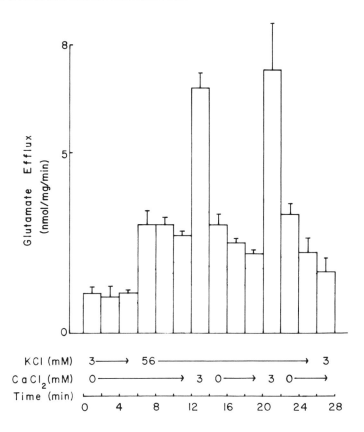

Fig. 2    Release of endogenous glutamate from slices of the molecular layer of the dentate gyrus evoked by chemical stimulation.
Elevation of the K concentration to 56 mM stimulates efflux.  Addition of 3 mM Ca further increases efflux (from Hamberger et al,
1977a).

were prepared and placed in a small chamber having the provision
for stimulating and superfusing the slices.  Electrical pulses (10
V square waves, 5 msec duration, 100 Hz for 15 sec) were applied
between silver electrodes and the release of glutamate was monitored.  A brief electrical pulse in the presence of Ca causes an
immediate stimulation of glutamate efflux which is approximately
6-8 times higher than baseline efflux (Fig. 3).  In order to
determine whether this efflux is dependent on Ca as required for
neurotransmitter release, Ca was removed and 25 mM Mg included in
the superfusion medium.  This nearly abolishes the stimulated
glutamate efflux (dashed line Fig. 3).
    Thus the release of glutamate in the dentate molecular layer
appears to parallel the properties expected of a transmitter: its
release is stimulated by electrical or chemical depolarization in a

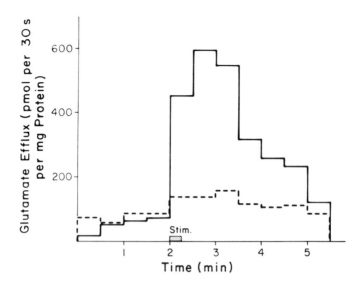

Fig. 3     Time course of glutamate efflux from a slice of the dentate gyrus evoked by electrical stimulation in the presence and
absence of Ca.   Solid lines: glutamate efflux into normal medium
containing 2 mM free Ca.  Dashed lines: glutamate efflux into Ca
free medium containing 25 mM MgCl₂.  (From White et al, 1977).

Ca-dependent manner.   Barium will substitute for Ca and Mg will
inhibit Ca dependent release.  Moreover, release is measured as
rapidly as the present perfusion systems allows and a substantial
portion of the total glutamate in the slice is released.  The Ca-
dependent release stimulated by tissue depolarization is specific
to certain small molecules.  Exogenously loaded proline (a putative
transmitter in other brain areas) and leucine (an unlikely neurotransmitter in the hippocampus) are not released in a Ca-dependent
manner (Nadler et al, 1977; Sandoval et al, 1977).  In addition,
glutamine (an important glutamate precursor) is not released in a
Ca-dependent manner (Fig. 4).  The glutamine data are particularly
significant because as will be shown in a later section in this
chapter glutamine enters the nerve ending and serves as a major
precursor for transmitter glutamate.
        In order to determine whether release is specific to afferents
originating from the entorhinal cortex, entorhinal cortex was
destroyed unilateraly and glutamate release from slices of dentate
gyrus prepared from the control and denervated sides examined at
various times after the lesion.  Ca-dependent release of endogenous
glutamate is markedly reduced (Nadler et al, 1976; Hamberger et
al, 1977).  At 4 days after destruction of the entorhinal cortex,
release is depressed about 70% and does not recover by 14 days

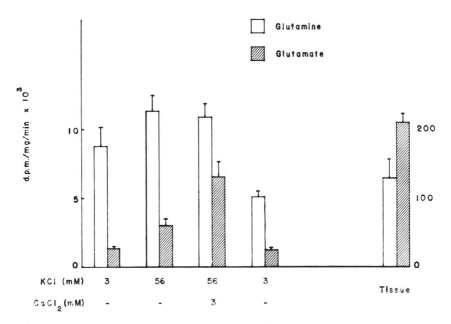

Fig. 4    Comparison of the efflux of radioactive glutamate and
radioactive glutamine from slices of the molecular layer of the
dentate gyrus.  Slices were loaded with [14]C glutamine and the efflux
of glutamine and radioactively derived glutamate were monitored.
Glutamate release (shaded bars) is stimulated by addition of Ca,
but glutamine efflux (clear bars is not.  (From  Hamberger et al,
1977c).

after the lesion.  In contrast Ca-dependent release of aspartate is
slightly increased (Nadler et al, 1976).  Baseline glutamate efflux
is not significantly different on the two sides.  Thus destruction
of the entorhinal cortex specifically reduced the Ca-dependent
release of glutamate.

Subcellular fractionation was used in order to determine the
structure from which glutamate release originates (Sandoval et
al, 1977).  Synaptosomes release glutamate in a manner which is
stimulated by high K and is dependent on Ca.  In so far as it is
possible to determine, Ca-dependent release is specific to synaptosomes.  Isolated microsomes accumulate exogenously loaded glutamate
and GABA but do not release it in a Ca-dependent manner.  Moreover, when the release of glutamate from a crude mitochondrial
fraction (consisting of synaptosomes, mitochondria, myelin and
membrane fragments) is compared to the release from a purified

synaptosomal fraction, the Ca-dependent release of exogenously
loaded glutamate is approximately 3 fold enriched in the synaptosomal fraction (Fig. 5). The absolute amount of endogenous glutamate released which is Ca-dependent is the same in both fractions,
but percent release is higher in the synaptosomal fraction. Ca-
dependent GABA release is also concentrated in the synaptosomal
fraction. K-stimulated, Ca-independent release is higher in the
crude mitochondrial fraction.

## POSTSYNAPTIC ACTION OF GLUTAMATE

In general iontophoretically applied glutamate has a powerful
excitatory effect on hippocampal neurons (Biscoe and Straughan,
1966; Segal, 1976; Spencer et al, 1976). Moreover, the glutamate
analog, glutamic acid diethyl ester, reversibly antagonizes excitations produced by iontophoretically applied glutamate but not
those produced by acetylcholine on CAl pyramidal cells in hippocampal slices. The nature of the responses to applied substances
is virtually identical in the intact animal and in the in vitro
slice preparation (Spencer et al, 1976).
Recently we examined the effect of the glutamate antagonist
2-amino-4-phosphonobutyric acid (APB) on the perforant path responses
in the hippocampal slice preparation (White et al, 1977). When
applied to invertebrate muscle fibers, APB competitively and
reversibly antagonizes the action of iontophoretic glutamate and
bath application of 2.5 mM APB inhibits neuromuscular transmission
(Cull-Candy et al, 1976; Clements and May, 1974). Since invertebrate motor neurons almost certainly use glutamate as their
transmitter (Gerschenfeld, 1973), APB appears to inhibit synaptic
transmission mediated by glutamate. Accordingly, we stimulated the
perforant path fibers in the presence and absence of APB and
recorded the extracellular field potentials in the molecular layer
of the dentate gyrus. The results of a typical experiment are
shown in Fig. 6. When the perforant path fibers are continuously
stimulated at 0.2 Hz a sizable negative potential is recorded (Fig.
6a) whose amplitude declines somewhat over the 22 min period
probably as a result of habituation. Introduction of APB into the
perfusion media substantially reduces the amplitude of the potential within one min and the amplitude recovers just as rapidly
upon return to normal media and finally reaches the habituated
level (Fig. 6b). Overall APB is maximally effective within 3 min
and at 2.5 mM effects a 46% reduction in the amplitude of the field
potential. 5 mM APB causes an 80% reduction which again is
reversible. APB has no affect on the orthodromic perforant path
fiber volley or on antidromic activation of the granule cells.
In a separate set of experiments hippocampal slices were used
to determine if APB affects glutamate release or uptake. APB does
not affect release of glutamate and does not alter glutamate uptake
(White et al, 1977). These results strengthen the contention that

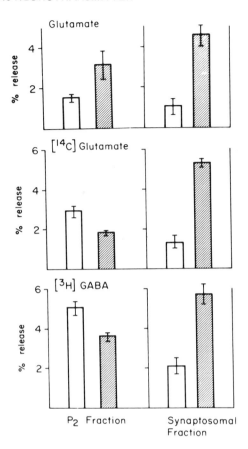

Fig. 5    $K^+$ stimulated Ca-dependent release (shaded bars) and $K^+$ stimulated efflux (unshaded bars) of endogenous glutamate, $^{14}C$ glutamate and $^3H$ GABA from hippocampal $P_2$ and synaptosomal fractions. (From Sandoval and Cotman, 1977).

glutamate may be the transmitter of the perforant path.[*]

INACTIVATION: Properties of the Na-dependent, high-affinity uptake system for glutamate

It is generally believed that the inactivation of amino acid neurotransmitters in brain occurs by way of a high-affinity Na dependent uptake process. Presumably, transmitters are swept from the cleft into presynaptic boutons and/or glial cells in order to

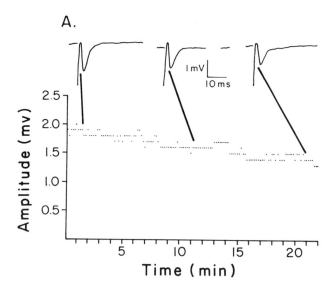

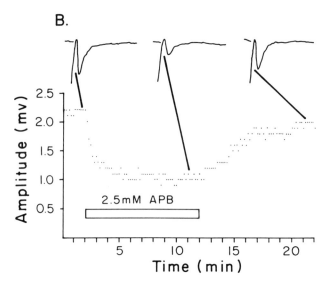

Fig. 6    Reduction of perforant path responses by APB recorded
extracellularly in slices of the hippocampus.  Perforant path
fibers were stimulated continuously at 0.2 Hz and at an intensity
just below that which evoked a population spike. (A).  Amplitude
of every second synaptic potential (dots) in a single experiment
without drug. (B).  Results of an experiment in which APB (2.5 mM)
was present in the period shown by the open bar.  The response is
rapidly reduced in the presence of the drug and rapidly recovers
when the drug is removed.  (From White et al, 1977).

terminate their synaptic action.

$^{14}$C-glutamate is accumulated by high-affinity processes into hippocampal synaptosomes (Sandoval et al, 1977). The high affinity system is Na-dependent and has a $K_m$ of about 3 x 10$^{-6}$ M which is in the range of the high affinity uptake systems for other putative neurotransmitters and for glutamate in the cerebral cortex and spinal cord (Logan and Snyder, 1972). Glutamate and aspartate do not appear to be differentiated by this transport system. Glutamate uptake does not differ greatly in various hippocampal sub-fields. The $V_{max}$ and $K_m$ for glutamate uptake are very similar in P$_2$ fractions prepared both regio superior and regio inferior of the dentate gyrus suggesting that the overall transport is not highly localized to one particular cell type. However, uptake does appear related to specific afferents. Recently Storm-Mathisen (this volume) has shown that the high-affinity Na-dependent uptake of glutamate displays a laminar organization of pyramidal and granule cells. The entorhinal zone on the granule cells displays significant uptake but the commissural-associational zone shows the greatest accumulation perhaps because this system also employs glutamate or aspartate as a transmitter (Nadler et al, 1976).

In order to determine if uptake of glutamate in the entorhinal zone is into afferent fibers originating from the entorhinal cortex, the entorhinal cortex was lesioned and uptake was studied at 8 days after lesion (Nadler et al, 1976). In the dentate gyrus, high-affinity glutamate uptake is significantly reduced whereas it is not significantly changed in regio superior. This observation, since confirmed (Storm-Mathisen, 1977), suggests that at least a portion of the glutamate is transported into the fibers of the perforant path. However, in as much as the reduction in uptake is not as large as the corresponding reduction in release, transport probably occurs into other compartments as well. It is known that shortly following an entorhinal lesion there is hypertrophy of astrocytes and a proliferation of microglial cells (Lynch et al, 1975). Assuming these glial cells have glutamate transport properties similar to glial cells elsewhere, they would accumulate more glutamate and obscure to some degree the reduction of glutamate uptake due to nerve fiber destruction. Also, and perhaps more importantly, commissural and/or associational boutons still present after entorhinal lesion may employ aspartate as their transmitter (Nadler et al, 1976). Because glutamate would be accumulated into these boutons the reduction would not be complete. These arguments are consistent with the presence of an uptake system related to the perforant path afferents which may serve as an inactivation mechanism for released glutamate.

[*]A note of caution should be interjected. In preliminary experiments the excitatory effect of iontophoretically applied glutamate was not markedly antagonized by iontophoretically applied APB.

Accordingly we tested the effects of D-aspartate, a glutamate uptake inhibitor, to determine if release from slices is larger in the absence of reuptake. Ca-dependent release of glutamate is increased very little if at all in the presence of D-aspartate (Hamberger et al, 1977c). It would appear that the perfusion technique effectively removes glutamate and reuptake is not effective in capturing the relatively large quantities of glutamate released. It is possible that under physiological conditions the situation is different.

### RELEASE OF ACCUMULATED GLUTAMATE

Exogenous glutamate is accumulated and released in a Ca-dependent manner from either slices or synaptosomes. The release though is different from endogenous glutamate in that it fatigues rapidly, and only a small portion of the total accumulated stores are released (Fig. 7). In slices loaded with $^{14}$C gluta-mate and stimulated repetitively with Ca in the presence of high K endogenous glutamate release remains relatively constant over at least 5 pulses. In contrast, release of accumulated gluta-mate rapidly declines after the first test pulse. Approximately 10% of the total $^{14}$C-glutamate is released in a Ca-dependent manner over a period of a few minutes.

Thus most of the accumulated glutamate is inaccessible to releasable pools. Structures other than nerve endings that can accumulate glutamate do not release it in a Ca-dependent fashion and probably even nerve endings release only a fraction of the accumulated glutamate. In isolated synaptosomes only about 5% of the total accumulated stores are released over the first minute. After an initial peak release drops off rapidly so that very little additional release is seen (Sandoval et al, 1977). It would appear that uptake is not specifically resupplying releasable glutamate stores. Most is metabolized or inaccessible to releasable pools.

This conclusion agrees with results obtained with other transmitters. GABA release falls off rapidly and in fact exogen-ously loaded GABA is not preferentially released unless the synaptosomes are previously stimulated. Once stimulated, accumu-lated GABA is much less available for release (Levy et al, 1973). And with GABA and as well for catecholamines only a few percent of stores are released in a manner dependent on Ca (Cotman et al, 1976). There are other indications that much of the accum-ulated transmitter is inaccessible to releasable stores. Cer-tain subcellular fractions accumulate, but do not release gluta-mate or other neurotransmitters (Sandoval et al, 1977; Levy et al, 1973; Cotman et al, 1976). Moreover, in the cerebellum after neonatal X-irradiation and loss of most granule cells, glutamate uptake is little if at all affected whereas release is reduced (Sandoval and Cotman, 1977). It would appear that uptake

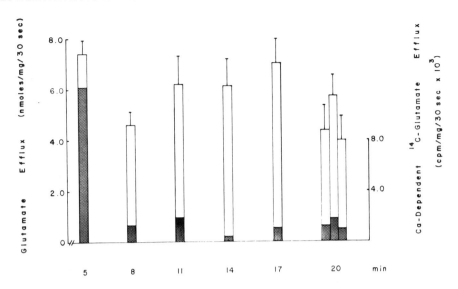

Fig. 7    Ca-dependent release of endogenous glutamate and exogenously loaded glutamate from slices of the dentate gyrus.  Slices were preloaded with 0.4 um $^{14}C$ glutamate and superfused with Kreb's Ringer medium containing 56 mM KCl and 0.4 mM glutamine.  Release was stimulated by 30 sec pulses of Ca.  Endogenous glutamate was released in simular quantities with each Ca pulse whereas $^{14}C$ glutamate release rapidly declined (Hamberger, Denner, and Cotman, Unpublished observations).

is not related simply to the inactivation and recovery of transmitter but must have other functions.

    After slices or subcellular fractions are labeled with exogenous glutamate elevated K produces efflux of a higher specific activity than that released in response to Ca (Sandoval et al, 1977; Nadler et al, 1977).  As previously suggested this may be due to a direct effect of K on the carrier (Nadler et al, 1977; Haycock et al, 1977).  High K appears to reverse carriers so as to stimulate flux in an outward direction (Martin, 1975).

### PREFERENTIAL RELEASE OF NEWLY SYNTHSIZED GLUTAMATE

    So far we can conclude that glutamate displays many of the properties expected of a neurotransmitter.  It is released in a Ca-dependent manner under depolarizing conditions, a high affinity uptake mechanism exists and the postsynaptic action and pharmacology are consistent with a neurotransmitter role.  This we feel provides a sufficient case in order to undertake a study

of the regulation of glutamate synthesis related to a transmitter
function.

Although a great deal is known about the metabolism of
glutamate in brain, relatively little is known specifically
about the metabolism in presynaptic endings that regulates the
releasable pools.  Glutamate may be synthesized directly from
glutamine via the enzyme glutaminase or may be synthesized from
glocose by a series of reactions (Fig. 8).  The relative importance of precursors such as glucose and glutamine is a key issue
in understanding the metabolism of glutamate (Berl et al, 1975).
In brain, glutamate is metabolized in at least two distinct
compartments due to the presence of two tricarboxylic acid
cycles distinguished by their choice of precursors (Van den Berg
and Garfinkel, 1971).  One compartment which has a preference
for glucose is probably neuronal.  For example, synaptosomes
will rapidly oxidize glucose and manufacture glutamate which
upon electrical or chemical stimulation in the presence of
calcium is discharged into the medium (de Belleroche and Bradford, 1972).  The other compartment is assigned to glial cells
and is characterized by an ability to use many precursors (ace-

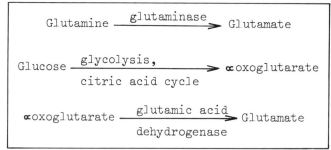

Fig. 8    Major pathways for the synthesis of glutamate.

tate, pyruvate, amino acids including glutamate, etc) and produce glutamine which is released into the extracellular space of
the brain.  Nerve terminals seem to lack glutamine synthetase
(Salganicoff and De Robertis, 1965) so they cannot synthesize
glutamine.  However, they do have a high activity of glutaminase
which, in the presence of glutamine catalyzes the synthesis of
substantial quantities of synaptosomal glutamate (Bradford and
Ward, 1976).

Glial cells then may act a sink for glutamate released
from the terminals (as well as other amino acids and precursors)
and return glutamic to the extracellular space where it is
taken up into the terminals and used as a glutamate precursor
(Van den Berg and Garfinkel, 1971; Benjamin and Quastel, 1972).
The glutamine concentration is about 0.4 mM in the cerebral
spinal fluid (Plum, 1974) and consequently may be the major

glutamate precursor in nerve endings (Bradford and Ward, 1976).

At present, however, it is not known whether glucose or glutamine (or perhaps even another precursor) is responsible for
the synthesis of the readily releasable pool of glutamate at
glutamatergic synapses. Initially, then we evaluated the relative contribution of glucose and glutamine as precursors for
glutamate in slices prepared from the molecular of the dentate
gyrus. Which precursor appears to be the most essential in
maintaining the readily releasable glutamate pools? And what
are the control mechanisms in the synthesis of glutamate derived
from that precursor?

Glucose as a glutamate precursor

Glutamate biosynthesis was studied in the presence of 3 mM
[14]C glucose and each of three different ionic media (low K, high
K and high K plus Ca; Table 1). Incubations were carried out for
15 min with intermittent media changes, and the amount of
glutamate released into the media and that remaining in the
slice were determined at the end of the experiment. In the
presence of 56 mM KCl and in the absence of Ca there is a small
increase of endogenous and radioactive glutamate in the medium.
In the 56 mM KCl, 3 mM $CaCl_2$ medium there is an increase in
endogenous glutamate release as well as radioactive glutamate over
and above that seen in the other two conditions. The tissue
displays a large increase in glutamate production but newly synthesized glutamate is not preferentially released since the specific
activity in the tissue is higher than that in the medium. The
incorporation of glucose into tissue glutamate is most affected by
the high K Ca stimulus.

The endogenous glutamate released is taken from tissue
stores because there is little net increase in endogenous glutamate in the tissue plus the medium combined. Glutamate levels in
the tissue are depleted and not replaced. However, glutamate
synthesis is stimulated, and based on the specific activity of the
glutamate released compared to that of the precursor most of the
glutamate is derived from the [14]C glucose. (Note the specific
activity of glutamate derived from U-([14]C) glucose must be multiplied by 2.5 to 3 in order to correct for the metabolism of
glucose converted to glutamate).

The release of prelabeled glutamate was also studied.
Glutamate was labeled for 15 min in the presence of [14]C glucose,
the radioactive precursor was removed and replaced by unlabeled
glucose. Slices were further incubated in the low K medium for 15
min and then stimulated with the high K medium followed by the
high K, Ca medium (Fig. 9). In the period following the incubation
a stable release of labeled and unlabeled glutamate was seen.
Instroduction of the high K medium has little if any effect on the
efflux of endogenous or [14]C glutamate with these procedures.

TABLE I. GLUTAMATE IN DENTATE SLICES AND MEDIA AFTER INCUATION WITH $^{14}$C-GLUCOSE

| Media | Glutamate (nmol/mg) | | | Radioactive glutamate (dpm/mg x $10^3$) | | | Specific radioactivity (dpm/nmol x $10^3$) | |
|---|---|---|---|---|---|---|---|---|
| | Tissue | Medium | Total | Tissue | Medium | Total | Tissue | Medium |
| 3 mM KCl | 90±2 | 11±2 | 101 | 758±63 | 183±71 | 944 | 8.4 | 16.4 |
| 56 mM KCl | 54±2 | 30±3 | 84 | 970±46 | 327±37 | 1,297 | 17.8 | 10.9 |
| 56 mM KCl, 3 mM CaCl$_2$ | 51±4 | 71±5 | 122 | 1,224±68 | 1,144±45 | 2,368 | 24.2 | 16.2 |

Slices of dentate gyrus were incubated in media for 15 min with $^{14}$C glucose (100 μCi/ml) and glucose (3 mM) in 0.2 ml/3 min at 37°C. Medium was pooled for analysis to give total glutamate during the 15 min incubation. Subsequently slices were extracted and analyzed for glutamate and radioactive glutamate. Means ± SEM for 3 experiments in each group. S.A. = specific radioactivity. P < 0.05 for slice radioactivity 3 mM KCl vs 56 mM KCl. SA for glucose in incubation medium 7.24 x $10^4$ dpm/nmol. (From Hamberger et al, 1977b).

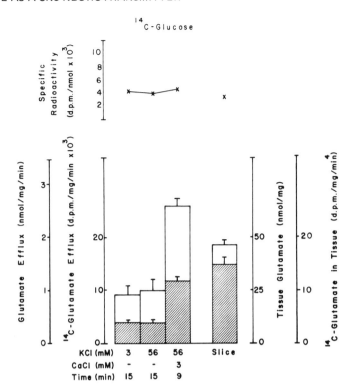

Fig. 9 Efflux of prelabeled glutamate derived from $^{14}$C glucose. Slices from the molecular layer were incubated for 15 min in the presence of 3 mM U-($^{14}$C)-glucose in low K medium. The isotope was removed and the release of glutamate (clear bars) and $^{14}$C glutamate (shaded bars) monitored during the sequence of ionic conditions indicated. The specific activity of released glutamate is indicated at the top of the figure. (From Hamberger et al, 1977b).

Introduction of Ca, however, causes and increase in endogenous and $^{14}$C glutamate efflux. Ca-evoked release has a specific activity insignificantly different from that of the glutamate in the slice measured at the end of the experiment.

Thus, $^{14}$C glutamate derived from $^{14}$C glucose is rapidly made and released into the medium, but neither newly synthesized (Table 1) nor prelabeled glutamate (Fig. 9) that is released is derived from a pool which has a specific activity higher than that of tissue glutamate. Moreover, the glutamate released appears to be largely at the expense of tissue glutamate stores since there is little net increase in total glutamate production at the end of the experiment (Hamberger et al, 1977b).

Glutamine as a Glutamate Precursor

     The difference between release in the presence of glucose and
in the presence of glucose plus glutamine is most striking.  This
can be seen in an experiment where slices are incubated in the
presence or absence of glutamine for 20 min and the total efflux
of glutamate is measured.  In the presence of glutamine, endogenous
glutamate efflux is markedly higher even in the low K medium (Fig.
10).  In the high K medium, efflux increases and in the high K-Ca
medium release is higher than that in the high K medium alone.
Release in high K-Ca medium amounts to a total of about 350 nmoles
of glutamate/mg protein in 20 min or approximately 10% of the
slice content of glutamate is released per minute.  Whereas the sum
of the tissue plus medium glutamate is similar in all media in the
absence of glutamine, in the presence of glutamine the sum of
tissue and medium glutamate increases with increasing amounts
released into the medium.  In high K-Ca medium there is approximately
a 4 fold increase in total glutamate production over a 20 min
period.  It is most striking to note that about 80% of the glutamine
derived glutamate is released into the medium (Hamberger et al,
1977a).
     The synthesis of glutamate from radioactive glutamine was
examined in order to 1) evaluate the control of glutamate synthesis derived from glutamine, 2) quantitate the amount glutamate
derived directly from glutamine, and 3) determine if glutamate
derived from glutamine is preferentially released.  Glutamate
biosynthesis was studied in the presence of radioactive glutamine
in each of the 3 media (Hamberger et al, 1977b).  Tissue was
incubated in the presence of radioactive glutamine for a total of
six minutes with intermitant media changes and the total amount of
glutamate released and remaining in the tissue at the end of the
experiments was determined (Table 2).  As in the previous experiment the total amount of glutamate produced increases in the high
K-Ca medium relative to the low K medium.  Moreover, the synthesis
of radioactive glutamate derived from radioactive glutamine is
similarly stimulated particularly in the high k-Ca medium.  The
specific activity in the medium is higher than that in the slice
indicating a preferential release of newly synthesized glutamate in
all three conditions.  The specific activity of released glutamate
is highest in the low K medium where it is approximately equal to
the specific activity of the precursor.  In the high K-Ca medium,
the specific activity is approximately 70% of that of the precursor
indicating that approximately this amount of the glutamate released
is newly synthesized from glutamine.
     The incorporation of glutamine into tissue glutamate was
little affected by the high K Ca medium.  In contrast the same
condition markedly stimulated the incorporation of glucose into
tissue glutamate (see Table 1 and Table 4).  This distinction
illustrates the difference in the compartmentation of glutamate
and shows that glutamine most specifically serves the synthesis of

TABLE II. GLUTAMATE IN DENTATE GYRUS SLICES AND MEDIA AFTER INCUBATION WITH $^{14}$C-GLUTAMINE

| Media | Glutamate (nmol/mg) | | | Radioactive glutamate (dpm/mg x 10$^3$) | | | Specific radioactivity (dpm/nmol x 10$^3$) | |
|---|---|---|---|---|---|---|---|---|
| | Tissue | Medium | Total | Tissue | Medium | Total | Tissue | Medium |
| 3 mM KCl | 104±7 | 35±12 | 139 | 85±14 | 108±41 | 193 | 8.2 | 30.8 |
| 56 mM KCl | 100±9 | 61±4 | 161 | 68±11 | 157±11 | 225 | 6.8 | 25.7 |
| 56 mM KCl, 3 mM CaCl$_2$ | 73±6 | 138±28 | 211 | 66±26 | 260±42 | 326 | 9.0 | 18.8 |

Incubation was carried out in 0.2 ml/2 min Krebs Ringer bicarbonate medium in 95% $O_2$: 5% $CO_2$ at 37°C. Media were changed every two minutes, giving a total volume of 0.6 ml for the 6 min incubation. Glucose concentration was 10 mM and $^{14}$C glutamine was 0.4 mM. Means ± SEM of 6 experiments. Specific activity for glutamine in the incubation medium was 2.65 x 10$^3$ dpm/nmol. (From Hamberger et al, 1977b).

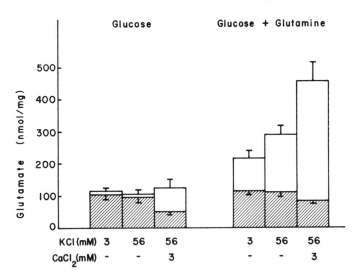

Fig. 10    Total and slice content of glutamate after incubation in
media with different ionic compositions.  Slice of the molecular
layer of the dentate gyrus were incubated in 0.2 ml of Krebs Ringer
bicarbonate medium for 20 min with media changes every two min.  The
glutamate content in the pooled media and tissue slices were determined.  Incubations were performed in media containing either 10 mM
glucose (left) or 10 mM glucose, 0.4 mM glutamine (right) with the
ionic composition indicated (bottom).  The portion of the glutamate (open bars) which was present in the tissue slice at the end
of the experiment is indicated by the shaded area (From Hamberger
et al, 1977a).

glutamate released via stimulus secretion coupling processes.
        The efflux of prelabeled glutamate was also studied in the
paradigm described above for studying glutamate efflux derived
from glucose.  In this way it is possible to examine the release of
performed glutamate under conditions where it is not replenished
from external radioactive glutamine.  Tissue was labeled for 15
min in the presence of $^{14}C$ glutamine; the label was removed and
replaced with unlabeled glutamine.  After a period of time in low
K medium, the tissue was stimulated with high K medium then high
K-Ca medium and efflux was monitored.  After the labeling period
glutamine is rapidly lost from the slice so that approximately 6
times more radioactivity chromatographs with glutamate than with
glutamine in the low K medium following the pulse.  Moreover, in
the high K medium there is a 20% increase in $^{14}C$ glutamine efflux
over low K medium.  The addition of Ca evokes no further increase
in $^{14}C$ glutamine efflux.
        Two features of Ca-dependent glutamate release are particu-
larly different from the previous paradigm where labeling is
continuous: 1) less radioactive glutamate is available for release

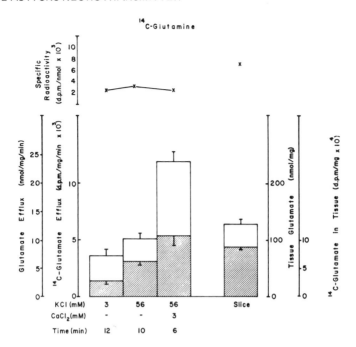

Fig. 11    Efflux of prelabeled glutamate derived from $^{14}$C glutamine.
Slices were incubated for 15 min in the presence of radioactive
glutamine.  The isotope was removed and the release of endogenous
glutamate (clear bars) and radioactive glutamate (shaded bars) monitored for the sequence of ionic media indicated.  The specific activity of glutamate is indicated above. (From Hamberger et al, 1977b).

and 2) the specific activity of glutamate released is nearly the
same in all 3 conditions and each is lower than that in the tissue.
Glutamate released to K stimulation shows a particularly rapid
turnover whereas the Ca pool retains its label longer since the
specific activity of release glutamate does not fall off as
rapidly in response to Ca (Fig. 11).

The release of glutamate rapidly responds to extracellular
glutamate.  Slices were superfused in glucose medium in the
presence of high K (zero Ca) to establish a baseline and glutamine
was added to the medium.  As shown in Fig. 12, efflux increases
almost immediately and a new efflux rate of radioactive and
endogenous glutamate is established which is about 5 times greater
than in the absence of glutamine.  Similarily, upon removal of
glutamine from the medium efflux decreases to a low level within
minutes and rapidly increases again upon reintroduction of glutamine.  The profile of radioactive glutamate follows that for
endogenous glutamate quite closely (Hamberger et al, 1977b).

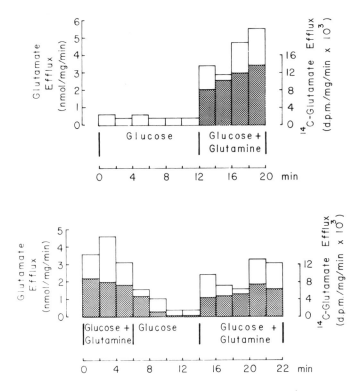

Fig. 12     Effect of 0.4 mM glutamine containing $^{14}$C glutamate on
the efflux of glutamate (clear bars) and glutamate associated
radioactivity (shaded bars).  Glutamine was added to the medium
as indicated.  Media contained 56 mM KCl throughout both experiments. (From Hamberger et al, 1977b).

     Ca-evoked release of newly synthesized glutamate appears
associated at least in path with the entorhinal input (Hamberger
et al, 1977b).  At 4 or 14 days after a unilateral entorhinal
lesion, Ca dependent release of $^{14}$C glutamate derived from either
precursor is reduced approximately 60% on the lesioned side.

## Dependence of glutamate biosynthesis derived from $^{14}$C glucose in the presence of glutamine

     The results described so far show that tissue in the presence
of glutamine can synthesize more glutamate for release than in the
presence of glucose alone; the quantities of glutamate released
are larger and the tissue is more able to sustain its output.  In
the absence of glutamine most of the glutamate is derived from
glucose but release is lower and not sustained as effectively.
Glutamate derived from glucose is not preferentially released.

However, glutamate synthesized from glutamine is preferentially
released.  About 70% of the glutamate release is newly synthesized
from glutamine.  The remaining 30% might come from glucose or
existing stores.
    Accordingly, the incorporation of $^{14}$C glucose into glutamate
in the presence of glutamine was examined in order to see if
readily releasable glutamate not synthesized from glutamine was
derived from glucose.  Slices were incubated in the presence of
radioactive glucose with and without glutamine (Table 3).  In the
low K medium $^{14}$C glucose incorporation into glutamate increases,
and in the high K or high K-Ca medium there is a 2 - 3 fold
stimulation in the incorporation of glucose into the glutamate
which is released into the medium.  With Ca in the medium there is
a net increase in glutamate production in the presence of glutamine (Hamberger et al. 1977b).  The radioactivity in slice glutamate in the high K and high K-Ca glutamine media is similar to
that in the high K-Ca medium without glutamine.  Thus most of the
stimulation is in releasable glutamate.
    Glutamine probably makes certain steps in the biosynthesis
of glutamate less rate limiting so that the overall oxidation of
glucose can proceed more rapidly.  The mechanism may be related to
the stimulation of pyruvate kinase by ammonia (Hawkins, 1973) and
could also be related to the availability of ammonia so that α-
oxoglutarate is converted more rapidly to glutamic acid by way of
glutamic dehydrogenase.
    In the presence of glutamine, glutamate derived from glucose
accounts for most if not all the glutamate released which is not
synthesized from glutamine.  Thus most of the readily releaseable
glutamate is in fact newly synthesized.

## REGULATION OF GLUTAMATE BIOSYNTHESIS IN THE READILY RELEASABLE POOL

    We have shown that glutamine is the most important precursor
for the readily releasable pool of glutamate and that it is
preferentially released.  Consequently, we next turned to an
analysis of the kinetics and mechanisms underlying the increased
synthesis of glutamate derived from glutamine.
    Initially we sought to determine how rapidly synthesis is
stimulated during release.  Accordingly, slices were stimulated
for a prolonged period of time in the presence of Ca while release
was monitored (Fig. 13).  The total endogenous glutamate efflux
increases upon addition of Ca in the presence of high K and decreases over time.  Radioactive glutamate, on the other hand, rapidly
rises and is sustained at a nearly constant level during the
period of release.  This suggests that the onset of the stimulatory effect is very rapid, as soon as can be measured, and
continues over the period studied.  The rate of glutamate synthesis
appears to decrease again rapidly after removal of the Ca stimulus.

TABLE III. COMPARISON OF MEDIUM AND TISSUE CONTENT OF GLUTAMATE AND $^{14}C$-GLUTAMATE AFTER INCUBATION IN $^{14}C$-GLUCOSE WITH AND WITHOUT 0.4 mM GLUTAMINE

| | 3 mM glucose | | | 3 mM glucose + 0.4 mM glutamine | | |
|---|---|---|---|---|---|---|
| | Glutamate nmol/mg | $^{14}C$ glutamate dpm/mg x $10^3$ | Specific Radioactivity dpm/rmol x $10^3$ | Glutamate nmol/mg | $^{14}C$ glutamate dpm/mg x $10^3$ | Specific Radioactivity dpm/nmol x $10^3$ |
| 3 mM KCl $^{14}C$ Glucose | 11±3 | 183±70 | 16.4 | 121±23 | 290±78 | 2.4 |
| Slice | 90±2 | 758±63 | 8.4 | 130±18 | 862±86 | 6.6 |
| 56 mM KCl $^{14}C$ Glucose | 30±2 | 327±37 | 10.9 | 245±24 | 982±151 | 4.0 |
| Slice | 55±2 | 971±46 | 17.8 | 87±23 | 1,325±145 | 15.2 |
| 56 mM KCl 3 mM CaCl$_2$ $^{14}C$ Glucose | 71±5 | 1,144±45 | 16.2 | 416±33 | 1,735±127 | 4.2 |
| Slice | 51±4 | 1,223±68 | 24.2 | 92±21 | 1,362±142 | 14.9 |

Slices were prepared from the whole dentate gyrus (molecular layer plus granule cells) and incubated in 0.2 ml/3 min for 15 min in Krebs-Ringer bicarbonate medium 95% $O_2$; 5% $CO_2$ at 37°C. Means ± SEM for 3 experiments in each group. $^{14}C$ glucose in media was 7.24 x $10^2$ dpm/nmol. (From Hamberger et al, 1977b).

How is glutamate synthesis regulated? There are two possibilities: one is that glutamine uptake is increased and the other
is that there is an activation of the enzyme glutaminase.

Control of glutamine uptake

Is the stimulation of glutamate synthesis due to an enhancement of glutamine uptake and retention? Slices were incubated for
6 min in the presence of glutamine and the amount of glutamine
accumulated in the slice determined. A 6 min incubation time was
chosen since glutamine uptake is linear over this period (Balcar
and Johnston, 1975). As shown in table 4 tissue glutamine is
lower in the high K an high K Ca media than in the low K medium.
However, when the amount of glutamine present in the tissue plus
the amount of radioactive glutamate released into the medium and
present in the tissue is added to the amount of glutamine in the
tissue, there is an increase in the total glutamine accumulated
in the high K-Ca condition. Thus glutamine uptake is stimulated
under conditions of Ca-stimulated glutamate release. Hence part
of the stimulation of glutamate synthesis appears to be due to
precursor availability. The notion that glutamine availability is
limiting is consistent with the finding that under conditions of
enhanced glutamate synthesis, the tissue content of glutamine is
lowest.

Glutamine efflux from the tissue is very rapid as previously
discussed, but it could be shown that the rate of efflux is not
substantially enhanced in the high K vs high K-Ca media. Relative
to the low K condition more glutamine is lost from the tissue (see
Fig. 4). Thus the increased accumulation of glutamine appears to
be due to an increase in uptake rather than an increase in retention.

TABLE IV. UPTAKE OF $^{14}$C GLUTAMINE INTO DENTATE SLICES IN VARIOUS MEDIA

| Medium | Radioactivity (dpm/mg x $10^3$) | | | |
|---|---|---|---|---|
| | Tissue Glutamine | Tissue Glutamate | Medium Glutamate | Tissue Glutamate & Glutamine & Medium Glutamate |
| 3 mM KCl | 112±7 | 101±11 | 78±6 | 352±19 |
| 56 mM KCl | 75±5 | 79±07 | 198±26 | 291±20 |
| 56 mM KCl 3 mM CaCl$_2$ | 57±2 | 78±07 | 312±37 | 448±31 |

Slices were incubated for six min in the presence of 0.4 mM $^{14}$C glutamine
(2.65 x $10^5$ dpm/nmol) in oxygenated Kreb's Ringer bicarbonate medium.
Means ± SEM for six experiments. (From Hamberger et al, 1977c).

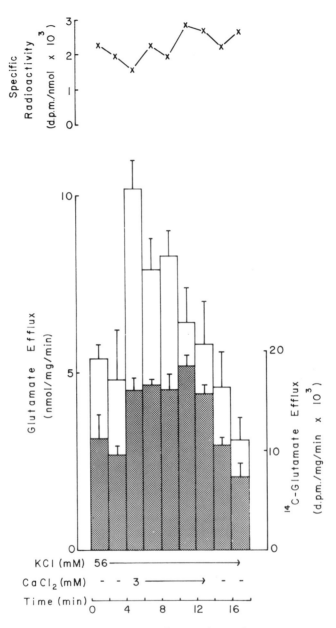

Fig. 13    Effect of prolonged stimulation with 3 mM CaCl$_2$ in the presence of 56 mM KCl on glutamate synthesis.    $^{14}$C glutamine was included throughout the experiment.    Total glutamate is shown by the white bars and radioactive glutamate by the dark bars (From Hamberger et al, 1977c).

## Regulation of glutaminase activity

The following experiment was designed to test whether glutaminase is regulated by the concentration of its end product glutamate as previously has been shown for the isolated enzyme (Weil-Malherbe, 1969; Krebs, 1935). Slices were loaded with glutamate by incubating them in the presence of 2 mM glutamate in the medium (Table 5). This results in a tripling in slice glutamate content under all ionic conditions and a marked inhibition of $^{14}$C glutamate formation from $^{14}$C glutamine in the high KCl medium (48%) and the high KCl Ca medium (56%). Less inhibition is observed in the low K medium (26%).

The experiment described above, shown in Table 5, also provides another demonstration of the increase of glutamine uptake in the high K-Ca medium as shown in Table 4. After summing the total radioactivity (tissue glutamine and glutamate plus medium glutamate) there is an increase in the total radioactivity

TABLE V.  EFFECTS OF L-GLUTAMATE (2mM) ON GLUTAMATE CONTENTS IN DENTATE SLICES AND MEDIA AFTER INCUBATION WITH 0.4mM $^{14}$C-GLUTAMINE

| Medium | Control | | L-Glutamate | |
|---|---|---|---|---|
| 3mM KCl | Tissue | Medium | Tissue | Medium |
| Glutamate | | | | |
| nmol/mg | 114±14 | - | 379±84 | - |
| dpm/mg x 10³ | 107±22 | 76±12 | 36±4 | 99±19 |
| Glutamine | | | | |
| dpm/mg x 10³ | 113±9 | - | 158±28 | - |
| 56mM KCl | | | | |
| Glutamate | | | | |
| nmol/mg | 120±4 | - | 292±24 | - |
| dpm/mg x 10³ | 93±3 | 151±10 | 30±5 | 96±7 |
| Glutamine | | | | |
| dpm/mg x 10³ | 85±3 | - | 113±10 | - |
| 56mM KCl, 3mM CaCl₂ | | | | |
| Glutamate | | | | |
| nmol/mg | 84±8 | - | 276±24 | - |
| dpm/mg x 10³ | 81±15 | 310±79 | 23±2 | 143±40 |
| Glutamine | | | | |
| dpm/mg x 103 | 57±2 | - | 332±92 | - |

Slices were incubated in 0.2ml/2min for 6 min in Krebs Ringer bicarbonate medium in 95% O$_2$:5% CO$_2$ at 37°. The glutamate group was incubated with 2 mM glutamate during the 20 min perincubation period as well as during the 6 min labelling period. Means ± S.E.M. for 3 experiments in each group. (From Hamberger et al, 1977c).

due to glutamine accumulation. The total radioactivity in the
control and the L-glutamate treated sample is similar but the
distribution of radioactivity is markedly different. Glutamine
accumulates in the tissue in the high K-Ca condition to a similar
extent even though glutamate synthesis decreases and the tissue
content of glutamate is different. This shows that the stimulation of glutamine transport is independent of the tissue glutamate
content and the amount of glutamate synthesized and released.
Glutamine uptake is not stimulated by Ca in the low K medium. The
stimulation of glutamine uptake appears related to the presence of
Ca and depolarization.

Glutaminase activity was measured in freeze-thawed homogenates in order to determine if the different ionic media have a
direct effect on the enzyme. Glutaminase activity is not significantly different in low K, high K or high K - Ca media (data
not shown). Thus the enzyme is not regulated directly by an
effect of the ions, rather it is regulated by a consequence of
the ions on other processes. One of these it appears is end
product inhibition.

### SUMMARY OF GLUTAMATE SYNTHESIS IN THE RELEASABLE POOL

We can summarize our findings on the biosynthesis of glutamate (Fig. 14). The synthesis of glutamate derived from glucose
or glutamine increases when the nerve terminals release glutamate
in response to depolarization and Ca influx. Glutamate release
from this compartment is reduced by a unilateral entorhinal
lesion so that it appears related to perforant path afferents to
the dentate gyrus. Nearly all of the releasable glutamate is
newly synthesized. 70% is derived from glutamine and the remainder from glucose. Glutamate synthesized from glutamate is preferentially released over and above tissue stores. In fact almost
all the glutamate produced from glutamine is released into the
medium. The control of glutamate synthesis derived from glutamine
is in part due to an increase in glutamine uptake which is related
to the presence of Ca and depolarization. In addition glutaminase
activity is regulated by end product inhibition: when the glutamate levels fall glutaminase activity increases.

### IS GLUTAMATE A TRANSMITTER IN THE DENTATE GYRUS?

We can now return to the question initially posed in this
chapter and evaluate the evidence that glutamate is a neurotransmitter in the molecular layer of the dentate gyrus.

1. Release. Glutamate release is dependent on Ca, antagonized by Mg and stimulated by depolarizing conditions. The
depolarization conditions can be high K, veratridine or electrical
pulses and in each case there is a robust, rapid efflux of glutamate. These properties are indistinguishable from those of GABA,
a known transmitter in the molecular layer. On the basis of

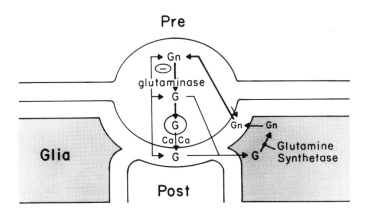

Fig. 14    Summary of the proposed regulation of glutamate synthesis
and cellular interactions at a glutamatergic synapse.  Depolarization
and Ca influx triggers a substantial glutamate release which lowers
the pool of glutamate.  This relieves presynaptic glutaminase from
end product inhibition and results in an activation of the enzyme.
Ca dependent release of glutamate also stimulates glutamine influx
from the extracellular space.  The glutamate released is recaptured
from the presynaptic ending via high affinity transport systems and
made available again for release.  In addition, glutamate probably
enters glial cells where it is converted into glutamine which is
released into the extracellular space and made available to the
boutons to serve again as a glutamate precursor.  (From Hamberger
et al, 1977c).

subcellular fractionation studies, glutamate release appears to
originate from nerve endings and is dramatically reduced by
destruction of the perforant path input to the dentate granule
cells.
     2.  Postsynaptic response.  The postsynaptic response elicited
by stimulation of the perforant path is antagonized by amino
phosphonobutyric acid, a presumptive glutamate antagonist.  We
have not yet, however, shown that the permeability changes in the
postsynaptic membrane and the metabolic responses created by
natural stimulation are identical to those created by applied
glutamate.
     3.  Inactivation.  The molecular layer contains a powerful
glutamate transport system which can rapidly sequester extracellular glutamate.  Destruction of the perforant path appears to
reduce glutamate transport so that at least a portion of the
uptake is associated with the integrity of these fibers.
     4.  Storage and Synthesis.  Glutamate is effectively stored
in the tissue, rapidly synthesized, and made available for release
upon depolarization and Ca influx.  The presynaptic terminals can

store and control the synthesis of glutamate.

These data then support our contention that glutamate may be the transmitter of the perforant input to the granule cells. However, additional work is still necessary particularly on the nature of the postsynaptic response and on the specificity of the secretory process for glutamate. Research is presently continuing along these lines.

DISCUSSION

Glutamate synthesis and release share many properties in common with those of other transmitters. Like ACh or catecholamines, newly synthesized glutamate is preferentially released. Similarly, glutamate and ACh synthesis are regulated in part through the increased accumulation of its precursor. In addition, glutamate synthesis appears regulated by end product inhibition, similar to one of the processes regulating tyrosine hydroxylase in the biosynthesis of catecholamines.

Glutamate metabolism is unique in that it appears to be linked to glial cells in a tight conservation cycle (Fig. 14). Our studies show that glutamine is of vital importance for sustaining releaseable glutamate pools. Glutamine is not transported from the blood (Sokoloff, 1976) but rather appears to be synthesized in glial cells after which it is released into the extracellular space and made available to glutamatergic nerve terminals. In turn those boutons synthesize and release glutamate. A part of the extracellular glutamate is recaptured and made available for release again (Sandoval et al, 1977) or metabolized within the neuron; another part most likely is captured by glial cells where it is rapidly converted to glutamine. In fact, it has been suggested that glial cells effectively utilize many precursors which they convert into glutamine (Benjamin and Quastel, 1972). Studies on glutamate metabolism in brain appear most readily interpretable in terms of two general compartments, one neuronal and one glial. Glial metabolism involving glutamate is largely biosynthetic using various precursors (e.g. acetate, glutamate and GABA) to generate glutamine which is released into the extracellular space. Neuronal metabolism, on the other hand, uses glucose for energy production and glutamine for central metabolism and the synthesis of certain transmitters. Based on computer modeling studies (van den Berg and Garfinkel, 1971) it appears as if glutamate metabolism in neurons and glial cells is linked: glutamine is supplied to neurons and GABA is returned to glial cells. GABA, however, is unlikely to provide the link in all cases. In the molecular layer of the dentate gyrus. for example, GABAnergic neurons are very sparse. In the overall balance of metabolism in brain GABA and glutamine may be coupled, but in the domain of glutamatergic boutons the metabolic intertwining

would be expected to be between glutamine and glutamate. Tissue
glutamine is rapidly lost to the medium and glutamate efflux
drops drastically within minutes after glutamine is removed.
Thus the relatively high levels of extracellular glutamine in the
brain (0.4 mM in the cerebral spinal fluid) are probably necessary
for an adequate supply in terminals because no high affinity
system for glutamine has been found in synaptosomes (Roberts and
Keen, 1974). Glial cells then serve as a metabolic helper to
glutamatergic boutons by supplying glutamine and in turn receiving
glutamate and probably other metabolites from the neurons.
Glutamatergic boutons operate with the aid of the glia in a
relatively interdependent manner. This interaction is likely to
be regulated. Glutamine efflux appears to increase in response to
elevated K$^+$, and if from glia this may indicate one level of
responsive interaction between synaptic activity and the glial
nutrient role in the surround of the glutamatergic bouton.

In the operation of a glutamatergic neuron, glutamate
uptake probably serves a particularly key role beyond its presumptive role of inactivation. In fact, uptake as an inactivation
mechanism in the CNS remains hypothetical in that prolongation of
an electrophysiological response as a consequence of reuptake
blockage -- as readily shown for cholinergic neurons when their
inactivation process is blocked -- has not yet been demonstrated.
A number of facts indicate that reuptake should be considered in
a broader context. As described in this symposium (see chapters
by Cuenod, McGeer and Chan-Palay) uptake occurs at all or nearly
all structures of the neuron -- terminals, cell body and dendrites. And as described in this chapter, very little of the
accumulated transmitter is available for release prior to its
degradation. It may be that uptake is a general function usually
relegated to a neuron which releases that substance as a find of
conservation and protective mechanism. Some transmitters --
particularly the amino acids -- have a carbon skelton very useful
to intermediary metabolism so their conservation would benefit
the neuron or glial cell. In glutamatergic neurons, for example,
uptake of glutamate as discussed above provides additional intermediates to fuel cellular metabolism. Moreover, in order for
cells to signal effectively, the extracellular space must normally
contain low levels of transmitter. This may be achieved by high
affinity transport systems in neurons releasing the substance
and, in some cases, with the aid of other surrounding glial
cells. In the absence of a "clear" extracellular environment,
feedback modulation such as seen at catecholaminergic neurons
would not be possible.

In contrast to catecholamines, members of the amino acid
transmitter group, particularly glutamate, occur as continuous
concentrations throughout the nervous system and are contained in
many structures not directly involved in neurotransmission.
Nonspecific increases of glutamic acid in the extracellular space

might cause detrimental effects so that effective uptake systems throughout the CNS are probably very critical. Even though the direct inactivation of the glutamate released by neurotransmission is probably largely done by reuptake into the presynaptic compartment, uptake is also probably necessary to maintain low glutamate levels throughout the CNS. Our findings show that in the presence of glutamine, much of the synthesized glutamate "leaks" into the medium even in the absence of stimulation. Accordingly, a breakdown of the glial or neuronal uptake system would lead to an immediate increase in extracellular glutamate which, in addition to general excitation, might even cause death of nerve cells. High levels of glutamate are cytotoxic to certain neurons. A malfunction of the high-affinity uptake system leading to high extracellular glutamate levels has actually been proposed as a cause in neuropathological conditions associated with cell death (Olney, 1974). Thus we would suggest that reuptake be considered in a broader context: in addition to inactivation it serves as a metabolic conservation mechanism and a protection process.

## ACKNOWLEDGEMENT

This work was supported by grants from NIH and NIMH. CWC is receipent of Research Scientist award from NIDA. We are grateful to Dr John Haycock for helpful comments on the manuscript and Miss Julene Mueller for secretarial aid.

## REFERENCES

Alger, B.E. and Teyler, T.J. (1976) Brain Res., 110, 463-480.
Balcar, V.J. and Johnston, G.A.R. (1975) J. Neurochem., 24, 875-879.
Benjamin, A.M. and Quastel, J.H. (1972) Biochem J., 128, 631-646.
Berl, S., Clarke, D.D. and Schneider, D. (1975) In: Metabolic Compartmentation and Neurotransmission; relation to brain structure and function, Plenum Press, New York.
Biscoe, T.J. and Straughan, D.W. (1966) J. Physiol., Lon. 183, 341-359.
Bliss, T.V.P. and Gardner-Medwin, A.R. (1973) J. Physiol., Lond., 232, 357-374.
Bliss, T.V.P. and Lomo, T. (1973) J. Physiol., Lond., 232, 331-356.
Blackstad, T.W., Fuxe, K. and Hökfelt, T. (1967) Z. Zellforsch, 78, 463-473.
Bradford, H.F. and Richards, C.D. (1976) Brain Res., 105, 168-172.
Bradford, H.F. and Ward, H.F. (1976) Brain Res., 110, 115-125.
Cotman, C.W., Haycock, J.W. and White, W.F. (1976) J. Physiol., 254, 475-505.
Clements, A.N. and May, T.C. (1974) J. Exp. Biol., 61, 421-442.
Crawford, I.L. and Conner, J.D. (1973) Nature (Lond) 244, 442-443.

Cull-Candy, S.G., Donnellan, J.F., James, R.W. and Lunt, G.G. (1976) Nature, Lond. 262, 408-409.

Curtis, D.R., Duggan, A.W., Felix, D., Johnston, G.A.R., Tebécis, A.K. and Watkins, J.C. (1972) Brain Res., 41, 283.

Curtis, D.R. and Watkins, J.C. (1965) Pharmacol. Rev., 17, 342.

Davidson, N. (1976) In: Neurotransmitter Amino Acids, Academic Press, London; New York; San Francisco, pp. 6-38.

de Belleroche, J.S. and Bradford, H.F. (1972) J. Neurochem., 19, 585-602.

Douglas, R.M. and Goddard, G.V. (1975) Brain Res., 86, 205-215.

Dudar, J.D. (1974) Neuropharmacol., 13, 1083-1089.

Gerschenfeld, H.M. (1973) Physiol. Rev., 53, 1-119.

Hamberger, A.C., Chiang, G.H., Nylén, E.S., Scheff, S.W. and Cotman, C.W. (submitted).

Hamberger, A.C. Chiang, G.H., Sandoval, M.E. and Cotman, C.W. (submitted).

Hawkins, R.A., Miller, A.L., Nielsen, R.C. and Veech, R.L. (1973) Biochem. J., 134, 1001-1008.

Haycock, J.W., Levy, W.B., Denner, L. and Cotman, C.W., J. Neurochem., (in press).

Johnson, J.L. (1972) Brain Res., 37, 1-17.

Krebs, H.A. (1935) Biochem. J., 29, 1951-1961.

Levy, W.B., Redburn, D.A. and Cotman, C.W. (1973) Science, 181, 676-678.

Logan, W.J. and Snyder, S.H. (1971) Nature (Lond.) 234, 297-299.

Logan, W.J. and Snyder, S.H. (1972) Brain Res., 42, 413-431.

Lynch, G.S., Rose, G., Gall, C. and Cotman, C.W. (1975) Golgi Centennial Symposium Proceedings (Antini, M., ed.) Raven Press, New York.

McBride, W.J., Aprison, M.H. and Kusano, K. (1976) J. Neurochem., 26, 867-971.

McIlwan, H., Harvey, J.A. and Rodriguez, G. (1969) J. Neurochem., 16, 363-370.

Martin, D.L. (1975) In: GABA in Nervous System Function Roberts, E., Chase, T.N. and Tower, D.B., eds.) pp. 347-386, Raven Press, New York.

Matthews, D.A., Cotman, C.W. and Lynch, G. (1976) Brain Res., 115, 1-21.

Mays, L.E. and Best, P.J. (1975) Expl. Neurol., 47, 268-279.

Moore, R.Y. and Halaris, A.E. (1975) J. Comp. Neuro., 164, 171-183.

Nadler, J.V., Vaca, K.W., White, W.F., Lynch, G.S. and Cotman C.W. (1976), Nature, 260, 538-540.

Nadler, J.V., White, W.F., Vaca, K.W., Redburn, D.A. and Cotman, C.W. (1977) J.Neurochem., 29, 279-290.

Olney, J.W. (1974) In: Heritable Disorders of Amino Acid Metabolism (Nyhan, W.L., ed) pp. 501-509, Wiley, New York.

Pickel, V.M., Segal, M. and Bloom, F.E. (1974) J. Comp. Neuro. 155, 15-20.

Plum, C.M. (1974) J. Neurochem., 23, 595-600.

Roberts, P.J. and Keen, P. (1974) Brain Res., 67, 352-357.

Salganicoff, L. and De Robertis, E. (1965) J. Neurochem., 12, 287-309.

Sandoval, M.E. and Cotman, C.W. (1977) Neuroscience, in press.

Sandoval, M.E., Horch, P. and Cotman, C.W. (submitted).

Segal, M. and Bloom, F.E. (1974) Brain Res., 72, 99-114.

Segal, M. (1976) Br. J. Pharmac., 58, 341-345.

Sokoloff, L. (1976) In: Basic Neurochemistry (Siegel, G., Albers, R.W., Katzman, R. and Agranoff, B.W., ed) 2nd Ed., pp. 388-413, Brown and Co., Boston.

Spencer, H.J., Gribkoff, V.K., Cotman, C.W. and Lynch, G.S. (1976) Brain Res., 105, 471-481.

Storm-Mathisen, J. (1976) In: GABA in Nervous System Function (Roberts, E., Chase, T.N. and Tower, D.B., eds.) pp 148-168. Raven Press, New York.

Storm-Mathisen, J. (1977) Brain Res., 120, 379-386.

Takeuchi, A. and Takeuchi, N. (1963) Nature, 198, 490-491.

Teyler, T.J. and Alger, B.E. (1976) Brain Res., 115, 413-425.

Van Baumgarten, R., Bloom, R., Oliver, F.E. and Salmoirkiglu (1963) Arch. Gen. Physiol., 277, 125-135.

Van den Berg, C.J. and Garfinkel, D.A. (1971) Biochem. J., 123, 211-218.

Watkins, J.C. (1973) Biochem. Soc. Symp., 36, 33-47.

Weil-Malherbe, H. (1969) J. Neurochem., 16, 855-864.

White, W.F., Nadler, J.V. Hamberger, A., Cotman, C.W., and Cummins, J. (1977) Nature, in press.

Yamamoto, C. and Matsui, S. (1976) J. Neurochem., 26, 487-491.

Young, A.B., Oster-Granite, M.L., Herndon, R.M. and Snyder, S.H. (1974) Brain Res., 73, 1-13.

# ROLE OF GABAERGIC AND GLYCINERGIC TRANSMISSIONS IN THE SUBSTANTIA NIGRA IN THE REGULATION OF DOPAMINE RELEASE IN THE CAT CAUDATE NUCLEUS

A. Chéramy[*], A. Nieoullon and J. Glowinski
([*]Research worker of la Société des Usines Chimiques Rhône-Poulenc)
Groupe NB, INSERM U.114,Collège de France, Paris 5e -F

## INTRODUCTION

It is well known that the substantia nigra contains numerous GABAergic terminals (Fonnum et al.,1974 ; Kataoka et al., 1974 ; Bak et al., 1975 ; Ribak et al., 1976). Most of these originate from the striatum (Feltz, 1971 ; Precht and Yoshida, 1971 ; Crossman et al., 1973 ; Fonnum et al., 1974 ; Kataoka et al.,1974; Bak et al., 1975; Dray et al.,1976) and/or the globus pallidus (Hattori et al.,1973,1975). According to electrophysiological studies, some of the striato-nigral inhibitory neurons projecting into the substantia nigra are involved in the regulation of the activity of an important nigro-thalamic pathway (Albe-Fessard et al.,1975 ; Deniau et al.,1976). It is also generally assumed that descending GABAergic neurons contribute to the control of the acti- vity of the nigro-striatal dopaminergic neurons. Several electro- physiological (Aghajanian and Bunney, 1975), biochemical (Anden and Stock, 1973; Lloyd et al., 1977) and pharmacological (Tarsy et al.,1975) studies have suggested that these GABAergic neurons exert a direct inhibitory action on the dopaminergic neurons. Besides this direct inhibitory input on dopaminergic neurons, other GABAergic neurons projecting into the pars reticulata could indi- rectly exert a facilitatory control on dopaminergic neurons by inhibiting nigral inhibitory interneurons (Dray and Straughan,1976; Fahn, 1976 ; Chéramy et al., 1977c). We postulated that the inhibi- tory interneurons were glycinergic since high amounts of glycine are present in the substantia nigra (Perry et al.,1971). Further- more, as revealed in microiontophoretic studies, glycine inhibited the activity of numerous nigral cells in the pars reticulata and in the pars compacta and its effects were specifically antagonized

by strychnine (Crossman et al.,1973; Dray and Gonye, 1975; Dray et
al., 1976).

An in vivo model was used in our studies on the role of GABA-
ergic and glycinergic transmissions on the regulation of the nigro-
striatal dopaminergic pathway at the substantia nigra level. Changes in the activity of the dopaminergic neurons were estimated by
measuring the release of $^3$H-dopamine continuously formed from L-
3,5-$^3$H-tyrosine which was administered with a push-pull cannula
implanted in the caudate nucleus of the cat. GABA, glycine and
agonists or antagonists of their receptors as well as related
compounds were usually introduced into the substantia nigra by
means of a second push-pull cannula, although in some cases drugs
were injected at the periphery.

## METHODOLOGICAL CONSIDERATIONS

The experiments were performed with "encéphale isolé" adult
cats. Physiological monitoring, push-pull cannula (Nieoullon et al.
1977a), perfusion procedure (Chéramy et al., 1977a,b) and biochemical analysis (Giorguieff et al., 1976) have been extensively
described previously. Briefly, a discrete area of the left caudate
nucleus was continuously superfused with an artificial cerebrospinal fluid containing L-3,5-$^3$H-tyrosine (40 Ci/mM, 40 μCi/ml,
500 μl/15 min). This allows the continuous synthesis of $^3$H-dopamine
in the dopaminergic nerve terminals since tyrosine hydroxylase,
the first enzyme involved in the biosynthesis of dopamine, is only
present in catecholaminergic neurons. The spontaneous release of
newly synthesized $^3$H-dopamine is easily detected in superfusates.
It reaches a steady state level (about 2nCi/15 min  fraction ;
about 100 times the blank value) after a short labelling period
(about 90 min)(Nieoullon et al.,1977a). This spontaneous release
can be modulated by a variety of physical or pharmacological treatments applied to the ipsilateral substantia nigra. For instance,
it is inhibited by the electrocoagulation or by the cooling of the
substantia nigra (Nieoullon et al.,1977a) and more specifically
during the nigral application of dopamine ($10^{-7}$M)(Chéramy et al.,
1977e) which reduces the firing of dopaminergic neurons by acting
on dopaminergic autoreceptors (Aghajanian and Bunney, 1975). On
the contrary the release of $^3$H-dopamine in the caudate nucleus is
increased during electrical or mechanical stimulation of the
substantia nigra (Nieoullon et al., 1977a). A similar effect is
seen during the superfusion of the substantia nigra with $K^+$ (30mM)
(Chéramy et al., 1977c) or substance P ($10^{-8}$M)(Chéramy et al.,
1977e). The release of $^3$H-dopamine from dopaminergic terminals is
thus dependent on the firing rate of dopaminergic neurons (Davies
and Dray, 1976).

## THE DIRECT GABAERGIC INHIBITORY INPUT ON THE NIGRO-STRIATAL DOPAMINERGIC PATHWAY

If a striato-nigral GABAergic descending system exerts an inhibitory role on the activity of the dopaminergic neurons, the interruption of GABAergic transmission by a GABAergic blocker should increase the firing of the dopaminergic neurons. Results obtained with picrotoxin support this hypothesis. Injected at the periphery, picrotoxin (0.25 to 2.5 mg/kg ip) stimulated the release of $^3$H-dopamine. The effect was particularly striking 90 min after the drug injection. However, this treatment induced seizures with important modifications of electroencephalogram pattern. Therefore, picrotoxin was introduced for 15 to 60 min into the substantia nigra through a second push-pull cannula. Under these conditions no seizure was observed and the various physiological parameters recorded, including the electroencephalogram and the blood pressure, were not altered. The results obtained were similar to those observed when the drug was injected at the periphery, i.e. the release of $^3$H-dopamine was markedly enhanced during the nigral application of the GABAergic antagonist. This effect was only seen when the push-pull cannula was precisely located in the substantia nigra, and the rate of release returned to control levels shortly after the removal of the drug from the superfusion medium.

According to electrophysiological studies, diazepam, a tranquillizing benzodiazepine, prevents the suppressing effect of bicuculline on the inhibitory potential evoked in the cat substantia nigra by the stimulation of the caudate nucleus (Schaffner and Haefely, 1975). Such an effect on GABAergic transmission has also been observed in other brain areas (Polc et al., 1974 ; Polc and Haefely, 1976). It has been postulated that diazepam could act at a presynaptic level by enhancing GABA release (Costa et al., 1975 ; Haefely et al., 1975). We thus injected diazepam before or after the injection of picrotoxin. The picrotoxin induced release of $^3$H-dopamine in the caudate nucleus was prevented or reversed by the peripheral injection of diazepam (10 mg/kg ip). However, diazepam by itself did not modify the spontaneous release of the transmitter. These results provided strong arguments in favor of a tonic inhibitory control of the GABAergic neurons on the nigro-striatal dopaminergic pathway. To complete these experiments we examined the effects of the nigral application of GABA and other GABAergic agonists on the release of $^3$H-dopamine. To our surprise the expected immediate inhibition of the activity of the dopaminergic neurons was not seen.

STIMULATION OF $^3$H-DOPAMINE RELEASE IN THE CAUDATE NUCLEUS DURING
THE NIGRAL APPLICATION OF GABA AND RELATED COMPOUNDS

In a first series of experiments, either GABA ($10^{-5}$M) or
muscimol ($10^{-6}$M) or GABAcholine ($10^{-5}$M), two GABAergic agonists,
were introduced during 15 min into the substantia nigra. Surprisingly, these treatments stimulated the release of $^3$H-dopamine in
the caudate nucleus in a way comparable to that obtained with
picrotoxin. Similar effects were seen with compounds such as gamma-
hydroxybutyrate ($10^{-5}$M) and baclofen ($10^{-6}$M). Furthermore, in
contrast to the observations in the rat in which the peripheral
injection of gamma-hydroxybutyrate reduced the firing of dopaminergic neurons, the intraperitoneal injection of gamma-hydroxybutyrate
in the cat stimulated the release of $^3$H-dopamine regardless of the
dose used from 30 to 300 mg/kg ip. Although the mechanisms of
action of gamma-hydroxybutyrate and baclofen are not yet well established, these drugs have generally been shown to mimick the effect
of GABA (Edwards and Kuffler, 1959 ; Anden and Stock, 1973). An
activation of $^3$H-DA release was also seen during the application
of aminooxyacetic acid which is an inhibitor of GABA transaminase,
the enzyme involved in the inactivation of GABA. However, the effect
was not immediate ; it developed as a function of time. Since GABA
inhibits the activity of various cells in the substantia nigra
including the neurons of the pars compacta which is particularly
rich in dopaminergic cell bodies, the stimulating effect of GABA
and other compounds tested on the release of $^3$H-dopamine must be
indirect. This suggests that a GABAergic inhibitory input in the
substantia nigra is exerting a facilitatory effect on the release
of $^3$H-dopamine from dopaminergic terminals through polysynaptic
pathways.

The facilitatory effect of GABA on $^3$H-dopamine release into
the caudate nucleus was antagonized when picrotoxin was added with
GABA into the superfusion medium of the push-pull cannula inserted
into the substantia nigra. This was surprising since a summation
of the stimulating effects of picrotoxin and GABA was expected.
Whatever the mechanisms involved, this antagonism indicates that
the GABA-induced release of $^3$H-dopamine is mediated by an interaction of GABA with GABAergic receptors.

Although GABA, muscimol, GABAcholine, gamma-hydroxybutyrate
and baclofen initially stimulated the release of $^3$H-dopamine in
the caudate nucleus, the temporal pattern in the changes in the
$^3$H-transmitter release induced by these compounds was different
when they were introduced during one hour into the substantia
nigra. A transient inhibition of $^3$H-dopamine which followed the
initial stimulation was observed with GABA ($10^{-5}$M) and GABA-
choline ($10^{-5}$M) but not with the other compounds. This inhibitory
phase could correspond to the direct inhibitory effect of GABA

on dopaminergic neurons. These results demonstrate the complexity
of the GABAergic mechanisms occurring in the substantia nigra and
reveal that muscimol, gamma-hydroxybutyrate and baclofen exhibit
some properties distinct from those of GABA. It cannot be excluded
that two types of GABAergic receptors present in the substantia
nigra exhibit slight differences in their affinity for GABA and
for muscimol or GABA related compounds. In fact, on the basis of
electrophysiological data, it has been claimed, that the cells
distributed in the pars reticulata were more sensitive to the
microiontophoretic application of GABA than the dopaminergic cells
located in the pars compacta (Aghajanian and Bunney, 1975 ; Dray
et al., 1976).


POSSIBLE CONTROL OF THE NIGRO-STRIATAL DOPAMINERGIC NEURONS BY
                NIGRAL GLYCINERGIC INTERNEURONS

     According to the data discussed previously, some GABAergic
neurons projecting into the substantia nigra exert a direct inhibitory effect on dopaminergic neurons, but others indirectly facilitate the release of $^3$H-dopamine in the caudate nucleus. This
indirect facilitation could result from an inhibitory influence
of GABAergic neurons on nigral inhibitory interneurons in contact
with the dopaminergic neurons. Such a circuit has already been
postulated by other authors (Dray and Straughan, 1976 ; Fahn,1976).
These interneurons could be glycinergic (Chéramy et al.,1977c) ;
high levels of glycine are found in the substantia nigra (Perry
et al., 1971). The microiontophoretic application of glycine
results in the inhibition of cells both in the pars compacta and
the pars reticulata (Dray et al.,1976). Furthermore, according to
Crossman et al.(1973) and to Dray and Gonye (1975), the inhibiting
effect of glycine was antagonized by strychnine but not by picrotoxin  or bicuculline.

     A slight sustained inhibition of the release of $^3$H-dopamine
was observed in the ipsilateral caudate nucleus when glycine
($10^{-5}$M) was introduced into the substantia nigra. The inhibiting
effect of glycine ($10^{-5}$M) on $^3$H-dopamine release cannot be attributed to an unspecific action on GABA receptors, since GABA induces
an opposite effect. This inhibition was no longer seen when strychnine, a specific glycinergic antagonist (Curtis and Johnston,1974;
Krnjevic, 1974) was added with glycine to the push-pull cannula
introduced into the substantia nigra. The nigral application of
strychnine alone resulted in a progressive activation of $^3$H-dopa-
mine release from the caudate nucleus. Similar results were obtained when strychnine (1 mg/kg ip) was injected at the periphery.
This suggests the presence of a tonic glycinergic inhibitory influence on the dopaminergic neurons. Obviously, further experiments
are required to confirm the hypothesis of an involvement of glyci-

nergic interneurons in the control of the activity of the dopaminergic neurons.

## POSSIBLE CONTROL OF [3]H-DOPAMINE RELEASE BY GABAERGIC NEURONS THROUGH EXTRANIGRAL POLYSYNAPTIC PATHWAYS

One of the advantages of our approach is that any influence
on the dopaminergic neurons is easily visualized by the direct in
vivo estimation of the transmitter released from nerve terminals.
However, as others this method has some limitations which should
be taken into consideration in interpreting the data obtained. In
contrast to electrophysiological studies, our method does not enable
us to evaluate changes in the range of the millisecond since the
superfusate fractions are collected every 10 or 15 minutes. The
second push-pull cannula introduced into the substantia nigra
allowed the determination of the effects of limited and well-
defined concentrations of transmitters and of agonists or antagonists of their receptors. The extent of the diffusion from the
tip of the cannula is rather limited. For instance,no stimulating
effect of picrotoxin on [3]H-dopamine release was seen when the tip
of the cannula was not in the substantia nigra but only in its
close surroundings (Chéramy et al., 1977a). Nevertheless, the
applied compounds may simultaneously act on a great number of un-
identified cells and the resulting effect observed could represent
the summation of several processes. Besides the dopaminergic neurons, other neuronal pathways originating both in the pars compacta
(Chan-Palay, 1977) and the pars reticulata (for a review see Usunoff
et al., 1976) may be influenced by descending GABAergic neurons.
Some of these pathways could also be involved in the regulation of
[3]H-dopamine release in the caudate nucleus. For instance, GABAergic
neurons could inhibit the activity of the nigro-thalamic pathway
originating in the pars reticulata (Deniau et al.,1976) and influence [3]H-dopamine release through the thalamo-striatal projection or
the thalamo-cortico-striatal loop (for a review see Tebecis,1974).
In this case, the change in [3]H-dopamine release from nerve terminals
would not be related to an increased firing of dopaminergic neurons,
but to a presynaptic regulation of the transmitter release. In fact,
the electrical stimulation of the nucleus centromedianus of the
thalamus (McLennan, 1964) and the electrical stimulation of the
motor cortex (Nieoullon et al., 1977b) resulted in an activation of
dopamine release in the caudate nucleus. These effects could be
mediated by thalamo-striatal cholinergic neurons (Wagner et al.,
1975 ; Simke and Saëlens, 1977) and by cortico-striatal glutamatergic neurons (Divac et al., 1977) respectively. Both acetylcholine and glutamic acid stimulate the release of newly synthesized
[3]H-dopamine in striatal slices (Giorguieff et al., 1977). The
cholinergic and glutamatergic neurons could act directly on dopaminergic terminals in the caudate nucleus. Indeed, the stimulating

effect of acetylcholine (Giorguieff et al., 1976) and L-glutamic acid (Giorguieff et al., 1977) on $^3$H-dopamine release was still seen in the presence of tetrodotoxin, suggesting the presence of cholinergic and glutamatergic presynaptic receptors on dopaminergic terminals. Finally, such polysynaptic pathways could be involved in the stimulatory effects of the nigral application of GABA and related compounds on the release of $^3$H-dopamine in the caudate nucleus.

## CONCLUSION

There are converging biochemical data in the literature which indicate that the interuption of GABAergic transmission (McGeer et al., 1976 ; Garcia-Munoz et al., 1977 ; DiChiara et al., 1977 ; Racagni et al., 1977 ; Chéramy et al., 1977a) induces an activation of the nigro-striatal dopaminergic neurons. They support the hypothesis of a direct tonic inhibitory influence of descending GABAergic neurons on the activity of nigral dopaminergic cells made in several electrophysiological and anatomical studies (Aghajanian and Bunney, 1975 ; Hattori et al., 1975). There is still a discrepancy concerning the direct effect of GABA, GABA agonists or related compounds on the regulation of the activity of dopaminergic neurons. This has been extensively discussed in the present chapter since under our experimental conditions such treatments favor the release of $^3$H-dopamine in the caudate nucleus. These results are not necessarily in contradiction with the hypothesis of the direct inhibitory control of GABAergic neurons on dopaminergic cells. We propose that some descending GABAergic neurons, which may correspond to a distinct GABAergic pathway, exert an effect on the control of dopamine release in the caudate nucleus through indirect mechanisms. They could either act on nigral inhibitory interneurons in contact with the dopaminergic cells or influence neuronal systems acting on dopaminergic terminals through polysynaptic pathways. As discussed extensively elsewhere (Chéramy et al., 1977d), the respective role of those GABAergic direct inhibitory and indirect facilitatory inputs on dopaminergic transmission in the caudate nucleus could be dependent on the state of activity of the dopaminergic neurons.

## ACKNOWLEDGMENT

This study was supported by grants from DRME (contract n° 76. 329) and la Société des Usines Chimiques Rhône Poulenc. We acknowledge Mrs M.L. Kemel for her excellent assistance.

REFERENCES

Aghajanian, G.K., and Bunney, B.S., 1975, Dopaminergic and non-dopaminergic neurons of the substantia nigra : differential responses to putative transmitters, in :"Neuropsychopharmacology", pp 442-452 (J.R. Boissier, H. Hippius, & P. Pichot, eds) Excerpta Medica, Amsterdam & American Elsevier Pub.Co. Inc. N.Y.

Albe-Fessard, D., Deniau, J.P., Feger, J., Lackner, D., Jacquemin, J., and Ohye, C., 1975, Reciprocal connections between the striatum, the substantia nigra and the ventrolateral nucleus of the thalamus, in :"Neuropsychopharmacology" pp 434-443 (J.R. Boissier, H. Hippius and P. Pichot, eds),Excerpta Medica, Amsterdam & American Elsevier Pub.Co.Inc. N.Y.

Anden, N.E., and Stock, G., 1973, Inhibitory effect of gamma-hydroxybutyric acid and gamma-aminobutyric acid on the dopamine cells in the substantia nigra. Naunyn-Schmiedeberg's Arch. Pharmacol. $\underline{279}$: 89-92

Bak, I.J., Choi, W.B., Hassler, R., Usunoff, K.G., and Wagner, A., 1975, Fine structural synaptic organization of the corpus striatum and substantia nigra in rat and cat, in:"Advances Neurol".Vol.$\underline{9}$, pp 25-41 (D.B. Calne, T.N. Chase & A. Barbeau, eds) Raven Press, N.Y.

Chan-Palay, V., 1977, Cerebellar dentate nucleus : organization, cytology and transmitters, p.202, Springer Verlag, Berlin

Chéramy, A., Nieoullon, A., and Glowinski, J., 1977a, Effects of peripheral and local administration of picrotoxin on the release of newly synthesized [3]H-dopamine in the caudate nucleus of the cat. Naunyn Schmiedeberg's Arch.Pharmacol. $\underline{297}$:31-37

Chéramy, A., Nieoullon, A., and Glowinski, J., 1977b, Blockade of the picrotoxin-induced in vivo release of dopamine in the cat caudate nucleus by diazepam, Life Sciences, $\underline{20}$: 811-816

Chéramy, A., Nieoullon, A., and Glowinski, J., 1977c, In vivo changes in dopamine release in the caudate nucleus and the substantia nigra of the cat induced by nigral application of various drugs including GABAergic agonists and antagonists, in:"Interactions among putative neurotransmitters in the brain" (S. Garattini, J.F. Pujol & R. Samanin, eds) Raven Press, N.Y. (in press)

Chéramy, A., Nieoullon A., and Glowinski, J., 1977d, Stimulating effects of gamma-hydroxybutyrate on dopamine release from the caudate nucleus and the substantia nigra of the cat. J. Pharmacol. exp. Ther. (in press)

Chéramy, A., Nieoullon, A., Michelot, R.,and Glowinski, J., 1977e, Effects of intranigral applications of dopamine and substance P.on the in vivo release of newly synthesized [3]H-dopamine in the ispilateral caudate nucleus of the cat. Neurosci.Letters, $\underline{4}$: 105-109

Costa, E., Guidotti, A., Mao, C.C., and Suria, A., 1975, New
    concepts on the mechanism of action of benzodiazepines, Life
    Sci. 17: 167-186

Crossman, A.R., Walker, R.J.,and Woodruff, G.N., 1973, Picrotoxin
    antagonism of gamma-aminobutyric acid inhibitory responses and
    synaptic inhibition in the rat substantia nigra. Brit.J.
    Pharmacol. 49: 696-698

Curtis, D.R., and Johnston, G.A.R., 1974, Amino acid transmitters
    in the mammalian central nervous system, Rev. Physiol., 69:
    96-188

Davies, J., and Dray, A., 1976, Substance P in the substantia
    nigra, Brain Research, 107: 623-627

Deniau, J.M., Feger, J., and Le Guyader, C., 1976, Striatal evoked
    inhibition of identified nigro-thalamic neurons, Brain Research,
    104: 152-156

DiChiara, G., Porceddu, M.L., Spano, P.F., and Gessa, G.L., 1977,
    Haloperidol increases and apomorphine decreases striatal
    dopamine metabolism after destruction of striatal dopamine-
    sensitive-adenylate cyclase by kainic acid, Brain Research,
    130: 374-382

Divac, I., Fonnum, F., and Storm-Mathisen, J., 1977, High affinity
    uptake of glutamate in terminals of cortico-striatal axons,
    Nature, 266: 377-378

Dray, A., and Gonye, T.J.,1975, Effects of caudate stimulation and
    microiontophoretically applied substances on neurons in the
    rat substantia nigra.J.Physiol.(Lond.) 246: 88-89

Dray, A., Gonye, T.J., and Oakley, N.R., 1976, Caudate stimulation
    and substantia nigra activity in the rat. J. Physiol.(Lond.)
    259: 825-849

Dray, A., and Straughan, D.W., 1976, Synaptic mechanisms in the
    substantia nigra, J.Pharm.Pharmacol.,28: 400-405

Edwards, C., and Kuffler, S.W., 1959, The blocking effect of  Ɣ-
    aminobutyric acid (GABA) and the action of related compounds
    on single nerve cells. J. Neurochem. 4: 19-30

Fahn, S., 1976, Biochemistry of the basal ganglia, in:"Advances in
    Neurology", Vol.14 , pp 59-88 (R.Eldridge & S. Fahn, eds) Raven
    Press, N.Y.

Feltz, P., 1971, Gamma-aminobutyric acid and a caudate-nigral inhi-
    bition, Can.J.Physiol.Pharmacol. 49: 1113-1115

Fonnum, F., Grofova, I., Rinvik, E., Storm-Mathisen, J., and
    Walberg, F., 1974, Origin and distribution of glutamate decar-
    boxylase in substantia nigra of the cat, Brain Research, 71:
    77-92

Garcia-Munoz, M., Nicolaou, N.M., Tulloch, I.F, Wright, A.K. and
    Arbuthnott, G.W., 1977, Feedback loop or output pathway in
    striato-nigral fibers ? Nature, 265: 363-365

Giorguieff, M.F., Le Floc'h, M.L., Westfall, T.C., Glowinski, J.,
    and Besson, M.J., 1976, Nicotinic effect of acetylcholine on
    the release of newly synthesized $^3$H-dopamine in rat slices
    and cat caudate nucleus, Brain Research, 106: 117-131
Giorguieff, M.F., Kemel, M.L., and Glowinski, J., 1977, Presynaptic
    effect of L-glutamic acid on the release of dopamine in rat
    striatal slices. Neurosci.Lett. (in press)
Haefely, W., Kulcsar, A., Möhler, H., Pieri, L., Polc, P., and
    Schaffner, R., 1975, Possible involvement of GABA in the
    central actions of benzodiazepines, Adv. Biochem. Psycho-
    pharmacol. 10: 131-152
Hattori, T., McGeer, P.L., Fibiger, H.C., and McGeer, E.G, 1973,
    On the source of GABA containing terminals in the substantia
    nigra: electron microscopic autoradiographic and biochemical
    studies, Brain Research, 54: 103-114
Hattori, T., Fibiger, H.C., and McGeer, P.L., 1975, Demonstration
    of a pallido-nigral projection innervating dopaminergic neu-
    rons, J. Comp. Neurol. 162: 487-504
Kataoka, K., Bak, I.J., Hassler, R., Kim, J.S.,and Wagner, A., 1974,
    L-glutamate decarboxylase and choline acetyltransferase acti-
    vity in the substantia nigra and the striatum after surgical
    interruption of the striato-nigral fibers of the baboon,
    Exp. Brain Research, 19: 217-227
Krnjevic, K., 1974, Chemical nature of synaptic transmission in
    vertebrates, Physiol.Rev. 54: 418-540
Lloyd, K.G., Shemen, L., and Hornykiewicz, O., 1977, Distribution
    of high affinity sodium-independent ($^3$H)-gamma-aminobutyric
    acid (($^3$H)GABA) binding in the human brain : alterations in
    Parkinson's disease, Brain Research, 127: 269-278
McGeer, E.G., Innanen, V.T., and McGeer, P.L., 1976, Evidence on
    the cellular localization of adenyl cyclase in the neostriatum
    Brain Research, 118: 356-358
McLennan, H., 1964, The release of acetylcholine and 3-hydroxy-
    tyramine from the caudate nucleus, J. Physiol.(Lond.) 174:
    152-161
Nieoullon, A., Cheramy, A., and Glowinski, J., 1977a, An adaptation
    of the push-pull cannula method to study the in vivo release
    of $^3$H-dopamine synthesized from $^3$H-tyrosine in the cat caudate
    nucleus : effects of various physical and pharmacological treat-
    ments. J. Neurochem. 28: 819-828
Nieoullon, A., Chéramy, A., and Glowinski, J., 1977b, Release of
    dopamine evoked under punctate electrical stimulations of the
    motor and visual areas of the cerebral cortex in both caudate
    nucleus and in the substantia nigra in the cat. Brain Research,
    (in press)
Perry, T.L., Berry, K., Hansen, S., Diamond, S., and Mok, C., 1971,
    Regional distribution of amino-acids in human brain obtained at
    autopsy, J. Neurochem. 18: 513-519

Polc, P., Möhler, H., and Haefely, W., 1974, The effect of diazepam
      on spinal cord activities : possible site and mechanisms of
      action. Naunyn Schmiedeberg's Arch. Pharmacol. 284: 319-337
Polc, P., and Haefely, W., 1976, Effects of two benzodiazepines,
      phenobarbitone, and baclofen on synaptic transmission in the
      cat cuneate nucleus, Naunyn Schmiedeberg's Arch.Pharmacol.
      294: 121-131
Precht, W. and Yoshida, M., 1971, Blockade of caudate-evoked inhi-
      bition of neurons in the substantia nigra by picrotoxin,
      Brain Research, 32: 229-233
Racagni, G., Bruno, F., Maggi, A., Cattabeni, F., and Groppetti,A.,
      1977, Functional interactions between dopamine and GABA in
      the nigro-striatal system. 6th International meeting of the
      International Society for Neurochemistry, Satellite Symposium,
      on dopamine, Southampton.
Ribak, C.E., Vaughn, I.E., Saito, K., Barker, R., and Roberts, E.,
      1976, Immunocytochemical localization of glutamate decarboxy-
      lase in rat substantia nigra, Brain Research, 116: 287-298
Schaffner, R., and Haefely, W., 1975, The effects of diazepam and
      bicuculline on the strio-nigral evoked potentials, Experientia
      (Basel) 31: 732
Simke, J.P., and Saelens, J.K., 1977, Evidence for a cholinergic
      fiber tract connecting the thalamus with the head of the
      striatum of the rat. Brain Research, 126: 487-495
Tarsy, D., Pycock, C., Meldrum,B., and Marsden, C.D., 1975, Rotatio-
      nal behavior induced in rats by intranigral picrotoxin, Brain
      Research, 89: 160-165
Tebecis, A.K., 1974, Transmitters and identified neurons in the
      mammalian central nervous system, Scientechnica Ltd, Bristol
Usunoff, K.G., Hassler, R., Romansky, K., Usunova, P., and Wagner,
      A., 1976, The nigrostriatal projection in the cat, Part 1,
      Silver impregnation method. J. Neurol. Sci. 28:265-288
Wagner, A., Hassler, R., and Kim, J.S., 1975, Striatal cholinergic
      enzyme activities following discrete centromedian nucleus
      lesion in cat thalamus, Trans. int. Soc. Neurochem. (Barcelona)
      abst.59, p.116

# THE INTERACTION BETWEEN GABA-ERGIC DRUGS AND DOPAMINERGIC STIMULANTS

J. Arnt, A.V. Christensen and J. Scheel-Krüger

Department of Pharmacology, Royal Danish School of Pharmacy, DK-2100 Copenhagen, Denmark, (A.V.C.) Department of
Pharmacology and Toxicology, H. Lundbeck & Co., Copenhagen
and (J.S.K.) Psychopharmacological Research Laboratory
Sct. Hans Mental Hospital, Roskilde.

In the human brain there is evidence for a functional dysba-
lance between γ-aminobutyric acid (GABA) and dopamine in Parkinson's
disease and Huntington's chorea (McGeer and McGeer, 1976). In both
diseases there are a pronounced decrease in GABA and its synthesizing enzyme glutamic acid decarboxylase (GAD) in the basal ganglia
system. Dopamine is in addition decreased in parkinsonism. A useful new therapeutic strategy for these diseases might be a supplementary treatment with drugs which increase GABA receptor activity.
Obviously there is a need for methods measuring the specific pharmacological effects of GABA-ergic drugs in vivo. This lack has
consequently limited conclusions based on clinical trials with
apparently unspecific drugs like baclofen (Naik et al, 1976). As
a model compound we used muscimol which until now has shown to be
the most potent and selective GABA-agonist able to penetrate the
bloodbrain barrier (Naik et al, 1976; Scheel-Krüger et al, 1977 a).
We investigated the behavioural interactions of different putative
GABA-ergic drugs with morphine and different dopaminergic stimulants. As an animal model for dopaminergic activity we used the
stereotyped behaviour and locomotor activity induced by methylphenidate, apomorphine and cocaine. Similarly there are evidence that
morphine induced motility is associated with dopaminergic mechanisms (Scheel-Krüger et al, 1977 b; Scheel-Krüger et al, 1977 c).
Male mice of the NMRI-strain, weighing 18-25 g were used throughout. The motility was measured in groups of three in Motron activity cages. The stereotypy was assessed by placing groups of two
in perspex boxes placed on corrugated paper. After one hour the
gnawing intensity was scored according to a four-point rating scale

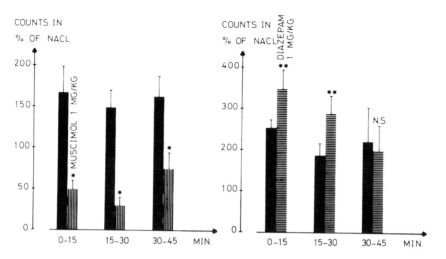

FIGURE 1.    The effect of muscimol and diazepam on cocaine motility.
All mice received cocaine 10 mg/kg i.p. 15 min after muscimol
1 mg/kg s.c. ( ▥▥▥ ); diazepam 1 mg/kg i.p. ( ▬▬ ) or saline ( ▬▬ ).
The motility was measured immediately and expressed in per cent of
mice receiving only saline.    Each value represents the mean ± s.e.m.
of 6 groups of 3 mice.    * P < 0,05 or ** P = 0,05 compared with
the saline-cocaine group according to Student's t-test.

as indicated in fig. 3.    The following drugs were used: Muscimol,
HBr; diazepam (valium-    ); baclofen; methylphenidate, HCl; apomorphine, HCl; cocaine, HCl and morphine, HCl.    All doses refer to
the salts.

       The locomotor stimulant effect of cocaine, methylphenidate
and apomorphine was pronounced inhibited by muscimol in a nonse-
dative dose of 1 mg/kg (Fig. 1, fig. 2).    The low motility was not
due to stereotypies but was observed to reflect true sedation beginning 5-10 min after injection of the stimulant and lasting 45-
60 min.    Muscimol also antagonized morphine induced hypermotility
(Fig. 2).    This sedative action of the drug combination is remarkable, since muscimol not only reduced the hypermotility induced by
the stimulants to control values but furthermore depressed the motility to a very low level.    Similar but less marked effects were
found with baclofen (Fig. 2).    In contrast we found that diazepam
in a slightly ataxic dose surprisingly increased the cocaine motility.    These data show a pharmacological differentiation between a
benzodiazepine and a GABA-ergic drug.    This has not been observed
in most other pharmacological models (Haefely et al, 1975; Naik et
al, 1976).

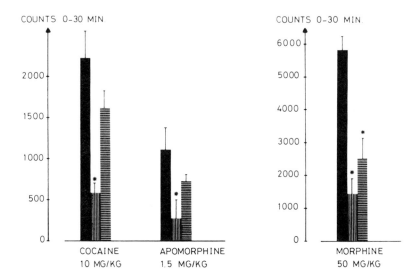

FIGURE 2.  The effect of muscimol and baclofen on hypermotility induced by various stimulants.  Cocaine (i.p.) and apomorphine (s.c.) was
injected 15 min after muscimol 1 mg/kg s.c. ( ||||| ), baclofen 5 mg/
kg i.p. ( ▦ ) or saline ( ■ ).  Morphine (i.p.) was injected 15
min before GABA-agonist or saline.  The motility was measured immediately for 30 min.  Each value represents the mean ± s.e.m. of at
least 4 groups of 3 mice.  * P < 0,05 compared with the saline-sti-
mulant group according to Student's t-test.


     The combined treatment of muscimol (0,63 and 1 mg/kg) with me-
thylphenidate (10 mg/kg) or cocaine (30 mg/kg) induced an intense
stereotyped gnawing in the corrugated paper (Fig. 3).  We consider
this effect as a strong increase in stereotypy since this behaviour
is only seen after high doses of methylphenidate (30-60 mg/kg) (Pedersen and Christensen, 1972).  Concerning cocaine muscimol induce
a facilitation of the occurrence of stereotyped gnawing.  Even high
doses of cocaine (30-60 mg/kg) induce by itself only a weak or no
gnawing response.  Higher doses of muscimol (2 mg/kg) induce heavy
sedation, which inhibits the occurrence of strong gnawing induced
by the drug combination.  (Scheel-Krüger et al, submitted).

     The present results emphasize that GABA-ergic mechanisms not
exclusively depress all behavioural elements dependent on dopaminergic activity since the motility was completely inhibited whereas

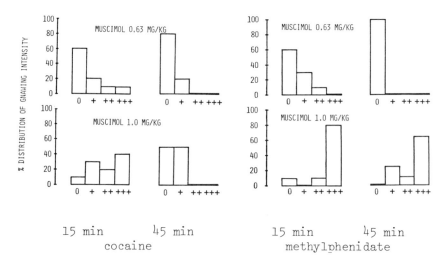

FIGURE 3. Stereotyped gnawing in mice induced by combined treatment of muscimol with methylphenidate or cocaine. Muscimol 0,63 or 1,0 mg/kg s.c. was injected 15 or 45 minutes before methylphenidate 10 mg/kg s.c. or cocaine 30 mg/kg i.p. The gnawing intensity was scored on corrugated paper after one hour as follows: 0: No gnawing; +: weak gnawing ; ++: moderate gnawing; +++: strong gnawing. Each figure represents the gnawing distribution in per cent in 5-10 groups of 2 mice.

the development of stereotypy was facilitated by muscimol. This pharmacological profile is also found with THIP, a new specific analogue of GABA (Krogsgaard-Larsen et al, 1977); results in preparation. The nature of this differential interaction with dopaminergic stimulants is not certain but exactly the same effects are observed when muscimol is injected into the nucleus accumbens of rats treated systemically with apomorphine (Scheel-Krüger et al, submitted). Similarly, it has been shown that muscimol antagonized the dopamine-dependent locomotor activity of ergometrine after injection into nucleus accumbens (Scheel-Krüger et al 1977 d). Furthermore, muscimol by itself produce a strong stereotypy after injection into substantia nigra (Scheel-Krüger et al, 1977 a). However, it had to be considered that the muscimol induced increase in methylphenidate and cocaine stereotypy could be secondary to an increased synthesis of neostriatal dopamine, which in turn changes the dopaminergic stereotypy. This biochemical effect is well-known after drugs inhibiting impulse flow in the nigrostriatal dopaminergic neurones and has also been found with muscimol (in preparation).

This alternative, however is unlikely since inhibition of dopamine synthesis with α-methyltyrosine did not attenuate the gnawing activity induced by muscimol and methylphenidate or cocaine (Scheel-Krüger et al, submitted). This suggests that the stereotypy-facilitating action of muscimol depends on a direct GABA-mechanism influencing stereotyped behavior.

The mechanism of action of baclofen and benzodiazepines still needs further clarification. In our model baclofen acts like muscimol although less pronounced. In contrast, diazepam had the opposite effect on the cocaine-induced motility. Other workers have found baclofen unspecific, while diazepam had strong GABA-like activity (Haefely et al, 1975; Naik et al, 1976). These discrepancies may be due to different GABA systems and/or different ways of interaction with GABA neurones resulting in differences in pharmacological profile. These complex GABA-dopamine interactions severiously challenge the generally accepted hypothesis of GABA as mainly or only controlling behavioural inhibition and emphasize the need for models evaluating the functions of GABA in the central nervous system.

Acknowledgements. We are grateful to Dr. P. Krogsgaard-Larsen, Department of Chemistry, The Royal Danish School of Pharmacy for the generous supply of muscimol for this study.

## REFERENCES

Haefely, W., Kulcsar, A., Möhler, H., Pieri, L., Polc, P., and Schaffner, R., 1977, Possible involvement of GABA in the central actions of benzodiazepines, in "Mechanism of Action of Benzodiazepines" (E. Costa and P. Greengard, eds.), pp. 131-151, Raven Press, New York.

Krogsgaard-Larsen, P., Johnston, G.A.R., Lodge, D., and Curtis, D.R., 1977, A new class of GABA agonist, Nature 268:53-55.

McGeer, P.L., and McGeer, E.G., 1976, Enzymes associated with the metabolism of catecholamines, acetylcholine and GABA in human controls and patients with Parkinson's disease and Huntington,s chorea, J. Neurochem 26:65-76.

Naik, S.R., Guidotti, A. and Costa, E, 1976, Central GABA receptor agonists: Comparison of muscimol and baclofen, Neuropharmacology 15:479-484.

Pedersen, V. and Christensen, A.V., 1972, Antagonism of methylphenidate - induced stereotyped gnawing in mice, Acta Pharmacol Toxicol. 31:488-496.

Scheel-Krüger, J., Arnt, J., and Magelund, G., 1977 a, Behavioural
    stimulation induced by muscimol and other GABA agonists in-
    jected into the substantia nigra, Neuroscience Letters 4:
    351-356.
Scheel-Krüger, J., Bræstrup, C., Nielsen, M., Golembiowska, K. and
    Mogilnicka, E., 1977, Cocaine: Discussion of the role of dopa-
    mine in the biochemical mechanism of action, in "Cocaine and
    other stimulants" (E.H. Ellinwood and M.M. Kilbey, eds.),
    pp. 373-407, Plenum Press, New York.
Scheel-Krüger, J., Golembiowska, K., and Mogilnicka, F., 1977,
    Evidence for increased apomorphine sensitive dopaminergic
    effects after acute treatment with morphine, Psychopharmaco-
    logy, 53:55-63.
Scheel-Krüger, J., Cools, A.R., and Honig, W., 1977, Muscimol an-
    tagonizes the ergometrine-induced locomotor activity in nuc-
    leus accumbens: Evidence for a GABA-dopaminergic interaction,
    Europ. J. Pharmacol 42:311-313.

GLUTAMATE DECARBOXYLASE, PROPERTIES AND THE

SYNAPTIC FUNCTION OF GABA

Ricardo Tapia and Manuel Covarrubias

Departamento de Biología Experimental, Instituto
de Biología, Universidad Nacional Autónoma de México
Apdo. Postal 70-600, México 20, D. F., México

Among the factors involved in the function of chemical
synapses, the synthesis of the neurotransmitter to be released is
a crucial event. This is particularly important in view of recent
evidence indicating that in the case of catecholamines (Glowinski,
1975), acetylcholine (Molenaar and Polak, 1975) and GABA (Ryan
and Roskoski, 1975; Tapia, 1976), there is a pool of newly
synthesized transmitter from which it is preferentially released.
The knowledge of the regulatory mechanisms controlling the
activity of the neurotransmitter synthesizing enzymes is thus
fundamental for the understanding of synaptic phenomena. In the
present paper I will deal with some properties of glutamate
decarboxylase (GAD) relevant to the synaptic function of GABA.

PYRIDOXAL PHOSPHATE, GABA SYNTHESIS AND NEURONAL EXCITABILITY

GAD catalyzes the one-step synthesis of GABA. This enzyme in
brain tissue is particularly sensitive to deficiencies of
pyridoxal 5'-phosphate (PLP), both in vitro (Roberts et al., 1964;
Tapia et al., 1967) and in vivo (Tapia et al., 1969; Tapia and
Pasantes, 1971). Furthermore, this dependence on PLP
concentration in vivo has been demonstrated to occur in synaptic
terminals (Pérez de la Mora et al., 1973). The relationships
between the role of PLP in controlling GAD activity and the
transmitter function of GABA at inhibitory synapses seems to be
fairly well established, since the results of several kinds of
experiments indicate that GAD activity is a critical factor for
controlling neuronal excitability (Tapia, 1974; 1975). An
inhibition of this enzyme results in the appearance of seizures,

TABLE I.   CORRELATION BETWEEN GAD INHIBITION AND SEIZURES AT
           DIFFERENT GABA LEVELS IN MICE

| Treatment | % change | | | Seizures |
|---|---|---|---|---|
| | GABA | GAD[a] | DOPA-D | |
| Glutamyl hydrazide | +35 | -54 (-6) | —— | Yes |
| + PLP 30, 60 and | +70 | -56 (-8) | —— | Yes |
| 90 min later | +195 | -52 (-2) | —— | Yes |
| PLP-glutamyl hydrazone | -61 | -63 (0) | -64 | Yes |
| $\alpha$-methyl-DOPA | —— | 0 | -72 | No |

The doses used were: glutamyl hydrazide, 1 g/kg; PLP, 50 mg/kg;
PLP-glutamyl hydrazone, 80 mg/kg; $\alpha$-methyl-DOPA, 400 mg/kg.
Data from Tapia et al., 1967; Tapia and Pasantes, 1971; Tapia
et al., 1975.

[a]Measured in the absence of exogenous PLP.  In parentheses it is
shown the change when 0.1 mM PLP was added to the incubation
mixtures.

even after the levels of GABA have been previously increased.
This is well exemplified by experiments in which the concentration
of GABA was initially augmented by inhibition of GABA-amino-
transferase and subsequently GAD was inhibited secondarily to a
decrease of PLP levels (Table I).  Under these experimental
conditions all animals showed convulsions.  Among several other
$B_6$-enzymes tested in brain, only DOPA decarboxylase was inhibited
by the combination of drugs used in the latter experiments (Tapia
and Pasantes, 1971).  However, it has been demonstrated that a
70% inhibition of DOPA decarboxylase does not produce convulsions
when GAD activity is not affected (Table I).

The foregoing data led us to postulate that the activity of
GAD is a regulatory mechanism of cerebral excitability through a
coupling of the synthesis and the release of GABA, and further,
that the concentration of PLP played a key role in such mechanism
(Tapia, 1974; 1975; Tapia et al., 1975).  With these considerations
in mind, we recently carried out some experiments aimed at
obtaining information on two points centrally connected with the
above postulation.  The first refers to the kinetics of GAD with
respect to its interactions with PLP, glutamate and the Schiff base
PLP-glutamate, and the second to the possibility that GAD may bind
to membranes.  The latter point is particularly relevant for
explaining the coupling between the synthesis and the secretion of
GABA, and seemed possible in view of the findings of Salganicoff
and De Robertis (1965) and Fonnum (1968) that GAD is capable of
binding to nervous tissue membranes in the presence of $Ca^{2+}$.

### KINETIC STUDIES OF GAD: A FREE PLP-INDEPENDENT AND A FREE PLP-DEPENDENT FORMS OF ACTIVITY

Since we were interested in the regulation of GAD activity by PLP, we decided to study kinetically the effect on the enzyme of several structural analogs of the glutamate-PLP Schiff base, which on theoretical grounds should be useful for obtaining information on the properties of the active site. The main results of these experiments, using the reduced Schiff bases aminooxyacetate-PLP (PLPAOA), GABA-PLP, cysteinesulfinate-PLP and glutamate-PLP, indicate that two forms of GAD activity exist in brain, one dependent on and the other independent of free PLP (Tapia and Sandoval, 1971; Bayón et al., 1977a). Part of these results are summarized in Fig. 1. It is evident that the enzyme cannot be inhibited by PLPAOA more than about 2/3 of its maximal activity when saturated with PLP. Because of the structure of PLPAOA, we concluded that the glutamate-PLP Schiff base analogs could inhibit only the free PLP-dependent form of GAD activity (Tapia and Sandoval, 1971; Bayón et al., 1977a). A detailed kinetic study of the interactions of GAD with glutamate, PLP and the glutamate-PLP Schiff base in the absence of inhibitors confirmed the existence of a free PLP-dependent and a free PLP-independent GAD activities, and indicated, in agreement with the inhibition studies, that the Vmax ratio free PLP-dependent/free PLP-independent was close to 3 (Fig. 2) (Bayón et al., 1977b).

These studies also permitted to conclude that the glutamate-PLP Schiff base cannot be a substrate of the enzyme, and therefore that the trapping of PLP in the form of Schiff bases by glutamate, by amines or by other amino acids, including GABA itself, might contribute to the regulation of the free PLP-dependent GAD activity in nerve terminals, in vivo. The free PLP-independent GAD activity would not be susceptible to this type of regulation and this might play a role in maintaining a basal rate of GABA synthesis. The possibility of regulation by the formation of the PLP-GABA Schiff base is particularly interesting in view of the high concentration of GABA in GABAergic terminals (Fonnum and Walberg, 1973), which is in the same order of magnitude as the dissociation constant of the GABA-PLP Schiff base (about 40 mM, Bayón, Possani, Rode and Tapia, unpublished). In this respect it is also possible that the GABA taken up by the synaptic terminals might contribute to the trapping of PLP.

### BINDING OF GAD TO PHOSPHOLIPID MEMBRANES

For the hypothesis of the synthesis-secretion coupling of GABA the finding that GAD may be bound to membranes in the presence of $Ca^{2+}$ (Salganicoff and De Robertis, 1965; Fonnum, 1968) was of particular importance. In order to develop an experimental model

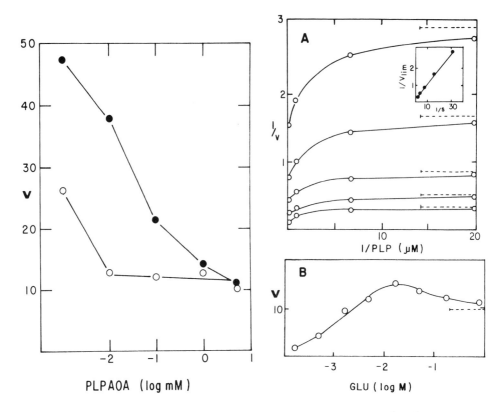

PLPAOA ( log mM )

I/PLP ( μM )

GLU ( log M )

FIGURE 1.  Effect of PLPAOA on GAD activity in mouse brain.  v,
μmoles/h/g.  The first point in each curve indicates the value in
the absence of inhibitor.  Glutamate concentration was 33 mM.  O,
in the absence of exogenous PLP; ●, with 0.1 mM PLP added.  Data
from Tapia and Sandoval (1971) (see also Bayón et al., 1977a).

FIGURE 2.  A, double reciprocal plots of GAD activity vs PLP
concentrations, at several fixed glutamate concentrations.  v,
μmoles/h/g.  The glutamate concentrations used for each curve
were, from top to bottom (mM): 0.031, 0.062, 0.12, 0.25 and 0.5.
The dashed lines show the estimated asymptotes for each curve;
these values, which correspond to the free PLP-independent
activity, were replotted as $1/V_{lim}$ vs 1/S (glutamate) in the
inset.  B, plot of v vs glutamate concentration at very low PLP
concentration (0.5 μM).  The dashed line indicate the estimated
asymptote to the curve, which again indicates the free PLP-
independent activity, because the free PLP has been trapped by
glutamate.  The data were taken from Bayón et al., 1977b.

for studying the synthesis-secretion coupling, we have studied the effect of $Ca^{2+}$ on the binding of soluble GAD to phosphatidylcholine-phosphatidylserine liposomes (Bangham, 1972). As shown in Figs. 3 and 4, in the absence of $Ca^{2+}$ practically no enzyme is bound to the liposomes, but with 0.5 mM $Ca^{2+}$ some enzyme binds and with 2 mM 35% sediments with the liposomes. With 4 or 8 mM $Ca^{2+}$, more than 50% of GAD binds to the phospholipid membranes. Most interestingly, the form of the binding curve is very similar to that reported by Fonnum (1968) using a disrupted synaptosomes fraction (Fig. 3). In contrast to the binding of GAD, and also similarly to the results of Fonnum, $Ca^{2+}$ did not cause any binding of lactate dehydrogenase to the liposomes. This enzyme remained soluble at all $Ca^{2+}$ concentrations used.

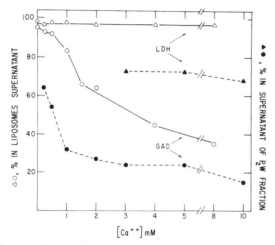

FIGURE 3. Calcium-dependent binding of GAD to phospholipid membranes. Multilamellar phosphatidylcholine-phosphatidylserine (4:1) liposomes (30 mg) were incubated at 37° for 20 min with supernatant (approx. 20 mg protein) of a high-speed centrifugation (100,000 g, 1 h) of mouse brain water homogenates, in the presence of 0.1 mM PLP and the indicated concentrations of $Ca^{2+}$. The control without calcium contained 1 mM EGTA. After incubation the mixture was centrifuged at 100,000 g for 45 min, the pellet was resuspended in 0.4% Triton-X-100 containing 0.1 mM PLP and GAD and lactate dehydrogenase (LDH) activity was measured in the resuspended pellet and in the supernatant. The values refer to the percent of recovered activity. Each point is the mean value of 4-6 independent experiments. The filled symbols refer to the values reported by Fonnum (1968) in the supernatant after the addition of $Ca^{2+}$ to osmotically shocked synaptosomes (fraction $P_2W$).

   That the binding of GAD to the liposomes is not the result of
unspecific binding of protein is demonstrated by the graphs shown
in Fig. 4, which express the binding as relative specific activity
(RSA, % of GAD bound/% of protein bound), both in the supernatant
and in the liposomes pellet.  In the pellet, the RSA increased
more than 5-fold from 0 to 4 or 8 mM $Ca^{2+}$, whereas the
corresponding decrease was observed in the supernatant.  With 1.5
and 2 mM $Ca^{2+}$ the RSA was well above 1.  The form of the curve is
again very similar to the specific activity curve found by
Salganicoff and De Robertis (1965) for the binding of $Ca^{2+}$ to a
membrane and synaptic vesicles fraction (Fig. 4).  In contrast,
the RSA of lactate dehydrogenase in the liposomes pellet is very
low and tends to decrease with increasing $Ca^{2+}$ concentrations,
while in the supernatant there is a corresponding increase.

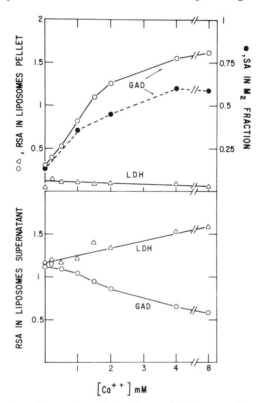

FIGURE 4.  Calcium-dependent binding of GAD to phospholipid
membranes, expressed as relative specific activity (RSA = % of
recovered enzyme activity/% of recovered protein).  The
experimental details were as described in the legend to Fig. 3.
The filled symbols refer to the specific activity (SA) values
reported by Salganicoff and De Robertis (1965) in the membranes
and synaptic vesicles fraction ($M_2$) after the addition of $Ca^{2+}$
to osmotically shocked synaptosomes.

SUMMARY AND FINAL COMMENT

The data shown in the present paper emphasize the importance of the knowledge of GAD properties for the understanding of the function of GABA synapses. The studies in vivo have shown that GAD activity is a crucial factor in the control of neuronal excitability, and that it is very much dependent on PLP concentration. The kinetic approach, on the other hand, indicate that this regulation of GAD activity by PLP is exerted only upon one type of enzyme activity, since a free PLP-independent form also exists. Furthermore, the trapping of PLP in the form of Schiff bases might participate in the control of free PLP concentration. By means of this mechanism, the intraterminal GABA could act as a product inhibitor and thus exert a negative feedback control of GAD activity.

If, as the in vivo experiments suggest, the secretion of GABA is coupled to its synthesis, the binding of the synaptoplasmic GAD to membranes, in the presence of low $Ca^{2+}$ concentrations, might represent a fundamental event for the release of the newly synthesized GABA (Tapia, 1974). The finding that this phenomenon occurs with phospholipid vesicles in close parallelism to the binding previously reported with brain membranes, and that it seems to be relatively specific for GAD, provides an experimental model that may be useful for the study of the postulated synthesis-secretion coupling of GABA.

REFERENCES

Bangham, A.D., 1972, Lipid bilayers and biomembranes, Ann. Rev. Biochem. 41:753-776.

Bayón, A., Possani, L.D., and Tapia, R., 1977a, Kinetics of brain glutamate decarboxylase. Inhibition studies with N-(5'-phosphopyridoxyl)amino acids, J. Neurochem. in press.

Bayón, A., Possani, L.D., Tapia, M., and Tapia, R., 1977b, Kinetics of brain glutamate decarboxylase. Interactions with glutamate, pyridoxal 5'-phosphate and glutamate-pyridoxal 5'-phosphate Schiff base, J. Neurochem. in press.

Fonnum, F., 1968, The distribution of glutamate decarboxylase and aspartate transaminase in subcellular fractions of rat and guinea-pig brain, Biochem. J. 106:401-412.

Fonnum, F., and Walberg, F., 1973, An estimation of the concentration of $\gamma$-aminobutyric acid and glutamate decarboxylase in the inhibitory Purkinje axon terminals of the cat, Brain Res. 54:115-127.

Glowinski, J., 1975, Properties and functions of intraneuronal monoamine compartments in central aminergic neurons, in "Handbook of Psychopharmacology", Vol. 3 (L.L. Iversen, S.D. Iversen and S.H. Snyder, eds.), pp. 139-167, Plenum, New York.

Molenaar, P.C., and Polak, R.L., 1975, Preferential release of
    newly synthesized acetylcholine by cortex slices from rat
    brain, in "Metabolic Compartmentation and Neurotransmission"
    (S. Berl, D.D. Clarke and D. Schneider, eds.), pp. 641-649,
    Plenum Press, New York.
Pérez de la Mora, M., Feria-Velasco, A., and Tapia, R., 1973,
    Pyridoxal phosphate and glutamate decarboxylase in subcellular
    particles of mouse brain and their relationship to convulsions,
    J. Neurochem. 20:1575-1587.
Roberts, E., Wein, J., and Simonsen, D.G., 1964, $\gamma$-Aminobutyric
    acid ($\gamma$ABA), vitamin $B_6$, and neuronal function- A speculative
    synthesis, Vitam. Horm. 22:503-559.
Ryan, L.D., and Roskoski, R., Jr., 1975, Selective release of
    newly synthesised and newly captured GABA from synaptosomes by
    potassium depolarisation, Nature 258:254-256.
Salganicoff, L., and De Robertis, E., 1965, Subcellular
    distribution of the enzymes of the glutamic acid, glutamine
    and $\gamma$-aminobutyric acid cycles in rat brain, J. Neurochem.
    12:287-309.
Tapia, R., 1974, The role of $\gamma$-aminobutyric acid metabolism in
    the regulation of cerebral excitability, in "Neurohumoral
    Coding of Brain Function" (R.D. Myers and R.R. Drucker-Colín,
    eds.), pp. 3-26, Plenum Press, New York.
Tapia, R., 1975, Biochemical Pharmacology of GABA in CNS, in
    "Handbook of Psychopharmacology", Vol. 4 (L.L. Iversen, S.D.
    Iversen and S.H. Snyder, eds.), pp. 1-58, Plenum Press,
    New York.
Tapia, R., 1976, Evidence for a synthesis-dependent release of
    GABA, in "Transport Phenomena in the Nervous System" (G. Levi,
    L. Battistin and A. Lajtha, eds.), pp. 385-394, Plenum Press,
    New York.
Tapia, R., and Pasantes, H., 1971, Relationships between
    pyridoxal phosphate availability, activity of vitamin $B_6$-
    dependent enzymes and convulsions, Brain Res. 29:111-122.
Tapia, R., and Sandoval, M.E., 1971, Study on the inhibition of
    brain glutamate decarboxylase by pyridoxal phosphate oxime-0-
    acetic acid, J. Neurochem. 18:2051-2059.
Tapia, R., Pérez de la Mora, M., and Massieu, G., 1967,
    Modifications of brain glutamate decarboxylase activity by
    pyridoxal phosphate- $\gamma$ -glutamyl hydrazone, Biochem.
    Pharmacol. 16:1211-1218.
Tapia, R., Pérez de la Mora, M., and Massieu, G., 1969,
    Correlative changes of pyridoxal kinase, pyridoxal
    5'-phosphate and glutamate decarboxylase in brain, during
    convulsions, Ann. N.Y. Acad. Sci. 166:257-266.
Tapia, R., Sandoval, M.E., and Contreras, P., 1975, Evidence for
    a role of glutamate decarboxylase activity as a regulatory
    mechanism of cerebral excitability, J. Neurochem. 24:1283-1285.

THE POSSIBLE INVOLVEMENT OF GABA AND ITS COMPARTMENTATION IN THE

MECHANISM OF SOME CONVULSANT AND ANTICONVULSANT AGENTS

J. D. Wood, E. Kurylo and S. J. Peesker

Department of Biochemistry, University of Saskatchewan

Saskatoon, Canada

## GABA METABOLISM AND SEIZURE ACTIVITY

### Lack of a Simple Correlation between Seizure Activity and any Single Parameter of GABA Metabolism.

Several research groups have demonstrated that there is no simple relationship between seizure activity and any single parameter of GABA metabolism in brain, be it the concentration of GABA, the activity of glutamate decarboxylase (GAD), the activity of GABA-$\alpha$-oxoglutarate aminotransferase (GABA-T), or the uptake of GABA (see review by Wood, 1975). Typical results with respect to GABA content and GAD activity are shown in Table I which indicates that there is a wide variation in GABA content and GAD activity at the onset of seizures. A close perusal of the data in this table reveals, however, the establishment of a definite pattern with respect to the changes in GABA level relative to the changes in GAD activity at the onset of seizures. Specifically, the greater the inhibition of GAD activity, the greater the GABA content of brain at the onset of seizures. These results suggest that a decrease in GAD activity may be the major factor involved in the induction of the seizures, but that this effect is modulated by the GABA level in the brain, elevations in GABA content counteracting the convulsant action of low GAD activities. A minor role is ascribed to the effect of GABA level in this respect since very great changes in the concentration are required to counteract much smaller changes in GAD activity.

TABLE I.   CHANGES IN GABA CONTENT AND IN GAD ACTIVITY OF BRAIN
AT THE ONSET OF SEIZURES.

| Species | Convulsant agent | GABA (%) | GAD (%) |
|---------|------------------|----------|---------|
| [1]Mouse | Pyridoxal phosphate-glutamyl hydrazone | -34 | -42 |
|  | Glutamic acid-γ-hydrazide | +265 | -82 |
|  | Aminooxyacetic acid | +40 | -64 |
| [2]Rat | Hydrazine | +30 | -86 |
|  | Monomethylhydrazine | -45 | -57 |
| [3]Mouse | Hydrazine | +91 | -69 |
|  | Unsymmetrical dimethylhydrazine | -25 | -49 |
|  | Isonicotinic acid hydrazide | -31 | -45 |

[1]Tapia et al. (1969);   [2]Medina (1963;   [3]Wood and Peesker (1974)

### Development of an Equation Relating Brain Excitability to Changes in GABA Metabolism.

The above observations suggested to us that the excitable
state of the brain might be related to a function containing
GAD activity as the major factor and GABA level as the minor
factor.   This possibility was therefore examined in detail and
the following equation was formulated (Wood and Peesker, 1974).

$$RE_{GABA} = 100 + \frac{\Delta GAD + 0.4\ \Delta(\sqrt{GABA})}{1.4}$$

where $RE_{GABA}$ is the effectiveness of the GABA system with respect to its modulation of brain excitability under particular
experimental conditions and $\Delta GAD$ and $\Delta(\sqrt{GABA})$ are the percentage
changes in GAD activity and in the square root of the GABA con-
tent respectively brought about by the experimental conditions.
The $RE_{GABA}$ value is thus expressed in percent and can be considered a quantitative measure of brain excitability in as much
as it is influenced by the GABA system.

Where there are no changes in GAD activity or GABA level,
i.e. the brain GABA metabolism is functioning normally, the
$RE_{GABA}$ value will be 100%.   On the other hand a complete lack of
function would give a value of 0%.   If the assumption that the
overall level of GABA metabolism is related to the excitable
state of the brain is correct, a hyperexcited state should exist
in the brain in situations where the $RE_{GABA}$ values are less than
100%.   An extension of this mode of thought leads to the conclusion that seizures should occur if the $RE_{GABA}$ value drops to
some definite critical low value.   The demonstration that the
same critical $RE_{GABA}$ value exists with respect to the action of

TABLE II.   $RE_{GABA}$ VALUES AT THE ONSET OF DRUG-INDUCED SEIZURES IN MICE.

| Exp. | Drug (mmol/kg) | Mean time (or range) to onset of seizures (min) | $RE_{GABA}$ (%) |
|------|----------------|--------------------------------------------------|-----------------|
| 1[1] | Hydrazine (2.5) | 65 | 61 |
|      | Hydrazine (4.0) | 20 | 62 |
|      | Unsymm. dimethylhydrazine (6.0) | 60 | 61 |
| 2[1] | Isonicotinic acid hydrazide (2.2) | 34 | 63 |
| 3[1] | Hydrazine (4.0) | 20 | 62 |
| 4[1] | Isonicotinic acid hydrazide (3.0) | 28 | 62 |
| 5[1] | Allylglycine (6.0) | 49 | 64 |
|      | Hydrazine (4.0) | 19 | 64 |
|      | Isonicotinic acid hydrazide (2.2) | 30 | 60 |
| Tapia | PALP-glutamyl hydrazone (0.2) | (30-45) | 64 |
| et al. | Glutamic acid-$\gamma$-hydrazide (12.4) | (120-210) | 67 |
| (1969) | Aminooxyacetic acid (3.7) | (10-20) | 60 |

[1]Data from Wood and Peesker (1974) and Wood and Peesker (unpublished).

different convulsant agents, would provide strong support for the validity of the equation and the concepts embodied in it. The results of such a test are described below.

### Test of the Validity of the Equation.

The data in Table I, together with other unpublished data by Wood and Peesker were used to calculate the $RE_{GABA}$ value in mouse brain at the onset of seizures induced by various chemical agents at different dosage levels (Table II). The $RE_{GABA}$ value existing at the onset of convulsions was remarkably reproducible and constant, not only for different dosages of the same convulsant agent, but also for the different convulsant agents. The above results therefore support the validity of the equation and its inherent hypothesis. In other words, it would appear that the disruption of GABA metabolism by chemical agents can lead to seizures which are a direct result of the deranged GABA metabolism.

The validity of the expression was also supported by data obtained with anticonvulsant agents such as hydroxylamine, aminooxyacetic acid and hydrazine (although these compounds are convulsant agents at high dosage levels, they exhibit an anticonvulsant effect when administered in lesser amounts). The delay in onset of seizures brought about by these agents was related to their ability to maintain the $RE_{GABA}$ value above the critical

level for seizures (Fig. 2 of Wood and Peesker, 1975). The data
presented in this previous publication also allowed determination
of a critical $RE_{GABA}$ value based not just on the action of a
single convulsant agent, but based rather on the actions and
interactions of a variety of convulsant and anticonvulsant agents.
This value was 63% which is in excellent agreement with the values
obtained by its direct determination (Table 2). It must be pointed
out that in order to analyze the anticonvulsant data quantitatively
using $RE_{GABA}$ values, both convulsant and anticonvulsant agents
must act via the GABA system. The presence of a non-GABA mechanism
in either action negates the use of such an approach.


## COMPARTMENTATION OF GABA AND THE EFFECT OF AMINOOXYACETIC ACID

The observed relationship between brain excitability and a
single function containing changes in an enzyme activity and a
metabolite level can only be explained by invoking the concept of
compartmentation of GABA metabolism in brain. We suggest that the
$RE_{GABA}$ value reflects events at a specific subcellular location in
the cell, namely, the GABA concentration in the synaptic cleft.
That changes in GAD activity are the major factor (in the equation)
influencing the functioning of the total GABA system is in accord
with the preferential location of that enzyme in the nerve endings
where it would be in a prime location to influence the concentration of its product (GABA) in the synaptic cleft. In contrast,
GABA-T is a mitochondrial enzyme and elevation in GABA levels resulting from an inhibition of this enzyme might initially be remote
from the synaptic cleft. Very high levels of GABA might therefore
be needed before the effect is transmitted to the GABA concentration
in the cleft, either by a leakage into the latter location, or by
a decrease in the rate of uptake of GABA from the cleft into the
cell. Either phenomenon is in harmony with the minor role ascribed
in the equation to GABA levels.

A knowledge of the distribution of GABA in brain tissue at the
subcellular level and the effect of drugs on this distribution are
critical to a complete understanding of the role of GABA in brain.
Unfortunately, real or putative technical difficulties have hindered
research in this area. Specifically, it has been claimed that the
observed distribution of GABA after subcellular fractionation does
not reflect the in vivo situation, due to the loss of GABA from
the organelles during either the homogenization process or centrifugation procedures, or due to the extensive redistribution of
GABA during fractionation ( Neal and Iversen, 1969, Tachika, et al.,
1972).

Is it possible, however, that the situation is not as serious
as predicted, and that subcellular studies can provide meaningful

results?  For example, we found that the observed GABA content of
synaptosomes and mitochondria was not influenced by exogenous GABA
in the homogenizing medium in concentrations up to 1 mM (isotonic,
sodium-free homogenizing medium;  2°C).  This suggests that extensive redistribution did not take place.  Moreover, Neal and
Iversen (1969) reported that the loss of GABA from the particulate
material did not occur when the homogenate in isotonic, sodium-free
sucrose medium was kept at 0°C for 2 hours, but that the loss occurred only when the preparation was "exposed" to centrifugation, and/or
hypertonic sucrose.  However, these data were not expressed on a per
mg. protein basis, and the loss might not be due to a leakage from
more-or-less intact organelles, but rather to a disintegration of
organelles with release of their contents.  In the latter case,
determination of GABA in the remaining particles could still reflect the in vivo situation.

     In view of this possibility we fractionated brain tissue from
control and aminooxyacetic acid (AOAA) treated mice and determined
the GABA content of the synaptosomal mitochondrial, and supernatant
fractions (Table III).  The AOAA-induced increase in GABA was
greater in the synaptosomes than in the mitochondria, but by far
the greatest percentage increase was in the supernatant fraction.
One explanation, apropos the technical problems outlined above, is
that the AOAA induced increase in GABA occurred in the particles,
but that it was released during fractionation.  An equally plausible
explanation is that the in vivo accumulation of GABA occurred in the
cytoplasm.  Since synaptosomes did not show this magnitude of increase, the data suggest that the increased GABA concentration
occurred in the cytoplasm of neuronal cell bodies or of glia.  This
postulate is in harmony with the minor role ascribed GABA levels in
the $RE_{GABA}$ equation, since the cytoplasmic elevation in GABA would
not be in the best situation to influence GABA levels in the

TABLE III.   EFFECT OF AOAA ON THE SUBCELLULAR DISTRIBUTION OF GABA
             IN MOUSE BRAIN.

| Fraction | GABA (nmol/mg protein) | | $\Delta$GABA (%) |
| | Untreated | AOAA-treated[1] | |
| --- | --- | --- | --- |
| Synaptosomal | 29.7 ± 0.9 (12) | 64.5 ± 6.9 (6) | 117 |
| Mitochondrial | 10.6 ± 0.2 (12) | 16.1 ± 1.3 (6) | 52 |
| Supernatant | 44.6 ± 2.3 (3) | 233.7 ± 6.8 (3) | 424 |

[1] Six hours after the intramuscular administration of 0.23 mmol
AOAA/kg.  Values are mean ± S.E.M. for the number of samples
shown in parenthesis.  GABA was analyzed by the method of
Balcom et al. (1974).  Synaptosomal and mitochondrial enriched
fractions were prepared by the method of Cotman (1974).  Supernatant fractions were prepared by centrifuging 0.32M sucrose
homogenate at 100,000 g for 1 hour.

synaptic cleft compared, for example, with events in the nerve
endings.  AOAA treatment caused no change in the distribution of
protein among the fractions.

In summary, we are of the opinion that subcellular fractionation studies with respect to GABA metabolism are worth performing,
and might well provide a better understanding of the role of GABA
in brain.  It is possible that an extensive accumulation of data
on this topic may help to unravel the real from the artefactual
situations.

## ACKNOWLEDGMENT

This research was supported by the Medical Research Council
of Canada Grant No. MT 3301.

## REFERENCES

Balcom, G. J., Lenox, R. H., and Meyerhoff, J. L., 1975, Regional
    γ-aminobutyric acid levels in rat brain determined after
    microwave fixation. J. Neurochem. 24:  609-613.
Cotman, C. W., 1974, Isolation of synaptosomal and synaptic plasma
    membrane fractions, in "Methods in Enzymology", Vol. 31
    (S. Fleischer and L. Packer, eds.) p.p. 445-452, Academic
    Press, New York.
Medina, M. A., 1963, The in vivo effects of hydrazines and vit-
    amin $B_6$ on the metabolism of gamma-aminobutyric acid.  J.
    Pharmac. Exp. Ther. 140:  133-137.
Neal, M. J., and Iversen, L. L., 1969, Subcellular distribution
    of endogenous and [³H] γ-aminobutyric acid in rat cerebral
    cortex, J. Neurochem. 16:  1245-1252.
Tachiki, K. H., De Feudis, F. V., and Aprison, M. H.  1972.  Studies
    on the subcellular distribution of γ-aminobutyric acid in
    slices of rat cerebral cortex, Brain Res. 36:  215-217.
Tapia, R., De la Mora, M. P., and Massieu, H., 1969,  Correlative
    changes of pyridoxal kinase, pyridoxal-5'-phosphate and
    glutamate decarboxylase in brain, during drug induced con-
    vulsions, Ann. N. Y. Acad. Sci. 166:  257-266.
Wood, J. D., 1975, The role of γ-aminobutyric acid in the mechan-
    ism of seizures, Progress in Neurobiol. 5:  77-95.
Wood, J. D., and Peesker, S. J., 1974, Development of an expression
    which relates the excitable state of the brain to the level
    of GAD activity and GABA content, with particular reference
    to the action of hydrazine and its derivatives, J. Neurochem.
    23:  703-712.
Wood, J. D., and Peesker, S. J., 1975, The anticonvulsant action
    of GABA-elevating agents:  a re-evaluation, J. Neurochem.
    25:  277-282.

# THE GABA RECEPTOR ASSAY: FOCUS ON HUMAN STUDIES

S.J. Enna

Depts. of Pharmacology and Neurobiology & Anatomy

Univ. of Tex. Med. Sch. PO Box 20708 Houston, Tx 77025

Recently a biochemical technique for labeling the synaptic receptor site for γ-aminobutyric acid (GABA) in mammalian brain has been reported (Zukin et al., 1974; Enna and Snyder, 1975; Enna and Snyder, 1977). This procedure has proven to be a versatile new tool for studying the biochemical, pharmacological and neurobiological characteristics of this neurotransmitter receptor site. Among other things, important new information has been obtained about the neuropathological characteristics of certain neurological disorders (Enna et al., 1976a; Enna et al., 1976b; Lloyd et al., 1977), and new insights gained into the neuronal connections which exist in the normal human brain. Furthermore, this receptor binding assay has been used to develop a rapid, simple and sensitive radioreceptor assay capable of measuring trace quantities of GABA in biological tissues and fluids (Enna and Snyder, 1976; Enna et al., 1977e). This ability to measure GABA in human cerebrospinal fluid has resulted in a better understanding of the relationship between brain GABA and central nervous system disorders (Enna et al., 1977c).

The GABA receptor binding assay has also been used as a simple method for studying the structure-activity relationships of this binding site (Enna et al., 1977b) in an attempt to discover more potent and specific chemical agents which may be used to treat neurological and psychiatric disabilities involving GABA. As a result of these studies, recent reports have indicated that there may be two or more pharmacologically distinct receptor sites for this neurotransmitter (Enna et al., 1978; Mohler and Okada, 1977).

The present communication is a brief review of some of the ways in which the GABA receptor binding technique has been used to better understand this important transmitter system. Emphasis is

445

placed on studies involving human subjects and tissues and on the
relationship between GABA, GABA receptors and human disease.

## I.    METHODOLOGY OF GABA RECEPTOR BINDING

The GABA receptor binding technique most commonly used for
human studies has been the method originally described by Zukin
et al. (1974) as modified by Enna and Snyder (1975).  Briefly,
rat or human brain membrane fragments (1 mg protein) are incubated
in 2 ml of 0.05 M Tris-citrate buffer (pH 7.1 at 4°C) containing
8 nM $^3$H-GABA (34 Ci/mmole) in the presence or absence of a high
concentration of unlabeled GABA (1 mM) or bicuculline (0.1 mM),
compounds which are known to interact specifically with this neurotransmitter receptor site.  This suspension is incubated at 4°C
for 5 min, centrifuged at 48,000 x g for 10 min and the resultant
pellet rinsed rapidly and superficially with 15 ml ice cold water
prior to analysis for the amount of $^3$H-GABA bound.  Under these
conditions, membranes which have been treated with 0.05% Triton
X-100 prior to assay contain approximately 8,000 cpm/mg protein
when incubated with $^3$H-GABA alone but only 1,000 cpm/mg protein
when incubated with $^3$H-GABA in the presence of unlabeled GABA or
bicuculline (Enna and Snyder, 1977).  The difference between these
two values, 7000 cpm/mg protein, represents the amount of $^3$H-GABA
which can be displaced by the unlabeled substances and is termed
specifically bound GABA.  Studies on the brain subcellular and regional distribution of this specifically bound GABA suggest that
it represents attachment to the synaptic GABA receptor site (Zukin
et al., 1974; Enna and Snyder, 1975; Enna et al., 1975; Enna et al.,
1977a).  In addition, further evidence that this binding is to the
biologically relevant site is provided by the fact that only these
amino acids and drugs which are known to interact neurophysiologically with the synaptic GABA receptor have any significant potency
in displacing the specifically bound isotope (Enna and Snyder,
1975; Enna and Snyder, 1977).  Thus, these findings suggest that
this binding assay is a valid procedure for studying the GABA receptor site in mammalian brain tissue.

## II.   RECEPTOR BINDING IN HUMAN BRAIN

Important advances in understanding the neurochemical abnormalities present in neurological and psychiatric disorders have
been made by studying autopsy material obtained from individuals
who had suffered with these disorders.  Prior to the advent of receptor binding assays, these investigations centered upon  neurotransmitter and neurotransmitter metabolite levels and on enzyme
activities.  A classical example of the utility of these studies
was the discovery of a dopamine deficit in Parkinson's disease
(Ehringer and Hornykiewicz, 1960) which led to the successful
treatment of this disorder with the neurotransmitter precursor,

levodopa.

However, for drug therapy to be effective it is necessary that the receptor for the drug be unaltered by the disease.  Thus, by studying receptor binding in postmortem brain tissue, it may be possible to determine why some agents are ineffective in certain disorders and to predict what type of drugs may be of benefit.  In addition, the most useful information of this type can be obtained by investigating several neurotransmitter receptor sites simultaneously in order to determine the relationships between the various systems.  For example, with regard to Parkinson's disease, recent receptor binding studies have revealed that, in the caudate nucleus, those neurons which possess receptor sites for dopamine are degenerating in this disorder (Reisine et al., 1977), providing an explanation for the relative ineffectiveness of dopamine receptor agonists in advanced stages of the disease (Table I).  Furthermore, this study revealed significant changes in serotonin, and cholinergic muscarinic receptors in certain areas of the Parkinson brain, changes which are undoubtedly related so some of the symptoms of this disorder.  With respect to the GABA receptor, no alterations in GABA receptor binding were observed in the caudate, putamen or globus pallidus of the Parkinson brain, but a decrease in GABA binding was noted in the substantia nigra (Lloyd et al, 1977).

Huntington's disease, a neurological disorder characterized by a profound degeneration of GABA- and acetylcholine-containing neurons in the basal ganglia (Enna et al., 1977d), has also been studied in this way.  Because of the known deficit of cholinergic cells, attempts have been made to treat Huntington's disease by increasing the brain acetylcholine content (Growdon et al., 1977; Shoulson and Chase, 1975).  Unfortunately, these attempts have met with only limited success.  Receptor binding studies on Huntington brain have suggested that the ineffectiveness of this therapy may be related to the fact that there is a significant reduction in the number of cholinergic muscarinic receptors in the basal ganglia of Huntington patients (Hiley and Bird, 1974; Enna et al., 1976a; Enna et al., 1976b).  Like the cholinergic muscarinic receptor binding, receptors for serotonin are reduced in this disease, but β-adrenergic receptors are unchanged.

Though GABA levels are reduced in Huntington's disease, GABA receptor binding is unchanged or enhanced suggesting that appropriate GABA-mimetic agents may be useful therapy.  Along these lines it has been recently reported that muscimol, a GABA receptor agonist, does not improve the symptoms of Huntington's disease (Shoulson et al., 1977).  This negative finding may be indicative of different pharmacological populations of GABA receptors, with the muscimol receptor not being involved in this disease, or may indicate that for significant improvement, both the GABA and the remaining cholinergic receptors must be activated simultaneously.

Studies such as these provide not only important information

TABLE I

NEUROTRANSMITTER RECEPTOR BINDING IN HUNTINGTON'S
AND PARKINSON'S DISEASE[a]

| Neurotransmitter receptor | Receptor Binding (% of control) | | | | | | | |
|---|---|---|---|---|---|---|---|---|
| | Caudate | | Putamen | | Globus Pallidus | | Substantia Nigra | |
| | H[b] | P[c] | H | P | H | P | H | P |
| GABA | 83 | 76 | 109 | 88 | 130 | 64 | 183* | 31* |
| Muscarinic cholinergic | 45* | 102 | 46* | 129* | 47* | 88 | 107 | -- |
| Serotonin | 50* | 90 | 75* | 93 | 23* | 102 | --- | -- |
| β-Adrenergic | 77 | -- | 73 | -- | 53* | --- | --- | -- |
| Dopamine | -- | 77* | -- | 93 | -- | 57 | --- | -- |

a  Data adapted from Enna et al. (1976a); Wastek et al. (1976);
   Enna et al. (1976b); Lloyd et al. (1977); Reisine et al. (1977).
b  Huntington brain
c  Parkinson brain
*P > .05

about receptor alterations in central nervous system disorders,
but may also yield insights into neuronal connections present in
the normal brain.  For example, the decrease in GABA receptor binding in the Parkinson substantia nigra, where dopamine cells have
degenerated, provides direct evidence for the theory that the GABA-
ergic system modulates the nigro-striatal dopamine pathway (Okada,
1976).  In contrast, the finding that GABA receptors are unchanged
in the Parkinson striatum and globus pallidus, in the face of a
severe deficiency in dopamine terminals, suggests that the receptors for GABA in this brain area are not primarily localized to
dopamine nerve endings.  Also, the loss of cholinergic muscarinic
receptor binding in Huntington's disease supports the notion that
cholinergic receptors are located upon GABA cells in the striatum
since the GABA-containing cells have degenerated in this area.

    The decrease in serotonin receptor binding in Huntington's di-
sease suggests that the receptors for this neurotransmitter may be
localized to either GABAergic or cholinergic cells since these cell
types are missing in this disorder.  However, the significant reduction in serotonin receptors in the Parkinson globus pallidus

indicates that serotonin most likely modulates the cholinergic
system in this brain area since GABA cells are intact in Parkinson's
disease, but there is a significant reduction in pallidal cholinergic cells in this disorder (Reisine et al., 1977). Further support for a serotonergic-cholinergic interaction in the globus pallidus is provided by the finding of a highly positive correlation
between the reduction in serotonin receptors and the loss of cholinergic cells in Parkinson's disease (Reisine et al., 1977).

Other neuronal interactions have been implicated in these
studies, implications which may be of value in designing effective
treatment for not only Parkinson's and Huntington's disesase, but
other central nervous system disorders as well.

### III. RADIORECEPTOR ASSAY FOR ENDOGENOUS GABA

Another application for the GABA receptor assay technique has
been as a simple and sensitive procedure to measure endogenous
levels of this amino acid in biological tissues and fluids (Enna
and Snyder, 1976; Enna et al., 1977e). The principle of this
assay is based on the fact that the amount of $^3$H-GABA specifically
bound to brain membranes is inversely related to the concentration
of unlabeled GABA present in the incubation medium. Thus, to
measure the GABA content of brain it is necessary only to homogen-
ize the frozen tissue in water and, and centrifugation, to place
a small quantity of the aqueous supernatant into the receptor binding incubation tubes and determine the amount of $^3$H-GABA bound in
the presence of the brain extract. Similarly, the measurement of
GABA in biological fluids such as cerebrospinal fluid (CSF), can be
readily accomplished using the assay technique simply by placing
small quantities of untreated CSF into the incubation medium and
comparing the amount of $^3$H-GABA bound in the presence of the CSF
to the isotope bound in the present of known concentrations of unlabeled GABA. Because of the relatively high affinity of GABA for
the receptor site (16 nM), this assay can reliably detect as little
as 10 pmoles of GABA present in a 2 ml incubation volume. Studies
have indicated that the only naturally occurring substance in either
brain or CSF which will displace specifically bound $^3$H-GABA, at the
concentration of tissue or CSF normally used, is GABA itself (Enna
and Snyder, 1976; Enna et al., 1977e).

With the advent of this procedure, it is now possible to rapidly determine the GABA content in very small amounts of tissue.
In addition, prior to the development of the radioreceptor assay,
extensive purification procedures and sophisticated analytical
equipment were necessary to measure the small quantities of GABA in
CSF (Glaeser and Hare, 1975; Grossman et al., 1976). While exquis-
itly sensitive and accurate, these procedures tend to be laborious
and time consuming relative to the radioreceptor assay technique.

Analysis of CSF GABA using the radioreceptor assay has sug-

gested that the CSF content of this amino acid reflects the brain
levels of GABA (Enna et al., 1977e) and thus by studying the GABA
content in CSF it may be possible to learn which neurological and
psychiatric abnormalities involve this neurotransmitter.  Furthermore, when a disorder is known to be characterized by a deficiency
of brain GABA, CSF GABA analysis may be useful as a diagnostic aid.
For example, it has recently been reported that cerebrospinal fluid
GABA levels are significantly reduced in most individuals who have
been diagnosed as having Huntington's disease (Table II) (Enna et
al., 1977c).  Interestingly, no correlation was found between the
level of GABA in the CSF and the duration of the illness suggesting that cerebrospinal fluid GABA levels may be reduced in Huntington patients prior to the onset of symptoms.  Since this disease
is an autosomal dominant disorder, this finding suggests that it
may be possible to predict which individuals are carrying the
Huntington gene before symptoms of the disability appear.

TABLE II

CEREBROSPINAL FLUID GABA CONTENT IN
VARIOUS NEUROLOGICAL DISORDERS[a]

| Disorder | CSF GABA Content (% of controls)[b] |
|---|---|
| Huntington's Disease[c] | 50* |
| Parkinson's Disease[c] | 91 |
| Alzheimer's Disease[c] | 52* |
| Myoclonic Epilepsy | 68* |
| Tourettes Syndrome | 92 |

[a]     In all cases, CSF GABA was determined using the radiore-
        ceptor assay as described in the text.
[b]     The control value was 220 pmole GABA/ml CSF
[c]     Adapted from Enna et al. (1977c)
*P >.05

Using the radioreceptor assay, it has also been determined
that cerebrospinal fluid GABA levels are normal in Parkinson patients treated with levodopa, but may be reduced in individuals
diagnosed as having Alzheimer's disease (Enna et al., 1977c). This
apparent decrease in the cerebrospinal fluid GABA content found in
Alzheimer patients is important since some of the symptoms of this

disorder are similar to those observed in Huntington's disease
making a differential diagnosis difficult. Thus, it appears that
cerebrospinal fluid GABA content, in itself, may not be sufficient
for diagnosing either disability.

Other studies have indicated that while the level of GABA in
the CSF appears normal in Gilles de la Tourette syndrome, it is
abnormally low in patients having myoclonic epilepsy (Table II).
This finding substantiates the theory that brain GABA abnormalities
may be causally related to certain types of epilepsy (Tower, 1976).

## IV.   PHARMACOLOGY OF THE GABA RECEPTOR BINDING SITE

Since GABA is thought to be one of the more important inhibitory neurotransmitters in the mammalian central nervous system
(Iversen and Bloom, 1972) and since alterations in the GABAergic
system appear to be involved in a variety of disease states, the
development of chemical agents which will specifically activate
postsynaptic GABA receptor sites after systemic administration
would be a boon to both the basic scientist and clinician. In the
past, neurophysiological and behavioral techniques were the primary methods used to demonstrate the relative activity and specificity of GABA receptor agonists and antagonists. While these methods are indispensible for demonstrating biological activity, they
do not readily lend themselves to routine screening of hundreds of
potentially active agents. However, since it has been shown that
only those drugs which activate GABA receptors neurophysiologically
will inhibit specific $^3$H-GABA receptor binding, the receptor binding assay can be used as a rapid preliminary screen to discover
GABA-mimetic agents. Due to the simplicity of the binding assay,
hundreds of compounds can be tested in a few days and those which
show promise as GABA receptor agents can then be tested neurophysiologically and behaviorally to determine biological potency.

Further evidence that the GABA binding procedure is an accurate reflection of the biologically relevant synaptic receptor
site is provided by the finding that a series of phthalideisoquin-
olines displaces membrane-bound $^3$H-GABA in a manner consistent with
their reported neurophysiological potencies (Enna et al., 1977b).
Similarly, a series of bicyclophosphates were shown to be relatively potent in displacing specifically bound GABA, their potencies
paralleling their neurophysiological and convulsant activities. It
was also found that muscimol, a potent GABA agonist neurophysiologically, is more potent than GABA in displacing $^3$H-GABA (Enna et
al., 1977b). As a result of this discovery, muscimol is now being
used as a ligand for studying the GABA receptor and may be useful
as a probe for identifying subpopulations of this neurotransmitter
site (Enna et al., 1978). Also, $^3$H-bicuculline has been successfully used to label GABA receptors (Mohler and Okada, 1977) and
the characteristics of $^3$H-bicuculline binding are slightly different from those found for $^3$H-GABA binding to the receptor. By using

different ligands such as these, it may be possible to better define the precise pharmacological characteristics of this receptor
site by, for example, determining the relationships between the
agonist and antagonist conformations of this site.  Also, different ligands should reveal whether pharmacologically distinct GABA
receptors exist and, by exploiting these differences, more specific GABAergic agents can be developed to treat GABA—related disorders.

### V    REGIONAL DISTRIBUTION OF GABA RECEPTOR IN BRAIN

It is generally held that the functional importance of any
neurotransmitter system in the brain is related to the concentration and turnover rate of the transmitter in a given brain area.
However, these measurements are primarily presynaptic and it likely
that the functional importance of a neurotransmitter system in
different areas of the brain is related not only to presynaptic
innervation but also to the density of the postsynaptic receptors
present in that brain area.  This proposition is supported by the
finding that norepinephrine-sensitive adenylate cyclase, presumably associated with the norepinephrine receptor site, is most
enriched in cerebellum, an area which has relatively little norad-
renergic innervation (Rall and Gilman, 1970).  Furthermore, the
densities of muscarinic cholinergic, serotonin and β-adrenergic
binding sites show only a limited correlation with levels of the
endogenous neurotransmitters (Table III).

The regional distribution of specifically bound $^3$H-GABA in
human brain also shows only a limited correlation with the regional distribution of glutamic acid decarboxylase (GAD), GABA content,
and the high affinity neuronal GABA uptake system, markers for presynaptic innervation.  Specific $^3$H-GABA receptor binding is most
enriched in the cerebellum, an area with low uptake and enzyme
activity.  Conversely, areas of the brain which contain the highest GABA levels and GAD activity possess only moderate amounts of
GABA receptor binding.  These include the caudate, putamen, globus
pallidus and substantia nigra (Table III).  Information such as
this may be an important clue as to the possible side-effects that
may be encountered with GABA agonist therapy.  Also, if the number
of membrane receptors is modulated by the amount of neurotransmitter released, as seems to be the case (Hartzell and Fambrough,
1972; Mickey et al., 1975; Enna et al., 1976a; Creese et al., 1977),
then these regional distributions may be sensitive indicators of,
not only postsynaptic receptor content, but also presynaptic terminal activity.

Thus, the ability to quantitate neurotransmitter receptor
sites provides a different perspective with regard to the functional activity of neurotransmitter systems in different brain regions.
Since binding assays can be adapted to measure receptor densities
in small amounts of tissue, it is now possible to study receptor

TABLE III

NEUROTRANSMITTER RECEPTOR BINDING IN

SELECTED AREAS OF THE HUMAN BRAIN[a]

| Region | Receptor Binding (% of Caudate)[b] | | | |
|---|---|---|---|---|
| | GABA | Serotonin | Muscarinic Cholinergic | β-Adrenergic |
| Frontal cortex | 175 | 230 | 61 | 73 |
| Hippocampus | 211 | 162 | 41 | 86 |
| Amygdala | 83 | 156 | 62 | 133 |
| Thalamus | 94 | 47 | 38 | 80 |
| Putamen | 44 | 108 | 98 | 85 |
| Globus pallidus | 39 | 132 | 13 | 99 |
| Caudate | 100 | 100 | 100 | 100 |
| Substantia nigra | 28 | 106 | 4 | 110 |
| Cerebellar hemisphere | 864 | 23 | 0 | 67 |
| Pontine tegmentum | 33 | 58 | 3 | 184 |
| Medullary tegmentum | 25 | 26 | -- | 249 |

a    Adapted from Enna et al. (1977a)

b    Values for receptor binding in the caudate as follows
     (fmole/ mg protein):  GABA, 36; serotonin, 66; muscarinic
     cholinergic, 480; β-adrenergic, 105.

concentrations in discreet brain regions, such as on specific nuclei, which will provide even more precise information about the
synaptic relationships between neurotransmitter systems.

ACKNOWLEDGEMENTS

Portions of this work were supported by a Pharmaceutical Man-
ufacturers Association Research Starter Grant, the Huntington's
Chorea Foundation, USPHS grant MH-29739 and by Eli Lilly and Merck
Sharp and Dohme.  The author thanks Drs. Melvin VanWoert and Ian
J. Butler for their assistance and Ms. Barbara Block for her sec-
retarial support.

REFERENCES

Creese, I., Burt, D. and Snyder, S., 1977, Dopamine receptor bind-
    ing enhancement accompanies lesion-induced behavioral super-
    sensitivity, Science 197:596-598.
Ehringer, H. and Hornykiewicz, O., 1960, Verteilung von noradrena-
    lin und dopamin (3-hydroxytyramin) im gehirn des menschen und
    ihr verhalten bei erkrankungen des extrapyramidalen systems,
    Klin. Wsch. 38:1236-1239.
Enna, S.J., Beaumont, K. and Yamamura, H., 1978, Comparison of $^3$H-
    muscimol and $^3$H-GABA receptor binding in rat brain, in
    "Amino Acids as Chemical Transmitters", (F. Fonnum, ed.),
    Plenum Press, New York.
Enna, S.J., Bennett, J., Bylund, D., Creese, I., Burt, D., Charness,
    M., Yamamura, H., Simantov, R. and Snyder, S., 1977a, Neuro-
    transmitter receptor binding: regional distribution in human
    brain, J. Neurochem. 28:233-236.
Enna, S.J., Bennett, J., Bylund, D., Snyder, S., Bird, E. and
    Iversen, L., 1976a, Alterations of brain neurotransmitter re-
    ceptor binding in Huntington's Chorea, Brain Res. 116:531-537.
Enna, S.J., Bird, E., Bennett, J., Bylund, D., Yamamura, H., Iver-
    sen, L. and Snyder, S., 1976b, Huntington's Chorea: Changes
    in neurotransmitter receptors in the brain, New Eng. J. Med.
    294:1305-1309.
Enna, S.J., Collins, J. and Snyder, S., 1977b, Stereospecificity
    and structure-activity requirements of GABA receptor binding
    in rat brain, Brain Res. 124:185-190.
Enna, S.J., Kuhar, M. and Snyder, S., 1975, Regional distribution
    of postsynaptic receptor binding for γ-aminobutyric acid
    (GABA) in monkey brain, Brain Res. 93:168-174.
Enna, S.J. and Snyder, S., 1975, Properties of γ-aminobutyric acid
    (GABA) receptor binding in rat brain synaptic membrane frac-
    tions, Brain Res. 100:81-97.
Enna, S.J. and Snyder, S., 1976, A simple, sensitive and specific
    radioreceptor assay for endogenous GABA in brain tissue, J.
    Neurochem. 26:221-224.
Enna, S.J. and Snyder, S., 1977, Influences of ions, enzymes, and
    detergents on γ-aminobutyric acid receptor binding in synaptic
    membranes of rat brain, Mol. Pharmacol. 13:442-453.

Enna, S.J., Stern, L., Wastek, G. and Yamamura, H., 1977c, Cerebro-
    spinal fluid γ-aminobutyric acid variations in neurological
    disorders, Arch. Neurol., in press.
Enna, S.J., Stern, L., Wastek, G. and Yamamura, H., 1977d, Neuro-
    biology and pharmacology of Huntington's disease, Life Sci.
    20:205-212.
Enna, S.J., Wood, J. and Snyder, S., 1977e, γ-aminobutyric acid
    (GABA) in human cerebrospinal fluid: radioreceptor assay,
    J. Neurochem. 28:1121-1124.
Glaeser, B. and Hare, T., 1975, Measurement of GABA in human
    cerebrospinal fluid, Biochem. Med. 12:274-282.
Grossman, R., Beyer, C., Shannon, G., Kelly, P. and Haber, B.,
    1976, Monoamine oxidase, catechol-o-methyl transferase, LDH
    and γ-aminobutyric acid in human ventricular fluid following
    brain injury, Proc. Soc. Neurosci. 2:763.
Growdon, J., Cohen, E. and Wurtman, R., 1977, Huntington's disease:
    clinical and chemical effects of choline administration,
    Ann. Neurol. 1:418-422.
Hartzell, H. and Fambrough, D., 1972, Acetylcholine receptors.
    Distribution and extrajunctional density in rat diaphragm
    after denervation correlated with acetylcholine sensitivity,
    J. Gen. Physiol. 60:248-262.
Hiley, C. and Bird, E., 1974, Decreased muscarinic receptor con-
    centration in post-mortem brain in Huntington's Chorea,
    Brain Res. 80:355-358.
Iversen, L. and Bloom, F., 1972, Studies of the uptake of $^3$H-GABA
    and $^3$H-glycine in slices and homogenates of rat brain and
    spinal cord by electron microscopic autoradiography, Brain
    Res. 41:131-143.
Lloyd, K. Shemen, L. and Hornykiewicz, O., 1977, Distribution of
    high affinity sodium-independent $^3$H-gamma-aminobutyric acid
    ($^3$H-GABA) binding in human brain: Alterations in Parkinson's
    disease, Brain Res. 127:269-278.
Mickey, J., Tate, R. and Lefkowitz, R., 1975, Subsensitivity of
    adenylate cyclase and decreased β-adrenergic receptor binding
    after chronic exposure to (-)-isoproterenol in vitro, J. Biol.
    Chem. 250:5727-5729.
Mohler, H. and Okada, T., 1977, GABA receptor binding with $^3$H-bic-
    culline methiodide in rat CNS, Nature 267:65-67.
Okada, Y., 1976, Role of GABA in the substantia nigra, in "GABA in
    Nervous System Function", (E. Roberts, T. Chase and D. Tower,
    eds.), Raven Press, New York.
Rall, T. and Gilman, A., 1970, The role of cyclic AMP in the ner-
    vous system. Neurosci. Res. Bull. 8:223-232.
Reisine, T., Fields, J., Yamamura, H., Bird, E., Spokes, E.,
    Schreiner, P. and Enna, S.J., 1977, Neurotransmitter receptor
    alterations in Parkinson's disease, Life Sci., in press.
Shoulson, I. and Chase, T., 1975, Huntington's disease, Ann. Rev.
    Med. 26:419-426.

Shoulson, I., Goldblatt, D., Charlton, M. and Joynt, R., 1977,
    Huntington's disease: treatment with muscimol, a GABA-mimetic
    drug, Ann. Neurol. 1:506.
Tower, D., 1976, GABA and seizures: clinical correlates in man, in
    "GABA in Nervous System Function", (E. Roberts, T. Chase and
    D. Tower, eds.), Raven Press, New York.
Wastek, G., Stern, L., Johnson, P. and Yamamura, H., 1976, Hunt-
    ington's disease: regional alteration in muscarinic cholin-
    ergic receptor binding in human brain, Life Sci. 19:1033-1040.
Zukin, S., Young, A. and Snyder, S., 1974, Gamma-aminobutyric acid
    binding to receptor sites in the rat central nervous system,
    Proc. Nat. Acad. Sci. 71:4802-4807.

[3]H-GABA BINDING TO MEMBRANES PREPARED FROM POST-MORTEM HUMAN

BRAIN : PHARMACOLOGICAL AND PATHOLOGICAL INVESTIGATIONS

K.G. Lloyd and S. Dreksler

Department of Neuropharmacology
Synthélabo, F 92220 Bagneux, France
                and
Department of Psychopharmacology
Clarke Institute of Psychiatry
Toronto, Canada M5T 1R8

Recently the study of receptors for neurotransmitters and other biologically active compounds has been greatly facilitated by the use of radiolabelled-ligand binding to membrane preparations. In our laboratories we have been interested for some time in the physiological state of GABA neurons in both pathological conditions such as Parkinson's disease (Lloyd and Hornykiewicz, 1973 ; Lloyd et al., 1977a) and in relation to the use of neuroleptic drugs (Lloyd et al., 1977b). We have adapted the [3]H-GABA binding technique (cf Enna and Snyder, 1977 ; Young et al., 1976) for use in human material and have studied the state of GABA receptors in both normal tissues and in pathological conditions (Lloyd et al., 1977c and d).


METHODS AND MATERIALS

Distinct regions were dissected from frozen human brains as previously described (Lloyd and Hornykiewicz, 1972). The high affinity, sodium-independent [3]H-GABA binding to membranes prepared from frozen human material was measured as described by Enna and Snyder (1975) as modified by Lloyd et al. (1977d). Drugs were dissolved in deionized water (when possible) and the $IC_{50}$'s estimated over a dose range of 1mM-1nM (0.01nM in the case of muscimol). When drugs were insoluble in water, [3]H-GABA binding was compared to membrane preparations containing an equal concentration of diluent. L-glutamic acid decarboxylase (GAD) activity was estimated as described by Lloyd and Hornykiewicz (1973). Proteins were estimated by the method of Lowry et al. (1951).

TABLE 1.    DISTRIBUTION OF $^3$H-GABA BINDING IN HUMAN BRAIN.

| REGION | $^3$H-GABA binding | | GAD activity |
|---|---|---|---|
| | $\dfrac{\text{fmol GABA}}{\text{mg protein}}$ | $\dfrac{\text{fmol GABA}}{\text{mg tissue}}$ | $\dfrac{\text{nmol CO2}}{\text{100 mg protein x 2 hr}}$ |
| Cerebral Cortex and Cerebellum | | | |
| Cerebellar Cx. | 328.1±50.1 (10) | 13.10±2.06 | 780±149 (12) |
| Hippocampus | 204.6±18.6 ( 8) | 12.11±1.12 | 290± 53 ( 4) |
| Insular Cx. | 202.7±18.5 ( 3) | 10.31±3.85 | --- |
| Temporal Cx. | 187.8±27.6 (12) | 9.27±1.68 | 1024±154 (13) |
| Parietal Cx. | 169.4±32.4 (11) | 8.80±1.86 | 789±161 ( 5) |
| Occipital Cx. | 140.0±20.9 ( 5) | 6.74±0.60 | 592±126 ( 5) |
| Frontal Cx. | 133.9±28.1 ( 9) | 4.01±0.59 | 1048±161 ( 7) |
| Olfactory Cx. | 122.9±32.0 ( 3) | 4.32±1.31 | --- |
| Cingulate Cx. | 67.2±15.8 ( 4) | 2.58±0.69 | --- |
| Dentate Nucleus | 15.3± 7.8 ( 7) | 1.08±0.70 | 1481±410 ( 4) |
| Substantia Alba | 1.7± 1.7 ( 5) | 0.12±0.12 | 30± 8 (12) |
| Subcortical Nuclei | | | |
| Amygdala | 74.5±22.3 ( 5) | 3.89±1.49 | 336          ( 2) |
| Putamen | 67.8±13.7 (17) | 6.36±1.35 | 1243±220 (13) |
| Caudate Nucleus | 66.3± 8.2 ( 9) | 4.20±0.84 | 1381±186 (13) |
| Accumbens | 58.1±29.0 ( 4) | 5.09±3.69 | ---- |
| Substantia Nigra | 30.8± 5.0 (11) | 3.09±0.55 | 1273±297 (13) |
| Thalamus | 24.7± 5.5 ( 5) | 1.66±0.39 | 364± 77 ( 8) |
| Pallidum-Internal | 17.6± 5.7 ( 7) | 1.79±0.80 | 1492±675 ( 7) |
| Pallidum-External | 15.5± 3.0 ( 6) | 0.94±0.28 | 1106±306 ( 8) |
| Red Nucleus | 4.9± 2.2 ( 4) | 0.65±0.37 | 302± 32 ( 5) |

All values are expressed as mean ± S.E.M. Number of estimations in parentheses. Values from Lloyd et al (1977d) and
Lloyd (1972).

RESULTS AND DISCUSSION

The sodium-independent binding of $^3$H-GABA to membranes prepared
from different regions of frozen human brain is shown in Table 1.
The high density of $^3$H-GABA binding seen in the cerebellar cortex
correlates well with the occurence of at least 4 neurons (Purkinje

cells, basket cells, Golgi Type II cells and stellate cells) which
utilize GABA as the inhibitory transmitter (Hökfelt and Ljungdahl,
1972 ; Ito, 1976 ; Obata, 1972). Similarly, the hippocampus is also
innervated by GABA interneurons (Storm-Mathisen, 1976), and it has
been estimated that more than 20 percent of cerebral cortical interneurons may be GABAergic (Bloom and Iversen, 1971). In spite of this
close relationship between [3]H-GABA binding and morphological and
electrophysiological observations, [3]H-GABA binding does not correspond well with the distribution of GAD in the human brain (Table 1).
The likely reason for this is that [3]H-GABA binding represents postsynaptic GABA receptors (and therefore correlates with the distribution of GABA nerve terminals and synapses) whereas GAD activity
occurs not only in GABA terminals but also in GABA cell bodies, glial
elements and other cells (cf Baxter, 1976).

The specificity of the [3]H-GABA binding in the human cerebellar
cortex and rat brain has been examined and compared with similar
data from the rat brain. In both species the cerebellum exhibits the
greatest [3]H-GABA binding (present results ; Enna and Snyder, 1975).
The Kd's and $IC_{50}$'s for unlabelled GABA are similar for both species
(0.3-0.5 μM, Table 2 ; Enna and Snyder, 1975a and b ; Lloyd et al.,
1977d). In either species, treatment of the membranes with 0.05
percent Triton-X-100 lowers the $IC_{50}$ by a factor of 10 (Enna and
Snyder, 1977 ; Lloyd, unpublished data). In human material the [3]H-
GABA binding is stable between 4 and 24 hours post-mortem and is not
altered by storage at -45°C for up to 68 months. The [3]H-GABA binding
is also independent of patient age over a span of at least 14-80
years (Lloyd, unpublished results).

The pharmacology of the [3]H-GABA binding to membranes prepared
from control human cerebellar cortices is reported in Table 2. Only
those compounds which are known to be potent GABA mimetics (Johnson,
1976) exhibit a potent inhibition ($IC_{50}$ <5 μM) of [3]H-GABA binding
(Table 2). Of the drugs tested, muscimol was the most potent. The
$IC_{50}$ of 0.014 corresponds well with the value of 0.05 μM for muscimol
in frozen rat brain (Enna and Snyder, 1977). The potency of 3-amino-
propane sulfonic acid is also in agreement with studies in the frozen
rat brain (Enna and Snyder, 1975, 1976). Imidazoleacetic acid, another
potent GABA mimetic (cf Johnson, 1976) and 3-hydroxy-GABA have been
reported in the rat brain to have $IC_{50}$'s similar to that of GABA,
(Enna and Snyder, 1976, 1977). In the present study, these compounds
exhibited $IC_{50}$'s significantly greater than GABA, indicating a somewhat lower potency. However, they are still among the most potent
compounds tested in the present series. δ-Amino-valeric acid has not
been studied on [3]H-GABA binding in the rat brain preparation, but
has been reported to be an inhibitor of GABA uptake (Johnson, 1976).
The inhibition of GABA uptake cannot explain the present activity
as other potent GABA uptake inhibitors are either ineffective
(chlorpromazine) or much less potent (diaminobutyric acid) on [3]H-

TABLE 2. PHARMACOLOGY OF $^3$H-GABA BINDING IN HUMAN CEREBELLUM.

| DRUG | $IC_{50}$ (µM) | Ratio $IC_{50} \dfrac{GABA}{drug}$ | $IC_{50}$ Rat (µM) (Enna and Snyder 1976, 1977) |
|------|------|------|------|
| Muscimol | 0.014 | 16.5 (< 0.01) | 0.05 |
| 3-Aminopropane-Sulfonic Acid | 0.083 | 2.81 | 0.24 |
| GABA | 0.233 | 1.00 | 0.20 |
| Imidazole Acetic Acid | 1.42 | 0.16 (< 0.01) | 0.30 |
| δ-Amino-n-Valeric Acid | 2.73 | 0.085 (< 0.01) | - |
| Dl-4-Amino-3-Hydroxy butyric Acid | 2.91 | 0.080 (< 0.01) | - |
| (±)-Bicuculline | 17.7 | 0.0131 | (+) = 4.0 (-) = 300 |
| Strychnine $SO_4$ | 33.2 | 0.0070 | 100 |
| Homocarnosine | 43.3 | 0.0054 | - |
| Pimozide | 59.0 | 0.0039 | - |
| Clozapine | 65.0 | 0.0036 | - |
| Thioridazine | 87.0 | 0.0027 | - |
| β-Alanine | 162 | 0.0014 | 80 |
| Perphenazine | 191 | 0.0012 | - |
| Glutamic Acid | 200 | 0.0012 | - |
| Apomorphine | 267 | 0.0009 | - |
| DL-2,4-Diaminobutyric Acid | 329 | 0.0007 | >1000 |
| p-Chloromercuriphenyl Sulfonic Acid | 340 | 0.0007 | - |
| d-Tubocurarine | 450 | 0.0005 | 38 |

Drugs were added "in vitro" to membranes prepared from control brains as decribed in the text. All values are the means of at least three experiments.

GABA binding (see below ; Enna and Snyder, 1975).

Several compounds exhibited an $IC_{50}$ for $^3$H-GABA binding between 10 and 500 µM (Table 2). Bicuculline, a blocker of GABA receptors (Johnson, 1976), in the present study exhibited a potency slightly lower than in the rat (Enna and Snyder, 1976). However, assuming that the (-) isomer has negligible activity, the $IC_{50}$ of the active isomer, (+) bicuculline, in the present system would be approximately 8 µM, approaching that reported for rat brain (4 µM, Enna and Snyder, 1977). Homocarnosine (GABA-histidine) and d-tubocurarine are less active in the present preparation than in the rat brain (Enna and

Snyder, 1975, 1976). Conversely, dl-2,4-diaminobutyric acid and glutamic acid have some slight activity in the present study whereas they were inactive when tested on rat brain membranes (Enna and Snyder, 1975, 1977).

Interestingly, a group of neuroleptics (pimozide, clozapine, thioridazine and perphenazine) exhibited some activity. Although chlorpromazine and haloperidol were inactive under the present conditions, in the rat brain chlorpromazine displaces ³H-GABA binding with an $IC_{50}$ similar to that presently seen for perphenazine (Enna and Snyder, 1975). Also, it has been demonstrated that after intraperitoneal injection haloperidol interferes with ³H-GABA binding in the rat brain (Lloyd et al., 1977b). Although the concentrations are quite high as compared to their affinity for the neuroleptic or dopamine receptor (Seeman et al., 1976 ; Snyder, 1976), this property may be of some importance upon chronic neuroleptic administration, as these drugs are known to accumulate in tissue (cf Brucke et al., 1969). The physiological importance of such a mechanism is not known at present, but could possibly be related to the lowering of seizure thresholds by neuroleptic drugs (cf Byck, 1975) or possibly to their neuroleptic effects.

In addition of the selectivity shown for ³H-GABA binding by direct acting GABA mimetics (Table 2), the specificity of this binding in human cerebellar cortex is also demonstrated by the wide variety of inactive substances. Thus, compounds which inhibit the metabolism of GABA (aminooxyacetic acid, sodium dipropylacetate ; Collins, 1973 : Godin et al., 1969), alter the chloride ion conductance associated with the GABA receptor (picrotoxin ; Takeuchi and Takeuchi, 1969) or have undefined GABA-mimetic properties (p-chloro-beta-phenyl-GABA, diazepam ; Chase and Walters, 1976: Costa et al., 1976) do not alter ³H-GABA binding ($IC_{50} > 1000$ μM). Similarly substances which attach to receptors for other putative neurotransmitters (arecoline, atropine, glycine, taurine, haloperidol, chlorpromazine, amantadine, diphenhydramine, methysergide) are inactive on ³H-GABA binding. Furthermore, local anesthetics, analgesics, narcotics, convulsants (other than bicuculline), anticonvulsants and phosphodiesterase inhibitors are also inactive.

These two groups of data (regional distribution and pharmacology) support the contention that the ³H-GABA binding as presently studied in human brain material is closely associated with the physiologically active GABA receptor. With this in mind, it is possible to meaningfully examine the ³H-GABA binding in different pathological conditions in order to assess the state of GABA receptors.

It is well known that in Parkinson's disease the major neurochemical - neuropathological deficits are a loss of the neuromelanin-containing dopamine cell bodies in the pars compacta of the substantia

nigra and a severe loss of dopamine and related enzymes and metabolites in the substantia nigra, caudate nucleus and putamen
(Berheimer et al., 1973 ; Lloyd et al., 1975). Other neurotransmitter
systems are also diminished in Parkinson's disease, including GAD
activity in striatum and substantia nigra (Lloyd et al., 1977a). In
most brain regions studied from Parkinsonian patients [3]H-GABA binding
was not diminished (Table 3). However in the hippocampus and substantia nigra [3]H-GABA binding was significantly decreased. In the
substantia nigra the only consistent cell loss in Parkinson's disease
occurs for neuromelanin-containing  dopamine cell bodies (cf
Bernheimer et al., 1973). From these observations, together with the
strong evidence for the existence of a striato-nigral GABA pathway
(cf Dray and Straughan, 1976) the conclusion may be drawn that most
of the [3]H-GABA binding sites (likely GABA receptors) in the substantia nigra are on dopamine cell bodies or their dendrites.

Huntington's chorea markedly differs from Parkinson's disease
clinically, morphologically and biochemically (cf Barbeau et al.,
1973 ; Bernheimer et al., 1973). Neuropathologically there is severe
degeneration and cell loss in the caudate nucleus, putamen and
cerebral cortex (Bernheimer et al., 1973 ; Earle, 1973 ; Heathfield,
1973). The [3]H-GABA binding in the cerebral cortex of the present
series of Huntington's patients is unchanged as compared to controls
(Table 4). In contrast, the [3]H-GABA binding is greatly decreased in
both caudate nucleus and putamen of these patients (Lloyd et al.,
1977c, Table 4). These changes are highly significant ($p < 0.01$)
when analyzed by either the two-tailed t-test or the Mann-Whitney
non-parametric U-test. When expressed as fmol/mg protein the results
for the caudate are unchanged : for the putamen, the binding is
slightly less severely decreased, but still is statistically significant ($p < 0.02$, Lloyd et al., 1977c). The present changes observed
in [3]H-GABA binding in the striatum are somewhat at variance with
the earlier findings of Enna et al. (1976a and b) in which a smaller
change in the caudate was observed without a similar change in the
putamen. Although the differences cannot presently be explained, it
is worth nothing that in the study of Enna et al. (1976b) some of
the [3]H-GABA binding values for the caudate nucleus in Huntington's
patients are very similar to those of the present study.

The present changes in the [3]H-GABA binding observed with striatal nuclei are consistent with the well-known atrophy and generalized
cell loss in these regions in Huntington's chorea (Bernheimer et al.,
1973 ; Earle, 1973 ; Heathfield, 1973). It is also, perhaps significant that to date there has been a singular lack of effectiveness
of GABA-mimetic compounds (imidazoleacetic acid ; dipropylacetate)
in Huntington's chorea (Chase and Walters, 1976 ; Shoulson et al.,
1975, 1976). These observations may, unfortunately, be related to
the low [3]H-GABA binding (loss of GABA receptors ?) in the striatum
in these patients. However, high potency GABA-mimetics which readily

TABLE 3.   SPECIFIC BINDING OF ³H-GABA TO MEMBRANES PREPARED FROM
           PARKINSONIAN PATIENTS.

| Region | ³H-GABA binding (fmol/mg protein) | | | Percent | Stat. |
| | Mean | S.E.M. | N | control | sign. |
| --- | --- | --- | --- | --- | --- |
| Pallidum-External | 61.3 | | 1 | 348.3 | -- |
| Pallidum-Internal | 42.4 | | 1 | 273.5 | -- |
| Cerebellar Cortex | 654.8 ± | 242.6 | 3 | 199.4 | NS |
| Frontal Cortex | 236.7 ± | 30.8 | 3 | 177.3 | <0.05 |
| Putamen | 91.7 ± | 19.6 | 8 | 135.3 | NS |
| Temporal Cortex | 240.8 ± | 14.8 | 5 | 128.5 | NS |
| Caudate Nucleus | 70.6 ± | 9.4 | 8 | 106.6 | NS |
| Hippocampus | 121.5 ± | 10.2 | 6 | 59.4 | <0.01 |
| Substantia Nigra | 9.7 ± | 2.9 | 6 | 31.4 | <0.01 |

Data from Lloyd et al., 1977c.


TABLE 4.   DISTRIBUTION OF ³H-GABA BINDING IN SELECTED REGIONS FROM
           BRAIN OF CONTROL PATIENTS AND PATIENTS WITH HUNTINGTON'S
           CHOREA.

| Brain region | ³H-GABA binding | | Percent |
| | Controls fmol/mg tissue | Huntington's chorea fmol/mg tissue | control |
| --- | --- | --- | --- |
| Cerebellar Cortex | 11.60±1.59 (15) | 22.48±3.42 (12) | 193.8 |
| Parietal Cortex | 8.8 ±1.86 (11) | 7.28±1.52 ( 6) | 82.7 |
| Caudate Nucleus | 3.88±0.72 (11) | 0.86±0.26 ( 9) | 22.2 |
| Putamen | 5.89±1.25 (19) | 1.47±0.25 (10) | 25.0 |

Data from Lloyd et al., 1977c.  Data expressed as Mean $\pm$ S.E.M.
Number of brains examined in parentheses.


enter the brain may still be of clinical benefit in Huntington's
chorea (see below).

In contrast to the above changes observed in the striatum,
an increased ³H-GABA binding appears to occur in the cerebellar
cortex (Table 4). This is associated with a highly significant
(p <0.001) ten fold decrease in the Kd (controls : 0.213 µM ;
Huntington's = 0.040 µM) and $IC_{50}$ (controls : 0.335 µM ; Huntington's
= 0.025 µM) for unlabelled GABA. This may be interpreted as an
increased affinity of the binding site for GABA. If such an increase
were to occur in other regions the potential for successful clinical
therapy with GABA-mimetics would be greatly increased.

In summary, the technique of sodium-independent ³H-GABA binding serves as a useful and informative marker for the state of GABA receptors in frozen post-mortem human brain tissue. The distribution, kinetics and pharmacology of this [3]H-GABA binding corresponds well with similar studies in the rat brain and also with electrophysiological data. To date in human brain material these binding studies have shown the existence of [3]H-GABA binding sites on nigral dopamine cell bodies (or dendrites) as well as alterations in Parkinson's disease and Huntington's chorea.

## ACKNOWLEDGEMENTS

This study was supported by the Clarke Institute of Psychiatry and grants from the National Institute of Mental Health, U.S.A. (M.H. 200500-5) and the Hospital for Sick Children Foundation, Toronto, S.D. is an undegraduate student in the Faculty of Dentistry, University of Toronto. The authors thank Dr E. Costa (Washington) for the gift of muscimol.

## REFERENCES

Barbeau, A., Chase, T.N. and Paulson, G.W., 1973 "Advances in Neurology, Vol. 1", Raven Press, New York.

Baxter, C.F., 1976, Some recent advances in studies of GABA-metabolism and compartementation, in "GABA in Nervous System Function" (E. Roberts, T.N. Chase and D.B. Tower, eds.), pp. 61-87, Raven Press, New York.

Bernheimer, H., Birkmayer, W., Hornykiewicz, O., Jellinger, K. and Seitelberger, F., 1973, Brain dopamine and the syndromes of Parkinson and Huntington, J. Neurol. Sci., 20:415-455.

Bloom, F.E. and Iversen, L.L., 1971, Localizing [3]H-GABA in nerve terminals of rat cerebral cortex by electron microscopic autoradiography, Nature, 229:628.

Brücke, E. Th. U., Hornykiewicz, O. and Sigg, E.B., 1969, "The Pharmacology of Psychotherapeutic drugs", Springer-Verlag, Heidelberg.

Byck, R., 1975, Drugs and the treatment of psychiatric disorders, in "The pharmacological Basis of Therapeutics", Fifth Edition, (L.S. Goodman and A. Gilman, eds), pp. 152-200, Macmillan, New York.

Chase, T.N. and Walters, J.R., 1976, Pharmacologic approaches to the manipulation of GABA mediated synaptic function in Man, in "GABA in Nervous System Function", (E. Roberts, T.N. Chase, and D.B. Tower, eds), pp. 497-513, Raven Press, New York.

Collins, G.G.S., 1973, Effect of aminooxyacetic acid, thiosemicarbazide and haloperidol on the metabolism and half-lives of glutamate and GABA in rat brain, Biochem. Pharmacol., 22:101-111.

Costa, E., Guidotti, A., and Mao, C.C., 1976, A GABA hypothesis for the action of benzodiazepines, in "GABA in Nervous System Function", (E. Roberts, T.N. Chase and D.B. Tower, eds), pp. 413-426, Raven Press, New York.

Dray, A. and Straughan, D.W., 1976, Synaptic mechanisms in the substantia nigra, J. Pharm. Pharmacol., 28:400-405.

Earle, K.M., 1973, Pathology and experimental model of Huntington's chorea, in "Advances in Neurology, Vol. 1", (A. Barbeau, T.N. Chase and G.W. Paulsen, eds), pp. 341-351, Raven Press, New York.

Enna, S.J. and Snyder, S.H., 1975, Properties of γ-aminobutyric acid (GABA) receptor binding in rat brain synaptic membrane fractions, Brain Research, 100:81-97.

Enna, S.J. and Snyder, S.H., 1976, A simple, sensitive and specific radioreceptor assay for endogenous GABA in brain tissue, J. Neurochem. 26:221-224.

Enna, S.J. and Snyder, S.H., 1977, Influences of ions, enzymes and detergents on γ-aminobutyric acid-receptr binding in synaptic membranes of rat brain, Molec. Pharmacol., 13:442-453.

Enna, S.J., Bird, E.D., Bennett, J.P., Bylund, D.B., Yamamura, H.I., Iversen, L.L. and Snyder, S.H., 1976b, Huntington's chorea: changes in neurotransmitter receptors in the brain, New Eng. J. Med. 294:1305-1309.

Enna, S.J., Bennett, J.P., Bylund, D.B., Snyder, S.H., Bird, E.D., and Iversen, L.L., 1976a, Alterations of brain neurotransmitter receptor binding in Huntington's chorea, Brain Research, 116: 531-537.

Godin, Y., Heiner, L., Mark, J., and Mandel, P., 1969, Effects of Di-n-propylacetate, an anticonvulsive compound, on GABA metabolism, J. Neurochem., 16:869-873.

Heathfield, W.G., 1973, Huntington's chorea: a centenary review, Postgrad Med., 49:32-45.

Hökfelt, T., and Ljungdahl, A., 1972, Autoradiographic identification of cerebral and cerebellar cortical neurons accumulating labelled Gamma-aminobutyric acid (³H-GABA), Exp. Brain Res. 14:354-362.

Ito, M., 1976, Roles of GABA neurons in integrated functions of the vertebrate CNS, in "GABA in Nervous System Function", (E. Roberts, T.N. Chase and D.B. Tower, eds), pp. 427-448, Raven Press, New York.

Johnston, G.A.R., 1976, Physiologic pharmacology of GABA and its antagonists in the vertebrate nervous system, in "GABA in Nervous System Function" (E. Roberts, T.N. Chase and D.B. Tower, eds.), pp. 395-411, Raven Press, New York.

Lloyd, K.G., 1972, "Biogenic amines and related enzymes in the Human and animal brain", Ph.D. Thesis, University of Toronto.

Lloyd, K.G. and Horhykiewicz, O., 1972, Occurrence and distribution of aromatic L-amino acid (L-DOPA) decarboxylase in the human brain, J. Neurochem. 19:1549-1559.

Lloyd, K.G. and Hornykiewicz, O., 1973, L-Glutamic acid decarboxylase in Parkinson's disease: effect of L-Dopa therapy, Nature, 243: 521-523.

Lloyd, K.G., Davidson, L. and Hornykiewicz, O., 1975, The neurochemistry of Parkinson's disease: effect of L-Dopa therapy, J. Pharmacol. Exp. Therap., 195:453-464.

Lloyd, K.G., Möhler, H., Bartholini, G. and Hornykiewicz, O., 1977a, Pathological alterations in glutamic acid decarboxylase acitivity in Parkinson's disease, in "Advances in Parkinsonism" 'W. Birkmayer and O. Hornykiewicz, eds.), pp. 186-197, Editions Roche, Basel.

Lloyd, K.G., Shibuya, M., Davidson, L., and Hornykiewicz, O., 1977b, Chronic neuroleptic therapy: tolerance and GABA systems, in "Advances in Biochemical Psychopharmacology", Vol. 16, (E. Costa and G.L. Gessa, eds.), pp. 409-415, Raven Press, New York.

Lloyd, K.G., Dreksler, S. and Bird, E.D., 1977c, Alterations in $^3$H-GABA binding in Huntington's chorea., Life Sciences, In press.

Lloyd, K.G., Shemen, L., and Hornykiewicz, O., 1977d, Distribution of high affinity sodium-independent ($^3$H) Gamma-aminobutyric acid ($^3$H-GABA) binding in the human brain. Alterations in Parkinson's disease, Brain Res, 127:269-278.

Lowry, O.H., Rosebrough, N.J., Raff, A.L., and Randall, R.J., 1951, Protein Measurement with the folin phenol reagent, J. Biol. Chem. 193:265-275.

Obata, K., 1972, The inhibitory action of Gamma-aminobutyric acid, a probable synaptic transmitter, Int. Rev. Neurobiol., 15:167-187.

Seeman, P., Lee, T., Chan-Wong, M. and Wong, K., Antipsychotic drug doses and neuroleptic/dopamine receptors, Nature, 261:717-719.

Shoulson, I., Chase, T.N., Roberts, E. and Van Balgooy, J.N.A., 1975, Huntington's disease: treatment with imidazole-4-acetic acid, New Eng. J. Med. 293:504-505.

Shoulson, I., Kartzinel, R. and Chase, T.N., 1976, Huntington's disease: treatment with dipropylacetic acid and gamma-aminobutyric acid, Neurology, 26:61-63.

Snyder, S.H., 1976, The dopamine hypothesis of schizophrenia: focus on the dopamine receptor, Amer. J. Psychiat. 133:197-202.

Storm-Mathisen, J., 1976, Distribution of the components of the GABA system in neuronal tissue: cerebellum and hippocampus effects of axotomy, in "GABA in Nervous System Function", (E. Roberts, T.N. Chase and D.B. Tower, eds.), pp. 149-168, Raven Press, New York.

Takeuchi, A., and Takeuchi, N., 1969, A study of the action of picrotoxin on the inhibitory neuromuscular junction of the crayfish, J. Physiol. (Lond), 205:377-391.

Young, A.B., Enna, S.J., Zukin, S.R., and Snyder, S.H., Synaptic GABA receptor in mammalian CNS, in "GABA in Nervous System Function", (E. Roberts, T.N. Chase and D.B. Tower, eds.), pp. 305-317, Raven Press, New York.

# STUDIES ON THE GAMMA-AMINOBUTYRIC ACID RECEPTOR/IONOPHORE PROTEINS IN MAMMALIAN BRAIN

R. W. Olsen, D. Greenlee, P. Van Ness, and M. K. Ticku

Department of Biochemistry
University of California
Riverside, California  92521

Receptor-ionophore proteins which mediate postsynaptic membrane responses to neurotransmitters can be studied in vitro by suitable radioactive ligand binding assays. Radioactive ligands are most appropriate when they act as potent and specific agonists or antagonists on the synapse under study. Drugs or toxins meeting these specifications are available for identification of numerous neurotransmitter receptors (Changeux et al., 1975; Cuatrecasas, 1974); in other cases binding of the radioactive neurotransmitter itself has been utilized (Snyder & Bennett, 1976). In very few cases have ligands been available for potential identification of elements other than the neurotransmitter recognition site (receptor) involved in mediating postsynaptic membrane responses (Young & Snyder, 1974; Bon & Changeux, 1975; Eldefrawi et al. 1977). Identification of binding sites in vitro as physiologically relevant postsynaptic receptor-ionophore proteins requires that numerous criteria be met, such as suitable quantity, binding affinity, tissue and subcellular location, and chemical specificity of the binding sites. In practice this last criterion demands quantitative estimates of dose-effect relationships for drugs active on the tissue under study and at least one such drug which is very specific for the receptor-ionophore as opposed to other potential binding proteins. Following identification, receptor-ionophore proteins ought to be susceptible to biochemical characterization, purification, and functional analysis. Furthermore the binding assays can be useful for various studies of normal and abnormal brain function.

We have assayed GABA receptor sites in mammalian brain with radioactive GABA itself, differentiating the receptor sites from other binding proteins for the neurotransmitter by the method of

Zukin et al. (1974), in which most nonreceptor binding is eliminated by carrying out the assays in sodium-free buffer and by using well disrupted tissue.    Further studies by Enna and Snyder,
(1975, 1977); Enna et al. (1977); and Coyle & Enna (1976), suggest
that the properties of the sodium-independent GABA binding sites
thus detected are consistent with those expected of receptors.
Furthermore, these sites are below normal in quantity in hamster
cerebellum which has been depleted by virus of granule cells
(Simantov et al. 1976); these cells are known to receive inhibitory GABA-mediated innervation, and would therefore be expected to
contain GABA receptors.    The binding sites are also depleted in
the brain region (substantia nigra) of human Parkinsonism patients
known to contain subnormal levels of dopamine-containing cells
believed to receive GABA innervation (Lloyd et al. 1977).

    We have confirmed the observations of sodium-independent
binding sites for GABA in homogenates of mammalian brain, and
have  described conditions needed for tissue preparation suitable
for GABA binding assays.    This report summarizes our findings on
the quantity, binding affinity, subcellular and brain regional
distribution, and chemical specificity of the sodium-independent
GABA binding sites.    All the information is consistent with their
identification as receptor sites (Greenlee et al. 1977).    We also
report on some of the properties of sodium-dependent GABA binding
sites (Van Ness et al. 1978).

    We also investigated another aspect of GABA postsynaptic
action, namely, the mode of action of the convulsant plant product,
picrotoxin.    This drug is a relatively potent and specific antagonist of GABA synapses (Curtis & Johnston, 1974; Krnjević, 1974;
Johnston, 1978).    It inhibits GABA-stimulated chloride permeability in crustacean muscle (Ticku & Olsen, 1977) in an apparently
noncompetitive fashion (Takeuchi & Takeuchi, 1969), and picrotoxinin (the active ingredient in picrotoxin) does not inhibit the
binding of GABA to the presumed receptor sites in mammalian brain
(Olsen et al. 1977; Enna et al. 1977).    This suggests that picrotoxinin acts at some other element of the GABA postsynaptic
membrane receptor-ionophore complex, perhaps the ionophore.
Radioactive picrotoxinin might thus provide a probe for analysis
of these elements in vitro.

    We have synthesized a radioactive biologically active ana-
logue of picrotoxinin, α-dihydropicrotoxinin.    This ligand bound
to sites in rat brain (Ticku & Olsen, 1977b) and crayfish muscle
(Olsen et al. 1978) having properties consistent with a relationship to the physiological action of picrotoxinin at the GABA
synapse.    These binding sites showed a similar quantity, subcellular and regional distribution as the GABA receptor sites.    Inhibition of binding by picrotoxinin analogues correlated well with the
biological activity of these drugs.    Binding of α-dihydropicrotox-

inin was not inhibited by GABA even at high concentrations, consistent with separate sites of action.  The binding sites for the
two ligands could also be differentiated on the basis of selective
sensitivity to chemical treatments.  It is likely that this radioactive toxin will provide a useful tool in analyzing the postsynaptic mechanism of neurotransmitter action.


## GABA RECEPTOR SITES IN MAMMALIAN CNS


### Binding in the Absence of Sodium Ion

Specific binding of radioactive GABA to rat brain homogenates
was measured by a centrifugation assay, using disrupted tissue

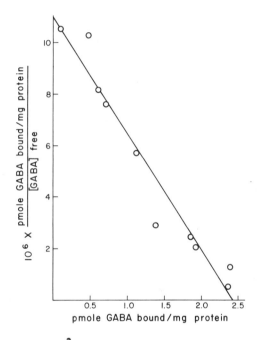

Figure 1.  Binding of [³H]GABA to Rat Brain Membranes:  Scatchard
Plot.  Rat brain particulate fractions (mitochondria plus microsomes) were prepared by osmotic shock, freezing and thawing, and
thorough washing in sodium-free buffer, 0.05 M Tris-citrate, pH
7.1.  Aliquots of 1.0 mg/ml protein in triplicate were incubated
at 0° with 10 nM [³H]GABA at 12.6 Ci/mmol. without (total binding)
or with (background) excess nonradioactive (0.1 mM) GABA.  GABA
concentrations were varied with nonradioactive ligand.  After
15 min, the tubes were centrifuged and decanted, the pellets
solubilized and radioactivity measured.

and sodium-free assay buffer as described by Zukin et al. (1974).
We observed that in order to obtain tissue samples showing maximal
binding which was stable with time and proportional to protein
concentration, one was required to use a more rigorous tissue
preparation. This was due to the presence in the CNS homogenates
of an endogenous inhibitor of binding, presumably GABA itself.
Several freeze-thaw steps and tissue washings by both distilled
water and assay buffer were necessary and sufficient to remove
this inhibitor, which was observed in all subcellular fractions
and no matter how vigorous the tissue disruption procedure (Greenlee et al. 1977).

Using suitably washed tissue, binding to rat brain membranes
in the absence of sodium showed saturation at 2-3 pmol/mg protein,
corresponding to 85 $\pm$ 15 pmol/g wet brain, and an apparent single
class of sites of $K_D$ 0.2 μM (Figure 1).

Over thirty structural analogues of GABA and a dozen other
neuroactive drugs were tested for their ability to inhibit these
sodium-independent GABA binding sites, and the concentrations
inhibiting 50% ($IC_{50}$ values) are given in Table 1, in order of
potency. An excellent correlation was observed between the
ability of a compound to inhibit binding and its activity as an
agonist or antagonist on GABA synapses.

The first five compounds have been reported to have activity
equal to or greater than GABA on several preparations studied
by electrophysiological techniques (Curtis & Johnston 1974;
Krnjević, 1974; Krogsgaard-Larsen et al. 1975). Compounds #7-10
and 13-17 have been reported to have GABA-like activity on various
preparations with potencies ranging from slightly to rather less
than GABA itself. Compounds 12 (strong), 18, and 19 (weak) are
probable GABA antagonists (perhaps competitive). Compounds 34-38
have also been reported to act as GABA antagonists (Johnston,
1978); their structures suggest a noncompetitive effect (except
for #36, which may require metabolic cleavage of the lactam
in vivo to produce an active GABA analogue). Compounds 30-33 may
have some effects on GABA synapses, but are not believed to
interact directly with GABA receptor sites.

Compounds inactive at GABA synapses were, without exception,
inactive at inhibiting GABA binding. In particular the compounds
(-)nipecotic acid and 2,4-diaminobutyrate, which specifically
inhibit GABA uptake but are inactive on GABA receptors (Johnston,
1978), did not significantly inhibit binding up to 100 μM.

The most potent inhibitors of binding, muscimol and homotau-
rine, are potent GABA agonists on all preparations studied (Curtis
& Johnston, 1974; Krogsgaard-Larsen et al. 1975; Wheal & Kerkut,

TABLE 1.   INHIBITORS OF GAMMA-AMINOBUTYRIC ACID RECEPTOR BINDING
           SITES IN RAT BRAIN

| Compound | $IC_{50}$ ($\mu M$) | Physiological Activity |
|---|---|---|
| 1.  Muscimol | 0.03 + 0.02 | ⎫ |
| 2.  Homotaurine | 0.07 + 0.02 | ⎪ |
| 3.  trans-Aminocyclopentane-3- | | ⎪ |
|       carboxylic acid | 0.27 + 0.03 | ⎬ > GABA |
| 4.  GABA | 0.34 + 0.06 | ⎪ |
| 5.  trans-4-Amino-crotonic acid | 0.43 + 0.20 | ⎭ |
| 6.  Homohypotaurine | 0.6 + 0.1 | Not tested |
| 7.  β-Hydroxy GABA | 0.7 + 0.3 | ⎫ |
| 8.  Imidazole acetic acid | 0.9 + 0.1 | ⎬ <GABA |
| 9.  β-Guanidino-propionic acid | 1.8 + 1.2 | ⎪ |
| 10. 3-Hydroxy,5-aminoethyl isoxazole | 3 + 1 | ⎭ |
| 11. N-Lauroyl GABA | 3 + 2 | Not tested |
| 12. (+) Bicuculline | 4 + 2 | Antagonist |
| 13. 4-Aminovaleric acid | 5 + 1 | ⎫ |
| 14. cis-Aminocyclopentane-3- | | ⎪ |
|       carboxylic acid | 5.2 + 0.8 | ⎬ <<GABA |
| 15. β-Alanine | 42 + 14 | ⎪ |
| 16. Taurine | 44 + 8 | ⎭ |
| 17. Homomuscimol | 50 + 10 | <GABA |
| 18. Benzyl pencillin | 50 + 30 | ⎫ Antagonist |
| 19. d-Tubocurarine | 85 + 25 | ⎭ |
| 20. L-Glutamic acid | 150 + 50 | Inactive |
| 21. 3-Hydroxy,4-methyl,5-aminomethylisoxazole | | ⎫ |
| 22. Azamuscimol | | ⎪ |
| 23. 5-Aminolevulinic acid | | ⎬ <<GABA |
| 24. β-p-(chlorophenyl) GABA (Lioresal) | | ⎭ |
| 25. 2,4-Diaminobutyric acid (DABA) | | ⎫ |
| 26. (-) Nipecotic acid | | ⎬ Inactive |
| 27. 2-Aminoethyl dithiocarbamic acid | | ⎫ |
| 28. 1-Piperidine propane sulfonic acid | >100 | ⎬ Not tested |
| 29. 6-Aminopenicillanic acid | | Inactive |
| 30. Chlorpromazine | | ⎫ |
| 31. Diazepam | | ⎪ |
| 32. Pentobarbital | | ⎬ Ambiguous |
| 33. Diphenylhydantoin | | ⎭ |
| 34. Pentylenetetrazole | | ⎫ |
| 35. Picrotoxinin | | ⎪ |
| 36. Caprolactam | | ⎬ Antagonists |
| 37. t-butyl Bicyclophosphate | | ⎪ |
| 38. Isopropyl Bicyclophosphate | | ⎭ |

The following substances had no effect up to 200 $\mu M$: Tetramethylenedisulfotetramine, Haloperidol, Imipramine, 3-Hydroxy-5-(1-aminopropyl) isoxazole, 3-Hydroxy-4-(2-aminoethyl)5-methyl isoxazole, D-Glutamic acid, Glycine.

1976; Ticku & Olsen, 1977a). Since muscimol has no effect on GABA
uptake except at concentrations of over 100 μM (Krogsgaard-Larsen
& Johnston, 1975; Olsen et al. 1977) and is not a substrate nor
inhibitor of glutamic acid decarboxylase (Olsen et al. 1977) nor
of GABA transaminase (Beart & Johnston, 1973), this "magic mush-
room" ingredient appears to provide the long-sought specific drug
suitable for GABA receptor identification in vitro. We found it
to inhibit GABA binding competitively with a $K_I$ value of 10-30 nM.
These sodium-independent sites thus show the chemical specificity
expected of receptor sites.

The structure-function analysis suggested by these binding
inhibition data are discussed by G.A.R. Johnston and by P. Krogsgaard-Larsen (this volume), who have generously provided us with
many of the compounds studied, as well as information on their
biological activity.

### Binding in the Presence of Sodium Ions

The binding of GABA to the receptor-like sites is best measured with thoroughly washed, frozen and thawed tissue, prepared
and assayed in sodium-free buffers. The binding detected was not,
however, an artifact of these procedures, as the same sites were
detectable in fresh tissue (adequate washing is required and
difficult to achieve) and in the presence of sodium ions.
Figure 2 depicts a Scatchard plot for GABA binding in the presence
of sodium ions. Under the conditions utilized (frozen and thawed,
thoroughly washed tissue, and low ligand concentration in binding
assays), more than half of the GABA cpm bound involved the receptor-like sites which can also be measured in the absence of
sodium. Thus a subclass of binding sites measured in sodium had
the same $K_D$ (0.3 μM) and number of tissue sites (2-3 pmol/mg
protein) as the sodium-independent sites. These high-affinity
sites were inhibited by low concentrations (10-100 nM) of muscimol
(Fig. 3), indicative of receptor sites.

Those sites measured in sodium which were not sensitive to
low concentrations of muscimol were inhibited only by much higher
concentrations of muscimol (over 100 μM), again supporting the
idea that this drug is specific for GABA receptor sites. These
muscimol-insensitive GABA binding sites measured in sodium had
lower affinity for GABA and were present in greater quantities
(amount bound at saturation). When assayed in the presence of 3μ
M muscimol to inhibit all the receptor sites, the residual binding
sites had a $K_D$ for GABA of 2-3 μM for one subclass and lower
affinity for one or more other site (Figure 2, insert). The
number of classes of binding sites is difficult to determine, but
it is reasonable that several should exist.

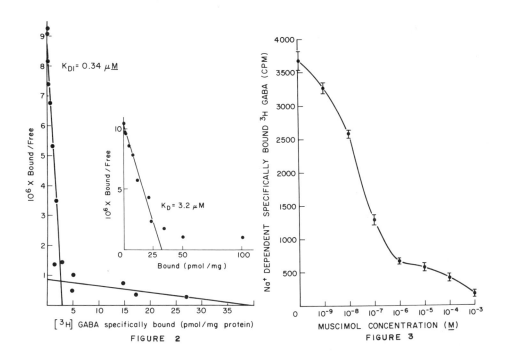

FIGURE 2

FIGURE 3

Figure 2. Binding of [³H]GABA to Rat Brain Membranes in the Presence of Sodium Ions: Scatchard Plot. Tissue was prepared and assayed as in Figure 1 except that the wash and assay buffer contained 0.2 M NaCl in addition to 50 mM Tris-citrate, pH 7.1. In the insert, tissue was prepared and assayed in the same manner with 0.2 M NaCl, except that the protein was increased to 2.2 mg/ml and all assays included 3 μM muscimol to inhibit the high-affinity, muscimol-sensitive (receptor) GABA binding sites. In these experiments the background was taken as that radioactive ligand associated with pelleted tissue which was not displaced by 1 mM nonradioactive GABA.

Figure 3. Inhibition by Varying Concentrations of Muscimol of GABA Binding in the Presence of Sodium Ions. Tissue was prepared and assayed as in Fig. 2, with 0.2 M NaCl, protein 2.0 mg/ml. The background as defined in Fig. 2 was subtracted from the total bound ligand to yield the amount of specifically bound GABA.

Binding of GABA in the presence of sodium was inhibited by analogues with a specificitv not consistent with any known binding protein related to receptor, transport, or enzyme. This is reasonable since a mixture of sites possibly related to all these proteins is being detected. If one measures GABA binding in the presence of sodium and inhibits the receptor sites with 3 μM muscimol, the residual non-receptor sites, in addition to having a lower affinity for GABA and very poor affinity for muscimol, have other differences from the GABA receptor sites, with respect to subcellular localization (discussed below), brain regional distribution, appearance in developing brain, and chemical specificity (VanNess et al. 1978). We have observed that a considerable portion of these sites (total brain) was inhibited by low concentrations of 2,4 diaminobutyrate (DABA) but not β-alanine, and another portion of the sites was inhibited by β-alanine but not DABA (Van Ness et al. 1978). It is thus possible that at least some of these sites are related to recognition sites for neuronal and glial transport systems which are known to be spcifically inhibited by DABA and β-alanine respectively (Iversen & Kelly, 1975).

## α-DIHYDROPICROTOXININ BINDING SITES

As mentioned above, picrotoxin generally inhibits GABA synapses rather potently (Curtis & Johnston, 1974; Krnjević,1974; Takeuchi, 1976). The drug has few if any other actions on the CNS at concentrations effective at blocking inhibitory synapses known or suspected to involve GABA (Johnston, 1978), and it seems to inhibit most, if not all, of these GABA synapses. Consistent with a chemical structure bearing no resemblance to GABA, picrotoxinin does not inhibit GABA binding to receptor sites (Enna et al., 1977; Olsen et al., 1977) and may inhibit GABA-mediated postsynaptic membrane chloride conductance in a manner which is noncompetitive with GABA (Takeuchi & Takeuchi, 1969). Where and how, then, does picrotoxinin act?

In an attempt to answer these questions, we prepared radioactive α-dihydropicrotoxinin by catalytic hydrogenation of picrotoxinin (Figure 4), and isolated a pure tritiated product (12 Ci/ mmol). α-Dihydropicrotoxinin (DHP) was reportedly only 5-fold weaker than picrotoxinin as a convulsant in mice (Jarboe et al. 1968), and we have confirmed that DHP is almost equal to picrotoxinin as a convulsant in mammals and in invertebrates (Table 2). Furthermore DHP is roughly equal to picrotoxinin at inhibiting either GABA-mediated inhibitory postsynaptic potentials in insect muscle (Table 2) or GABA-stimulated conductance in crayfish stretch receptor (Ikeda and Roberts, unpublished).

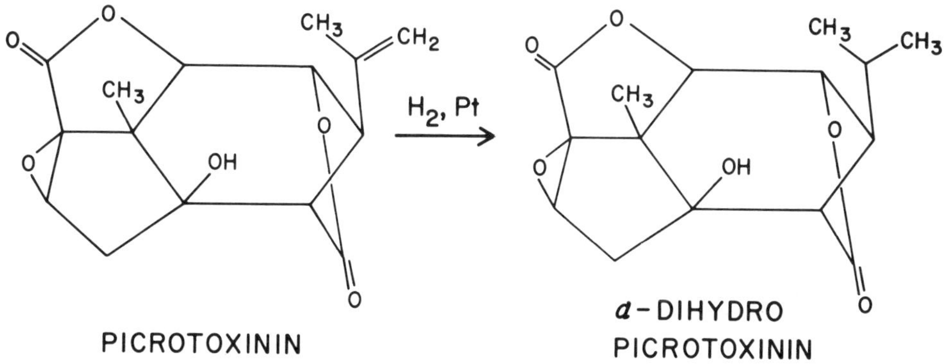

Figure 4.   Chemical Structures of Picrotoxinin and α-Dihydropicrotoxinin.

Using crayfish abdominal muscle fibers, we have previously shown (Ticku & Olsen, 1977a) that radioactive chloride ion flux could be stimulated by GABA.   This response involved the GABA receptor-ionophore, since it was specific for GABA and chloride and showed a dose-dependence on GABA which agreed remarkably well with microelectrode measurements done by Takeuchi & Takeuchi (1969) on crayfish muscle.   Picrotoxinin inhibited this GABA response with an $IC_{50}$ of 2-3 µM (Ticku & Olsen, 1977a); DHP did likewise with a just slightly weaker $IC_{50}$ of 4-5 µM (Table 2). This action of picrotoxin on GABA synapses can account for the convulsant action of the drug.

[3H]DHP binding to rat brain homogenates was measured by a centrifugation assay analogous to that employed with GABA.   Due to lower affinity for DHP binding than GABA receptor binding, detection of binding with the centrifugation assay was more difficult, yielding a signal-noise ratio of about 1:10; nevertheless binding was significant and reproducible.   Under the standard assay conditions (63 nM [3H]DHP, 12 Ci/mmol, see Fig. 5B), rat brain bound 3200 DPM/mg protein, while rat liver and lung showed no significant binding.   However, crayfish muscle, another tissue with GABA innervation, bound 6300 DPM/mg protein; the binding sites were shown to be localized to the sarcolemma fraction (Olsen et al., 1978).   DHP binding in rat brain was found to be rapid and reversible and proportional to protein concentration.   Binding was inhibited by trypsin treatment, but insensitive to phospholipase C and neuraminidase (Ticku & Olsen, 1977b).

Saturable specific binding of DHP was observed (Fig. 5A) when the concentration of [3H]DHP was varied.   Under optimal binding conditions, [3H]DHP binding was completely displaced by nonradio-

Table 2.  COMPARISON OF PICROTOXIN ANALOGUE ACTIVITY IN NEUROPHYSIOLOGY EXPERIMENTS AND INHIBITING BINDING OF [$^3$H]DHP

| Compound | Binding IC$_{50}$ (μM) | | [a] Mice: CD$_{50}$ (mg/kg) | [b] Crayfish: IC$_{50}$ (μM) | [c] Insects: Effective Concentration (μM) |
|---|---|---|---|---|---|
| | Rat Brain | Crayfish Muscle | | | |
| Picrotoxinin | 0.4 ± 0.2 | 0.5 ± 0.2 | 1.5 | 3 ± 1 | 1 |
| Tutin | 0.35 ± 0.2 | 0.5 ± 0.2 | 1.5 | --- | 1 |
| α-Dihydropicrotoxinin | 1.1 ± 0.2 | 1.1 ± 0.2 | 8 | 5 ± 1 | 1 |
| Picrotin | 70 ± 15 | 45 ± 15 | 80 | >10 | >10 |
| Picrotoxinin acetate | >200 | >200 | >272 | --- | >10 |
| Alkaline-hydrolyzed picrotoxinin | >200 | >200 | >300 | >100 | >10 |

Specific binding of [$^3$H]α-dihydropicrotoxinin was determined by a centrifugation assay as described in Figure 5, using 63 nM DHP, 12 Ci/mmol, and 2 mg/ml protein (mitochondria plus microsomes of rat brain or sarcolemma-enriched fraction of crayfish muscle [Meiners et al., 1978]). Background radioactivity not displaceable by 0.1 mM nonradioactive DHP was subtracted from total radioactivity associated with pelleted tissue. Varying concentrations of analogues were included in the binding assays (quadruplicates, done twice) to determine the concentrations inhibiting 50% of the specific binding (IC$_{50}$ values). a. Jarboe et al. (1968). b. GABA-stimulated $^{36}$Cl$^-$ flux assayed according to Ticku and Olsen (1977a). c. Causes convulsions when applied to the exposed insect nervous system and also at the same concentration inhibits GABA-mediated inhibitory postsynaptic potentials in insect muscle, assayed according to Olsen et al. (1976).

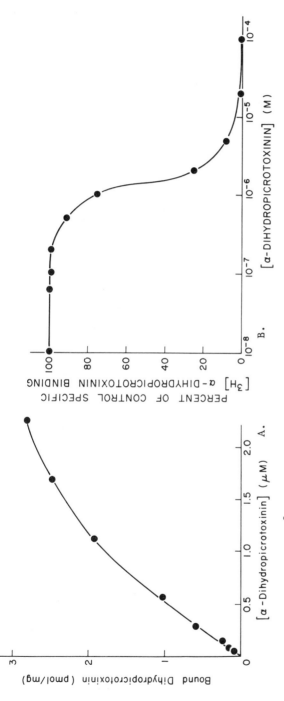

Figure 5. A. Binding of [$^3$H]α-Dihydropicrotoxinin to Rat Brain Membranes as a Function of Varying [$^3$H] Ligand Concentration. B. Displacement of [$^3$H]α-Dihydropicrotoxinin Binding by Nonradioactive Ligand. Fresh rat brain particulates (mitochondria plus microsomes) were incubated at 2.3 mg/ml protein in 0.2 M NaCl, 5 mM NaPO$_4$, pH 7.0, for 15 min at 0° with A. varying amounts of [$^3$H]DHP of 1.34 Ci/mmol or B. constant [$^3$H]DHP of 12 Ci/mmol and 63 nM but varying concentrations of nonradio-active DHP. Specifically bound ligand was determined by centrifuging in a manner analogous to that employed with GABA binding assays. Background was taken as that ligand which could not be displaced by 0.1 mM nonradioactive DHP. Each point is the mean of quadruplicates (variation less than 15%); experiments depicted are typical of three or more.

active DHP at 100 μM, with an $IC_{50}$ of 1.1 μM (Fig. 5B). The amount
of ligand bound at saturation was 3-4 pmol/mg protein (mitochondria plus microsomes of total brain) and 120 $\pm$ 20 pmol/g wet brain.

Other analogues of DHP also inhibited the binding (Table 2),
and the relative potency of inhibition agreed with the biological
activity of these substances, tutin and picrotoxinin being
slightly better than DHP in all cases, picrotin weaker than DHP,
and picrotoxinin acetate and alkaline-hydrolyzed DHP inactive.
GABA (0.2 mM) and muscimol (0.1 mM) did not inhibit DHP binding,
nor did numerous other neurotransmitter candidates and drugs.
Bicuculline inhibited weakly ($IC_{50}$ = 100-200 μM), compared to
an $IC_{50}$ to inhibit GABA receptor binding of 3-4 μM.

Chloride ion concentration (0-400 mM) had no dramatic effect
on DHP binding, either with rat brain or crayfish muscle tissue.
Despite one report that picrotoxin was more potent in low chloride
solution than in physiological saline at inhibiting the postsynaptic response to GABA in crayfish muscle (Takeuchi & Takeuchi, 1969)
there is no convincing evidence that picrotoxinin blockade of GABA-
mediated chloride conductance involves direct competition with the
anions. It appears, however, that the site of action of picrotoxinin is distinct from that of GABA, muscimol and bicuculline.

Table 3.  BRAIN REGIONAL DISTRIBUTION OF PICROTOXININ AND GABA
RECEPTOR BINDING SITES IN RAT BRAIN

|  | Picrotoxinin | GABA |
|---|---|---|
| Cerebellum | 6047 $\pm$ 190 | 13766 $\pm$ 2000 |
| Cerebral cortex | 4179 $\pm$ 690 | --- |
| Pyriform- | 3000 $\pm$ 124 | 3604 $\pm$ 900 |
| Neo- | 6759 $\pm$ 1307 | 8778 $\pm$ 800 |
| Hippocampus | 6539 $\pm$ 310 | 7505 $\pm$ 1100 |
| Corpus striatum | 5367 $\pm$ 482 | 5465 $\pm$ 540 |
| Hypothalamus | 3962 $\pm$ 388 | 3093 $\pm$ 590 |
| Brain stem | 2317 $\pm$ 441 | 2126 $\pm$ 360 |

Dissected regions of several fresh rat brains were stored in
0.32 M sucrose at -20°. After thawing, aliquots were washed in
0.2 M NaCl, 0.01 M $NaPO_4$, pH 7.1 and assayed at 2 mg/ml in that
buffer for DHP binding with 63 nM [$^3$H]DHP, 12 Ci/mmol by the centrifugation assay described in Figure 5. Other aliquots were
osmotically shocked, frozen and thawed, and thoroughly washed for
assay in 0.05 M Tris-citrate, pH 7.1 (sodium-free), at 1.0 mg/ml
protein with 10 nM [$^3$H]GABA of 12.6 Ci/mmol. Values given in
DMP bound/mg protein; average of 2-5 experiments in triplicate.

The quantity of binding sites for DHP varied with brain region (Table 3). Highest activity was found in cerebellum and some cerebral cortex regions including hippocampus. This distribution agreed well with that of GABA receptor (Table 3, also, Enna & Snyder, 1975), and also with the distribution of radioactive bicuculline binding sites (Mühler & Okada, 1977). We are likewise comparing the GABA and DHP binding sites in various cell types and fractions purified from cerebellum of normal and neurologically mutant mice, (Olsen et al., 1978a).

Table 4 gives the subcellular distribution in fractions of rat brain for DHP binding sites, GABA receptor sites, and the nonreceptor (muscimol-insensitive) sodium-dependent GABA binding sites. DHP binding sites were enriched in the synaptosome and light microsome fractions, as were the GABA receptor sites. Likewise, other neurotransmitter binding sites have been found to be enriched in these fractions (DeBlas & Mahler, 1976). Thus DHP and GABA receptor binding sites show a similar although not identical distribution which is consistent with a postsynaptic membrane location; (Ticku et al. 1978). The nonreceptor GABA-binding sites, which we believe involve a mixture of two or more binding sites, were also enriched in the crude mitochondrial fraction, but were higher in the myelin fraction than GABA receptor sites. Further characterization of the various subclasses of nonreceptor sites is in progress (VanNess et al., 1978).

Table 5 summarizes a comparison between DHP binding sites and GABA receptor sites. Both were found in approximately the same quantity in rat brain (and also in crayfish muscle, although the amount of each type of binding site was about 10-fold lower than in mammalian brain). The brain regional and subcellular distribution was similar for the two as shown above; (also in crayfish muscle the two types of sites were found in the same subcellular fractions, Olsen et al. 1978). This is consistent with a possible association of DHP binding sites and GABA receptors in the postsynaptic membrane.

Nevertheless, the drugs which inhibited the GABA binding site did not inhibit the DHP site and vice versa, indicating distinct sites. That GABA receptor sites and DHP binding sites are distinct was further supported by observations of differential sensitivity to chemical treatment. Exposure of the tissue to the histidine-specific reagent diethylpyrocarbonate partially inhibited the GABA receptor binding sites, but did not inhibit DHP sites, whereas the sulfhydryl group reagent N-ethyl maleimide and the detergent Triton X-100 had greater effects on DHP binding than on the GABA receptor sites (Table 5).

Table 4. SUBCELLULAR LOCALIZATION OF PICROTOXININ AND GABA BINDING SITES IN RAT BRAIN

| | PROTEIN | DHP BINDING | | GABA BINDING −Na⁺ | | GABA BINDING +Na⁺ | |
|---|---|---|---|---|---|---|---|
| | % of total | DPM/mg | % of total | DPM/mg | % of total | DPM/mg | % of total |
| Homogenate | 100 | 1858±96 | 100 | 2570±205 | 100 | 1026 | 100 |
| P₁ | 30 | 695±198 | 11 | 2387±260 | 24 | 786 | 23 |
| P₂ | 39 | 2489±303 | 50 | 2962±230 | 39 | 1306 | 50 |
| P₃ | 32 | 2405±314 | 40 | 3328±210 | 36 | 888 | 28 |
| | of P₂ | | of P₂ | | of P₂ | | of P₂ |
| Mitochondria | 49 | 695±54 | 23 | 1653±150 | 38 | 521 | 23 |
| Synaptosomes | 26 | 3058±224 | 55 | 4308±310 | 53 | 1709 | 40 |
| Myelin | 24 | 1368±108 | 23 | 891±97 | 9 | 1669 | 36 |

Fresh rat brain was fractionated according to established procedures (Whittaker & Barker, 1972). Protein was assayed according to Lowry et al. (1951). DHP binding and GABA binding were determined with samples that had been frozen and thawed, osmotically shocked, and thoroughly washed. Binding was measured by centrifugation assays under standard conditions, protein 2-2.5 mg/ml. DHP was incubated at 63 nM, 12 Ci/mmol, in 0.2 M NaCl, 5 mM NaPO₄, pH 7.0; GABA was incubated at 10 nM, 12.6 Ci/mmol in either sodium-free 0.05 M Tris-citrate, pH 7.1; or in 0.2 M NaCl plus 0.05 M Tris-citrate, pH 7.1 and also 3 µM muscimol to inhibit all the receptor binding (+Na⁺ columns). Assays were done in triplicate with variation less than 6%; results are average ± S.E.M. of four experiments, except for the +Na⁺ data done only twice.

Table 5.   COMPARISON OF GABA RECEPTOR AND PICROTOXININ BINDING
           SITES IN RAT BRAIN

|  | GABA Receptor Binding Sites | Picrotoxinin Binding Sites |
|---|---|---|
| Quantity of sites (pmol/g wet tissue) | 85 ± 15 | 120 ± 20 |
| Apparent $K_D$ (µM) | 0.2 | 1.1 |
| Brain regional distribution | very similar | |
| Subcellular localization | similar (synaptosomes, light microsomes) | |

Chemical treatment
A.  Diethylpyrocarbonate
    (0.8 mM, pH 6.5, 0°, 20 min)          +                    -

B.  N-Ethyl maleimide
    (1 mM, 0°, 20 min)                    -                    +

C.  Triton X-100
    (0.05%, 0°, 20 min)                   -                    +

D.  GABA
    muscimol        ⎱ 10 µM
    bicuculline     ⎰                     +                    -

(+) Signifies inhibition of at least 50%;
(-) Insignificant effect.


    In summary, the GABA binding sites in rat brain, detected
in sodium-free buffer with thoroughly disrupted and washed tissue,
have properties which satisfy the criteria mentioned above for
identification as receptor sites. These sites can also be detected
in sodium-containing buffers, and identified by their affinity for
GABA and receptor-specific drugs such as muscimol.  Several other
classes of GABA binding sites are dependent upon sodium ions; one
of these sites appears to be inhibited by low concentrations of
diaminobutyrate but not β-alanine, another by β-alanine but not
DABA.  These binding sites may be related to the sodium-dependent
transport systems for GABA in neurons and glial cells.

    Likewise, radioactive picrotoxinin (DHP) binds to saturable
sites in brain, and the quantity of DHP binding sites, the binding

affinity, the chemical specificity for picrotoxinin analogues, the tissue, brain region, and subcellular distribution all suggest a relationship to the physiological action of picrotoxinin at the GABA postsynaptic membrane. Since picrotoxinin does not act on the GABA receptor itself, the drug may prove to be a valuable probe for analyzing other aspects of postsynaptic response mechanisms, such as regulation of the chloride ionophore. Further studies are aimed at clarifying the relationship of DHP binding sites to GABA receptor-ionophore function. Likewise, other convulsant drugs, e.g. bicyclophosphates (Bowery et al. 1977), and anticonvulsant drugs, e.g. barbiturates (Bowery & Dray, 1976; Barker et al. 1977), may act at the level of GABA receptor-regulated chloride ionophores; the relationship of their site(s) of action to that of picrotoxinin is under investigation.

## HOW MANY GABA RECEPTOR CLASSES EXIST?

At the present time there is no evidence to prove or rule out the existence of more than one class of GABA receptor. Species and regional differences have been observed in electrophysiological studies of GABA action, both in vertebrates (Curtis & Johnston, 1974; Krnjević,1974) and invertebrates (Gerschenfeld, 1973; Takeuchi, 1976; Dudel & Hatt, 1976). These observed differences can be summarized as a. varying sensitivity to bicuculline of responses to GABA or to agonists (McLennan, 1973; Krnjević, 1974; Curtis & Johnston, 1974); b. inconsistent responses to agonists or antagonists in different regions responding to GABA (Curtis & Johnston, 1974; Krnjević, 1974); c. variation in desensitization of GABA response (Dudel & Hatt, 1976); or d. different equilibrium potentials and/ or ionic selectivity of responses to GABA (Gerschenfeld, 1973; Takeuchi, 1976; Barker et al. 1977; Yarowsky & Carpenter, 1976). All of these differences might be explained by reasons other than differences in GABA receptors, but the possibility of pharmacological variation in GABA receptors or ionophores is suggested.

At the level of binding studies, we observed apparently one class of GABA binding sites having the properties of receptors, but of course there could be more than one class of sites of similar affinity. Some support for this latter idea comes from our observations of a lack of strictly competitive inhibition of GABA receptor binding by bicuculline (Greenlee et al. 1977). Also, Möhler and Okada (1978) reported a "negatively cooperative" inhibition by GABA of radioactive bicuculline binding. Furthermore the binding of bicuculline (Möhler & Okada, 1977) and of picrotoxinin (Table 3) shows a partial but not perfect agreement with GABA receptor sites with respect to brain regional distribution. Further support for the multiple GABA receptor idea comes from the observation of two high-affinity receptor-like binding sites detected in brain membranes treated with the mild detergent Triton X-100 (Enna & Snyder, 1977; Wong & Horng, 1977). These properties could be artifacts of the treatment, but it is also possible that two populations of GABA receptors are present. The two populations might differ in bicuculline and/or picrotoxinin sensitivity, or all GABA receptors may not be coupled to the same antagonist and/or ionophore sites.

By analogy to the muscarinic acetylcholine receptors (Birdsall & Hulme, 1976), two classes of receptor binding sites may reflect two states for a single type of receptor: a physiologically functional, or "coupled" state (implying coupling in a functional manner to an ionophore), and a nonfunctional or "uncoupled" state, still maintaining high binding affinity; (the latter could be related to desensitization [Changeux et al., 1975]). The regulation of distribution between these two states of the receptor would then be very important with respect to synaptic plasticity.

Further information on these questions will undoubtedly come forth from neuro-physiological and -pharmacological studies on monosynaptic preparations, and from biochemical studies on purified receptor/ionophore proteins from defined brain regions or cultured cell populations.

## ACKNOWLEDGMENTS

Supported by NSF grant BNS 73-02078, NIH grants NS 12422 and Research Career Development Award NS 00224, and by the Alfred P. Sloan Foundation. We thank T. Miller for neurophysiology assistance, W. B. Levy, B. Meiners, and P. Kehoe for helpful discussions.

## REFERENCES

Barker, J. L., MacDonald, R. L. and Ransom, B. R. 1977. Post-synaptic pharmacology of GABA on CNS neurons grown in tissue culture. In "Iontophoresis and Transmitter Mechanisms in the mammalian CNS", (R. W. Ryall & J. S. Kelly, ed.) Elsevier, Amsterdam, in press.

Beart, P. M. and Johnston, G. A. R. 1973. Transamination of analogues of γ-aminobutyric acid by extracts of rat brain mitochondria. Brain Res. 49:459-462.

Birdsall, N. J. M. and Hulme, E. C. 1976. Biochemical studies on muscarinic acetylcholine receptors. J. Neurochem. 27:7-16.

Bon, C. and Changeux, J.-P. 1975. Ceruleotoxin:an acidic neuro-toxin from the venom of Bungarus caeruleus which blocks the response to a cholinergic agonist without binding to the cholingeric receptor site. FEBS Lett. 59:212-216.

Bowery, N. G. and Dray, A. 1976. Barbiturate reversal of amino acid antagonism produced by convulsant agents. Nature 264:276-278.

Bowery, N. G., Collins, J. F., Hill, R. G., Pearson, S. 1977. t-Butyl bicyclophosphate:a convulsant and GABA antagonist more potent than bicuculline. Br. J. Pharmacol. In press.

Changeux, J.-P., Benedetti, L., Bourgeois, J.-P., Brisson, A., Cartaud, J., Devaux, P., Grunhagen, H., Moreau, M., Popot, J.-L., Sobel, A., and Weber, M. 1975. Some structural properties of the cholinergic receptor protein in its membrane environment relevant to its function as a pharmacological receptor. Cold Spring Harbor Symp. Quant. Biol. XL:211-230.

Coyle, J. T. and Enna, S. J. 1976. Neurochemical aspects of the ontogenesis of GABAnergic neurons in the rat brain. Brain Res. 111:119-133.

Cuatrecasas, P. 1974. Membrane receptors. Ann. Rev. Biochem. 43:168-214.

Curtis, D. R. and Johnston, G. A. R. 1974. Amino acid transmitters in the mammalian central nervous system. Ergebn. Physiol. 69: 98-188.

DeBlas, A. and Mahler, H. R. 1976. Studies on nicotinic acetylcholine receptors in mammalian brain, VI: isolation of a membrane fraction enriched in receptor function for different neurotransmitters. Biochem. Biophys. Res. Commun. 72:24-32.

Dudel, J. and Hatt, H. 1976. Four types of GABA receptors in crayfish leg muscles characterized by desensitization and specific antagonists. Pflugers Arch. 364:217-222.

Eldefrawi, A. T., Eldefrawi, M. E., Albuquerque, E. X., Oliveira, A. C., Mansour, N., Adler, M., Daly, J. W., Brown, G. B., Burgermeister, W., and Witkop, B. 1977. Perhydrohistrionicotoxin: a potential ligand for the ion conductance modulator of the acetylcholine receptor. Proc. Nat. Acad. Sci. USA 74: 2172-2176.

Enna, S. J. and Snyder, S. H. 1975. Properties of γ-aminobutyric acid binding to receptor sites in rat central nervous system. Brain Res. 100:81-97.

Enna, S. J. and Snyder, S. H. 1977. Influence of ions, enzymes, and detergents on GABA receptor binding in synaptic membranes of rat brain. Mol. Pharmacol. 13:442-453.

Enna, S. J. Collins, J. F. and Snyder, S. H. 1977. Stereospecificity and structure-activity required of GABA receptor binding in rat brain. Brain Res. 124:185-190.

Gerschenfeld, H. M. 1973. Chemical transmission in invertebrate central nervous systems and neuromuscular junctions. Physiol. Rev. 53:1-119.

Greenlee, D. V., VanNess, P. C. and Olsen, R. 1977. Gamma-aminobutyric acid receptor binding sites in membrane fractions from mammalian brain. Submitted.

Iversen, L.L. and Kelly, J.S. 1975. Uptake and metabolism of γ-aminobutyric acid by neurones and glial cells. Biochem. Pharmacol., 24:933-938.

Jarboe, C.H., Porter, L.A. and Buckler, R.T., 1968. Structural aspects of picrotoxinin action. J. Med. Chem. 11:729-731.

Johnston, G. A. R. 1978. Neuropharmacology of amino acid inhibitory transmitters. Ann. Rev. Pharmacol. Toxicol. 18: In press.

Krnjević, K. 1974. Chemical nature of synaptic transmission in vertebrates. Physiol. Rev. 54:418-540.

Krogsgaard-Larsen, P. and Johnston, G. A. R. 1975. Inhibition of GABA uptake in rat brain slices by nipecotic acid, various isoxazoles and related compounds. J. Neurochem. 25:797-802.

Krogsgaard-Larsen, P., Johnston, G. A. R., Curtis, D. R., Game, C. J. A. and McCulloch, R. M. 1975. Structure and biological activity of a series of conformationally restricted analogues of GABA. J. Neurochem. 25:803-809.

Lloyd, K. G., Shermen, L. and Hornykiewicz, O. 1977. Distribution of high affinity sodium-independent ($^3$H) gamma-aminobutyric acid (GABA) binding in human brian: alterations in Parkinson's disease. Brain Res. 127:269-278.

Lowry, O. H., Rosebrough, N. J., Farr, A. L. and Randall, R. J. 1951. Protein measurement with the Folin phenol reagent. J. Biol. Chem. 193:265-275.

McLennan, H. 1973. γ-Aminobutyric acid antagonists in crustacea. Can. J. Physiol. Pharmacol. 51:774-775.

Meiners, B., Kehoe, P., Shaner, D. M. and Olsen, R. W. 1978. Preparation of plasma membranes from crayfish muscle enriched in gamma-aminobutyric acid uptake and binding sites. Submitted Biochim. Biophys. Acta.

Möhler, H. and Okada, T. 1977. GABA receptor binding with H(+) biculline methiodide in rat CNS. Nature 267:65-67.

Möhler, H. and Okada, T. 1978. Properties of GABA receptor binding with $^3$H(+) bicuculline-methiodide in rat cerebellum. Mol. Pharmacol. In press.

Olsen, R. W., Ban, M. and Miller, T. 1976. Studies on the neuropharmacological activity of bicuculline and related compounds. Brain Res. 102:283-299.

Olsen, R. W., Ticku, M. K., Van Ness, P. C. and Greenlee, D. 1977. Effects of drugs on gamma-aminobutyric acid receptors, uptake, release, and synthesis in vitre. Brain Res. In press.

Olsen, R. W., Mikoshiba, K. and Chanjeux, J.-P. 1978a. Gamma-cerebellum and depletion in agranular mutant mice. Submitted J. Neurochem.

Olsen, R. W., Ticku, M. K. and Miller, T. 1978b. Dihydropicrotoxinin binding to crayfish muscle sites possibly related to gamma-aminobutyric acid receptor-ionophores. Submitted Mol. Pharmacal.

Simantov, R., Oster-granite, M. L., Herndon, R. M. and Snyder, S. H. 1976. Gamma-aminobutyric acid (GABA) receptor binding selectively depleted by viral induced granule cell loss in hamster cerebellum. Brain Res. 105:365-371.

Snyder, S. H. and Bennett, J. P. 1976. Neurotransmitter receptors in the brain. Ann. Rev. Physiol. 38:153-175.

Takeuchi, A. and Takeuchi, N. 1969. A study of the action of picrotoxin on the inhibitory neuromuscular junction of the crayfish. J. Physiol. (London) 205:377-391.

Takeuchi, A. 1976. Studies of inhibitory effects of GABA on invertebrate nervous system. In "GABA in Nervous System Function" (E. Roberts, T. N. Chase, and D. B. Tower, eds.) Raven Press, New York, pp. 255-267.

Ticku, M. K. and Olsen, R. W. 1977a. γ-Aminobutyric acid-stimulated chloride permeability in crayfish muscle. Biochem. Biophys. Acta 464:519-529.

Ticku, M. K., Ban, M and Olsen, R. W. 1978b. Binding sites in rat brain for GABA synaptic antagonist, picrotoxin. Submitted.

Ticky, M. K., Van Ness, P. C., Haycock, J. W., Levy, W. B. and Olsen, R. W. 1978b. Picrotoxinin binding sites in rat brain: regional distribution, and ontogeny, compared to GABA receptors. Submitted Brain Res.

Van Ness, P. C., Greenlee, D. and Olsen, R. W. 1978. Gamma-aminobutyric acid binding sites in rat brain: comparison of sodium-dependent and -independent sites. In preparation.

Wheal, H. V. and Kerkut, G. A. 1976. The action of muscimol on the inhibitory postsynaptic membranes of the crustacean neuromuscular junction. Brain Res. 109:179-183.

Whittaker, V. P. and Barker, L. A. 1972. The subcellular fractionation of brain tissue with special reference to the preparation of synaptosomes and their component organelles. In "Methods in Neurochemistry", Vol. 2. (R. Fried, ed.) Marcel Dekker, New York, pp. 1-52.

Wong, D. T. and Horng, J. S. 1977. Na$^+$-independent binding of GABA to the Triton X-100 treated synaptic membranes from cerebellum of rat brain. Life Sci. 20:445-452.

Young, A. B. and Snyder, S. H. 1974. The glycine synaptic receptor: evidence that strychnine binding is associated with the ionic conductance mechanism. Proc. Nat. Acad. Sci. USA 71:4002-4005.

Yarowsky, T. and Carpenter, D. O. 1976. A comparison of ionophores activated by acetylcholine and γ-aminobutyric acid in Aplysia neurons. Fed. Proc. Fed. Am. Soc. Exp. Biol. 35:543.

Zukin, S. R., Young, A. B. and Snyder, S. H. 1974. Gamma-aminobutyric acid binding to receptor sites in rat central nervous system. Proc. Nat. Acad. Sci. USA 71:4802-4807.

# COMPARISON OF [3]H-MUSCIMOL AND [3]H-GABA RECEPTOR BINDING IN RAT BRAIN

S.J. Enna, K. Beaumont and H.I. Yamamura

Depts. of Pharmacology and Neurobiology & Anatomy

Univ. of Tex. Med. Sch. PO Box 20708 Houston, Tx. 77025

Muscimol (3-hydroxy-5-aminomethylisoxazole) has been reported to be a GABA receptor agonist in the mammalian central nervous system (Johnston, 1976; Krogsgaard-Larsen et al., 1975). Administration of this agent is known to cause both lethargy and hallucinations suggesting that muscimol penetrates the central nervous system. However, the specificity of this agent for central GABA receptors has yet to be conclusively demonstrated making it possible that these behavioral effects result from an interaction of muscimol with other neurotransmitter receptor sites.

Recently a specific, high affinity binding of [3]H-muscimol has been demonstrated in rat brain synaptic membranes (I. Beaumont, W. Chilton, H.I. Yamamura and S.J. Enna, in preparation). In the present communication the characteristics of this specific [3]H-muscimol binding are compared to those of [3]H-GABA binding which represents attachment to the biologically relevant synaptic GABA receptor site (Enna and Snyder, 1975; Enna and Snyder, 1977) in an attempt to determine the specificity of muscimol for the GABA receptor.

[3]H-muscimol was synthesized by decarboxylating ibotenic acid in the presence of tritiated water (Ott et al., 1975). The specific activity of the [3]H-muscimol is 0.3 Ci/mmole. For the binding studies, a portion (1 mg protein) of crude synaptic membranes prepared from rat brain (Enna and Snyder, 1975) was incubated in 6 ml of 0.05 M Tris-citrate buffer (pH 7.1  4oC) containing 2.0 nM [3]H-muscimol in the presence or absence of 10 μM unlabelled muscimol or 200 μM unlabelled GABA. After incubation at 4oC for 30 min, the mixture was centrifuged at 48 000 x g and the resultant pellet was rinsed rapidly and superficially with 15 ml of ice cold

distilled water and, after dissolution, the radioactivity in the
pellet was determined using liquid scintillation spectrometry.
Specifically bound $^3$H-muscimol is defined as the amount of isotope
displaced by the high concentration of unlabelled muscimol or GABA.
Saturation studies indicate that the binding of $^3$H-muscimol to rat
brain membranes is at equilibrium within 5 - 10 min and the specific binding is saturable with an apparent dissociation constant
of 2.2 nM.

### I.   SUBCELLULAR DISTRIBUTION OF $^3$H-MUSCIMOL AND $^3$H-GABA RECEPTOR BINDING

When the specific binding of both $^3$H-muscimol and $^3$H-GABA
was examined in various subcellular fractions of whole rat brain
it was found to be most enriched in the crude mitochondrial pellet
($P_2$).  In addition, after osmotic disruption of the $P_2$ pellet,
both $^3$H-muscimol and $^3$H-GABA binding were found to be 2 to 7 times
higher in the resultant crude synaptic membrane pellet than in the
mitochondrial-myelin fraction suggesting that the specific binding
of both isotopes is primarily associated with synaptic elements
(Zukin et al., 1974).

Like $^3$H-GABA, the specific binding of $^3$H-muscimol is not
found in tissues outside of the central nervous system.  Organs
which have been examined include the heart, stomach, small intes-
tine, liver and kidney.

TABLE I.   REGIONAL DISTRIBUTION OF SPECIFIC $^3$H-MUSCIMOL AND
$^3$H-GABA BINDING IN RAT CENTRAL NERVOUS SYSTEM

| Region | Specifically Bound Ligand (fmoles/mg protein) | |
| --- | --- | --- |
|  | $^3$H-Muscimol | $^3$H-GABA |
| Cerebral Cortex | 147 | 91 |
| Hippocampus | 60 | 51 |
| Corpus Striatum | 60 | 42 |
| Midbrain | 56 | 56 |
| Hypothalamus | 50 | 36 |
| Cerebellum | 280 | 194 |
| Medulla oblongata-pons | 20 | 37 |
| Spinal Cord | 17 | 5 |

Experiments were performed on previously frozen whole homogenate
particulate fractions prepared as described in the text.  Final
concentration of $^3$H-muscimol in the incubation medium was 2 nM.
The $^3$H-GABA data was adapted from Enna and Snyder, 1975.

## II.  REGIONAL DISTRIBUTION OF $^3$H-MUSCIMOL BINDING IN RAT BRAIN

Measurement of specifically bound $^3$H-muscimol in eight regions of the rat brain indicates  that the greatest number of receptors for this agent are found in the cerebellum which is twice as high as the next most enriched area, the cerebral cortex (Table I). The hippocampus, corpus striatum, midbrain and hypothalamus display roughly the same degree of specific binding for $^3$H-muscimol, about 20% of that observed in the cerebellum.  The brain regions with the least amount of $^3$H-muscimol binding were the medulla and spinal cord which have less than 10% of the cerebellar binding capacity.  This regional distribution for $^3$H-muscimol is virtually identical to that observed for $^3$H-GABA receptor binding in rat brain (Table I).

## III.  EFFECTS OF TRITON X-100 AND FREEZING ON SPECIFIC $^3$H-MUSCIMOL BINDING

Specific binding of $^3$H-GABA to the GABA receptor is enhanced in membranes which have been previously frozen and is increased even further if the membranes have been preincubated in 0.05% Triton X-100 (Enna and Snyder, 1977).  Similarily, specific $^3$H-muscimol binding is twice as high in tissue which has been frozen and is increased another 2 to 3-fold after treatment with 0.05% Triton X-100.

## IV.  PHARMACOLOGICAL CHARACTERISTICS OF $^3$H-MUSCIMOL BINDING IN RAT BRAIN

$^3$H-muscimol binding to Triton-treated membranes from whole rat brain is selectively inhibited by drugs and amino acids which are known to be GABA receptor agonists and antagonists (Table II). Thus GABA, 3-aminopropanesulfonic acid, trans-4-aminocrotonic acid and imidazoleacetic acid, all neurophysiological GABA receptor agonists, are all approximately equipotent to muscimol in displacing specifically bound $^3$H-muscimol.  In addition, $^3$H-muscimol binding is stereospecific in that trans-3-aminocyclopentane-1-carboxylic acid, the biologically active form of this agent, is more potent than the cis-form and (+)-bicuculline, which is more potent than (-)-bicuculline as a convulsant, is more potent in displacing the specifically bound isotope.  Furthermore, 1-methylimidazoleacetic acid, a very weak GABA receptor agonist neurophysiologically, is very weak in displacing $^3$H-muscimol.  Also, 2,4-diaminobutyric acid and (±) nipecotic acid, inhibitors of neuronal GABA uptake having little or no neurophysiological potency on GABA receptors, are also without activity in displacing the isotope.  The potency of other neurotransmitters and drugs on displacing $^3$H-muscimol binding has also been examined with none being found to have an $IC_{50}$ less than 10 µM. These include norepinephrine, dopamine, serotonin, histamine, phenobarbital, atropine, glycine, and diazepam. Qualitatively these results mimic the substrate specifically found for $^3$H-GABA binding to the GABA receptor (Table II). Quantitatively however, there are some interesting differences between the pharmacological profiles for $^3$H-muscimol and $^3$H-GABA binding. Most striking is the fact that while trans-3-aminocyclopentane-1-carboxylic acid is slightly more potent than GABA in displacing specifically bound $^3$H-GABA, it is about 10 times less potent than muscimol in displacing $^3$H-muscimol. Similarly, trans-4-aminocrotonic acid is about equipotent with muscimol on $^3$H-muscimol binding but is greater than 10 times more potent than GABA in displacing $^3$H-GABA binding. In contrast, the relative potencies of imidazoleacetic acid, 3-aminopropanesulfonic acid and bicuculline are similar in competing for $^3$H-muscimol and $^3$H-GABA binding.

TABLE II.  SUBSTRATE SPECIFICITY OF $^3$H-MUSCIMOL AND $^3$H-GABA BINDING TO RAT BRAIN MEMBRANES

| Compound | $IC_{50}$ (nM) | |
| --- | --- | --- |
| | $^3$H-muscimol | $^3$H-GABA |
| Muscimol | 5 | 3 |
| GABA | 8 | 20 |
| 3-Aminopropanesulfonic acid | 5 | 4 |
| trans-4-Aminocrotonic acid | 7 | 1 |
| Imidazoleacetic acid | 8 | 50 |
| (+)-trans-3-Aminocyclopentane-1-carboxylic acid | 80 | 5 |
| (+)-cis-3-Aminocyclopentane-1-carboxylic acid | 8000 | 3000 |
| (+)-Bicuculline | 2000 | 5000 |
| (−)-Bicuculline | >10,000 | >10,000 |
| 1-Methylimidazoleacetic acid | >10,000 | >10,000 |
| 2,4-Diaminobutyric acid | >10,000 | >10,000 |
| (±)Nipecotic acid | >10,000 | >10,000 |

Inhibition of specific ligand binding by various concentrations of the different compounds was determined using the standard assay procedure with previously frozen membrane preparations. $IC_{50}$ values, the concentration which inhibits specific $^3$H-ligand binding 50%, were calculated by log-probit analysis. The $^3$H-GABA displacement data was adapted from Enna and Snyder, 1977.

## V. DISCUSSION

The characteristics of high affinity ³H-muscimol binding in rat brain are very similar to those reported for ³H-GABA binding to the synaptic GABA receptor. Thus the distinctive effect of freezing and Triton X-100 treatment on enhancing ³H-GABA binding is also seen with ³H-muscimol binding. Similarly, the characteristic regional distribution of ³H-GABA binding in rat brain is observed for ³H-muscimol binding and both the brain subcellular and tissue distribution are the same for both ligands. Most convincing, however, is the fact that ³H-muscimol binding is inhibited by those drugs and amino acids which interact with ³H-GABA receptor binding, whereas other neurotransmitters and drugs have only a negligible affinity for the muscimol site, suggesting specificity of this agent for the synaptic GABA receptor. However, the present results do not conclusively demonstrate an absolute specificity of muscimol for the GABAergic system since it is possible that this alkaloid interacts with other, as yet untested, neurotransmitter processes. Nevertheless, the data does support the notion that muscimol is a potent and specific GABA receptor agent. Furthermore, the fact that certain GABA receptor agonists have distinctly different relative potencies in displacing ³H-GABA and ³H-muscimol from the GABA site suggests the existence of more than one type of GABA receptor.

## ACKNOWLEDGEMENTS

This work was supported in part by a Pharmaceutical Manufacturers Association Research Starter Grant, USPHS grant MH-29739, The Huntington Chorea Foundation and Merck Sharp and Dohme to S.J.E. and by USPHS grants MH-27257, MH-29840 and an NIMH RSDA (MH-00095) to H.I.Y. We thank Dr. W. Chilton for his assistance in preparing the ³H-muscimol.

## REFERENCES

Enna, S.J. and Snyder, S., 1975, Properties of γ-aminobutyric acid
    (GABA) receptor binding in rat brain synaptic membrane frac-
    tions, Brain Res. 100:81-97.

Enna, S.J. and Snyder, S., 1977, Influences of ions, enzymes and
    detergents on γ-aminobutyric acid receptor binding in synaptic
    membranes of rat brain, Mol. Pharmacol. 13:442-453.

Johnston, G., 1976, Physiologic pharmacology of GABA and its ant-
    agonists in the vertebrate nervous system, in "GABA in Nervous
    System Function,"(E. Roberts, T. Chase and D. Tower, eds.),
    Raven Press, New York.

Krogsgaard-Larsen, P., Johnston, G., Curtis, D., Game, C. and Mc-
    Culloch, R., 1975, Structure and biological activity of a
    series of conformationally restricted analogues of GABA, J.
    Neurochem. 25:803-809.

Ott, J., Wheaton, P. and Chilton, W., 1975, Fate of muscimol in
    the mouse, Physiol. Chem. and Physics 7:381-384.

Zukin, S., Young, A. and Snyder, S., 1974, Gamma-aminobutyric acid
    binding to receptor sites in the rat central nervous system,
    Proc. Nat. Acad. Sci. USA 71:4802-4807.

# GABA RECEPTOR IN RAT BRAIN: DEMONSTRATION

# OF AN ANTAGONIST BINDING SITE

H. Möhler and T. Okada

Pharmaceutical Research Department
F. Hoffmann-La Roche, 4002 Basle, Switzerland

A variety of evidence suggests that neurotransmitter receptors in the brain may exist in two interconvertible conformations, an agonist conformation with a selective high affinity for receptor agonists and an antagonist conformation with a selective high affinity for receptor antagonists. This hypothesis can be tested in binding studies using receptor agonists and antagonists as labelled ligands (Snyder and Bennett, 1976). For the GABA receptor, binding studies have so far been performed with GABA agonists as labelled ligands only (Enna et al. 1978). Thus, an attempt was made to identify biochemically the antagonist binding site of the GABA receptor by using the GABA antagonist (+)bicuculline-methiodide as labelled ligand. (+)Bicuculline and its chemically more stable N-methyl-derivative antagonise reversibly and, at low concentrations, rather specifically the synaptic inhibitory action of GABA in the CNS (Johnston et al., 1972) without affecting the uptake or release of GABA or enzymes metabolizing GABA (Beart and Johnston, 1972). Thus, $^3$H(+)BM should be a suitable ligand for binding studies of the synaptic GABA receptor.

Specific binding of $^3$H(+)BM was found to be saturable, stereospecific and maximally enriched in the synaptic membrane fraction; it showed an uneven regional distribution in the brain. Only GABA, GABA agonists and GABA antagonists were potent competitors for the (+)BM binding site. These characteristics of the (+)BM binding site are in agreement with the properties of the synaptic GABA receptor based on neurophysiological evidence. Thus, specific binding of $^3$H(+)BM seems to represent an ineraction with the synaptic GABA receptor.

Routine binding assays were performed by incubating previous-

ly frozen crude synaptic membrane fractions (2 mg protein) from
rat cerebellum prepared according to Zukin et al., with 5 nM
$^3$H(+)BM in the absence and presence of high concentrations of
GABA (50 µM) in 50mM Tris-HCl buffer pH 7.4 and 50 mM NaSCN. The
assay was terminated by centrifugation, the tubes washed and the
pellets dissolved to count the radioactivity bound. "Specific binding" of $^3$H(+)BM was obtained by subtracting from the radioactivity bound in the absence of GABA ("total binding") the amount
not displaceable by high concentrations of GABA ("non-specific
binding"). $^3$H(+)BM (specific activity 8.0 Ci/mmole) and $^3$H(-)BM
(13 Ci/mmole) were prepared by methylation of (+) and (-)bicucul-
line respectively with $^3$H-methyliodide (Möhler and Okada 1977a).
$^3$H(+)BM was not metabolized under the assay conditions used and
remained radiochemically pure for months under proper storage conditions (Möhler and Okada, 1977b).

I.   SATURATION AND SUBCELLULAR DISTRIBUTION OF (+)BM BINDING

      Specific binding of $^3$H(+)BM was saturable. Only a single po-
pulation of specific binding sites could be identified in crude
cerebellar synaptic membrane fractions showing an apparent dissociation constant $K_D$ = 0.38µM for (+)BM. The apparent total number
of binding sites was 4.5 pmole/mg protein, which corresponds to the
total number of $^3$H-GABA binding sites (3.9 pmole/mg protein) (Wong
and Horng, 1977). Other subcellular fractions of rat cerebellum
showed a much lower amount of $^3$H(+)BM specific binding except the
crude mitochondrial fraction ($P_2$) - containing intact synaptosomes-
with a capacity for $^3$H(+)BM specific binding similar to that of
the crude synaptic membrane fraction (Möhler and Okada, 1977a).

II.   STEREOSPECIFICITY OF (+)BM BINDING

      The inhibition of the synaptic action of GABA by bicuculline
is stereospecific with most of the activity residing in the (+)
isomer. This neurophysiological potency is reflected in the
$^3$H(+)BM binding: the inactive isomers (-)bicuculline and (-)BM
have only 1/800th and 1/400th the potency of the respective (+)iso-
mers in displacing $^3$H(+)BM from its binding site. Furthermore,
$^3$H(-)BM (5 nM) does not bind to the (+)BM binding site, since
$^3$H(-)BM could not be displaced by an excess of various GABA agonists and antagonists which were able to displace $^3$H(+)BM from its
binding site (Möhler and Okada, 1977a). Besides its GABA antagonistic action, BM elicits an excitatory effect in vivo, which so
far could not be associated with a molecular parameter. However,
the excitatory action of BM is not stereospecific (Collins and Hill,
1974) and is thus not reflected in the (+)BM binding presented
here.

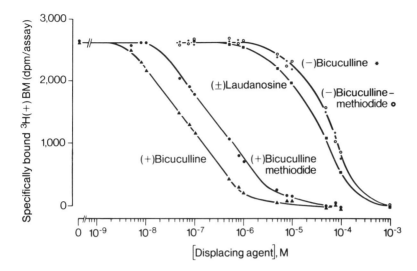

FIGURE I

STEREOSPECIFICITY OF $^3$H(+)BM SPECIFIC BINDING

Inhibition of specific $^3$H(+)BM binding by various concentrations of the compounds indicated was determined using standard assay conditions. (+)Laudanosine, although structurally
related to bicuculline, is neurophysiologically inactive.

III. LIGAND SPECIFICITY OF (+)BM BINDING

Only compounds considered to be GABA antagonists or GABA
agonists on neurophysiological evidence were found to be competitors for the specific binding site of (+)BM (Tab. 1). Among GABA
antagonists, (+)bicuculline had the highest displacing potency,
corresponding to the high in vivo potency of this compound (Curtis
et al., 1974). The in vitro inhibition of acetylcholine-esterase
by (+)bicuculline is not represented in the inhibition of $^3$H(+)BM
binding, since much higher concentrations of bicuculline are needed
to inhibit the enzyme ($K_i$ = 17$\mu$M) (Breuker and Johnston, 1975) than
(+)BM binding ($IC_{50}$ = 0.07$\mu$M). The lack of displacing potency of
picrotoxin and TETS (tetramethylene disulphotetramine) in $^3$H(+)BM
binding is attributed to the blockade of the chloride channel by
these compounds (Möhler and Okada, 1977b; Olsen 1978). The affi-

nity of strychnine to the GABA receptor is 1700 times less than that to the glycine receptor ($K_i$ = 2nM).

TABLE I

LIGAND SPECIFICITY OF $^3$H(+)BM BINDING

| Compound | $IC_{50}$ (nM) | | |
|---|---|---|---|
| (+)Bicuculline | 70 | $\pm$ | 2 |
| (+)Bicuculline methiodide | 222 | $\pm$ | 21 |
| Muscimol | 59 | $\pm$ | 7 |
| GABA | 430 | $\pm$ | 55 |
| 3-Aminopropanesulfonic acid | 500 | $\pm$ | 70 |
| Imidazole acetic acid | 3 900 | $\pm$ | 300 |
| $\beta$-Alanine | 60 000 | $\pm$ 6 | 000 |
| Strychnine | 3 600 | $\pm$ | 370 |
| ($\pm$)Laudanosine | 34 000 | $\pm$ 1 | 500 |
| (-)Bicuculline-methodide | 54 000 | $\pm$ 5 | 000 |
| (-)Bicuculline | 60 000 | $\pm$ 4 | 000 |
| Picrotoxin | no inhibition | | |
| TETS | " | | |
| D,L-2,4-Diaminobutyric acid | " | | |
| Nipecotic acid | " | | |

'No inhibition' refers to concentrations up to at least $10^{-5}$M. Further compounds without inhibitory effect up to $10^{-5}$M include: glutamate, asparate, $\alpha$-alanine, glycine, proline, taurine, aminooxyacetic acid, isoniazide, morphine, nialamide, kainic acid, chlordiazepoxide, diazepam, pentobarbital, baclofen, oxotremorin, physostigmin, haloperidol, chlorpromazine (Möhler and Okada 1977a).

IV.   REGIONAL DISTRIBUTION OF (+)BM BINDING

The capacity for specific binding of $^3$H(+)BM varied 10 fold in different rat brain regions with the highest levels in cerebral cortex and cerebellum and the lowest level in spinal cord (Möhler and Okada 1977a). The regional distribution is somewhat similar to that of $Na^+$-independent $^3$H-GABA-binding (Enna and Snyder, 1975). However, on the basis of the present data it cannot be decided if the regional variation is due to differences in the number of binding sites or in their affinity.

V.  COMPARISON OF (+)BM BINDING AND Na$^+$-INDEPENDENT GABA BINDING

   (+)BM binding as well as Na$^+$-independent GABA binding (Enna
and Snyder, 1975) seem to represent an interaction with the synaptic GABA receptor. It is striking that GABA agonists show a higher
affinity for the GABA binding site than for the (+)BM binding
site (e.g. GABA, $IC_{50}$ = 0.02 μM in GABA binding as compared to
$IC_{50}$ = 0.4 μM in (+)BM binding). The inverse relationship holds
for GABA antagonists (e.g. (+)bicuculline, $IC_{50}$ = 5.0 μM in GABA
binding as compared to $IC_{50}$ = 0.07 μM in (+)BM binding) (Table 1;
Enna and Snyder 1977). These findings may be explained by a GABA
receptor existing in two conformations, an agonist conformation
showing a high affinity for GABA agonists  and a low affinity for
GABA antagonists, while the inverse relationship holds for the
antagonist conformation (Fig. 2).

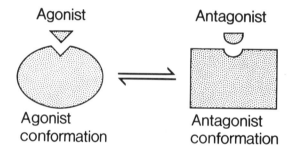

FIGURE 2

A MODEL OF GABA RECEPTOR FUNCTION

   The different assay conditions required for (+)BM binding and
Na$^+$-independent GABA binding may be interpreted on the basis of a
conformational change of the GABA-receptor: High affinity binding
of GABA is shown only after treating the membranes with Triton
(Enna and Snyder, 1977), which may induce a conformational change
of the GABA receptor from the antagonist to the agonist conformation, possibly by removing a phospholipid (Johnston, 1978). On the
other hand SCN$^-$, ClO$_4^-$ or I$^-$ seem to have a specific effect on the
antagonist conformation (Enna and Snyder, 1977; Möhler and Okada
1977b). However, more evidence is needed to support the GABA receptor model presented, especially in view of a possible hetero-
geniety of GABA receptors (Enna et al. 1978).

REFERENCES

Breuker, E. and Johnston, G.A.R., 1975, Inhibition of acetylcholinesterase by bicuculline and related alkaloids, J. Neurochem.
25: 903-904.
Beart, P.M. and Johnston, G.A.R., 1972, Bicuculline and GABA metabolizing enzymes, Brain Res. 38: 226-227.
Collins, J.F. and Hill, R.G., 1974, (+) and (-)bicuculline methochloride as optical isomers of a GABA antagonist, Nature
249: 845-846.
Curtis, D.R., Johnston, G.A.R., Game, C.J.A. and McCulloch, R.M.,
1974, Central action of bicuculline, J. Neurochem. 23:
605-606.
Enna, S.J. and Snyder, S.H., 1975, Properties of $\gamma$-aminobutyric
acid (GABA) receptor binding in rat brain synaptic membrane
fractions, Brain Res. 100: 81-97.
Enna, S.J. and Snyder, S.H., 1977, Influences of ions, enzymes and
detergents on $\gamma$-aminobutyric acid receptor binding in synaptic membranes of rat brain, Molec. Pharmac. 13: 442-453.
Enna, S.J., Beaumont, K. and Yamamura, H.I., 1978, Comparison of
$^3$H-muscimol and $^3$H-GABA receptor binding in rat brain, in
"Amino acids as chemical transmitters", Fonnum, F. ed.,
Plenum Press (this volume).
Johnston, G.A.R., Beart, P.M., Curtis, D.R., Game, C.J.A., McCul-
loch, R.M. and MacLachlan, R.M., 1972, Bicuculline methochlo-
ride as a GABA antagonist, Nature New Biol. 240: 219-220.
Johnston, G.A.R., 1978, in "Amino acids as chemical transmitters",
Fonnum, F. ed., Plenum Press (this volume).
Möhler, H. and Okada, T., 1977a, GABA receptor binding with $^3$H(+)bi-
cuculline methiodide in rat CNS, Nature, 267: 65-67.
Möhler, H. and Okada, T., 1977b, Properties of GABA receptor bin-
ding with $^3$H(+)bicuculline methiodide in rat cerebellum,
Molec. Pharmac., (in press).
Olsen, R.W., 1978, in "Amino acids as chemical transmitters",
Fonnum, F. ed. Plenum Press (this volume).
Snyder, S.H. and Bennett, J.P., 1976, Neurotransmitter receptors
in the brain: Biochemical identification, Ann. Rev. Physiol.,
38: 153-175.
Wong, D.T. and Horng, J.S., 1977, Na-independent binding of GABA
to the Triton X-100 treated synaptic membranes from cerebellum of rat brain, Life Sciences, 20: 445-452.
Zukin, S.R., Young, A.B. and Snyder, S.H., 1974, $\gamma$-Aminobutyric
acid binding to receptor sites in the rat central nervous
system, Proc. Nat. Acad. Sci., U.S.A., 71: 4802-4807.

# A STUDY OF THE GABA RECEPTOR USING [3]H-BICUCULLINE METHOBROMIDE

J.F. Collins* and G. Cryer

Department of Chemistry
City of London Polytechnic
31 Jewry Street
London EC3N 2EY

γ-aminobutyric acid (GABA) is now considered to be a major inhibitory neurotransmitter in the CNS (Kelly and Beart, 1975). The post-synaptic receptor for GABA has been previously studied using [3]H-GABA (Zukin, Young and Snyder, 1974; Enna and Snyder, 1975; Enna, Snyder and Collins, 1977). However, GABA, as well as binding to the post-synaptic receptor, also binds to glial and neuronal uptake sites. Thus it has been suggested that only the $Na^+$ independent [3]H-GABA binding is associated with receptor binding (Enna and Snyder, 1975). A better approach to a study of the receptor might be to use a specific radio labelled GABA antagonist or agonist.

The phthaleidoisoquinoline alkaloid bicuculline (1) is now widely accepted as a selective GABA antagonist (Curtis and Johnston, 1973). However, in practice certain disadvantages attend the use of bicuculline in a study of the post-synaptic GABA receptor. In particular solutions of bicuculline at neutral pH gradually lose their ability to antagonise GABA (Olsen, 1975). Bicuculline methiodide (II X = $I^-$), prepared from bicuculline and iodomethane, has also been found to be a potent antagonist (Pong and Graham, 1973). Although this compound is water soluble it is unstable and decomposes quite rapidly at room temperature to yield an inactive, water insoluble oil. Johnston et al. (1972) have shown that bicuculline methochloride (II, X = $Cl^-$) is a stable, water soluble GABA antagonist. The preparation of the methochloride is, however, quite lengthy, and requires relatively sophisticated chemical facilities.

In contrast, bicuculline methobromide is very easily prepared from bicuculline and bromomethane. It is a white, crystalline compound, which is stable indefinitely in aqueous solution at room temperature. Radioactive bicuculline methobromide of high specific activity (> 2 Ci/m mole) has now been prepared and has been shown to be stable for long periods in aqueous solution. We have used this compound in a study of its binding to the GABA receptor.

Bowery and Dray (1976) have shown that both in vivo and in vitro pentobarbitone reverses GABA antagonism produced by bicuculline methobromide and other GABA antagonists. We now report that the inhibition of $^3$H-GABA binding produced by bicuculline methobromide can be reversed using pentobarbitone.

## METHODS AND MATERIALS

(+) Bicuculline (Sigma, 500 mg) was dissolved in acetone (15 cm$^3$) and bromomethane from a cylinder was bubbled into the cooled solution until saturation was reached. The reaction mixture was set aside for three hours at room temperature. At the end of this time the white crystalline solid which had precipitated was filtered off and dried to yield bicuculline methobromide (570 mg, 95%). Crystallisation of the methobromide could be effected from acetone-methanol, but this was rarely necessary.

$^3$H-Bicuculline methobromide was prepared by the quarternisation of bicuculline with $^3$H-bromomethane in acetone solution. The product was purified by paper chromatography (The Radiochemical Centre, Amersham). The purified bicuculline methobromide had a specific activity of 2.1 Ci/m mol and was found to be radiochemically pure (> 98%) as judged by thin layer chromatography on cellulose in 3 different systems:

(i)    n-butanol: water: acetic acid (12:5:3)
(ii)   n-butanol: ethanol: water (104:66:30)
(iii)  iso-propanol: ethanol: IN hydrochloric acid (3:3:2)

and also by thin layer chromatography on silica gel in:

(iv)   chloroform: methanol: acetic acid (8:1:1)
(v)    n-butanol: water: acetic acid (12:5:3).

The R$_f$ values corresponded to those of inactive (+) bicuculline. The solution of (+) bicuculline methobromide was re-analysed at monthly intervals and no significant decomposition has yet been detected.

(-) Bicuculline was synthesised by the method of Teitel et al. (1972) and was converted into the (-) methobromide as described above.

$^3$H-GABA was obtained from the Radiochemical Centre, Amersham and had specific activity of 12.6 Ci/m mole.


## Preparation of Synaptosomal Fractions

Membranes were prepared by a modification of the method described by Zukin et al. (1974).

Three rats (Sprague - Dawley, 300-350 g) (male or female) were killed and their brains rapidly removed and homogenised in 15 volumes of ice-cold 0.32M sucrose solution using a Potter-Elvehjem glass homogeniser fitted with a Teflon pestle. The homogenate was centrifuged at 1000 x g for 10 minutes; the pellet was discarded and the supernatant was centrifuged at 20,000 x g for 20 min. The pellet was dispersed in cold distilled water using a X-1020 high speed stirrer. The suspension was centrifuged at 8000 x g for 20 min. The supernatant was collected and the pellet, a bilayer with a soft, buffy upper coat, was rinsed carefully with the supernatant to collect the upper layer. The combined supernatant fraction was then centrifuged at 48,000 x g for 20 min. The final crude fraction was suspended in water and centrifuged at 48,000 x g for 10 min. twice and then stored at - 30°C for at least 24 hours.

The assay. The frozen pellet was allowed to thaw and then suspended in 25 mls distilled water and left for 30 min. at room temperature. A sample was removed for the Lowry protein determination. The suspension was adjusted in volume to give a concentration of 1 mg of protein/ml. The suspension was then transferred in 1 ml aliquots to the appropriate number of 1.5 ml Eppendorf tubes and then centrifuged at 11,500 x g for 2 min. using a Microfuge B. The supernatant was removed and discarded. Each pellet was then resuspended in 0.05M Tris-citric acid buffer pH 7.1 and incubated at room temperature with the appropriate drug for 10 min. followed by incubation for 10 min. with either $^3$H-GABA (7.4 nM) or $^3$H-(+)-bicuculline (5 nM). Incubation was terminated by centrifugation at 11,500 x g for 5 min. The supernatant was rapidly removed and the tubes carefully dried. The pellets were dissolved overnight in soluene tissue solubiliser. After neutralisation of the soluene by 1.5M hydrochloric acid the samples were made up to 11 mls with Toluene-Triton X-100 scintillant containing PPO (0.5%) and POPOP (0.05%) and counted using an ICN 2700 liquid scintillation counter at a counting efficiency of 28%.

Determinations were done in triplicate or sextuplicate.  In
triplicate determinations only assays which gave groups of values
which differed by less than 10% from the mean were used.  In
sextuplicate determinations values which differed by more than the
standard deviation from the mean were discarded.  Specific binding
was obtained by subtracting from the total bound radioactivity the
amount not displaced by high concentrations of GABA (1 mM) or
bicuculline methobromide (.1 mM).  Protein was determined by the
Lowry Method (Lowry, 1951).

X = I, Cl or Br

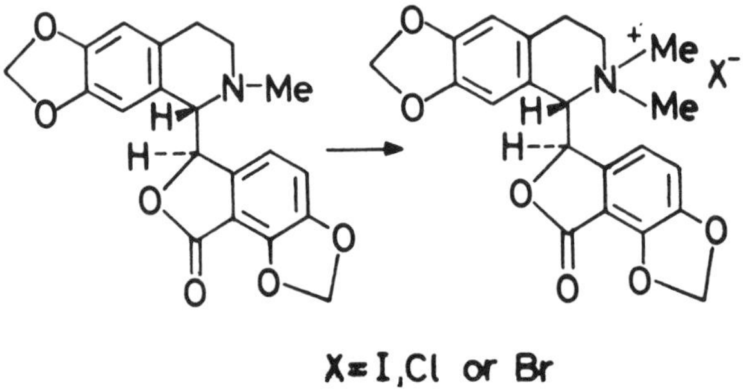

Fig. 1.   The preparation of (+)-bicuculline methosalts.

RESULTS

(+) [3]H-bicuculline methobromide binding:  The results obtained
are shown in figure 2.  Clearly, (+) bicuculline methobromide at
.1 mM concn is able to displace about 16% of the [3]H-bicuculline
methobromide binding while (−) bicuculline methobromide was very
much less efficient at this process, only being able to displace
about 5.8% of the binding.  However, it is of considerable interest
that a high concentration (1 mM) GABA is not very effective in
displacing the [3]H-bicuculline methobromide binding.

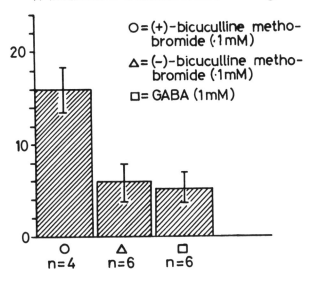

Fig. 2. Bicuculline methobromide binding to synaptosomal membranes.
Membranes were prepared as indicated in Methods, n= number of
experiments carried out. The height of the histogram is the mean
percentage of these experiments. The concentration of (+)-$^3$H-bicu-
culline methobromide was 5.0 nM. Error bars represent ± the S.E.M.
All experiments were conducted in the absence of added cations or
anions.

Pentobarbitone reversal of counts displaced by bicuculline:
In figure 3 the results obtained in the study using $^3$H-GABA are
shown. In agreement with the results obtained previously by Zukin
et al. (1974) pentobarbitone (.1 mM) has no effect on the total
$^3$H-GABA binding, while both GABA (1 mM) and (+)-bicuculline
methobromide displace $^3$H-GABA binding. However, when pentobarbitone
(.1 mM) is added to incubations containing (+) bicuculline
methobromide, there is a significant decrease in the number of
counts displaced as a percentage of the total GABA binding. In

some experiments the effect was such that no counts whatever were
displaced, i.e. a total reversal of the effect had occurred.

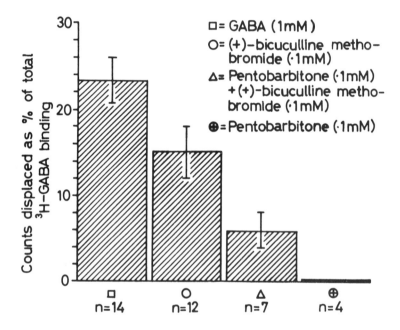

Fig. 3:  The effect of pentobarbitone on the displacement of $^3$H-GABA
elicted by (+) bicuculline methobromide.  Membranes were prepared
as described in the Methods.  n = number of experiments carried out.
The height of the histogram is the mean of these experiments.  The
concentration of $^3$H-GABA was 7.4 nM.  Error bars represent ± S.E.M.
All experiments were conducted in the absence of added cations or
anions.

No uptake of $^3$H-bicuculline methobromide into brain slices
could be observed (Bowery and Neal – unpublished observations).

## DISCUSSION

Very recently Möhler and Okada (1977) have described the
characteristics of the binding of $^3$H-bicuculline methiodide to
synaptosomal fragments. They found that the binding was specific,
saturable, stereospecific and was reversed by unlabelled (+)
bicuculline methiodide, (+) bicuculline and GABA but not by (-)
bicuculline methiodide. However, their binding studies were always
conducted in the presence of 50 mM sodium thiocyanate, as they were
unable to detect any specific binding in its absence (Möhler -
personal communication). Enna and Snyder (1977) have recently
reported that the anions thiocyanate, iodide and nitrate increase
the potency of bicuculline ten-fold in inhibiting $Na^+$-independent
GABA receptor binding without affecting the potency of GABA agonists.
All these ions are defined as being highly chaotropic (Hatefi and
Hanstein, 1969), i.e. inter alia, they tend to promote chain
unfolding in proteins. It may well be, therefore, that these
agents subtly change the conformation of the GABA receptor and
thus promote the binding of $^3$H-bicuculline methiodide. Different
binding sites have been postulated to exist on the post-synaptic
receptor (Möhler, 1977) for agonists and antagonists. Our results
tend to support this theory. In particular the failure of 1 mM
GABA to reverse the $^3$H-bicuculline methobromide binding suggests
the existence of different sites. Again, the reversal by .1 mM
pentobarbitone of the inhibition of $^3$H-GABA binding produced by
bicuculline methobromide while pentobarbitone is itself without
effect would also support this theory.

REFERENCES

Bowery, N.G. and Dray, A., 1966, Barbiturate reversal of amino acid antagonism produced by convulsant agents, Nature, 264:276.

Curtis, D.R. and Johnston, G.A.R., 1973, Amino acids as transmitters in the mammalian central nervous system, Ergebn. Physiol., 69:97-187.

Enna, S. and Snyder, S.H., 1975, Properties of GABA receptor binding in rat brain synaptic membrane fractions, Brain Res., 100: 81-97.

Enna, S., Snyder, S.H. and Collins, J.F., 1977, Stereospecificity and structure-activity requirements of GABA receptor binding in rat brain, Brain Res., 124:185-190.

Enna, S. and Snyder, S.H., 1977, Influence of ions, enzymes and detergents on GABA receptor binding in synaptic membranes of rat brain, Mol. Pharm., 13:442-453.

Hatefi, Y. and Hanstein, 1969, Solubilization of particulate proteins and non electrolytes by chaotropic agents, Proc. Nat. Acad. Sci., 62:1129-1136.

Johnston, G.A.R., Beart, P.M., Curtis, D.R., Game, C.G.A. and McClachlan, R.W., 1972, Bicuculline methochloride a GABA antagonist, Nature New Biol., 240:219-220.

Kelly, J.S. and Beart, P.M., 1975, Amino acid receptors in the CNS. II. GABA in supraspinal regions. In "Handbook of Psychopharmacology", Vol. 5 (L.L. Iversen, S.D. Iversen and S.H. Snyder, eds.), Plenum Press, New York.

Lowry, O.H., Rosebrough, N.J., Farr, A.L. and Randall, R.J., 1951, Protein measurement with the Folin phenol reagent, J. Biol. Chem, 265-275.

Möhler, H. and Okada, T., 1977, GABA receptor binding with $^3$H(+) bicuculline methiodide in rat CNS, Nature, 267:65-67.

Olsen, R.W., Ban, M., Miller, T. and Johnston, G.A.R., 1975, Chemical instability of the GABA antagonist bicuculline under physiological conditions, Brain Res., 98:383-387.

Pong, S.F. and Graham, L.T., 1973, A simple preparation of bicuculline methiodide, a water soluble GABA antagonist, Brain Res., 58:266-267.

Teitel, S., O'Brien, J. and Brossi, A., 1972, Conversion of (-) β-Hydrastine into (-) Bicuculline and related phthaleido isoquinolines, J. Org. Chem., 37:1879-1881.

Zukin, S.R., Young, A.B. and Snyder, S.H., 1974, GABA binding to receptor sites in the rat central nervous system, Proc. Nat. Acad. Sci., 71:4802-4807.

# GABA RECEPTORS AND PHOSPHOLIPIDS

Graham A.R. Johnston and Sue M.E. Kennedy

Department of Pharmacology

Australian National University, Canberra, Australia

The sodium-independent binding of GABA to certain membrane preparations from rat brain exhibits many of the properties of the interaction of GABA with postsynaptic receptors anticipated from *in vivo* studies (see papers by Enna and Olsen, this meeting). Enna and Snyder (1975) found that, while sodium-independent GABA binding could be detected in homogenates of fresh brain tissue, freezing and thawing the membrane preparation led to a 2-fold increase in observed sodium-independent binding. Subsequently these authors reported that treatment of the membranes with 0.05% Triton X-100 further increased binding up to 5-fold, and also increased the apparent potencies of various GABA agonists (Enna and Snyder, 1977). Wong and Horng (1977) reported that treatment with 0.5% Triton X-100 increased both the apparent affinity and the apparent density of sodium-independent GABA binding from the values obtained using membranes prepared by extensive freezing and thawing.

In connection with our work on structure-activity properties of GABA analogues (see Krogsgaard-Larsen, this meeting), we have substantiated many of the findings of Enna and Snyder (1975, 1977), and of Wong and Horng (1977). Some of our results are summarised in Table I with respect to the potencies of GABA and the GABA agonists, muscimol and isoguvacine, in displacement of radioactive GABA bound to membranes prepared from rat brain in 1 of 3 ways: (i) "freeze-thaw" membranes prepared as described by Enna and Snyder (1975) and thoroughly washed at least 3 times by a routine of suspension in Tris-citrate buffer, freezing overnight, thawing, centrifuging (48,000 g, 20') and removal of the supernatant; (ii) "0.05% Triton" membranes prepared from (i) by treatment suspended in buffer at a concentration of 5 mg protein/ml with 0.05% v/v

Triton X-100 at 37°C for 30', followed by centrifugation and
washing of the membrane pellet several times by suspension in
buffer, centrifugation and removal of the supernatant; and (iii)
"0.5% Triton" membranes prepared as for (ii) using 0.5% Triton
X-100. The binding of radioactive GABA was measured using the
centrifuge assay of Enna and Snyder (1975) with 1 mM unlabelled
GABA to correct for non-specific binding. Electron microscopic
examination of the 3 types of membrane preparation by Dr M.C.W.
Minchin using phosphotungstic acid staining (Bloom and Aghajanian,
1968) showed the presence of synaptic junctional complexes
particularly enriched in the 0.5% Triton preparations.

Many investigators have used Triton treatment to give membrane
fractions enriched in junctional complexes (e.g. Fiszer and
De Robertis, 1967; Cotman, Levy, Banker and Taylor, 1971; Davis
and Bloom, 1973). Our results (Table I) show that Triton treatment
appreciably increases the potencies of muscimol, GABA and isoguvacine in the displacement of radioactive GABA bound to the
membranes. In agreement with Enna and Snyder (1977), Triton
treatment appeared to increase the potencies of all GABA agonists
studied. In agreement with Wong and Horng (1977), our 0.5% Triton
membrane preparation had a readily observable GABA binding site
with an apparent dissociation constant for GABA of 21 nM and an
apparent density of 4.2 pmole/mg protein, together with a less
readily observable site of higher affinity ($K_D$ approx. 6 nM) and
lower density (1 pmole/mg) which really needs radioactive GABA of
higher specific activity than is presently available in order to
be studied with any accuracy.

TABLE I

$IC_{50}$ FOR DISPLACEMENT OF RADIOACTIVE GABA ($\mu$M ± SEM)

| Inhibitor | Membrane preparation | | |
|---|---|---|---|
| | Freeze-thaw | 0.05% Triton | 0.5% Triton |
| Muscimol | 0.024 ± 0.003 | 0.0076 ± 0.0005 | 0.0041 ± 0.0002 |
| GABA | 0.34 ± 0.01 | 0.028 ± 0.001 | 0.014 ± 0.0006 |
| Isoguvacine | 1.4 ± 0.01 | 0.12 ± 0.01 | 0.059 ± 0.004 |

ENDOGENOUS INHIBITORS OF GABA BINDING

The apparent increases in the potencies of GABA and related compounds in displacing radioactive GABA bound to Triton-treated membrane preparations led us to investigate the possible existence of membrane-bound endogenous inhibitors that could be liberated by detergent extraction. The supernatants obtained after centrifugation of the various membrane preparations that had been subjected to Triton extraction, and also those obtained from freeze-thaw preparation, were shown to inhibit potently GABA binding. Extensive washings of the membrane preparations with Tris-citrate buffer were necessary to remove the inhibitory factor(s) and to obtain membranes that showed maximal and constant specific binding to radioactive GABA.

The supernatant extracts were analysed for GABA itself using (i) ion exchange chromatography in an automated amino acid analyser, (ii) the double-labelled dansyl amino acid thin layer chromatographic assay of Snodgrass and Iversen (1973), and (iii) the radioreceptor binding assay of Enna and Snyder (1976). All three methods indicated the presence of GABA in the supernatant extracts, but the two chromatographic methods indicated much less GABA (approx. 50% in most cases) than did the radioreceptor assay. The Triton-labile, membrane-bound GABA may be GABA "in the occult form" of Elliott and Van Gelder (1958), and may represent a storage or inactivated form of GABA.

There was clearly a factor other than GABA in the supernatant extracts that could inhibit the binding of radioactive GABA to the membrane receptors. This situation is somewhat reminiscent of the Factor I problem, where the inhibitory effect of certain nerve extracts on crayfish stretch receptor neurones was much more potent than could be accounted for by the GABA content of the extracts. GABA accounted for some 35% of the inhibitory effect of extracts of mammalian brain, while aspartate, glutamate and taurine accounted for a further 30%: the remaining 35% "must be due to the presence of other blocking compounds" (Koidl and Florey, 1975). Aspartate, glutamate and taurine at 10 μM do not influence GABA binding in the radioreceptor assay which is reputed to be highly specific for GABA (Enna and Snyder, 1976): nonetheless something other than GABA in the detergent extracts of rat brain membranes inhibited GABA binding.

PHOSPHOLIPIDS

Our attention was directed towards phospholipids as likely endogenous inhibitors of GABA binding by the work of Giambalvo and Rosenberg (1976) on the binding of GABA to junctional complexes

prepared from rat cerebellum by a procedure that included treatment
with 0.12% Triton X-100. These authors showed that incubation of
the membranes with phospholipase C split off the polar head groups
of endogenous phospholipids in the junctional complexes and
increased GABA binding. This would suggest that the phospholipid
polar head groups are associated with modifying the binding
characteristics of GABA receptors. At a chemical level it had been
shown that Triton treatment of junctional complexes from rat brain
results in differential solubilization of membrane protein,
phospholipid and sialic acid (Cotman *et al.*, 1971), and examination
of our supernatant extracts for phospholipids by thin layer
chromatographic procedures indicated clearly the presence of
relatively high concentrations of phosphatidylcholines and
phosphatidyethanolamines, with lesser concentrations of phosphatidyl-
serines.

Giambalvo and Rosenberg (1976) showed that sonicated exogenous
phospholipids could inhibit GABA binding to junctional complexes,
and that phosphatidylethanolamine was more potent than phosphatidylcholine. We were able to show that homogenising our 0.5% Triton
membrane preparations with 0.1 mM dipalmitoyl L-α-phosphatidyl-
ethanolamine could reduce specific GABA binding by 50% without
influencing non-specific binding, and that the equivalent
phosphatidylcholine and phosphatidylserine derivatives had no
significant effect under these conditions (Table II). The added
concentration of phosphatidylethanolamine in our experiments, and
in those of Giambalvo and Rosenberg (1976), may seem high at
0.1 mM, but it appears from studies using radioactive dansyl
phosphatidylserine that only about 1% of the added phospholipid is
bound to the membranes after homogenisation (Abood and Takeda, 1976),
and all of the bound exogenous phospholipid would not necessarily
be associated with GABA binding sites. While certain phospholipids
are known to bind *nor*-adrenaline (Formby, 1967), acetylcholine
(Izumi and Freed, 1974) and morphine (Abood and Hoss, 1975), the
observed inhibition of specific GABA binding by phosphatidylethanolamine is unlikely to be due to this phospholipid binding
radioactive GABA and thus reducing the amount of radioactive
GABA available to be bound to the membrane, since the amount of
radioactivity non-specifically bound is not altered (Table II).

These studies demonstrate that Triton treatment of brain
membranes releases phosphatidylethanolamine into the supernatant
medium, and that the supernatant medium contains factors other than
GABA that inhibit the binding of GABA to Triton-treated membranes.
Since exogenous dipalmitoyl phosphatidylethanolamine can inhibit
GABA binding, it seems highly likely that at least one of the
endogenous factors that modify GABA binding is phosphatidylethanolamine. It is not possible to quantify this hypothesis as yet due
to the difficulties in adding phospholipids back to the Triton-

treated membranes and a lack of knowledge regarding the fatty acid
substituents of the endogenous phosphatidylethanolamine(s).  From
the work of Abood *et al.* (1977) on the enhancement of opiate
binding by various molecular forms of phosphatidylserine, it is
likely that the fatty acid substituents of phosphatidylethanolamine
would play important roles in any interaction with GABA receptors.
Ethanolamine and ethanolamine-0-phosphate did not influence GABA
binding at 0.1 mM concentrations.

TABLE II

EFFECT OF EXOGENOUS PHOSPHOLIPIDS ON GABA BINDING

| Membrane homogenised with 0.1 mM exogenous phospholipid | $^3$H-GABA (DPM) bound to 0.5% Triton membranes from rat brain (values are means of triplicates which differed by less than 5%) | | |
|---|---|---|---|
| | Total | Non-specific | Specific |
| Control | 59208 | 5213 | 53995 |
| Phosphatidylethanolamine | 32503 | 5274 | 27229 |
| Phosphatidylcholine | 59663 | 4942 | 54721 |
| Phosphatidylserine | 64902 | 5531 | 59371 |

     With respect to GABA and phospholipids, it is interesting to
note that intracisternal injection of GABA inhibits the *in vivo*
incorporation of $^{33}$Pi into rat brain phospholipids (Friedel,
Slotnick and Bombardt, 1977).  This effect of GABA on phospholipid
metabolism may be mediated via GABA postsynaptic receptors since
it can be antagonised by bicuculline.  No specific effects of
GABA have been noted, however, on the metabolism of phosphatidylethanolamine, most of the phospholipid fractions being influenced
to a similar extent.

     Watkins (1965), noting the striking structural similarities
between the polar head groups of phospholipids and certain
neurotransmitters, proposed that neuronal membranes contain
phospholipid-protein complexes and "that the pharmacological
actions of acetylcholine, GABA and glutamic acid result from

dissociation of these complexes by the three substances and the
permeability changes ensuing therefrom".  GABA clearly resembles
phosphatidylethanolamine:

$$
\begin{array}{c}
O \\
\parallel \\
C-CH_2-CH_2-CH_2-NH_3^+ \\
\overset{\mid}{O}{}^-
\end{array}
$$

$$
\begin{array}{l}
\phantom{R''-}O \\
\phantom{R''-}\parallel \\
R'-C-O-CH_2 \qquad\qquad O \\
\phantom{R''-C-O-CH}\overset{\mid}{\phantom{}}{}_2 \qquad \parallel \\
R''-C-O-CH-CH_2-O\!\!-\!\!P\!\!-\!\!O\!\!-\!\!CH_2-CH_2-NH_3^+ \\
\phantom{R''-}\parallel \qquad\qquad\quad \overset{\mid}{O}{}^- \\
\phantom{R''-}O
\end{array}
$$

GABA was proposed to cause dissociation of a phosphatidylethanol-
amine-protein complex by either associating with the protein or
with the phospholipid.  The results of Giambalvo and Rosenberg
(1976) and the present results provide some support for this
aspect of Watkin's hypothesis, and indicate that GABA neuronal
receptors are normally associated with phosphatidylethanolamine
and that some of this phosphatidylethanolamine can be extracted
from neuronal membranes by treatment with Triton X-100 resulting
in an apparent increased affinity of GABA for the binding sites
and in an apparent increased density of binding sites on the
membranes.  The membrane-bound phosphatidylethanolamine may act
to control the availability of the GABA binding sites and may be
an integral part of physiologically active GABA receptors.

## HUNTINGTON'S DISEASE

GABA and its synthesising enzyme GAD are found in lower
concentration in the substantia nigra, putamen-globus pallidus and
caudate nucleus of autopsied brains from patients who suffered
from Huntington's disease as compared to autopsied brains from
neurologically normal subjects (Perry, Hansen and Kloster, 1973;
Bird and Iversen, 1974).  These findings suggest degeneration of
GABA neurones in these brain areas during Huntington's disease.
When GABA receptor binding was assayed on membranes prepared from
these brain areas by freezing and thawing, there was no apparent
difference between Huntington's and normal tissues from the
putamen-globus pallidus and caudate nucleus.  In the substantia
nigra, however, the binding of radioactive GABA (8 nM in medium)
was twice as high in the Huntington's tissue (Enna *et al*., 1976).
It was suggested that this apparent increase in GABA receptor
binding may reflect a "denervation supersensitivity phenomenon".

Significantly elevated levels of glycerophosphoethanolamine were found in the three brain regions from Huntington's patients (Perry *et al.*, 1973). This perhaps indicates that the metabolism of phosphoethanolamine is altered in Huntington's disease, and suggests that it may be profitable to study phospholipid metabolism in Huntington's patients in some detail particularly with respect to possible association with GABA receptors. The apparent increase in GABA receptor binding in membrane from Huntington's substantia nigral tissue may reflect a decreased association of phosphatidylethanolamine with GABA binding sites.

## DRUGS AND PHOSPHOLIPIDS

Cuthbert (1967) in a review on membrane lipids and drug action made the following comment: "Generally it is believed that drugs active on the cell membrane bring about a conformational change in a membrane protein, the receptor, which acts as a trigger for subsequent events which may involve the lipids. It is interesting to speculate that a second order involvement of membrane lipids in drug action provides another dimension for the diversity of drug action". It seems likely that the effect of diazepam in increasing the apparent affinity of GABA binding to membrane receptors (Guidotti, this meeting) represents an example of a second order involvement of membrane lipids as envisaged by Cuthbert (1967). It is known from studies using radioactive diazepam that diazepam binding sites on membranes are sensitive to Triton extraction (H. Möhler, unpublished) and that the effect of diazepam on the apparent affinity of GABA binding is less in Triton-treated membranes than in freeze-thaw membrane preparations (A. Guidotti, unpublished). These observations indicate that diazepam binds to a Triton-labile membrane component in such a way as to alter the apparent binding affinity of GABA to a relatively Triton-stable membrane component. A likely diazepam binding site would be fatty acid side chains of phosphatidylethanolamines which are associated with GABA binding sites, such interaction decreasing association of ethanolamine head groups with GABA binding sites and thus reducing any competition between such head groups and GABA for the binding sites. Benzodiazepines, such as diazepam, are relatively lipophilic substances and fatty acid moieties are likely sites of action for these drugs. A similar mechanism could operate for other lipophilic drugs that appear to modify GABA synapses, e.g. certain barbiturates, hydantoins and related drugs. This rationale would mean that it would be wise to study the possible effects of drugs, and perhaps also GABA agonists, on GABA receptors *in vitro* using preparations in which any phospholipid association was preserved, in addition to preparations treated to exhibit maximal GABA binding affinity.

CONCLUSIONS

A possible association between certain phospholipids and
GABA binding sites could provide a basis for a better understanding
of the postsynaptic action of GABA.  Such phospholipids may represent sites whereby the postsynaptic responses of GABA might be
modified by lipophilic drugs, e.g. benzodiazepines.  Denervation
supersensitivity could be the result of less phospholipid being
associated with GABA binding sites and this would indicate that
presynaptic influences on postsynaptic events might involve
phospholipids.  It is possible that phospholipids are involved
in the synaptic action of other neurotransmitters.


*Acknowledgements* - The authors are grateful to Dr J.C. Watkins
for helpful discussions, to Dr K.G. Lloyd for drawing our attention
to the elevation of glycerophosphoethanolamine in Huntington's
disease, to Drs H. Möhler and A. Guidotti for unpublished results,
to Dr M.C.W. Minchin for electron microscopy, and to Mr B. Twitchin
for skilled assistance.

REFERENCES

Abood, L.G., and Hoss, W., 1975, Stereospecific morphine adsorption to phosphatidylserine and other membranous components of brain, *Europ. J. Pharmac.* 32:66–75.

Abood, L.G., Salem, N., Macneil, M., Bloom, L., and Abood, M.E., 1977, Enhancement of opiate binding by various molecular forms of phosphatidylserine and inhibition by other unsaturated lipids, *Biochim. Biophys. Acta.* 468:51–62.

Abood, L.G., and Takeda, F., 1976, Enhancement of stereospecific opiate binding to neural membranes by phosphatidylserine, *Europ. J. Pharmac.* 39:71–77.

Bird, E.D., and Iversen, L.L., 1973, Huntington's chorea. Post-mortem measurement of glutamic acid decarboxylase, choline acetyltransferase and dopamine in basal ganglia, *Brain* 97: 457–472.

Bloom, F.E., and Aghajanian, G.K., 1968, Fine structural and cytochemical analysis of the staining of synaptical junctions with phosphotungstic acid, *J. Ultrastruct. Res.* 22:361–375.

Cotman, C.W., Levy, W., Banker, G., and Taylor, D., 1971, An ultrastructural and chemical analysis of the effect of Triton X-100 on synaptic plasma membranes, *Biochim. Biophys. Acta* 249:406–418.

Cuthbert, A.W., 1967, Membrane lipids and drug action, *Pharmac Rev.* 19:59–106.

Davis, G.A., and Bloom, F.E., 1973, Isolation of synaptic junctional complexes from rat brain, *Brain Res.* 62:135–153.

Elliott, K.A.C., and Van Gelder, N.M., 1958, Occlusion and metabolism of γ-aminobutyric acid by brain tissue, *J. Neurochem.* 3: 28–40.

Enna, S.J., Bennett, J.P., Bylund, D.B., Snyder, S.H., Bird, E.D., and Iversen, L.L., 1976, Alterations of brain neurotransmitter receptor binding in Huntington's chorea, *Brain Res.* 116:531–537.

Enna, S.J., and Snyder, S.H., 1975, Properties of γ-aminobutyric acid (GABA) receptor binding in rat brain synaptic membrane fractions, *Brain Res.* 100:81–97.

Enna, S.J., and Snyder, .H., 1976, A simple, sensitive and specific radioreceptor assay for endogenous GABA in brain tissue, *J. Neurochem.* 26:221–224.

Enna, S.J., and Snyder, S.H., 1977, Influences of ions, enzymes and detergents on GABA receptor binding in synaptic membranes of rat brain, *Molec. Pharmac.* 13:442–453.

Fiszer, S., and De Robertis, E., 1967, Action of Triton X-100 on ultrastructure and membrane-bound enzymes of isolated nerve endings from rat brain, *Brain Res.* 5:31–44.

Formby, B., 1967, The binding of noradrenaline to phosphatidyl-serine. *In vitro* studies of an artificial model system of biological origin, *Molec. Pharmac.* 3:284–289.

Friedel, R.O., Slotnick, R.N., and Bombardt, P.A., 1977, Effects
    of γ-aminobutyric acid on [33]Pi incorporation into rat brain
    phospholipids *in vivo*, *Life Sciences* 20:235-242.
Giambalvo, C., and Rosenberg, P., 1976, The effect of phospholipase:
    and proteases on the binding of γ-aminobutyric acid to
    junctional complexes of rat cerebellum, *Biochim. Biophys. Acta.*
    436:741-756.
Izumi, F., and Freed, S., 1974, Binding of acetylcholine and
    cholinergic drugs to proteolipid fractions from rat cerebral
    cortex and to phospholipids from bovine brain, *FEBS Letters*
    42:319-322.
Koidi, B., and Florey, E., 1975, Factor I and GABA: resolution of
    a long-standing problem, *Comp. Biochem. Physiol.* 51C:13-23.
Perry, T.L., Hansen, S., and Kloster, M., 1973, Huntington's
    chorea deficiency of γ-aminobutyric acid in brain, *New
    Eng. J. Med.* 288:337-342.
Snodgrass, S.R., and Iversen, L.L., 1973, A sensitive double
    isotope derivative assay to measure release of amino acids
    from brain *in vitro, Nature New Biol.* 241:154-156.
Watkins, J.C., 1965, Pharmacological receptors and general
    permeability phenomena of cell membranes, *J. Theoret. Biol.*
    9:37-50.
Wong, D.T., and Horng, J.S., 1977, Na[+]-independent binding of GABA
    to the Triton X-100 treated synaptic membranes from
    cerebellum of rat brain, *Life Sciences* 20:445-452.

SECOND MESSENGER RESPONSES AND REGULATION OF HIGH AFFINITY RECEPTOR
BINDING TO STUDY PHARMACOLOGICAL MODIFICATIONS OF GABAERGIC
TRANSMISSION

A. Guidotti, G. Toffano[*], L. Grandison, E. Costa

Laboratory of Preclinical Pharmacology, National
Institute of Mental Health, Saint Elizabeths Hospital
Washington, D.C. 20032

[*]On leave from FIDIA Research Laboratories, Abano Terme,
Italy

One of the current research trends in neuropharmacology centers
on possible mechanisms whereby drugs modify GABA transmission (Costa,
1977; Johnston, 1976). This concern about new developments in the
pharmacology of GABA transmission stems from the direct or indirect
implication of GABA in the pathogenesis of Huntington's chorea
(Perry et al., 1973), Parkinson's disease (McGeer et al., 1971),
epilepsy (Wood and Peesker, 1974), senile dementia, schizophrenia,
anorexia nervosa and other neurological disorders (Roberts, 1976).

The need for drugs that modify GABA transmission by mechanism
other than direct activation of GABA receptors derives from the
ubiquity of GABA in brain and its involvement in various aspects of
CNS function. In fact, GABA acts as putative neurotransmitter in
substantia nigra (Fonnum et al., 1974; Perry et al, 1973; Ribak
et al., 1976), cerebellum (Eccles et al., 1967; Kuriyama et al.,
1966), hippocampus (Okada and Shimada, 1976), hypothalamus
(Kuriyama and Kimura, 1976) and spinal cord (Barker and Nicoll,
1973). This anatomical situation explains why direct GABA receptor
agonists can be readily used in therapy to elicit stimulation of a
selected population of GABA receptors. These drugs could not be
used without causing a number of collateral side effects deriving
from the stimulation of all GABA receptors in CNS.

517

Histoimmunofluorescence (Ribak et al., 1976), radioautography (Iversen and Neal, 1968) and electrophysiological (Precht and Yoshida, 1976) techniques have shown that GABA is present in glial cells and neurons. The uptake of GABA by neurons is blocked by nipecotic acid which fails to block the uptake of GABA by glial cells; conversely, beta-alanine blocks the uptake of GABA by glial cells and not by neurons (Johnston, 1976). Although this information has provided theoretical implications on the possible therapeutic value of GABA uptake blockers (Johnston, 1976), analogues of nipecotic acid which can cross the blood brain barrier have not yet become available for further experimentation.

The studies of GABA binding to postsynaptic receptors using radioactive GABA and synaptic membrane preparations from brain (Enna and Snyder, 1977) have revealed that specific high affinity receptor sites for GABA present a specific distribution pattern in different brain areas. It is not yet known whether these recognition sites for GABA are coupled to specific enzymes located on postsynaptic membranes, however, such a link is supported by several lines of indirect investigation. Natural candidates for such a role are enzymes which prime the membrane pump for $Cl^-$ exclusion and which may be inhibited following occupation of the high affinity sites for GABA binding at postsynaptic membranes. In fact, some investigators have shown that the simulation of GABA receptors changes the $Cl^-$ conductance across neuronal membrane at all sites (for references, see Roberts, 1974; and Roberts, 1976).

Though much evidence suggests that studies of GABA affinity binding should be coupled with the measurement of $Cl^-$ conductance, major technical problems limits the feasibility of these studies:

1. The increase of $Cl^-$ conductance is also elicited by other putative neurotransmitters (for example, glycine or taurine (Krnjevic and Puil, 1976); thus, unless one measures $Cl^-$ conductance with a preparation containing only GABA postsynaptic receptors, the interpretation of the results obtained becomes questionable.

2. Measurement of $Cl^-$ conductance in mammalian CNS are extremely difficult to perform. Up to now these measurements have been successfully applied only to GABA receptor function ininvertebrate neurons.

These considerations prompted us to study GABA receptor pharmacology by coupling the GABA high affinity binding studies (Enna et al., 1977; Enna et al., 1975; Enna and Snyder, 1975) with the measurement of a second messenger response which relates to the activation of GABA receptors. We have taken the latter as an index of the specific output changes which are triggered in post-synaptic cells by activation of postsynaptic GABA receptors.  In this report we use as a second messenger response the 3',5'-cyclic guanosine monophosphate (cGMP) content of rat cerebellar cortex (Biggio et al., 1977) or the 3',5'-cyclic adenosine mono-phosphate (cAMP) content of the anterior pituitary as a measure of the functional changes elicited by the activation of postsynaptic GABA receptors (Costa et al., 1975).  To elucidate the molecular nature of the mechanisms whereby drugs can facilitate the acti-vation of GABA receptors, we have used as a tool benzodiazepines which facilitate GABA transmission (Costa et al., 1975; Haefely et al., 1975) and muscimol which activates GABA receptors by mimicking the action of GABA (Costa, 1977; Naik et al., 1976).

There are a limited number of models that can be used to devel-op drugs that can enhance GABA function when the amount of GABA re-leased at synapses is decreased.  These models include GABA transaminase inhibitors, GABA uptake inhibitors and drugs that act on the regulation of the high affinity binding of GABA to post-synaptic receptors.  The experiments included in the present paper were prompted by our current hypothesis that the high affinity binding of GABA to receptors can be regulated by an allosteric site which is included in the supramolecular structure that mediates GABA receptor function at postsynaptic membranes.

I.  MEASUREMENT OF CYCLIC 3',5'-ADENOSINE MONOPHOSPHATE (cAMP) CON-TENT IN ANTERIOR PITUITARY AS AN INDEX OF GABA RECEPTOR ACTIVA-TION IN MEDIAN EMINENCE

The concentration of GABA, the density of GABA receptor binding sites and the activity of glutamic acid decarboxylase vary in different hypothalamic nuclei.  This suggests that postsynaptic GABA receptors may be more abundant in certain hypothalamic areas (Enna et al., 1975).  This suggestion is supported also by physiological findings that indicate that GABA synapses partici-pate in control of the activity of specific types of tuberoinfundi-bular neurosecretory neurons (Sawaki and Yagi, 1976).

Reports by Kuriyama et al. (Kuriyama and Kimura, 1976) and by Grandison et al. (Grandison and Guidotti, 1977) indicate that hypothalamic GABA synapses regulate feeding behavior and satiety.  Moreover, other reports (Guidotti et al., 1977; Makara and Start, 1974) have shown that when the synthesis of GABA is in-hibited  the decline of hypothalamic GABA content is associated with the activation of certain pituitary functions (Guidotti et al, 1977; Makara and Stark, 1974).  These hormonal actions can be recorded before generalized convulsions are elicited by GABA synthesis inhibitors.

It is well established that changes in the rate of neuropep-
tide secretion from median eminence regulates anterior pituitary
function.  The activation of pituitary hormone secretion by these
neuropeptides is associated with an activation of adenylate cyclase bound to membranes of pituitary cells (Labbrie et al.,
1975).  Thus, by measuring the cAMP content of the pituitary one
can evaluate the global activity of pituitary cell function.  From
such measurements can also infer how drugs or other stimuli change
the function of tuberoinfundibular neurons which secrete pituitary
hormone releasing factors.  Specifically, we have found (Guidotti,
el al., 1977)    that an increase in the cAMP content of the anterior pituitary is elicited "inter alia" by a reduction in the
function of dopaminergic or GABAergic synapses.  Reserpine, a drug
which depletes brain monoamine stores (Figure 1.) and isoniazid
(Figure 1.) or picrotoxin (not shown), which reduce the function
of GABAergic synapses (Costa et al., 1975; Guidotti et al.,
1977) cause a 4 to 5 fold increase in the cAMP content of anterior
pituitary.  Strychnine, a glycine receptor antagonist fails to
change the function of GABAergic or dopaminergic synapses and
leaves unchanged the cAMP content of either anterior pituitary or
hypothalamus (Guidotti et al., 1977).

That the mechanism whereby reserpine increases the cAMP content
of anterior pituitary may differ from that of isoniazid and picrotoxin is inferred also from the following experiments.  Pargyline,
an inhibitor of type A monoamine oxidase (Yand and Neff,
1973),       when given alone fails to alter the cAMP content of
anterior pituitary (Figure 1.) it reduces the increase in pituitary
cAMP content caused by reserpine but not that caused by isoniazid.
Muscimol, a potent GABA receptor agonist (Krogsgaard-Larsen
et al., 1975) reduces pituitary cAMP content (Figure 1.).  However,
it fails to block the increase of anterior pituitary cAMP content
induced by reserpine but antagonizes the elevation in anterior
pituitary cAMP content caused by isoniazid (Figure 1.).  Similarly,
diazepam (Costa et al., 1975) (Figure 1.)    or nipecotic acid
(Krogsgaard-Larsen and Johnston, 1975; Johnston,
1976) which facilitate the stimulation of GABA receptors by two
different mechanisms fail to prevent the reserpine elicited increase in pituitary cAMP content, but counteract the increase in
pituitary cAMP content caused by isoniazid (Figure 1.).

The action of GABA receptor agonists and antagonists on the
cAMP content of anterior pituitary probably depends on an action
of hypothalamic GABAergic synapses.  In fact, isoniazid and bicuculline injected directly in the medial basal hypothalamus increase the cAMP content of anterior pituitary (Table 1.).  Muscimol,
a direct GABA receptor agonist, fails to change the pituitary cAMP

TABLE 1

EFFECT OF VARIOUS DRUGS ACTING ON GABAergic TRANSMISSION ON THE cAMP CONTENT
OF ANTERIOR PITUITARY

| DRUG | DOSE ng/μl | cAMP (pmoles/mg/prot) | |
|------|-----------|-------|-------|
| | | SALINE | ISONIAZID (300 mg/kg, s.c.) |
| SALINE | 1 μl | 8.3 $\pm$ 1 | 35 $\pm$ 6 |
| MUSCIMOL | 100 | 6.8 $\pm$ 0.7 | 9.0 $\pm$ 0.7 |
| ISONIAZID | 5 x 10$^5$ | 25 $\pm$ 3* | - |
| BICUCULLINE | 80 | 40 $\pm$ 8* | - |

Rats were killed 45 minutes after muscimol or isoniazid were injected into
the medial-basal hypothalamus or 15 minutes after intrahypothalamic bicuculline. Subcutaneous isoniazid was injected 45 min before.

* P < 0.01 when compared with saline treated rats.

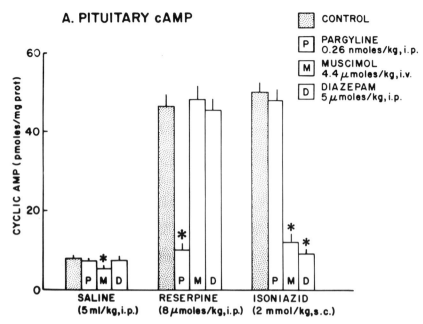

Figure 1.  Effect of different drugs on the increase in the cAMP
content of anterior pituitary elicited by reserpine and
isoniazid.  Pargyline was injected 30 min before reserpine or isoniazid, muscimol 5 min before.  Diazepam was
injected 30 min after reserpine or isoniazid.  The animals were killed 45 min after reserpine or isoniazid
with a microwave beam focussed to the head (Guidotti,
et al., 1974).      cAMP was determined as previously
described (Guidotti et al., 1974).  Each value is
the mean ± S.E. of 5 experiments.  *P < 0.01.

content when injected in the hypothalamus, but inhibits the increase of anterior pituitary cAMP content induced by systemic
isoniazid (Table 1.).  Thus, by measuring the second messenger
responses in anterior pituitary we have established a useful model
to study how drugs can modify the postsynaptic output in hypothalamic synapses regulated by GABA.  The type of GABAergic regulation appears to be one of tonic inhibition.  When this tonic
GABAergic inhibition is nullified by the injection of the GABA receptor blocker, bicuculline, or by the blockade of GABA synthesis,
the cAMP content of pituitary increases.  When the GABAergic control
is intact, the systemic injection of diazepam or muscimol fails to
decrease the cAMP increase elicited by reserpine.  Muscimol injected parenterally causes a modest decrease of pituitary cAMP content.  This effect must be indirect because it cannot be reproduced
by intrahypothalamically injected muscimol.

II.  MEASUREMENT OF CYCLIC 3',5'-GUANOSINE MONOPHOSPHATE (cGMP)
     CONTENT IN CEREBELLUM AS AN INDEX OF GABA RECEPTOR FUNCTION

       Cerebellum was used as another model to study in vivo the ac-
tion of drugs acting on GABA receptor function.  The cerebellum
consists of two parts: the cerebellar nuclei whose connections to
the various parts of the central nervous system coordinate muscle
movements and the cerebellar cortex which exerts an inhibitory influence on the cerebellar nuclei through the release of GABA from
Purkinje cells (Eccles et al., 1967).  The activity of the
Purkinje cells is regulated by two excitatory inputs to the cerebellar cortex - the climbing and mossy fibers - and by a neuronal
network within the cortex which inhibits the activity of Purkinje
cells through the release of GABA from interneurons (Eccles
et al., 1967).  The net activity of Purkinje cells appears to have
as a biochemical correlate a change in the content of cGMP.  The
concentration of this second messenger increases or decreases in
direct relation with the increase or decrease in the activity of
the climbing and mossy fibers.  The cGMP content of cerebellar
cortex also decreases when the GABA receptors are maximally activated.  When GABA receptor function is inhibited, the cGMP content
of cerebellar cortex increases (Biggio et al., 1977).  Thus,
unlike the hypothalamic pituitary system here GABA participates in
a continuous feed-back or feed-forward inhibition of Purkinje cells
by multineuronal loops which include GABAergic neurons.

       In order to increase the value that cerebellar cGMP content
measurements possess in assessing drug modification of GABAergic
mechanisms, we have dissected the various components involved in
the control of cerebellar cGMP content.  The participation of
climbing fiber activation in the action of a given drug can be
evaluated by the use of specific lesions of the climbing fiber by
3-acetylpyridine (for reference, see  Biggio and Guidotti,
1976).  Thus, the injection of high doses of this drug blocks the
increase in cerebellar cGMP content and the tremor induced by har-
maline (a stimulant of climbing fiber activity) (Biggio
and Guidotti, 1976).  When a drug increases the cGMP content of
cerebellar cortex in 3-acetylpyridine treated rats, it may act via
GABA receptor stimulation or mossy fiber activation.  These two
actions can be differentiated by comparing the cGMP content of
cerebellar cortex after intracerebellar, intrastriatal or parenteral injections of the drug under study.  Using this approach, we
have studied the site of action of diazepam, muscimol, haloperidol
and morphine which injected parenterally lowers the cGMP content of
cerebellar cortex (Figure 2.).  We could exclude climbing fibers
participation in mediating the decrease of cGMP content caused by
these four drugs because they still decrease the cerebellar cGMP
content after the climbing fibers have been destroyed by 3-acetyl-
pyridine (Biggio et al., 1977).

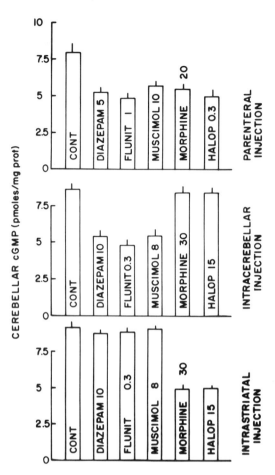

Figure 2.   Cerebellar cGMP content after intracerebellar or intra-
striatal injection of drugs that lower cerebellar cGMP
content of rat when injected parenterally.  All the
drugs, when injected intracerebrally were dissolved in
a volume of 1 µl; the molecular layer of the left cerebellar hemisphere or the head of the left nestriatum
were the sites of injection (Ribak, 1976).  Controls were injected with the solvents.  The animals were
killed with microwave (Guidotti et al., 1974) 30 min
after the injection.  Each bar shows the mean ± S.E. of
four determinations.  The numbers in the bars show drug
doses in µmoles for the parenteral injection (intraperitoneal except for muscimol which is given i.v.) or µg/µl
for the intracerebellar or in the striatal injections.
cGMP was determined as previously reported (Guidotti,
et al., 1974).

As shown in Figure 2, the intracerebellar injection of diazepam, flunitrazepam and muscimol decrease the cGMP content of
cerebellar cortex while haloperidol or morphine by such a route of
injection fail to change the cerebellar cGMP content. It can be
seen from Figure 2 that flunitrazepam is about 30-fold more active
than diazepam. Morphine and haloperidol but not diazepam or flunitrazepam decrease cerebellar cGMP content when injected into the
striatum (Figure 2.). These experiments indicate that the decrease
of cerebellar cGMP content induced by intraperitoneal injection of
diazepam and muscimol is due to a direct action of the drugs on
cerebellum. In contrast, haloperidol and morphine decrease cerebellar cGMP by activation of receptors located extracerebellarly.
Successive experiments have shown that the decrease of cerebellar
cGMP content elicited by parenteral morphine was antagnoized by
intrastriatal naltrexone (Biggio et al., 1977) and that the
decrease of cerebellar cGMP content elicited by parenteral haloperidol was antagnoized by intrastriatal apomorphine (Biggio and
Guidotti, 1977). The decrease of cerebellar cGMP content induced by parenteral muscimol was inhibited by neither naltrexone nor
apomorphine injected intrastriatally. Instead, the increase of
cerebellar cGMP content induced by the intracerebellar injection of
isoniazid was blocked by parenterally injected muscimol but not by
parenterally injected haloperidol or morphine (Biggio et al.,
1977). Thus, cerebellar cGMP measurements and intracerebellar or
intrastriatal injection of the drugs may represent a useful paradigm to study whether a drug acts on GABAergic transmission. However, the results of these experiments are only indicative and can
become more definitive when combined with direct experiments to
study whether the drug in question binds with high affinity to
specific GABA receptors. When such studies were conducted with
diazepam and muscimol, it became evident that the mechanism of action of the two drugs that appears to be similar on the basis of
their action on the cGMP content of cerebellum is indeed different.


III.  DIFFERENT MECHANISMS WHEREBY MUSCIMOL AND DIAZEPAM INFLUENCE
                GABAergic TRANSMISSION


Several lines of indirect investigation (Costa et al.,
1975; Costa, 1977; Haefely et al., 1975) suggest that a
modification of GABAergic transmission may participate in the action of benzodiazepines; probably, these drugs by an unknown molecular mechanism facilitate GABAergic transmission (Costa et al.,
1975; Costa, 1977). As reported in Figures 1. and 2., there
are striking similarities between the action of muscimol and diazepam on GABA mediated changes of cecond messenger content in the
anterior pituitary (Figure 1.) and cerebellum (Figure 2.). Diazepam, like muscimol, blocks the isoniazid-induced increase in
anterior pituitary cAMP content but does not block the cAMP increase

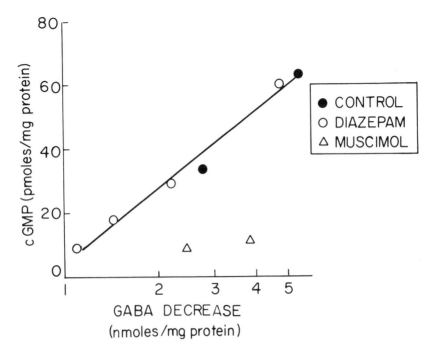

Figure 3.    Correlation between the decrease of GABA cerebellar
             content and the increase in cerebellar cGMP content in
             rats treated with saline, diazepam (3 mg/kg, i.p.) or
             muscimol, 2 mg/kg (i.v.).  Isoniazid (1.2 g, kg, s.c.)
             was injected immediately after saline, diazepam or mus-
             cimol.  The animals were sacrificed 25 min after iso-
             niazid.  There is a clear correlation between the de-
             crease of cerebellar GABA and the increase of cerebellar
             cGMP content in the case of saline or diazepam treated
             rats.  Muscimol decreases the cGMP content of cerebellum
             independently from the cerebellar GABA content.

elicited by reserpine.  Equally strong evidence for a similarity of
action between diazepam and muscimol was obtained in cerebellum
(Figure 2.).

    Based on this evidence, it was tempting to conclude that benzo-
diazepines and muscimol can be considered GABA-mimetic compounds.
However, further studies have suggested that despite the similar
pharmacological profiles, the two drugs probably act on GABAergic
transmission by different mechanisms.  For example, muscimol mimics
the GABA electrophysiologically (Costa et al., 1975) and binds
with high affinity to specific GABA receptors located in neuronal

membranes (Enna and Snyder, 1977).    In contrast, diazepam mimics GABA in several electrophysiological tests on Purkinje
cells    (Hoffer,    Personal Communication) but has little or no
affinity for specific GABA receptors (Snyder and Enna, 1977).
We have therefore decided to study further the difference
in the mode of action of diazepam and muscimol on cerebellar cGMP
content and on the binding of GABA to neural cerebellar membrane
preparations.

     Cerebellar GABA and cGMP content were determined at various
times after injection of high doses of isoniazid in rats pretreated
with muscimol or diazepam (Figure 3.).   Both drugs are known to
antagonize isoniazid-elicited convulsions (Costa et al., 1975;
Costa, 1977; Haefely et al, 1975; Naik et al., 1971).
The data of Figure 3. show that diazepam and muscimol antagonized
the isoniazid-induced increase in cerebellar cGMP content; however,
the mechanism involved is obviously different.   The protective
effect of diazepam appears to depend on the extent of GABA depletion (Figure 3.), in contrast, the action of muscimol against the
increase in cGMP content caused by isoniazid is independent from
the cerebral GABA content.

     Thus, despite the similar pharmacological profiles, diazepam
and muscimol act on GABA transmission by different mechanisms.
The data of Figure 3. is compatible with the view that diazepam
acts on GABA transmission by releasing GABA from presynaptic stores.
However, recent studies from our laboratory have made this view
untenable because diazepam rather than increasing it, lowers the
rate of synthesis of GABA in various brain structures (Mao
et al., 1977).   To explain the molecular mechanisms whereby benzodiazepines facilitate GABAergic transmission, we have then turned
our attention to the  possibility that bensodiazepines modify al-
losterically the affinity of GABA for its own postsynaptic receptors.   Thus, GABA receptors are seen as a multimolecular entity in
which the affinity of the natural agonist for the recognition site
can be modified by changes in the tertiary structure of a protein
which is part of the multi-molecular complex.   Indeed, diazepam
considerably influences the kinetic constants of GABA receptors
binding in cortex and cerebellar membrane preparations.   In these
preparations, diazepam concentrations from $5 \times 10^{-7}$ M to $5 \times 10^{-5}$ M
decrease the number of sites for the high affinity binding of GABA
(Figure 4) but, more important, they increase the affinity of the
receptor for GABA: the extent of this increase varies from 2 to 7
fold and depends on the concentration of diazepam (see Figure 4).
The effect of diazepam was duplicated by flunitrazepam, nitrazepam
and clonazepam.   Moreover, this site in which benzodiazepines act
to increase the high affinity binding of GABA is stereospecific.
In fact. Ro 11-3128/001 ((+)-5-(o-chlorophenyl)-1,3-dihydro-3-
methyl-7-nitro-2H-1,4-benzodiazepin-2-one) lowers the affinity con-

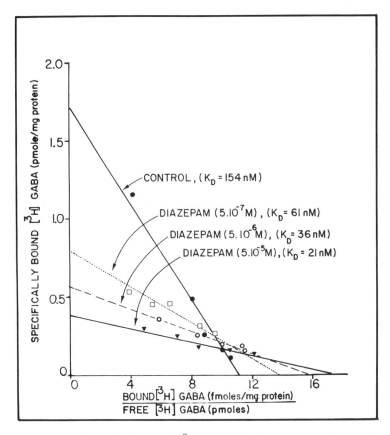

Figure 4. Specific binding of $^3$H-GABA to fresh, crude membrane preparation of rat cerebellum incubated with diazepam × 15 min at 0°C before the addition of $^3$H GABA. $^3$H GABA (3-200 nM) was incubated with a crude membrane preparation of rat cerebellum, in triplicate, with and without excess of cold GABA ($10^{-3}$ M). The specific binding was calculated by subtracting from the total binding, the binding which is not displaced by excess cold GABA. The method used is that of Enna and Snyder (1977). The data are transformed to Scatchard plots. The intercept of the ordinate give direct maximum binding/mg protein. The reciprocal of the slope value indicates the affinity constant ($k_D$).

stant for GABA but Ro 11-3624/000 ((-)-5-(o-chlorophenyl)-1,3-dihydro-3-methyl-7-nitro-2H-1,4-benzodiazepin-2-one) does not. We interpreted the results to suggest that the action of bensodiazepines on GABA binding is due to an allosteric activation of a regulatory site for the high affinity binding of GABA to postsynaptic receptors (Figure 4.). This possibility is in keeping with a recent report showing that the density of stereospecific binding for diazepam in different regions of CNS parallels the density of GABA receptors (Squires and Braestrup, 1977). It is possible that the allosteric activity of benzodiazepines on GABA receptors is part of the molecular mechanism whereby these anxiolytic drugs facilitate GABA transmission in vivo.

## REFERENCES

Barker, J.L. and Nicoll, R.A., 1973, J. Physiol., 228:259-277.

Biggio, G., Brodie, B.B., Costa, E. and Guidotti, A., 1977, Proc. Natl. Acad. Sci. USA, 74: in press.

Biggio, G., Costa, E. and Guidotti, A., 1977, J. Pharmacol. Exp. Ther., 200:207-215.

Biggio, G. and Guidotti, A., 1976, Brain Res., 107:365-373.

Biggio, G. and Guidotti, A., 1977, Nature, 265:240-242.

Biggio, G., Guidotti, A. and Costa, E., 1977, Naunyn-Schmiedeberg's Arch. Pahrmacol., 296:117-121.

Costa, E., Guidotti, A., Mao, C.C. and Suria, A., 1975, Life Sci., 17:167-186.

Costa, E., 1977, in Neuroregulators and Psychiatric Disorders (Usdin, E., Hamburg, D.A. and Barchas, J.D., eds.), Oxford Press, New York, pp. 372-380.

Eccles, J.C., Ito, M. and Szentagothai, J., 1967, The Cerebellum as a Neuronal Machine, Springer-Verlag, Berlin.

Enna, S.J., Collins, J.F. and Snyder, S., 1977, Brain Res., 124: 185-190.

Enna, S.J., Kuhar, J. and Snyder, S., 1975, Brain Res., 93:168-174.

Enna, S.J. and Snyder, S.H., 1975, Brain Res., 100:81-97.

Enna, S.J. and Snyder, S.H., 1977, Mol. Pharmacol., 13:442-453.

Fonnum, F., Grofova, I., Rinvik , E., Storm-Mathisen, J. and Walberg, F., 1974, Brain Res., 71:77-92.

Grandison, L. and Guidotti, A., 1977, Neuropharmacology, 16:533-536.

Guidotti, A., Cheney, D.L., Trabucchi, M., Doteuchi, M., Wang, C. and Hawkins, R.A., 1974, Neuropharmacology, 13:1115-1122.

Guidotti, A., Naik, S.R. and Kurosawa, A., Psychoneuroendocrinology, Vol. 2: In press.

Haefely, W., Kulisar, W.A., Möhler, H., Pieri, L., Polc, P. and Schaffner, R., 1975, Advan. Biochem. Psychopharmacol. (Costa, E. and Greengard, P., eds.), 14:131-152.

Hoffner, B., Personal Communication.

Iversen, L.L. and Neal, M.J., 1968, J. Neurochem., 15:1141-1149.

Krnjevic, K. and Puil, E., 1976, in Taurine (Huxtable, R. and Barbeau, A., eds.), Raven Press, New York, pp. 179-189.

Krogsgaard-Larsen, P. and Johnston, G.A., 1975, J. Neurochem., 25:797-802.

Krogsgaard-Larsen, P., Johnston, G.A.R., Curtis, D.A., Game, C.J.A. and McCulloch, R.M., 1975, J. Neruochem., 25:803-809.

Kuriyama, K., Haber, B., Sisken, B. and Roberts, E., 1966, Proc. Natl. Acad. Sci., 55:846-850.

Kuriyama, K. and Kimura, H., 1976, in GABA in Nervous System Function (Roberts, E., Chase, T.N. and Tower, D.B., eds.), Raven Press, New York, pp. 203-216.

Johnston, G.A.R., 1976, in GABA in Nervous System Function (Roberts, E., Chase, T.N. and Tower, D.B., eds.), Raven Press, New York, pp. 395-411.

Labbrie, F., Borgeat, P., Lemay, A., Lamaire, S., Barden, N., Drouin, J., Lemaire, I., Jolicoeur, P. and Belanger, A., 1975, in Advances in Cyclic Nucleotides Research, Vol. 5 (Drummond, G.I., Greengard, P. and Robison, G.A., eds.) p. 787, Raven Press, New York.

Makara, G.B. and Stark, E., 1974, Neuroendocrinology, 16:178-180.

Mao, C.C., Marco, E., Revuelta, A., Bertilsson, L. and Costa, E., 1977, J. Biol. Psychiatry, 12:359-371.

McGeer, P.L., McGeer, E.G., Wada, J.A. and Jung, E., 1971, Brain Res., 32:425-451.

Naik, S.R., Guidotti, A. and Costa, E., 1976, Neuropharmacology, 15:479-484.

Okada, Y. and Shimada, C., 1976, in GABA in Nervous System Function (Roberts, E. and Chase, T.N., eds.), Raven Press, New York, pp. 223-233.

Perry, T.L., Hansen, S. and Kloster, M., 1973, N. Engl. J. Med., 288:337-342.

Precht, W. and Yoshida, M., 1976, Brain Res., 32:229-233.

Ribak, C.E., Vaughan, J.E., Saito, K., Barber, R. and Roberts, E., 1976, Brain Res., 116:287-299.

Roberts, E., 1974, Biochem. Pharmacol., 23:2637-2649.

Roberts, E., 1976, in GABA in Nervous System Function (Roberts, E., Chase, T.N. and Tower, D.B., eds.), Raven Press, pp. 515-539.

Sawaki, Y. and Yagi, K., 1976, J. Physiol., 260:447-461.

Snyder, S.H. and Enna, S.J., in Advances in Biochem. Psychopharmacol., Vol. 14 (Costa, E. and Greengard, P., eds.), Raven Press, New York, pp. 81-92.

Squires, R.F. and Braestrup, C., 1977, Nature, 266:732-733.

Wood, J.D. and Peesker, S.J., 1974, J. Neurochem., 23:703-712.

Yang, H.-Y. and Neff, N.H., 1973, J. Pharmacol. Exp. Ther., 187:365-371.

GLYCINE:  INHIBITION FROM THE SACRUM TO THE MEDULLA

M. H. Aprison and N. S. Nadi

The Institute of Psychiatric Research
Departments of Psychiatry and Biochemistry
and the Department of Neurological Surgery
Indiana University School of Medicine
Indianapolis, Indiana 46202

I.  A SPECIAL INTEREST IN GLYCINE IN THE CNS


A.  Statement

From a theoretical point of view, the fact that glycine has
many metabolic roles as well as a functional role in the CNS is
extremely interesting to the neurobiologist.  Glycine does not
have an assymetric carbon atom nor is it an essential amino acid
(except in the chick).  It is found in most tissues and its synthesis has been demonstrated in animals, plants and microor-
ganisms.  It has also been shown to be present in varying amounts
in the tissues of the central nervous system.  Most standard textbooks of biochemistry indicate that glycine is metabolically active
and is utilized in the formation of proteins, heme, purines, glutathione, hippuric acid, creatine, glycocholic acid, serine, for-
mate (for the one-carbon pool), glucose and glycogen.  However,
although glycine is biosynthetically involved in these important
metabolic processes, in 1965 and shortly thereafter, a series of
papers from the laboratories of Aprison and Werman announced that
glycine was a segmental inhibitory transmitter in the cat spinal
cord and thus also had an important functional role in the CNS
(Aprison and Werman, 1965; Graham et al., 1967; Davidoff et al.,
1967a,b; Werman et al., 1967, 1968).  Thus, in addition to GABA,
the role of glycine had to be considered in studying inhibitory
processes of CNS functions.

## B.  Background

Since 1960, Aprison and co-workers have been interested in
the relationship between CNS transmitters and behavior (Aprison,
1965; Aprison and Hingtgen, 1970; Aprison et al., 1975).  A logical
expansion of this work was the development of a program which could
lead to the identification of new neurotransmitters in the CNS of
vertebrates.  Between 1965 and 1968, the data from these new experiments supported the suggestion that glycine was an inhibitory
transmitter in the cat spinal cord.  This transmitter function was
found as a result of a combined neurochemical and neurophysiological approach directed to the problem of the identification of
CNS transmitters (Aprison and Werman, 1968; Werman and Aprison,
1968).  It was made possible both by methodological advances in
allied disciplines and by the convergence of several lines of biochemical and physiological effort -- namely, the great impetus
given to the study of amino acids in small amounts of nervous tissue by the development of the technique to measure these substrates with enzymes (Graham and Aprison, 1966) and the application
of ion-exchange chromatography, as well as the development of iontophoresis and equilibrium potential measurements as tools to study
the effects of biochemical compounds applied onto synaptic membranes.

As these research techniques were applied in specific experiments, Aprison and Werman also attempted to establish minimal criteria for the proper proof for identification.  Thus, they suggested that a neurotransmitter candidate must fulfill three principal criteria before being accepted as the mediator of neuronal
signals in the CNS.  Their criteria state that:  (a) the putative
neurotransmitter should be present in the presynaptic terminals of
the junction studied; (b) the putative transmitter should repro-
duce the ionic membrane process evoked by the release of the natural
neurotransmitter, and (c) the transmitter candidate should be released into the extracellular fluid upon the stimulation of the
presynaptic nerve (Aprison and Werman, 1968; Werman and Aprison,
1968).  The first is called the Presynaptic Criterion and involves
the accumulation of neurochemical data whereas the second, the
Identity of Action Criterion, is satisfied by specific neurophysiological data (Werman, 1965).  When the third criterion, the Release
Criterion, is satisfied, the investigator will have provided both
neurophysiological and neurochemical data.

The data which satisfy these three criteria are considered of
primary importance in these kinds of investigations.  However, other
supportive data are also useful (Aprison, 1977).  Thus, in addition
to having a compound fulfilling the above criteria, investigators
should also try to obtain information on (a) the synthesis (and/or
transport), (b) the storage, (c) the mechanism of release of the
putative transmitter from the presynaptic ending, (d) its mode of

action at the postsynaptic receptor site, (i.e., the presence of specific receptor proteins for the transmitter compound in the postsynaptic membrane), (e) identification of pharmacological antagonists, (f) its action on second messengers, and finally (g) the manner in which the putative transmitter compound is inactivated once it is released (i.e., does it diffuse away, or is it hydrolyzed by an extracellular enzyme or is it taken up into the surrounding glia, the presynaptic nerve terminal or the postsynaptic cell). These points are illustrated in Figure 1.

In addition to identifying and studying the physiological and biochemical properties of a compound that is a transmitter, one

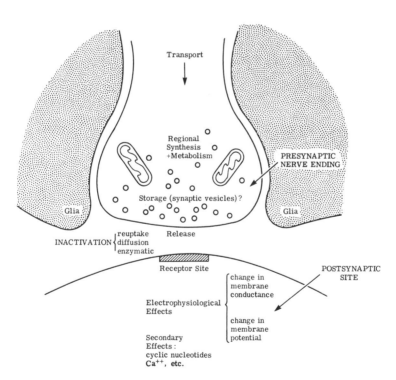

FIGURE 1. Diagrammatic sketch of a synapse indicating a number of presynaptic, postsynaptic and synaptic cleft events.

would like to know whether these findings made in the laboratory
animals have any applications to the human central nervous system.
Investigators should ask the following questions:  (a) Are there
cases of human disease(s) where a demonstrated imbalance in the
metabolic pathways of the putative transmitter such as glycine can
be linked to a disorder of the particular area of the central nervous system?; (b) If such cases do exist, can the alteration of
the levels of the transmitter help in alleviating the symptoms of
the disease?  The current treatment for myasthenia gravis which
involves increasing the number of acetylcholine molecules available in the cleft of the neuromuscular junction is a good example
of just such an approach.

In this chapter the evidence that glycine has an important
physiological role in the CNS will be briefly reviewed (also see
Aprison and Werman, 1968; Aprison et al., 1976) as will some other
supportive studies on the in vivo and in vitro metabolism of glycine, uptake of glycine, and strychnine blockade of glycine action
and receptor binding.  In addition, the role of glycine in several
neurological diseases now known to involve faulty metabolism of
this amino acid or disruption of neural connections utilizing
glycine as a transmitter will be briefly discussed.


II.  PRESYNAPTIC LOCALIZATION

In view of the extreme diversity of the CNS, and the techniques available at the present time, the investigator has a better chance of identifying new transmitters by the above criteria
if one chooses a region where the synaptic organization and physiology of neurons are known.  Thus, it was the relatively advanced
knowledge in the anatomy and the physiology of the lumbosacral
spinal cord physiology of the cat (Eccles, 1964) that led Aprison
and colleagues to choose this region of the CNS for their search
of new neurotransmitters.

The physiological studies of the spinal cord have demonstrated
that the majority of the inhibitory synapses in this area are mediated by interneurons which are relatively small cells, with short
axons (Eccles, 1964).  Careful examination of the cross section of
the spinal cord shows that these interneurons are located mainly
in the central portion of the dorsal and ventral gray.  Based on
this knowledge, Aprison and Werman (1965) predicted the distribution of the postsynaptic inhibitory neurotransmitter in the
spinal cord.  Since the interneurons are small in size, one would
expect that this putative transmitter, its synthesizing enzyme,
and its precursor would all be present in the gray matter.  Thus,
in the spinal cord a postsynaptic inhibitory neurotransmitter would
be expected to be found at higher levels in the gray matter, but

at lower levels in the white matter and roots.

The first group of compounds selected for study were the amino acids; this decision was based mainly on the fact that a number of amino acids had known pharmacological actions (inhibitory or excitatory). Although earlier studies (Crawford and Curtis, 1964; Curtis, 1963; Curtis et al., 1959, 1960; Curtis and Watkins, 1960, 1963, 1965) had shown that GABA and glycine were both inhibitory in their actions on neurons, the general conclusion by these investigators was that most of the amino acids including glycine were not transmitters, but acted nonspecifically on neurons (including motoneurons) in vertebrates. Aprison and Werman felt that these data were not sufficient to warrant such a conclusion. Therefore, they began their studies by measuring the content of a number of amino acids in the cat spinal cord. On the basis of the distribution of GABA and glycine in the gray and white matter from the cat spinal cord, both compounds appeared to be likely candidates as inhibitory transmitters (Aprison and Werman, 1965; Graham et al., 1967). The content of glycine in the gray matter was greater than GABA, but the ratio of the content in gray to that of roots favored GABA over glycine at the time of the initial studies (TABLE I). The distribution data for glycine in the spinal cord was confirmed by Johnston (cat; 1968) and Berger et al. (rabbit; 1977a).

Also of interest at the time were the findings that glutamic acid, an excitatory putative transmitter, and glutamine, an amino acid with no demonstrable effect on neurons, had entirely different distribution patterns (Aprison et al., 1965; Graham et al., 1967). Therefore, it was felt that the distribution patterns of glycine and GABA did reflect specific neuroanatomical difference in various regions of the spinal cord which suggested a possible functional role. Further studies were necessary.

On the basis of their distribution in the spinal cord, both GABA and glycine could be the inhibitory transmitter(s) acting on motoneurons. However, utilizing the technique of aortic occlusion to produce a selective loss of interneurons in the intermediate and ventral gray matter of the lumbosacral region of the cat spinal cord (Rexed's lamina V-IX), Davidoff et al. (1967a,b) found that the content of glycine but not that of GABA was significantly decreased. These data were interpreted to demonstrate that glycine is concentrated in the interneurons in the central and ventral gray regions of the spinal cord. Based on the higher levels of GABA in the dorsal gray of the spinal cord, and the data from the aortic occlusion experiment, it was suggested that GABA is probably the inhibitory neurotransmitter released from the interneurons in the dorsal horn of the spinal cord (Rexed's lamina I-IV). This conclusion correlates well with the recent immunocytochemical locali-

TABLE I.   DISTRIBUTION OF FOUR AMINO ACIDS IN FOUR AREAS OF THE CAT SPINAL CORD AND ROOTS

| Amino acids ($\mu$moles/g)[a] | Cord Areas | | | | Roots | |
|---|---|---|---|---|---|---|
| | dorsal white | dorsal gray | ventral gray | ventral white | dorsal | ventral |
| Glycine (9)[b] | 3.04±0.26 | 5.65±0.18 | 7.08±0.31 | 4.39±0.26 | 0.71±0.06(4) | 0.74±0.08(4) |
| GABA (8) | 0.43±0.05 | 2.18±0.25 | 1.04±0.10 | 0.44±0.06 | 0.06±0.01 | 0.08±0.01 |
| Glutamate(7) | 4.80±0.07 | 6.48±0.15 | 5.25±0.18 | 3.89±0.12 | 4.61±0.01(8) | 3.14±0.13(8) |
| Glutamine(3) | 3.59±0.17 | 5.31±0.40 | 5.35±0.12 | 3.81±0.19 | 1.98±0.24 | 1.93±0.22 |

[a] Mean ± SEM.
[b] Number of animals.

zation of glutamate decarboxylase obtained by McLaughlin et al.
(1975). In addition, data from Hökfelt and Ljungdahl (1971),
Matus and Dennison (1972), and Ljungdahl and Hökfelt (1973) have
demonstrated that when slices of spinal cord are incubated with
($^3$H)-glycine, the latter is localized primarily in the nerve
endings in the ventral spinal cord. Price et al. (1976) labelled
synapses in the ventral horn cells of the rat by direct microinjection of ($^3$H)-glycine into the spinal cord. Approximately 49%
of the labelled synapses were axosomatic and 37% axodendritic.
Presynaptic terminals were more densely labelled than axons, glia
and postsynaptic cells and many of the labelled terminals had
elliptical vesicles (Uchizono, 1965). Dennison et al. (1976) also
found that in cat spinal cord incubated in vivo with ($^3$H)glycine,
the radioactivity was distributed over all the cellular elements
but that in the synaptic regions, 82% of it was over synapses with
flat vesicles.

Using the same neurochemical-anatomical approach for the purpose of locating other areas of high glycine content, Aprison et
al. (1969) determined the distribution of glycine in ten areas of
the neuraxis in seven vertebrates (cat, rat, pigeon, caiman, bullfrog, catfish and boa constrictor). These data show that for each
species the medulla oblongata and spinal cord contain higher levels
of glycine than any other area of the brain. In any one species
the mean content of glycine in the medulla oblongata are three to
seven times higher than the mean content in either the cerebral
hemispheres or the cerebellum (TABLE II). The data on the different regions of the spinal cord (TABLE III) show that the mean
content of glycine in the cervical and lumbar enlargements (and in
the sacral cord when assayed) of the cat, rat, pigeon and caiman
was higher than in the midthoracic cord, and that glycine was uniformly distributed along the spinal cord of the snake and the catfish (animals without limbs). It is interesting to note that the
content of glycine is higher in the regions of the spinal cord
which innervate the limbs (cervical and lumbar enlargements), and
low in the thoracic region which has little musculature to supply. Thus, in the case of caiman which has powerful hind limbs
and tail, the content of glycine was highest in lumbar and sacral
spinal cord. In the pigeon which has a strong wing musculature,
levels of glycine were expected to be highest in the cervical cord.
This was indeed the case (TABLE III). In the case of the medulla,
the neurochemical evidence strongly pointed to this area as one
where glycine could function as a neurotransmitter. Neurophysiological evidence given below confirmed this suggestion.

It is of interest that Boehme et al. (1973) later measured the
glycine levels in five areas of the cervical, thoracic, and lumbar
human spinal cord. They also found that the highest levels were in
the lumbar ventral gray.

TABLE II. DISTRIBUTION OF GLYCINE IN THE BRAIN OF SEVEN VERTEBRATES

| Species[b] | Cerebral hemisphere | Diencephalon | Midbrain and tectum | Cerebellum | Pons | Medulla |
|---|---|---|---|---|---|---|
| Cat | 1.27 + 0.09 | 1.60 + 0.16 | 1.97 + 0.11 | 0.83 + 0.05 | 2.96 + 0.15 | 3.42 + 0.10 |
| Rat | 0.95 + 0.09 | 1.00 + 0.09 | 1.55 + 0.14 | 0.62 + 0.08 | 2.72 + 0.15 | 3.81 + 0.13 |
| Pigeon | 1.21 + 0.05 | 1.32 + 0.09 | 1.45 + 0.09 | 1.18 + 0.04 | 3.89 + 0.18 | 4.79 + 0.18 |
| Caiman | 1.16 + 0.09 | 1.17 + 0.11 | 1.19 + 0.19 | 1.00 + 0.15[d] | — | 4.03 + 0.35 |
| Bullfrog | 0.71 + 0.09 | 0.81 + 0.10 | 1.37 + 0.09 | 1.28 + 0.25[d] | — | 3.41 + 0.27 |
| Snake[c] | 0.65 + 0.13 | 0.84 + 0.06 | 1.38 + 0.12 | 1.32 + 0.48[e] | — | 4.19 + 0.13 |
| Catfish | 0.77 + 0.16 | 0.54 + 0.15 | 0.63 + 0.07 | 0.68 + 0.12 | — | 1.84 + 0.07 |

Area of Brain[a]

[a] Glycine data (mean + SEM) for each brain area are expressed as μmoles/g wet weight.
[b] N = 6 in all cases except where indicated to the contrary.
[c] N = 4.
[d] N = 5.
[e] N = 2.

TABLE III. DISTRIBUTION OF GLYCINE IN THE SPINAL CORD OF SEVEN VERTEBRATES[a]

| | Glycine content, μmol/g wet wt. | | | |
|---|---|---|---|---|
| Animals with limbs | Cervical enlargement | Middle thoracic cord | Lumbar enlargement | Sacral cord |
| Cat | 3.76 ± 0.15 | 2.13 ± 0.20 | 4.52 ± 0.20 | 4.53 ± 0.20 |
| Rat | 4.14 ± 0.20 | 3.43 ± 0.09 | 4.30 ± 0.23 | 4.08 ± 0.16 |
| Pigeon | 4.80 ± 0.29 | 3.20 ± 0.13 | 4.53 ± 0.32 | — |
| Caiman | 4.65 ± 0.24 | 3.83 ± 0.18 | 5.32 ± 0.27 | 4.91 ± 0.45 |
| Bullfrog | 3.89 ± 0.20 | 3.66 ± 0.21 | 4.08 ± 0.22 | — |
| Animals without limbs | First quarter | Second quarter | Third quarter | Fourth quarter |
| Snake | 3.26 ± 0.09 | 3.06 ± 0.11 | 3.02 ± 0.22 | 3.21 ± 0.10 |
| Catfish | 1.74 ± 0.13 | 1.83 ± 0.21 | 2.08 ± 0.15 | 1.99 ± 0.17 |

[a]From Aprison et al. (1969). Values represent the means ± SEM.

Presently there are at least four areas of the CNS where glycine is considered to have a functional role. Thus, in addition
to being a transmitter in the medulla and spinal cord, the two
regions of the CNS emphasized here, it should be pointed out that
glycine has been suggested to be a possible neurotransmitter in the
retina (Voaden, 1974; Berger et al., 1977b), and in the optic tectum
(Reubi and Cuenod, 1976).


III.  PHYSIOLOGY

As a renewed interest in glycine was initiated by the finding
that the distribution of glycine in the spinal cord fit that of
the postsynaptic inhibitory neurotransmitter, the effect of glycine
on spinal neurons was retested and found to be comparable to, or
in some cases better than GABA (Werman et al., 1966, 1967, 1968).
As these findings were later confirmed and extended (Curtis et al.,
1968a; Bruggencate and Engberg, 1968), other studies appeared which
reported that glycine was also inhibitory in the cuneate nucleus in
the medulla oblongata (Galindo et al., 1967; Kelly and Renaud,
1971, 1973), and several areas of the brainstem (Davis and Huffman,
1969; Hösli and Tebēcis, 1970; Tebēcis and DiMaria, 1972; Tebēcis
et al., 1971; Bruggencate and Engberg, 1971; Bruggencate and
Sonnhof, 1972).  Recently it was reported that the superfusion of
glycine to certain regions of the medulla of the cat are associated
with a profound drop in blood pressure (Guertzenstein and Silver,
1974).  A recent study of the effect of the microiontophoresis of
glycine, GABA and taurine on the bulbar respiratory neurons showed
that glycine had a more potent effect on these cells than did the
other two amino acids (Denavit-Saubie and Champagnat, 1975).

In order to obtain further critical evidence that glycine is
the inhibitory neurotransmitter in the spinal cord, Werman et al.
(1967, 1968) performed a detailed analysis of the effects of glycine on the membrane potential and the membrane conductance of
spinal motoneurons.  These studies showed that glycine caused an
increase in membrane potential (hyperpolarization) and a large fall
in membrane resistance, a phenomenon which could be expected if
there were a large increase in permeability of the chloride ion.
A supramaximal dose of glycine caused complete abolition of the
IPSP,i.e., the IPSP reached its equilibrium potential of glycine-
produced hyperpolarization and the inhibitory process.  When the
equilibrium potential is changed by passing hyperpolarizing current, a depolarizing IPSP is seen.  These data confirm the equi-
valence of the equilibrium potentials of glycine-produced hyperpolarization and the inhibitory process.  The identity of the two
actions was confirmed by showing that the reversal potentials of
glycine and the IPSP were changed in the same way by the injections
of two foreign anions (Werman, 1965; Werman et al., 1968).  These

observations on changes in the intracellular conductance in motoneurons were confirmed by Curtis et al. (1968a); Bruggencate and
Engberg (1968), Curtis et al.(1968b) and Belcher et al (1976).  Observations similar to those above were also made on spinal cord
cells grown in tissue culture (Hösli et al., 1971).  The findings
that glycine has potent electrophysiological activity in the medulla
and the spinal cord are in accord with the neurochemical-anatomic
observations.

Electrophysiological studies of glycine on cortical neurons
indicated that its potency on these cells was less than GABA and
other longer chain amino acids (Krnjević and Phillis, 1963).
Further studies on cortical neurons (Kelly and Krnjević, 1969;
Biscoe et al., 1972) have confirmed these earlier findings.  Cerebellar neurons also appear to be less sensitive to glycine than
they are to GABA (Kawamura and Provini, 1970).  The very weak
effects of glycine on the cortical and cerebellar neurons also agree
with the neurochemical data and these results support the suggestion
that glycine probably does not act as an inhibitory transmitter in
these two areas of the CNS unless it does so in a small group of
specialized cells.

During their study of the electrophysiological effects of glycine, Curtis et al.(1968a) reported that its action was blocked by
strychnine.  Since this drug is known to abolish spinal reflexes,
this was interpreted as further evidence that glycine is a natural
inhibitory transmitter in the spinal cord (Werman et al., 1967,
1968; Aprison and Werman, 1968).  These observations were confirmed
by Davidoff et al. (1969), Larson (1969) and DeGroat (1970).  Strychnine block of glycine inhibition has now been observed on neurons
in the spinal cord, on medullar reticular neurons (Tebēcis and
DiMaria, 1972; Hösli and Tebēcis, 1970), and on cells of the cuneate
nucleus (Hill et al., 1973, 1976; Galindo, 1969; Kelly and Renaud,
1971, 1973).  The data on the cerebral cortex indicates that there
is an insensitivity to moderate amounts of strychnine which is also consistent with the thought that there are probably very few
or no glycinergic neurons in the region (Brooks and Asanuma, 1965;
Crawford et al., 1963; Krnjević et al., 1966).  Structural analogs
of strychnine such as thelaine and bruceine also show a similar
ability to block glycine inhibition (Curtis et al., 1968).  However, it should be noted that the strychnine activity is by no
means specific.  It has been shown to block the action of other
short chain amino acids much as β-alanine and taurine, but not that
of GABA (Curtis et al.,(1968b)unless it is given in high doses.
Studies investigating other possible antagonists of glycine activity with tetramethylenedisulphotetramine (TETS) have shown that
this drug is not a specific antagonist of the glycine induced
hyperpolarization (Hill et al., 1976).  Physiological investigation
of the action of the barbiturate etomidate (+form) have shown it to

be half as active as glycine or GABA in depressing the neurons of the cuneate nucleus (Hill and Taberner, 1976).

Two other physiological studies involving the effect of glycine are of interest. Takano and Neumann (1972) have shown that intravenously injected glycine is capable of inhibiting the stretch reflex tension. Stern and Catovic (1975) reported that in the rat, intraperitoneal glycine reduced aggressiveness caused by water deprivation or forebrain septal lesion. Nalorphine and mephensin, drugs shown centrally to elevate glycine levels, acted similarly to systematically administered glycine. In mice made aggressive by prolonged isolation, glycine and mephenesin acted as tranquilizers.

## IV.  UPTAKE AND RELEASE

### A.  Uptake of Glycine by Nerve Terminals

There are several ways in which a neurotransmitter can be inactivated: (a) reuptake into the presynaptic cell (terminal), the postsynaptic cell, surrounding glia or any combination of these cells; (b) diffusion out of the synaptic cleft; and (c) catabolism by a degradative enzyme located in the membranes of the synapse. In 1963, Tsukada et al. (1963) and Lajtha and Toth (1963) reported that glycine, and several other amino acids are taken up by brain slices. It was also known that the concentration of glycine in CSF of several species was very low (Aprison and Werman, 1965; Humoller et al., 1966; Dickinson and Hamilton, 1966). The ratio of glycine in CSF to that in blood is one of the lowest of the amino acids measured. Based on these data, Aprison and Werman (1965, 1968) and Werman and Aprison (1968) postulated that the inactivation of glycine must occur by an uptake mechanism. Neal and Pickles (1969) then reported that labelled glycine was readily taken up by slices prepared from the rat spinal cord. Neal (1971) further showed that ($^{14}$C)glycine is taken up into slices of tissue prepared from various areas of the CNS as well as from spinal cord gray matter. But these latter studies did not distinguish between a "net" uptake of glycine or a simple exchange between the unlabelled glycine in the intracellular pools and labelled glycine. Johnston and Iversen (1971) and Logan and Snyder (1972) reported the presence of a low affinity and a $Na^+$ dependent high affinity transport system in the spinal cord of the rat; only the low affinity transport system was detected in the cerebral cortex. Similar data have been reported in the cat spinal cord (Balcar and Johnston, 1973). A $Na^+$ dependent high affinity uptake system for ($^3$H)glycine has also been demonstrated in spinal cord explants of the chick embryos grown in tissue culture (Cho et al., 1973).

The uptake of $(U-^{14}C)$glycine into crude synaptosomes $(P_2)$ prepared from the telencephalon and the spinal cord of the rat were studied by Aprison and McBride (1973). During the first 3 minutes the rates of $(U-^{14}C)$glycine $(8 \times 10^{-7}M)$ uptake by crude synaptosomal preparations $(P_2)$ from the spinal cord or telencephalon were estimated to be 0.100 and 0.0243 nmole/mg protein/min, respectively. The addition of either $10^{-5}M$ ouabain or $10^{-3}M$ DNP significantly inhibited the accumulation of $(U-^{14}C)$glycine. Approximately 85% of the radioactivity taken up by the incubated $P_2$ fraction, was found in the subfraction of $P_2$ containing synaptosomes. In order to circumvent the objection that an exchange of labelled and unlabelled glycine molecules occurred, Aprison and McBride (1973) then used unlabelled glycine in their uptake experiments. A net accumulation of unlabelled glycine was observed when the crude synaptosomal fraction $(P_2)$ was incubated at 37°C in the presence of increasing amounts of glycine (0.0375, 0.015 and 0.150 mM). In the preparation from spinal cord as well as from telencephalon, the uptake of glycine occurred against a large concentration gradient. The rate of uptake was more than 5 times larger from $P_2$ in the spinal cord than in $P_2$ from the telencephalon at 0.0375 mM. Thus, on the basis of the studies reported above, and physiological studies involving the effect of uptake inhibitors of amino acids, diaminobutyric acid (Curtis et al., 1976a), it is now generally accepted that the inactivation of the released glycine is largely due to a reuptake process.

## B. Release of Glycine

To properly satisfy the third criterion, one must demonstrate release of transmitter from presynaptic terminals after proper stimulation of a coherent input. Demonstrating such release of a transmitter has proven to be a very difficult task.

Jordan and Webster (1971) briefly reported that when the cat spinal cord was loaded with $(^{14}C)$glycine and the central canal perfused with artificial CSF fluid containing $10^{-5}M$ p-hydroxymercuribenzoate, increased release in vivo occurred after stimulation of femoral and sciatic nerves in four out of six attempts. Investigators soon turned to in vitro studies, as it became apparent that in vivo experiments were not very successful. Using a hemisectioned toad spinal cord and stimulating the dorsal roots while recording from the ventral roots, release of $(^{14}C)$glycine but not of labelled insulin was obtained (Figure 2). The $(^{14}C)$amino acids released into the medium were separated and analyzed by thin layer chromatography (Shank and Aprison, 1970b); only glycine and serine were labelled. Some correlation was observed between the amount of $(^{14}C)$glycine released and the number of stimuli applied to the dorsal roots (Aprison, 1970a,b; Aprison et al., 1976). Unfortunately,

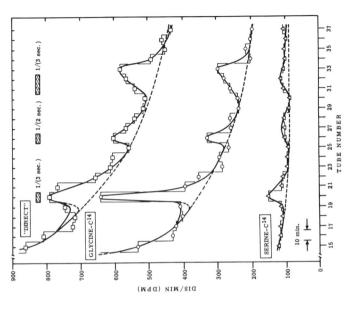

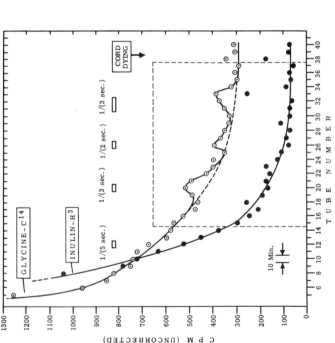

FIGURE 2. Left Side: Time course of efflux of ($^3$H)-inulin and ($^{14}$C)-glycine from hemisectioned toad spinal cord at rest and during stimulation. The rate of stimulation and the duration are shown. The samples within the dotted lines (No. 15-37) were used for chemical analysis. Right Side: Time course of efflux of ($^{14}$C)-glycine and ($^{14}$C)-serine from hemisectioned toad spinal cord at rest and during stimulation. Analysis of samples 15-37 showed that only glycine and serine of the amino acids assayed were radioactive. These data are replotted here along with the original data (direct). From Aprison et al. (1976).

success with this experiment was also unpredictable.

Roberts and Mitchell (1972) reported that ($^{14}$C)glycine could be released consistently from isolated hemisectioned frog or toad cords upon rostral stimulation after the tissue was first incubated in the presence of the labelled compound for 40 min. However, they failed to show release upon the stimulation of the ventral or dorsal roots. After stimulating the rostral cord, they also observed the release of ($^3$H)GABA, L-($^{14}$C)glutamate and L-($^{14}$C)-aspartate, but not of L-($^{14}$C)threonine, L-($^{14}$C)serine, L-($^3$H)leucine, ($^{14}$C)mannitol or ($^{14}$C)urea. It is not clear why dorsal root stimulation did not produce a release of amino acids. It should also be noted that Roberts and Mitchell (1972) did not find evidence of greater metabolism of the labelled amino acids when the cords were preincubated for 40 minutes in the presence of either ($^{14}$C)-glycine, L-($^{14}$C)serine or L-($^{14}$C)glutamate. For instance, in view of their positive results after the stimulation of the rostral cord, one would have expected ($^{14}$C)glycine to be released in their experiments in which incubations were carried out in the presence of L-($^{14}$C)serine, since the latter is readily converted to glycine (Shank and Aprison, 1970a; McBride et al., 1973). Mulder and Snyder (1974) have shown that a glycine pool labelled by the high affinity uptake system, is more efficiently released from rat spinal cord slices, than cortex slices upon stimulation in vitro by K$^+$.

More recently Beart and Bhilal (1976) have shown the K$^+$ stimulated release of ($^{14}$C)glycine synthesized from L-($^{14}$C)glucose and L-($^{14}$C)serine, by spinal cord slices. In addition, they reported that the specific activity of the glycine released upon incubation of the tissue with ($^{14}$C)glyoxylate and ($^{14}$C)pyruvate was lower; these data were interpreted to reflect a compartmentation of glycine within the nerve terminals.

Bradford and coworkers (Bradford, 1970; DeBelleroche and Bradford, 1973; Bradford et al., 1973; Osborne et al., 1973) studied the release of amino acids including glycine from subcellular fractions isolated from the telencephalon, medulla and spinal cord. Differential release of glutamate, aspartate, GABA and glycine occurred during electrical stimulation and when K$^+$ was increased in the medium.

Roberts (1974) was able to show that the in vivo stimulation of the cat medial lemniscus caused a significant increase in the release of both GABA and glycine, whereas only the release of GABA was increased when the dorsal tract was stimulated. Since the stimulation of the medial lemniscus causes the inhibition of the cuneothalamic relay system (Andersen et al., 1962, 1964), and that there is strychnine antagonism of the glycine effect but not that

of GABA in this nucleus (Hill et al., 1976), these findings are
suggestive of the fact that glycine may be the transmitter in
some of the interneurons of the cuneate nucleus.

Stimulus dependent release of ($^{14}$C)glycine was recently demonstrated after stimulation of the nucleus isthmi pars (parvocellularis) in the pigeon optic lobe (Reubi and Cuénod, 1976).  In addition, Ehinger and Lindberg-Baur (1976) and Voaden (1974) have reported release of glycine from the retina.

V.   METABOLISM OF GLYCINE

A.   In Vivo Studies

Glycine is a metabolically active amino acid and theoretically
can be derived from a number of precursors.  The levels of glycine
in the CNS might be maintained by the net flux of glycine from the
blood or by the net flux of serine into the CNS and its subsequent
conversion into glycine.  Current data support the concept that
glycine is derived mainly from serine and glucose and not from
such precursors as protein, choline, and glutathione.  Glyoxylate
has also been suggested as a precursor.

The investigations of the in vivo metabolism of glycine depend on a number of considerations:  (a) the CNS must ultimately
depend on the blood to receive its supply of glycine, or that of
a precursor to this compound; (b) serine and glyoxylate can be converted enzymatically to glycine in the CNS; (c) glucose is probably
the ultimate supplier of the carbon atoms in the pathway of glycine
synthesis; (d) there probably is a difference in the metabolic pathways of glycine in glycinergic versus non-glycinergic neurons, presumably reflecting a "compartmentation" of the neuronally used glycine, as opposed to the metabolically used glycine.

It can be reasoned that the rate at which labelled carbon atoms
from different precursors flow into CNS glycine may be a reflection
of the importance of different precursors in the maintenance of
neuronal glycine pools (Shank and Aprison, 1970a).  Uniformly
labelled glycine,serine and glucose were administered intraperitoneally, and the specific radioactivities of these substances
were determined in the blood and brain at various time intervals.
From these data, Shank and Aprison (1970a) calculated the net flux
of glycine in the CNS from each of these substances.  These investigators found that the net flux and/or exchange of glycine from
blood into brain is slow (0.03-0.15 µmol/g/h).  The biosynthesis of
glycine from serine was higher (1-3 µmol/g/h) as was the biosynthesis
of serine from glucose within the CNS (approximately 1.0 µmol/g/h);

these systems appear to be important factors in maintaining the
level of glycine in these tissues.

Radioactivity accumulated in glycine within the CNS after an
i.p. injection of (U-$^{14}$C)serine, and label accumulated in both
serine and glycine after an i.p. injection of (U-$^{14}$C)glucose was
also determined (TABLE IV). From data reported by Shank and
Aprison (1970a), it can be deduced that the accumulation of label
in glycine after the injection of ($^{14}$C)serine, and the accumulation of label in both serine and glycine after the injection of
($^{14}$C)glucose, was primarily the result of metabolism within the
CNS rather than metabolic conversion in other tissues and subsequent transport into the CNS. After an injection of (U-$^{14}$C)
glucose, the ratio of the total radioactivity in glycine to that
in serine (G/S) was similar to that ratio obtained after the administration of (U-$^{14}$C)serine (TABLE IV) in the medulla, spinal
cord, cerebellum and telencephalon. These similar G/S ratios provide a clear indication that the flow of carbons from glucose to
glycine in all four CNS areas is predominantly through serine.
The higher G/S ratios in the medulla and spinal cord (0.4-0.5)
as compared to those in the telencephalon and cerebellum (0.1-0.2)
can be attributed to the much higher content of glycine and lower
content of serine in the former areas. These studies appear to indicate that serine is probably the major precursor (and product)
of glycine metabolism in the CNS tissues (Shank and Aprison, 1970a;
Aprison et al., 1976).

Johnston and Vitali (1969a,b) were the first to show that
glyoxylate could be converted to glycine in homogenates of CNS
tissues. Shank and Aprison (1970a) confirmed this reaction when
they injected ($^{14}$C)glyoxylate into the cisterna magna and found
some label in glycine and little or no radioactivity appearing in
the rest of the amino acids. Although there are two major problems
in studying the role of glyoxylate as a precursor to glycine in
the CNS (its low content (10 nmole/g) normally found in CNS tissues
as reported by Liang (1962), Johnston (1970), Shank et al. (1973)
and the lack of sensitive analytical procedures to measure this
compound), it was important to determine whether this compound was
a precursor of one of the glycine compartments in glycinergic
nerve endings.

One approach toward the evaluation of glyoxylate as a precursor has been to inject labelled compounds into the cisterna
magna and determine whether glycine is synthesized preferentially
via the glyoxylate pathway or the serine pathway. In one such
study, Shank et al. (1973) used (1-$^{14}$C)glucose and (3,4-$^{14}$C)glucose,
and then measured the accumulation of label in different amino
acids following the injection of each of these compounds (TABLE V).
Through pathways involving serine, the 1-carbon is not incorporated

TABLE IV. MEAN TOTAL RADIOACTIVITY IN GLYCINE AND SERINE IN FOUR AREAS OF THE RAT CNS 20 MIN AFTER AN INJECTION (i.p.) OF (U-$^{14}$C)SERINE OR (U-$^{14}$C)GLUCOSE

| CNS areas | Metabolite injected | | | | | |
|---|---|---|---|---|---|---|
| | (U-$^{14}$C)Serine | | | (U-$^{14}$C)Glucose | | |
| | Glycine | Serine | G/S[a] | Glycine | Serine | G/S[a] |
| Telencephalon | 2870 | 23,170 | 0.12 | 650 | 4010 | 0.16 |
| Cerebellum | 5730 | 28,100 | 0.20 | 710 | 3060 | 0.23 |
| Medulla | 9410 | 21,650 | 0.43 | 1430 | 3250 | 0.44 |
| Spinal cord (gray) | 8900 | 18,230 | 0.49 | 1600 | 3190 | 0.50 |

[a] G/S is the ratio of the total radioactivity in glycine to that in serine. Of each metabolite, 25 µCi/100 g body wt. was injected into the peritoneal cavity; 20 min after the injection each rat was killed by an injection of pentobarbital into the heart. Each rat was perfused with 0.15 M NaCl to remove residual blood from CNS tissue. Values are given as d.p.m./g wet tissue; N = 4. From Shank et al. (1973).

TABLE V.  MEAN SPECIFIC RADIOACTIVITY OF SEVEN AMINO ACIDS IN THE
MEDULLA-PONS OF RATS AFTER AN INJECTION OF $(3,4-^{14}C)$GLUCOSE OR
$(1-^{14}C)$GLUCOSE INTO THE CISTERNA MAGNA[a]

| Amino Acid | Metabolite injected | |
| --- | --- | --- |
| | $(3,4-^{14}C)$Glucose  (2 µCi) | $(1-^{14}C)$Glucose (2 µCi)[b] |
| Glycine | 494 + 58 | 99 + 9 |
| Serine | 4590 + 1300 | 4,950 + 500 |
| Alanine | 3850 + 280 | 8,150 + 435 |
| Glutamate | 1220 + 39 | 34,300 + 1870 |
| Glutamine | 1780 + 52 | 29,600 + 1540 |
| GABA | 649 + 48 | 24,800 + 410 (40,400)[c] |
| Aspartate | 846 + 19 | 24,000 + 1200 |

[a]The $(^{14}C)$-glucose was dissolved in 0.15 M NaCl and the volume injected with 5 µl.  The rats were lightly anesthetized with ether
during the injection process; 30 min after the injection the animals were killed.  Values are given in d.p.m./µmol and represent
the mean + SEM (N=4).  From Shank et al. (1973).
[b]For $(1-^{14}C)$-glucose, 3 µCi were injected into each rat.  The
actual values were reduced by one-third to make them comparable to
the data for $(3,4-^{14}C)$-glucose.
[c]One of these four values was considerably higher than the other
three.  This value may be in error and is therefore reported
separately.  From Shank et al. (1973).

into glycine, whereas with pathways involving glyoxylate, this
carbon atom is incorporated into glycine (FIGURE 3).  On the other
hand, the carbon atoms from the $(3,4-^{14}C)$glucose are incorporated
into glycine via the serine pathways, but are lost as $CO_2$ via the
glyoxylate pathways.  Shank et al. (1973) found that five times
more label was accumulated into glycine from $(3,4-^{14}C)$glucose than
from $(1-^{14}C)$glucose.  Although these data could be interpreted as
20% of the CNS glycine is synthesized via glyoxylate, it was also
possible that $(1-^{14}C)$glucose could be incorporated into glycine
via serine through an indirect pathway.  This would involve the
formation of glycine from methylene tetrahydrofolate, ammonia and
carbon dioxide.  If this were true, it would mean that 80% or
even 100% of the glycine in the CNS is formed via serine.

In further studies to establish whether the glyoxylate to
glycine pathway is operative in the CNS, compounds which are considered to be direct precursors of glyoxylate were injected into

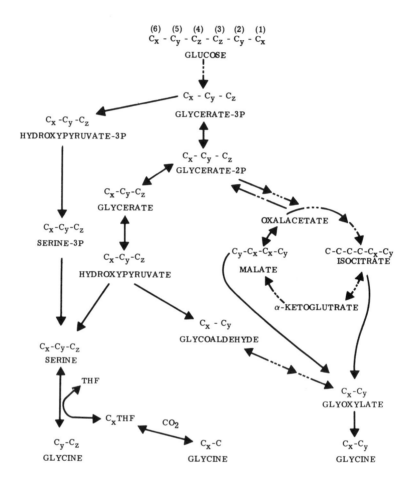

FIGURE 3. Simplified diagram showing pathways of carbon flow from glucose to glycine. Taken from Aprison et al. (1976).

the cisterna magna. Thus, after the administration of $(U-^{14}C)$
glycerate, $(1,5-^{14}C)$cistrate, and $(U-^{14}C)$aspartate, the label in
serine was higher than glycine, which was consistent with the trend
of thought that glycine is formed predominantly from serine. After
the intracranial injection of $(2-^{14}C)$ ethanolamine (which can be
converted into glyoxylate) no label was found in glycine. Data
as noted above and the facts that no major precursor for glyoxylate has been found in the CNS, and glyoxylate itself enters
the CNS slowly from the blood (Romano and Cerra, 1967), suggest
that glyoxylate is not a major precursor of glycine. However, it
is of interest to note that in cases of thiamine deficiency where
glyoxylate levels in the CNS have been shown to increase (Liang,
1962), the glycine levels in the CNS have also been found to increase (Gaitonde, 1975). Furthermore, recently Beart and Bhibal
(1976) reported that glycine synthesized from $(^{14}C)$glyoxylate as
a precursor in slices of spinal cord is released by high $K^+$ stimulation. Thus, it still remains to be conclusively shown whether
or not glyoxylate is a net precursor to neuronal glycine pools, or
whether glycine formation from glyoxylate is simply a non-specific
detoxification process.

## B. In Vitro Studies

Supportive evidence that glycine is a neurotransmitter comes
from the demonstration that the content of this amino acid is significantly higher in nerve ending fractions $(P_2)$ isolated from the
medulla and spinal cord (regions where the neurobiological evidence
suggests that it is an inhibitory transmitter) than in a similar
preparation from the telencephalon or cerebellum (areas where the
present evidence does not support that role). It is interesting
that except for glutamate, the levels of glycine in the synaptosomal preparations from spinal cord and medulla are the highest of
all the amino acid measured (Osborne et al., 1973; McBride et al.,
1973).

Studies on the subcellular distribution of $(U-^{14}C)$glycine and
$(U-^{14}C)$serine in incubated $P_2$ fractions show that both are readily
taken up by the crude $P_2$ synaptosomal preparations (Aprison and
McBride, 1973; McBride et al., 1973). After further subfractionation
of the incubated $P_2$ fractions into a myelin, a synaptosomal and a
mitochondrial fraction, 83 to 89% of the radioactivity taken up
after incubation with $(U-^{14}C)$glycine is in the synaptosomal fraction.
Glycine is readily converted to serine and serine is readily converted to glycine in these preparations (McBride et al., 1973).

## C. Enzyme Studies

Studies on the regional distribution of SHMT activity, GT

TABLE VI. DISTRIBUTION OF THE ACTIVITIES OF SERINE HYDROXYMETHYLTRANSFERASE, GLYCINE TRANS-AMINASE, THE GLYCINE CLEAVAGE SYSTEM, SUCCINATE DEHYDROGENASE AND THE CONTENT OF GLYCINE IN FIVE AREAS OF THE CNS OF THE RAT[a]

| Area of CNS | SHMT μmol/h/g (n = 6) | GT μmol/h/g (n = 6) | GCS activity nmol/h/g (n = 9) | SDH activity μmol/h/g (n = 3) | Glycine Content μmol/g (n = 4) |
|---|---|---|---|---|---|
| Telencephalon | 3.49 ± 0.14 | 19.8 ± 0.5 | 564 ± 30 | 322 ± 14 | 0.83 ± 0.05 |
| Midbrain | 3.78 ± 0.22 | 20.4 ± 0.3 | 146 ± 18 | 287 ± 31 | 1.50 ± 0.02 |
| Cerebellum | 4.80 ± 0.70 | 18.5 ± 0.3 | 258 ± 13 | 330 ± 9 | 0.68 ± 0.05 |
| Medulla-pons | 5.08 ± 0.27 | 19.2 ± 0.7 | 46 ± 9[b] | 241 ± 3 | 4.15 ± 0.18 |
| Spinal cord | 4.35 ± 0.09 | 13.7 ± 1.0 | 22 ± 9 | 161 ± 13 | 4.20 ± 0.25 |

Data are given as the mean ± S.E.M.
[a] Values from data in Daly and Aprison (1974a) and Daly, Nadi and Aprison (1976).
[b] n = 8.

activity, SDH activity and glycine content by Daly and Aprison
(1974a) indicate that these parameters varied differently among
the five different areas of brain and spinal cord (TABLE VI).  The
SHMT activity was highest in the spinal cord and medulla-pons,
followed in order to decreasing activity by the cerebellum, midbrain and telencephalon, whereas for the GT activities, the value
for the spinal cord was lowest and those of the four brain areas
were the same.  These investigators also found that SHMT is a
mitochondrial enzyme.  Daly and Aprison (1974a) found that a good
correlation exists between SHMT activity/mg-protein and glycine
levels when the cerebellar data were not considered (r = 0.997;
P<0.05).  However, when the SHMT activity per relative number of
mitochondria (SHMT/SDH) is calculated (Gregson & Williams, 1969)
excellent correlation with glycine levels was found for all five
areas studied.  Finally, there was no correlation between the GT
activity and glycine levels in the areas studied (r = -0.45;
P>0.05).

In subcellular distribution studies, the percentage distribution of SHMT in the primary subcellular fractions in each of the
five regions of the CNS was 96-99 percent of the total SHMT activity sediments in the particulate fractions ($P_1$ + $P_2$ + $P_3$).  A
similar distribution was noted for MAO.  Daly and Aprison found
that 90-97 percent of the total SHMT activity is in the $P_1$ and $P_2$
fractions.  It is of interest to note that the $P_1$ had a larger
percentage of SHMT activity than of MAO activity in all regions
studied.  However, when the distribution of LDH (a cytoplasmic
enzyme) was determined,it was found to be markedly different from
that noted for SHMT and MAO (Daly and Aprison, 1974a).  Thus,
these data support the fact that SHMT is mainly, if not exclusively,
a particulate enzyme in these areas of the CNS.

Since Shank & Aprison (1970a) had established that the glycine
content varies within the five areas of CNS of the rat, it is of
great interest to find that of the two suggested biosynthetic enzymes, only SHMT and not GT appears to be correlated to the levels
of glycine.  Furthermore, SHMT may play an important role in the
folate and one-carbon metabolism of the CNS in addition to its role
in the synthesis of glycine for the 'metabolic' pool(s) and the
transmitter pool.  Therefore, the high levels of SHMT in CB may reflect a greater need for folates, active carbons, and/or 'metabolic'
glycine in this region than in the others due to its higher cellular
density (Balázs et al., 1971).  These roles of SHMT in non-transmitter metabolism probably account for the largest portion of the
activity measured, and may also explain why the enzyme levels did
not extrapolate to zero activity at zero glycine content (Daly and
Aprison, 1974a).

There appear to be at least three pathways for glycine cata-

bolism within the CNS.  Since the conversion of serine to glycine
is readily reversible within the CNS, SHMT may function also as a
degradative enzyme for glycine (Bridgers, 1968; Shank & Aprison,
1970a; McBride et al., 1973).  In addition, D-amino acid oxidase
is present within the CNS and utilizes glycine as a substrate
(DiMarchi & Johnston, 1969).  Finally, the glycine cleavage system,
which has been postulated to be the major degradative mechanism for
glycine in some peripheral tissues (Kikuchi, 1973; Yoshida &
Kikuchi, 1973) has recently been measured within the CNS (Bruin
et al., 1973; Uhr, 1973; Yoshida & Kikuchi, 1973; Daly et al.,
1976).  The level of the GCS has been reported to be lower in the
spinal cord than in brain parts (cat: Uhr, 1973) (rat: Daly et al.,
1976) or whole brain (rat: Yoshida & Kikuchi, 1973).  Within the
CNS, the GCS is located in mitochondrial fractions (Bruin et al.,
1973; Uhr, 1973), as is SHMT (Daly & Aprison, 1974a; Burton &
Sallach, 1975).

When Daly et al. (1976) recently reported the regional distribution of the GCS activity in homogenates from various regions of
the CNS of the rat, they noted that it differed significantly among
these areas (TABLE VI) and does not appear to be linearly correlated (r = 0.74, P>0.05) with the SDH activity.  The 25-fold difference in GCS activity within the CNS is especially interesting
since the highest activity is found in the regions where the glycine
content is the lowest (telencephalon and cerebellum) and the lowest
activity is found in regions where the glycine content is the
highest (spinal cord and medulla-pons).  In agreement with studies
of the GCS activity in liver mitochondria (Kikuchi, 1973), Daly
et al. (1976) found that the formation of $^{14}CO_2$ from the carboxyl
carbon of glycine appeared to be coupled with the formation of
serine on a one-to-one basis in all the regions of the CNS.

The large range in the regional distribution of the GCS (5.64
nmol/h per g for telencephalon to 22 nmol/h per g for the spinal
cord) suggested the presence of an inhibitor(s) or controlling
mechanism in those regions of the CNS where the activity was low.
When telencephalon homogenates were incubated with homogenates
from each of the other regions under the standard conditions, a
significant non-additivity of the GCS activities was found (TABLE
VII).  The non-additivity appears to be greater in the regions
where the GCS activity is low (spinal cord and medulla-pons) than
in the region where GCS activity is higher (cerebellum).  When
similar experiments were performed measuring SHMT activity in the
homogenates, additivity was found between the telencephalon and
the other four regions of the CNS.

It remains to be seen whether this inhibition of the GCS has
any significance in the metabolic and/or transmitter roles of glycine in vivo.  Recent reports have described multiple forms of

TABLE VII.  APPARENT INHIBITION (NON-ADDITIVITY) OF THE GLYCINE
CLEAVAGE SYSTEM IN HOMOGENATES OF THE CNS OF THE RAT[a]

| Mixture of areas of CNS[b] | % Reduction of expected activity[c] |
|---|---|
| Telencephalon plus midbrain | $42 \pm 6$ |
| Telencephalon plus cerebellum | $24 \pm 6$ |
| Telencephalon plus medulla-pons | $50 \pm 6$ |
| Telencephalon plus spinal cord | $53 \pm 5$ |

[a]From Daly, Nadi and Aprison (1976).
[b]Mixtures contained $15.1 \pm 0.4$ mg of each area as homogenates in
  0.32 M-sucrose.
[c]Data are given as mean $\pm$ S.E.M.; N = 4.  The expected activity is
  the sum of the activities of the areas when assayed separately.

folates (Brody et al., 1975) and the soluble location of both
transmethylation and folate-interconverting enzymes within the CNS
of the rat (Burton & Sallach, 1975; Rassin & Gaull, 1975).  SHMT
and the GCS probably represent the major mechanism for the generation of the one-carbon pool (Burton & Sallach, 1975) and SHMT
appears to be the biosynthetic enzyme for glycine within the CNS
(Shank & Aprison, 1970a; Daly & Aprison, 1974a,b).The formation of
one-carbon units and glycine within the mitochondria, their utilization within the cytosol, and the necessity for strict control of
the levels of glycine in the transmitter pool emphasize the need
for regulation in both the metabolism and transport of these compounds within the mitochondrion (Aprison et al., 1976).  A substance inhibiting the activity of the GCS but not that of SHMT
would influence the degree of coupling in this enzymatic system.
A tightly coupled GCS and SHMT could rapidly degrade glycine without changing the levels of the one-carbon pool, whereas a loosely
coupled SHMT could mediate the synthesis of both glycine and one-
carbon units from the original carbon skeleton of glucose via
serine.

The properties of the GCS in homogenates of the rat telencephalon (Daly et al., 1976) appear to be similar to those described for the system in partially purified mitochondria isolated
from liver (Sato et al., 1969) and whole brain (Bruin et al., 1973).
The activity is not a typical amino acid decarboxylase in that it
is dependent on both NAD and THF.  In addition, Daly et al. (1976)
have shown that the liberation of the carboxyl carbon of glycine
is coupled with the formation of equimolar quantities of serine via

the condensation reaction between the alpha carbon and a second
molecule of glycine catalyzed by SHMT.  In liver mitochondria,
the GCS has been described as a complex of four proteins (Kikuchi,
1973) and together with SHMT is located within the inner membrane
fraction (Motokawa & Kikuchi, 1971).  Although the intra-mito-
chondrial localization of the GCS and SHMT within the CNS is not
known, the mitochondrial location of these enzymes (Bruin et al.,
1973; Uhr, 1973; Daly & Aprison, 1974a; Burton & Sallach, 1975) as
well as their metabolic coupling in vitro is consistent with the
suggestion that a close association exists in vivo.

### D.  The Glycine Receptor

In the past several years, Snyder and colleagues have conducted a detailed investigation of the glycine receptor by using
($^3$H)strychnine as a marker for the receptor.  They were able to
show that a) there is higher ($^3$H)strychnine binding in the spinal
cord and medulla than in other brain areas (Young & Snyder, 1973);
b) the binding of ($^3$H)strychnine in the spinal cord and medulla is
associated with the synaptic membrane portion (Young & Snyder,
1974a); c) glycine and strychnine appear to bind to two separate
sites of the same receptor, which are capable of mutually influencing each other (Young & Snyder, 1974b); d) the high affinity
uptake system of glycine and the ($^3$H)strychnine binding develop
between days 14 and 21 in the chick embryo (Zukin et al., 1975),
and these data are consistent with the time of emergence of electrophysiologically observable inhibition in the chick embryo spinal
cord (Stokes & Bignall, 1974; Oppenheim & Reitzel, 1975); e) the
($^3$H)strychnine binding site and the competition of different anions
with this site suggest a close association with the ionic conductance mechanisms of the receptor (Young & Snyder, 1974b), and f)
benzodiazepines have a similar potency in displacing ($^3$H)strychnine
from the receptor in vitro as glycine does, and that this may be
suggestive of these drugs exerting their muscle relaxant effects
through interference with the glycinergic system (Young et al., 1974).

Although the data described above correlate well in many
aspects with other findings in the glycine system, it should be
pointed out that, the benzodiazepine data obtained in vitro, was
not supported by in vivo physiological studies conducted by Curtis
et al.(1976b) indicating that caution must be exercised in the
extrapolation of in vitro data to in vivo conditions.  In these
experiments with cats, diazepam given intravenously did not affect
the strychnine induced loss of inhibition by glycine in the spinal
cord.  Similarly, in mice, diazepam which was intravenously administered failed to have any effect on the action of strychnine.

VI.  CLINICAL ASPECTS OF GLYCINE


A.  Genetic Disorders

A large number of genetic disorders involving amino acids
have been discovered.  In most cases, children bearing these diseases have some type of neurologic symptom.  In addition, severe
mental retardation appears to be associated with these disorders.
In this group of metabolic diseases involving amino acids, there
are two disorders in which glycine accumulates in appreciable
amounts in the blood of patients.

a)  Ketotic hyperglycinemia.  In the different disorders described in this category, the glycine metabolism is only indirectly
affected.  The primary defect appears to be the involvement of the
isoleucine and valine catabolism.  The hyperglycinemic episodes
are only intermittent in these cases, and are accompanied by protein induced ketoacidosis and hyperammonemia.  If the patients survive the severe metabolic imbalance in the early stages, they may
survive with intermittent ketoacidosis, or severe mental retardation
and seizures.  Although the defect in many of these pathways, and
the accumulation of glycine, propionic acid, or tiglic acid (in the
case of isoleucine metabolism) may be instrumental in causing the
neurotoxicity (Ando and Nylan, 1974), patients who have remained
neurologically intact while suffering similar diseases have also
been reported (Paulsen and Hsia, 1974).

b)  Nonketototic hyperglycinemia.  In these cases the primary
defect is in the major catabolic pathway of glycine, the glycine
cleavage system.  This disease is different from ketotic hyperglycinemia in that no ketosis is observed in these patients; they
usually exhibit an early onset of lethargy, hypotonia, myoclonic
jerks, and seizures that are unresponsive to anticonvulsant therapy
(Baumgartner et al., 1975).  If patients survive the early months,
mental retardation, decerebrate rigidity and hypertonus are observed in the later phases of their lives.  Tracer studies in some
of these patients show a normal glycine oxidation (Gerritsen et al.,
1969) and a block in the glycine cleavage system in both the brain
and the liver (Perry et al., 1975a; Tada et al., 1974; Trijbels et
al., 1974).  An increase in glycine levels of cerebrospinal fluid
and blood is also observed (Scriver et al., 1975; Perry et al.,
1975b).  The CSF to blood glycine ratio is higher than in control
subjects, which fits the criterion used by some physicians to
classify a disease as a genetic glycinemia, as opposed to other
syndromes which indirectly result in high blood glycine levels
(Applegarth and Poon, 1975).  Perry et al. (1975a) have noted that
in several cases of non-ketotic hyperglycinemia, in addition to the
above reported effects, the glycine levels in all areas of the
brain were also increased.  The cases of three brothers suffering
from "late onset" nonketotic hyperglycinemia, along with spasticity,

and a defect in the ventral and lateral lumbar spinal cord, an
apparent defect in the glycine cleavage system was noted (Bank and
Morrow, 1972).  Recently it has been reported that administration
of strychnine to a child with nonketotic hyperglycinemia produced
some recovery from the symptoms (Cuénod, personal communication).

Pathological studies on the nervous system of patients suffering from nonketotic hyperglycinemia have shown some bire-
fringent crystal inclusions, low myelination of white matter, and
spongioform degeneration of the cerebrum, cerebellum and the spinal
cord (Leupold et al., 1974).  A case of nonketotic hyperglycinemia
which was aggravated by valine, but somewhat alienated by sodium
benzoate treatment has also been reported by Krieger and Hart
(1974).  Hyperglycinemia also occurs in the nonketotic hyperglycinemia syndrome (Bank and Morrow, 1972).

Cases of hyperglycinemia have been described in which the
renal transport system for glycine has been impaired.  In such
cases patients are generally free of neurological symptoms (Greene
et al., 1973).

## B.  Tetanus Toxin

Tetanus toxin causes spastic and to a lesser extent paralytic
symptoms (for a review see Habemann and Wellhoner, 1974; also
Tarlov, 1967, 1974; Tarlov et al., 1973).  It achieves these effects
by affecting the organism at the neuromuscular junction and in the
central nervous system.  The protein tetanus toxin (tetraospamin)
can be transported into the CNS by retrograde intraaxonal transport from the site of the wound (Price et al., 1975).  In the CNS,
it is taken up and fixed by glycoproteins exclusively in the ventral
gray matter of the spinal cord (Dimpfel and Habermann, 1973).  Autoradiography of the spinal cord of rats injected with $(^{125}I)$-tetanus
toxin showed the highest accumulation of grains in the ventral spinal
cord in the region of the motoneurons (Dimpfel and Habermann, 1973)
and that it is the axosomatic synaptic area that is preferentially
labelled (Price et al., 1977).  Physiological studies have shown
that in early tetanus, gamma motoneurons, and in later phases both
gamma and alpha neurons are affected (Benecke et al., 1977).  On the
basis of these studies, it could be hypothesized that tetanus toxin
may act in one of two ways:  a) by binding to the postsynaptic site
and blocking the action of the neurotransmitter released or b) by
binding to the presynaptic site and preventing the release of the
neurotransmitter.  Working independently on this question, Curtis
and deGroat (1968) and Gushchin et al. (1969) established that on
the basis of its electrophysiological efforts, the toxin was producing its effects by binding to the presynaptic region of the
ventral cord where glycine probably acts as the inhibitory trans-

mitter. From the combined physiological data (Curtis and deGroat, 1968 and Gushchin et al., 1969) showing that the sensitivity of motoneurons to glycine is not impaired, and the biochemical data showing that: (a) electrically stimulated release of glycine (and other amino acids) was reduced in synaptosomes prepared from rats treated intramuscularly with tetanus 15 hr before death (Osborne et al., 1973), and (b) tetanus toxin did not deplete the glycine stores in the spinal cord (Fedinec and Shank, 1971; Johnston et al., 1969), it appears the best explanation is that the toxin must act by preventing the release of this transmitter. Recently Curtis et al. (1973) have shown that in addition to inhibiting the release of glycine, tetanus toxin also alters the release of GABA thus ex-plaining the suppression of prolonged presynaptic inhibition by tetanus toxin (Sverdlov et al., 1966). Thus it appears that there is a good correlation between the impairment of release mechanisms by glycinergic neurons in the spinal cord, and the effects of tetanus toxin on alpha and gamma motoneurons (Benecke et al., 1977; Curtis and deGroat, 1968; Gushchin et al., 1969).


C.  Experimental Spinal Spasticity

If glycine is indeed the segmental postsynaptic inhibitory transmitter, it would be reasonable to assume that in a condition involving the loss of segmental inhibition, such as spasticity (the release phenomenon frequently accompanying neurological injury in man), the content of glycine should fall in the gray matter of the spinal cord containing the interneurons. Perhaps it would not be unreasonable to predict that the level of other segmental trans-mitter candidates might also change. Two reports have been pub-lished by Aprison, Campbell and coworkers that support these sug-gestions (Hall et al., 1976; Smith et al., 1976). Experimental spasticity was induced in dogs following high thoracic spinal cord transections. The onset and degree of spasticity were assessed by observing the relative reflex activity of the hindlimbs and tail and by observing the relative monosynaptic and polysynaptic reflex responses. The tendon reflexes were used to assess monosynaptic activity and the response to noxious cutaneous stimuli to determine polysynaptic activity. The amino acids were measured in several areas of the spinal cord. Significant decreases in the levels of glycine and aspartate in ventral central gray occurred following spinal cord transection, and these changes followed the onset of spasticity. The decrease in glycine was thought to represent a loss of glycinergic inhibitory interneurons. A change in the level of GABA in the dorsal gray also occurred; the increase that was found correlates with the development of spinal spasticity and may represent a decreased release in GABA since this transmitter is thought to mediate presynaptic inhibition in this region (a decre-ment in presynaptic inhibition has been demonstrated in the clinical

condition).  The data in these preliminary studies indicate that
segmental inhibitory systems may be disrupted in spinal spasticity.
Perhaps the administration of glycine or glycine plus several other
compounds which will also modulate the levels of GABA and aspartate
will be helpful to the patient.  Certainly more work is necessary
in this important clinical area.

## ACKNOWLEDGMENT

These studies were supported in part by grants from the National
Science Foundation (GB28715X) and from the National Institute of
Mental Health (MH03225).

## REFERENCES

Andersen,P., Eccles, J.C., and Schmidt, R.F., 1962, Presynaptic in-
     hibition in the cuneate nucleus, Nature (Lond.) 194: 741-743.
Andersen, P., Eccles, J.C., Shima, K. and Schmidt, R.F., 1964,
     Mechanism of synaptic transmission in the cuneate nucleus,
     J. Neurophysiol. 27: 1096-1116.
Ando, T. and Nyhan, W.L., 1974, Proprionic acidemia and the ketotic
     hyperglycinemia syndrome, in "Heritable Disorders of Amino
     Acid Metabolism" (W.L. Nyhan, ed.), Wiley, New York.
Applegarth, D.A. and Poon, S., 1975, Interpretation of elevated
     blood glycine levels in children, Clin. Chim. Acta 63: 49-54.
Aprison, M.H., 1965, Research approaches to problems in mental
     illness: brain neurohumor-enzyme systems and behavior, Prog.
     Brain Res. 16: 48-80.
Aprison, M.H., 1970a, Evidence of the release of $^{14}$C glycine from
     hemisectioned toad spinal cord with dorsal root stimulation,
     Pharmacologist 12: 222.
Aprison, M.H., 1970b, Studies on the release of glycine in the iso-
     lated spinal cord of the toad, Trans. Am. Soc. Neurochem. 1: 25.
Aprison, M.H., 1977, Glycine as a neurotransmitter, in "Psycho-
     pharmacology: A Generation of Progress" (M.A. Lipton, A.
     Di Mascio and K.F. Killam, eds.) pp. 333-346, Raven Press,
     New York.
Aprison, M.H. and Hingtgen, J.N., 1970, Neurochemical correlates of
     behavior, Int. Rev. Neurobiol. 13: 325-341.
Aprison, M.H. and McBride, W.J., 1973, Evidence for the net accu-
     mulation of glycine into a synaptosomal fraction isolated from
     the telencephalon and spinal cord of the rat, Life Sci. 12:
     449-458.
Aprison, M.H. and Werman, R., 1965, The distribution of glycine in
     cat spinal cord and roots, Life Sci. 4: 2075-2083.

Aprison, M.H. and Werman, R., 1968, A combined neurochemical and neurophysiological approach to the identification of central nervous system neurotransmitters, in "Neurosciences Research", Vol. 1 (S. Ehrenpreis and O.C. Solnitzky, eds.) pp. 143-174, Academic Press, New York.

Aprison, M.H., Graham, Jr. L.T., Livengood, D.R. and Werman, R., 1965, Distribution of glutamic acid in the cat spinal cord and roots, Fed. Proc. Fed. Am. Soc. Exp. Biol. 24: 462.

Aprison, M.H., Shank, R.P. and Davidoff, R.A., 1969, A comparison of the concentration of glycine, a transmitter suspect, in different areas of the brain and spinal cord in seven different vertebrates, Comp. Biochem. Physiol. 28: 1345-1355.

Aprison, M.H., Hingtgen, J.N. and McBride, W.J., 1975, Serotonergic and cholinergic mechanisms during disruption of approach and avoidance behavior, Fed. Proc. Fed. Am. Soc. Exp. Biol. 34: 1813-1822.

Aprison, M.H., Daly, E.C., Shank, R.P. and McBride, W.J., 1976, Neurochemical evidence for glycine as a transmitter and a model for its intrasynaptosomal compartmentation, in "Metabolic Compartmentation and Neurotransmission" (S. Berl, D.D. Clarke and D. Schneider, eds.) pp. 37-63, Plenum Press, New York.

Balázs, R., Kovacs, S., Cocks, W.A., Johnson, A.L. and Eayrs, J.T., 1971, Effective thyroid hormone on the biochemical maturation of rat brain: postnatal cell formation, Brain Res. 25: 555-570.

Balcar, V.J. and Johnston, G.A.R., 1973, High affinity uptake of transmitters. Studies of the uptake of L-aspartate, GABA, L-glutamate, and glycine in cat spinal cord, J. Neurochem. 20: 529-539.

Bank, W.J. and Morrow, G., 1972, A familial spinal cord disorder with hyperglycinemia, Arch. Neurol. 27: 136-144.

Baumgartner, E.R., Bauchman, C., Brechbuhler, T. and Wick, H., 1975, Acute neonatal nonketotic hyperglycinemia: normal propionate and methylmalomate metabolism, Pediat. Res. 9: 559-564.

Beart, P.M. and Bhial, K.B., 1976, Compartmentation and release of glycine in vitro, Neuroscience Abst. 11: 594.

Belcher, G., Davies, J. and Ryall, R.W., 1976, Glycine mediated inhibitory transmission of group 1A-excited inhibitory interneurones by Renshaw cells, J. Physiol. (London) 256: 651-662.

Benecke, R., Takano, K., Schmidt, J. and Henatsch, H.D., 1977, Tetanus toxin induced actions on spinal Renshaw cells and Ia inhibitory interneurones during development of local tetanus in the cat, Exp. Brain Res. 27: 271-286.

Berger, S.J., Carter, J.G. and Lowry, O.H., 1977a, The distribution of glycine, GABA, glutamate and aspartate in rabbit spinal cord cerebellum and hippocampus, J. Neurochem. 28: 149-158.

Berger, S.J., McDaniel, M.L., Carter, J.G. and Lowry, O.H., 1977b, Distribution of four potential transmitter amino acids in monkey retina, J. Neurochem. 28: 159-163.

Biscoe, T.J., Duggan, A.W., and Lodge, D., 1972, Antagonism between bicuculline, strychnine, and picrotoxin and depressant amino-acids in the rat nervous system, Comp. Gen. Pharmacol. 3: 423-433.

Boehme, D.H., Fordice, M.W., Marks, N., and Vogel, W., 1973, Distribution of glycine in human spinal cord and selected regions of brain, Brain Res. 50: 353-359.

Bradford, H.F., 1970, Metabolic response of synaptosomes to electrical stimulation: Release of amino acids, Brain Res. 19: 239-247.

Bradford, H.F., Bennett, G.W. and Thomas, A.J., 1973, Depolarizing stimuli and the release of physiologically active amino acids from suspensions of mammalian synaptosomes, J. Neurochem. 21: 495-505.

Bridges, W.F., 1968, Serine transhydroxymethylase in developing mouse brain, J. Neurochem. 15: 1325-1328.

Brody, T., Shane, B., and Stokstad, E.L.R., 1975, Identification and subcellular distribution of folates in rat brain, Fed. Proc. Fed. Am. Soc. Exp. Biol. 34: 905.

Brooks, V.B. and Asanuma, H., 1965, Pharmacological studies of recurrent cortical inhibition and facilitation, Am. J. Physiol. 208: 674-681.

Bruggencate, G. Ten and Engberg, I., 1968, Analysis of glycine actions on spinal interneurones by intracellular recording, Brain Res. 11: 446-450.

Bruggencate, G. Ten and Engberg, I., 1971, Iontophoretic studies in deiters nucleus of the inhibitory actions of GABA and related amino acids and the interactions of strychnine and picrotoxin, Brain Res. 25: 431-448.

Bruggencate, G. Ten and Sonnhof, U., 1972, Effects of glycine and GABA and blocking actions of strychnine and picrotoxin in the hypoglossus nucleus, Arch. Ges. Physiol. 334: 240-252.

Bruin, W.J., Frontz, B.M. and Sallach, H.J., 1973, The occurrence of a glycine cleavage system in mammalian brain, J. Neurochem. 20: 1649-1658.

Burton, E.G. and Sallach, H.J., 1975, Methylenetetrahydrofolate reductase in the rat central nervous system: intracellular and regional distribution, Arch. Biochem. and Biophys. 166: 483-494.

Cho, Y.D., Martin, R.O. and Tunnicliff, G., 1973, Uptake of ($^3$H) glycine and ($^{14}$C) glutamate by cultures of chick spinal cord, J. Physiol. (London) 235: 437-446.

Crawford, J.M. and Curtis, D.R., 1964, The excitation and depression of mammalian cortical neurones by amino acids, Brit. J. Pharmacol. Chemotherap. 23: 313-329.

Crawford, J.M., Curtis, D.R., Voorhoeve, P.E. and Wilson, V.J., 1963, Strychnine and cortical inhibition, Nature (London) 200: 845-846.

Curtis, D.R., 1963, The pharmacology of central and peripheral in-
    hibition, Pharmacol. Rev. 15: 333-364.
Curtis, D.R. and DeGroat, W.C., 1968, Tetanus toxin and spinal in-
    hibition, Brain Res. 10: 208-212.
Curtis, D.R. and Watkins, J.C., 1960, The excitation and depression
    of spinal neurons by structurally related amino acids, J.
    Neurochem. 6: 117-141.
Curtis, D.R. and Watkins, J.C., 1963, Acidic amino acids with strong
    excitatory actions on mammalian neurones, J. Physiol. (London)
    166: 1-14.
Curtis, D.R. and Watkins, J.C., 1965, The pharmacology of amino acids
    related to gamma-aminobutyric acid, Pharmacol. Rev. 17: 347-392.
Curtis, D.R., Phillis, J.W. and Watkins, J.C., 1959, The depression
    of spinal neurones by γ-amino-n-butyric acid and β-alanine,
    J. Physiol. (London) 146: 185-203.
Curtis, D.R., Phillis, J.W. and Watkins, J.C., 1960, The chemical
    excitation of spinal neurones by certain acidic amino acids,
    J. Physiol. (London) 150: 656-682.
Curtis, D.R., Hösli, L., Johnston, G.A.R. and Johnston, I.H., 1968a,
    The hyperpolarization of spinal interneurones by glycine and
    related amino acids, Exptl. Brain Res. 5: 235-258.
Curtis, D.R., Hösli, L. and Johnston, G.A.R., 1968b, A pharma-
    cological study of the depression of spinal neurones by glycine
    and related amino acids, Exptl. Brain Res. 6: 1-18.
Curtis, D.R., Felix, D., Game, C.J.A. and McCulloch, R.M., 1973,
    Tetanus toxin and the synaptic release of GABA, Brain Res. 51:
    358-362.
Curtis, D.R., Game, C.J.A. and Lodge, D., 1976a, The in vivo in-
    activation of GABA and other inhibitory amino acids in the cat
    nervous system, Exp. Brain Res. 25: 413-428.
Curtis, D.R., Game, C.J.A. and Lodge, D., 1976b, Benzodiazepines and
    central glycine receptors, Br. J. Pharmac. 56: 307-311.
Curtis, D.R., Game, C.J.A., Lodge, D. and McCulloch, R.M., 1976c,
    A pharmacological study of Renshaw cell inhibition, J. Physiol.
    258: 227-242.
Daly, E.C. and Aprison, M.H., 1974a, Distribution of serine trans-
    hydroxymethylase and glycine transaminase in several areas of
    the central nervous system of the rat, J. Neurochem. 22: 877-
    885.
Daly, E.C. and Aprison, M.H., 1974b, Serine hydroxymethyltransferase,
    glycine transaminase, and the glycine cleavage system in the
    CNS of the rat, Trans. Am. Soc. Neurochem. 5: 131.
Daly, E.C., Nadi, N.S. and Aprison, M.H., 1976, Regional distribution
    and properties of the glycine cleavage system within the cen-
    tral nervous system of the rat: evidence for an endogenous in-
    hibitor during in vitro assay, J. Neurochem. 26: 179-185.
Davidoff, R.A., Shank, R.P., Graham, L.T., Jr., Aprison, M.H. and
    Werman, R., 1967a, Association of glycine with spinal inter-
    neurons, Nature (London) 214: 680-681.

Davidoff, R.A., Graham, L.T., Jr., Shank, R.P., Werman, R. and Aprison, M.H., 1967b, Changes in amino acid concentrations associated with loss of spinal interneurons, J. Neurochem. 14: 1025-1031.

Davidoff, R.A., Aprison, M.H. and Werman, R., 1969, The effects of strychnine on the inhibition of interneurons by glycine and γ-aminobutyric acid, Int. J. Neuropharmacol. 8: 191-194.

Davis, R. and Huffmann, R.D., 1969, Pharmacology of the brachium conjunctivum-red nucleus synaptic system in the baboon, Fed. Proc. Fed. Am. Soc. Exp. Biol. 28: 775.

DeBelleroche, J.S. and Bradford, H.F., 1973, Amino acids in synaptic vesicles from mammalian cerebral cortex: a reappraisal, J. Neurochem. 21: 441-451.

DeGroat, W.C., 1970, The effects of glycine, GABA and strychnine on sacral parasympathetic preganglionic neurones, Brain Res. 18: 542-544.

DeMarchi, W.J. and Johnston, G.A.R., 1969, The oxidation of glycine by D-amino acid oxidase in extracts of mammalian central nervous tissue, J. Neurochem. 16: 335-361.

Denavit-Saubie, M. and Champagnat, J., 1975, The effect of some depressing amino acids on bulbar respiratory and non-respiratory neurons, Brain Res. 97: 356-361.

Dennison, M.E., Jordan, C.C. and Webster, R.A., 1976, Distribution and localization of tritiated amino acids by autoradiography in the cat spinal cord in vivo, J. Physiol. (London)258: 55-56P.

Dickinson, J.C. and Hamilton, P.B., 1966, The free amino acids of human spinal fluid determined by ion exchange chromatography, J. Neurochem. 13: 1179-1187.

Dimpfel, W. and E. Habermann, 1973, Histoautoradiographic localization of $^{125}$I-labeled tetanus toxin in rat spinal cord, Naunyn-Schniedeberg's Arch. Pharmacol. 280: 177-182.

Eccles, J.C., 1964, "The physiology of synapses." Springer-Verlag, Berlin.

Fedineč, A.A. and Shank, R.P., 1971, Effect of tetanus toxin on the content of glycine, gamma-aminobutyric acid, glutamate, glutamine, and aspartic acid in the rat spinal cord, J. Neurochem. 18: 2229-2234.

Gaitonde, M.K., Fayein, N.A., and Johnson, A.L., 1975, Decreased metabolism in vivo of glucose into amino acids of the brain of thiamine-deficient rats after treatment with pyrithiamine, J. Neurochem. 24: 1215-1223.

Galindo, A., 1969, GABA-picrotoxin interaction in the mammalian central nervous system, Brain Res. 14: 763-767.

Galindo, A., Krnjević, K. and Schwartz, S., 1967, Micro-iontophoretic studies on neurones in the cuneate nucleus, J. Physiol. (London) 192: 359-377.

Galindo, A., Krnjević, K. and Schwartz, S., 1968, Patterns of firing
    in cuneate neurones and some effects of Flaxedil, Expt. Brain
    Res. 5: 87-101.
Gerritsen, T., Nyhan, W.L., Rehberg, M.L. and Ando, T., 1969, Meta-
    bolism of glyoxylate in nonketotic hyperglycinemia, Pediat.
    Res. 3: 269-274.
Graham, L.T., Jr. and Aprison, M.H., 1966, Fluorometric determination
    of aspartate, glutamate and γ-aminobutyrate in nerve tissue
    by using enzymic methods, Anal. Biochem. 15: 487-497.
Graham, L.T., Jr., Shank, R.P., Werman, R. and Aprison, M.H., 1967,
    Distribution of some synaptic transmitter candidates in cat
    spinal cord: glutamic acid, aspartic acid, γ-aminobutyric acid,
    glycine and glutamine, J. Neurochem. 14: 465-472.
Greene, M.L., Lietman, P.S., Rosenberg, L.E. and Seegmiller, J.E.,
    1973, Familial hyperglycinemia: new defect in renal tubular
    transport of glycine and amino acids, Am. J. Med. 54: 265-271.
Gregson, N.A. and Williams, P.L., 1969, A comparative study of brain
    and liver mitochondria from newborn and adult rats, J. Neuro-
    chem. 16: 617-626.
Guertzenstein, P.G. and Silver, A., 1974, Fall in blood presssure
    produced from discrete regions of the ventral surface of the
    medulla by glycine and lesions, J. Physiol. (London) 242: 489-
    503.
Gushchin, S., Kozhechkin, S.N. and Sverdlov, Y. S., 1969, Pre-
    synaptic nature of depression by tetanus toxin of postsynaptic
    inhibition, Doklady Akademii Nauk.(USSR) 187: 685-688.
Habermann, E. and Wellhomer, H.H., 1974, Advances in tetanus re-
    search, Klin. Wschr. 52: 255-265.
Hall, P.V., Smith, J.E., Campbell, R.L., Felten, D.L. and Aprison,
    M.H., 1976, Neurochemical correlates of spasticity, Life Sci.
    18: 1467-1472.
Hill, R.G. and Taberner, P.V., 1976, Some neuropharmacological pro-
    perties of the new non-barbiturate hypnotic etomidate (R(+)-
    ethyl-1-(α-methyl-benzyl) imidazole-5-carboxylate), Brit. J.
    Pharmac. 54: 241P.
Hill, R.G., Simmonds, M.A. and Straughan, D.W., 1973, Amino acid
    antagonists and the depression of cuneate neurones by γ-amino-
    butyric acid (GABA) and glycine, Brit. J. Pharmac. 47: 642-
    643P.
Hill, R.G., Simmonds, M.A. and Straughan, D.W., 1976, Antagonism of
    γ-aminobutyric acid and glycine by convulsants in the cuneate
    nucleus of cat, Br. J. Pharmac. 56: 9-19.
Hökfelt, T. and Ljungdahl, A., 1971, Light and electron microscopic
    autoradiography on spinal cord slices after incubation with
    labelled glycine, Brain Res. 32: 189-194.
Hösli, L. and Tebēcis, A.K., 1970, Actions of amino acids and con-
    vulsants on bulbar reticular neurones, Exp. Brain Res. 11:
    111-127.

Hösli, L., Andres, P.F. and Hösli, F., 1971, Effects of glycine on spinal neurones grown in tissue culture, Brain Res. 34: 399-402.

Humoller, F.L., Mahler, D.J. and Parker, M.M., 1966, Distribution of amino acids between plasma and spinal fluid, Int. J. Neuropsychiatry 2: 293-297.

Johnston, G.A.R., 1968, The intraspinal distribution of some depressant amino acids, J. Neurochem. 15: 1013-1017.

Johnston, G.A.R. and Iversen, L.L., 1971, Glycine uptake in the central nervous system slices and homogenates: evidence for different uptake mechanisms in spinal cord and cerebral cortex, J. Neurochem. 18: 1951-1961.

Johnston, G.A.R. and Vitali, M.V., 1969a, Glycine producing transaminase activity in extracts of spinal cord, Brain Res. 15: 471-472.

Johnston, G.A.R. and Vitali, M.V., 1969b, Glycine-2-oxoglutarate transaminase in rat cerebral cortex, Brain Res. 15: 201-208.

Johnston, G.A.R., DeGroat, W.C. and Curtis, D.R., 1969, Tetanus toxin and amino acid levels in cat spinal cord, J. Neurochem. 16: 797-800.

Jordan, C.C. and Webster, R.A., 1971, Release of acetylcholine and $^{14}$C-glycine from the cat spinal cord in vivo, Brit. J. Pharmacol. 43: 441P.

Kawamura, H. and Provini, L., 1970, Depression of cerebellar Purkinje cells by microiontophoretic application of GABA and related amino acids, Brain Res. 24: 293-304.

Kelly, J.S. and Krnjević, K., 1969, The action of glycine on cortical neurones, Exp. Brain Res. 9: 155-163.

Kelly, J.S. and Renaud, L.P., 1971, Postsynaptic inhibition in the cuneate blocked by GABA antagonists, Nature New Biol. 232: 25-26.

Kelly, J.S. and Renaud, L.P., 1973, On the pharmacology of the glycine receptors on the cuneothalamic relay cells of the cat, Brit. J. Pharmac. 48: 387-395.

Kikuchi, G., 1973, The glycine cleavage system: composition reaction mechanism and physiological significance, Mol. Cell Biol. 1: 169-187.

Krieger, I. and Hart, Z.H., 1974, Valine sensitive nonketotic hyperglycinemia, J. Pediat. 85: 43-48.

Krnjević, K. and Phillis, J.W., 1963, Iontophoretic studies of neurones in the mammalian cerebral cortex, J. Physiol. (London) 165: 274-304.

Krnjević, K., Randic, M. and Straughan, D.W., 1966, Pharmacology of cortical inhibition, J. Physiol. (London) 184: 78-105.

Lajtha, A. and Toth, J., 1963, The brain barrier system V: stereospecificity of amino acid uptake, exchange and efflux, J. Neurochem. 10: 909-920.

cinamie: klinik, diatetik, und pathologisch-anatomische veran-
derungen, Z. Kinderheilk., 116:95-114.

Liang, C.C., 1962, Studies on experimental thiamine deficiency.
Trends of keto acid formation and detection of glyoxylic acid,
Biochem. J., 82:429.

Ljungdahl, A. and Hökfelt, T.. 1973, Autoradiographic uptake patterns of ($^3$H) GABA and ($^3$H) glycine in central nervous tissues
with special reference to the cat spinal cord, Brain Res.,
62:587-590.

Logan, W.J. and Snyder, S.H., 1972, High affinity uptake systems
for glycine, glutamic and aspartic acids in synaptosomes of
rat central nervous tissues, Brain Res., 42:413-431.

Matus, I.I. and Dennison, M.E., 1972, An autoradiographic study of
uptake of exogenous glycine by vertebrate spinal cord slices
in vitro, J. Neurocytology, 1:27-34.

McBride, W.J., Daly, E. and Aprison, M.H., 1973, Interconversion of
glycine and serine in a synaptosome fraction isolated from the
spinal cord, medulla oblongata, telencephalon, and cerebellum
of the rat, J. Neurobiol., 4:557-566.

McLaughlin, B.J., Barber, R., Saito, K., Roberts, E. and Yu, J.Y.,
1975, Immunocytochemical localization of glutamate decarboxylase in rat spinal cord, J. Comp. Neurol., 164:305-321.

Motokawa, Y. and Kikuchi. G., 1971, Glycine metabolism in rat liver
mitochondria:  V. Intramitochondrial localization of the reversible glycine cleavage system and serine hydroxymethyltransferase, Arch. Biochem. Biophys., 146:461-466.

Mulder, A.H. and Snyder, S.H., 1974, Potassium induced release of
amino acids from cerebral cortex and spinal cord slices of
the rat, Brain Res., 76:297-308.

Neal, M.J., 1971, The uptake of ($^{14}$C) glycine by slices of mammalian
spinal cord, J. Physiol. (London), 215:103-117.

Neal, M.J. and Pickles, H., 1969, Uptake of ($^{14}$C) glycine by spinal
cord, Nature (London), 223:679.

Oppenheim, R.W. and Reitzel, J., 1975, Ontogeny of behavioral sensitivity to strychnine in the chick embryo: evidence for the
early onset of CNS inhibition, Brain Behav. Evol., 11:130-159.

Osborne, R.H., Bradford, H.F. and Jones, D.G., 1973, Patterns of
amino acid release from nerve endings isolated from spinal
cord and medulla, J. Neurochem., 21:407-419.

Paulsen, E.P. and Hsia, Y.E., 1974, Asymptomatic propionicacidemia:
variability of clinical expression in a Mennonite kindred,
Am. J. Hum. Genet., 26:66a.

Perry, T.L., Urquhart, N., MacLean, J., Evans, M.E., Hansen, S.,
Davidson, G.F., Applegarth, D.A., MacLeod, P.J. and Lock, J.E.,
1975a, Nonketotic hyperglycinemia: glycine accumulation due to
absence of glycine cleavage in the brain, New Engl. J. Med.,
292:1269-1273.

Perry, T.L., Urguhart, N., MacLean, J. and Hansen, S., 1975b, Response to a letter to the editor, New Engl. J. Med., 293:778.

Price, D.L., Griffin, J., Young, A., Peck, K. and Stocks, A., 1975, Tetanus toxin: direct evidence for retrograde intraaxonal transport, Sci., 188:945-947.

Price, D.L., Stocks, A., Griffin, J.W., Young, A. and Peck, K., 1976, Glycine specific synapses in rat spinal cord: identification by electron microscope autoradiography, J. Cell Biol., 68:389-395.

Price, D.L., Griffin, J.W. and Peck, K., 1977, Tetanus toxin: evidence for binding at presynaptic nerve endings, Brain Res., 121:379-384.

Rassin, D.K. and Gaull, G.E., 1975, Transmethylation and transsulfuration enzymes in rat brain: their subcellular distriution, Trans. Am. Soc. Neurochem., 6:134.

Reubi, J.C. and Cuenod, M., 1976, Release of exogenous glycine in the pigeon optic tectum during stimulation of a midbrain nucleus, Brain Res., 112:347-361.

Roberts, P.J., 1974, The release of amino acids with proposed neurotransmitter function from the cuneate and gracile nuclei of the rat in vivo, Brain Res., 67:419-428.

Roberts, P.J. and Mitchell, J.F., 1972, The release of amino acids from the hemisected spinal cord during stimulation, J. Neurochem., 19:2473-2481.

Romano, M. and Cerra, M., 1967, Further studies on the toxicity of glyoxylate in the rat, Gazz. Biochem., 16:354-358.

Sato, T., Kochi, H., Sato, N. and Kikuchi, G., 1969, Glycine metabolism by rat liver mitochondria, J. Biochem., 65:77-83.

Scriver, C.R., White, A., Sprague, W. and Horwood, S.P., 1975, Plasma-CSF glycine ratio in normal and nonketotic hyperglycinemic subjects, New Engl. J. Med., 293:778.

Shank, R.P. and Aprison, M.H., 1970a, The metabolism of glycine and serine in eight different areal of the rat central nervous system, J.Neurochem., 17:1461-1475.

Shank, R.P. and Aprison, M.H., 1970b, Method for multiple analyses of concentration and specific radioactivity of indivudual amino acids in nervous tissue extracts, Anal. Biochem., 35:136-145.

Shank, R.P., Aprison, M.H. and Baxter, C.F., 1973, Precursors of glycine in the central nervous system: comparison of specific activities in glycine and other amino acids after administration of (U-$^{14}$C) glucose, (3,4$^{14}$C) glycose, (1-$^{14}$C) glycose, (U-$^{14}$C) serine or (1,5$^{14}$C) citrate to the rat, Brain Res., 52:301-308.

Smith, J.E., Hall, P.V., Campbell, R.L., Jones, A.R. and Aprison, M.H., 1976, Level of gamma-aminobutyric acid in the dorsal grey lumbar spinal cord during the development of spinal spasticity, Life Sci., 19:1525-1530.

Stern, P. and Catović, S., 1975, Brain glycine and aggressive behavior, Pharmacol. Biochem. Beh. 3:723-726.

Stokes, B.T. and Bignall, K.E., 1974, The emergence of inhibition in the chick embryo spinal cord, Brain Res., 77:231-242.

Sverdlov, Y.S., Alekseeva, V.I., 1966, Effect of tetanus toxin on presynaptic inhibition in the spinal cord, Fed. Proc. Fed. Am. Soc. Exp. Biol., 25:931-935.

Tada, K., Corbeel, L.M., Eeckels, R., and Eggermont, E., 1974, A block in glycine cleavage reaction as a common mechanism in ketotic and nonketotic hyperglycinemia, Pediat. Res., 8:721-723.

Takano, K. and Neumann, K., 1972, Effect of glycine upon stretch reflex tension, Brain Res., 36:474-475.

Tarlov, I.M., 1967, Rigidity in man due to spinal interneuron loss, Arch. Neurol., 16:537-543.

Tarlov, I.M., 1974, Rigidity and primary motoneuron damage in tetanus, Exp. Neurol., 44:246-254.

Tarlov, I.M., Ling, H. and Yamada, H., 1973, Neuronal pathology in experimental local tetanus, clinical implications, Neurol. (Minneapolis), 23:580-591.

Tebécis, A.K. and DiMaria, A., 1972, Strychnine-sensitive inhibition in the medullary reticular formation: evidence for glycine as an inhibitory transmitter, Brain Res., 40:373-383.

Tebécis, A.K., Hösli, L. and Haas, H., 1971, Bicuculline and the depression of medullary reticular neurones by GABA and glycine, Experientia (Basel), 27:548.

Trijbels, J.M.F., Monnens, L.A.H., van der Zee, S.P.M., Vrenken, J.A.Th, Sengers, R.C.A. and Schretlen, E.D.A.M., 1974, A patient with nonketotic hyperglycinemia biochemical findings and therapeutic approaches, Pediat. Res., 8:598-605.

Tsukada, Y., Nagata, Y., Hirano, S. and Matsutani, T., 1963, Active transport of amino acid into cerebral cortex slices, J. Neurochem., 10:241.

Uchizono, K., 1965, Characteristics of excitatory and inhibitory synapses in the central nervous system of the cat, Nature (London), 207:642-643.

Uhr, M.L., 1973, Glycine decarboxylation in the central nervous system, J. Neurochem., 20:1005-1009.

Voaden, M.J., 1974, Light and spontaneous efflux of radioactive glycine from the frog retina, Exp. Eye Res., 18:467-475.

Yoshida, T. and Kikuchi, G., 1973, Major pathways of serine and glycine catabolism in various organs of the rat and cock, J. Biochem., 73:1013-1022.

Young, A.B. and Snyder, S.H., 1973, Strychnine binding associated with glycine receptors of the central nervous system, Proc. natn. Acad. Sci. U.S.A., 70:2832-2836.

Young, A.B. and Snyder, S.H., 1974a, Strychnine binding in rat spinal cord membranes associated with the synaptic glycine receptor: cooperativity of glycine interactions, Molec. Pharmac., 10:790-809.

Young, A.B. and Snyder. S.H., 1974b, The glycine synaptic receptor-evidence that strychnine binding is associated with the ionic conductance mechanism, Proc. natn. Acad. Sci. U.S.A., 71: 4002-4005.

Young, A.B., Zukin, S.R. and Snyder, S.H., 1974, Interaction of
    benzodiazepines with central nervous glycine receptors: pos-
    sible mechanism of action, Proc. natn. Acad. Sci. U.S.A.,
    71:2246-2250.
Werman, R., 1965, The specificity of molecular processes involved
    in neuronal transmission, J. Theoret. Biol., 9:471-477.
Werman, R. and Aprison, M.H., 1968, Glycine: the search for a spinal
    cord inhibitory transmitter, in "Structure and Functions of
    Inhibitory Neuronal Mechanisms" (C. von Euler, S. Skoglund and
    U. Soderberg, eds.) pp. 473-486, Pergamon Press, New York.
Werman, R., Davidoff, R.A. and Aprison, M.H., 1966, Glycine and
    postsynaptic inhibition in cat spinal cord, Physiologist,
    9:318.
Werman, R., Davidoff, R.A. and Aprison, M.H., 1967, Inhibition of
    motoneurones by iontophoresis of glycine, Nature (London),
    214:681-683.
Werman, R., Davidoff, R.A. and Aprison, M.H., 1968, Inhibitory
    action of glycine on spinal neurons in the cat, J. Neuro-
    physiol., 31:81-95.
Zukin, S.R., Young, A.B. and Snyder, S.H., 1975, Development of the
    synaptic glycine receptor in the chick embryo spinal cord,
    Brain Res., 83:525-530.

TAURINE AND OTHER SULFUR CONTAINING AMINO ACIDS:    THEIR FUNCTION IN

THE CENTRAL NERVOUS SYSTEM

D. K. Rassin and G. E. Gaull

Department of Human Development and Genetics
New York State Institute for Basic Research in Mental
Retardation, Staten Island, New York 10314
and
Departments of Pediatrics and Pharmacology
Mount Sinai School of Medicine of the City University
of New York, New York, New York 10029

Taurine and some of its metabolic precursors - cystathionine,
cysteine, cysteinesulfinic acid, cysteic acid and hypotaurine - have
been shown to have either biochemical, electrophysiological or behavioral properties that suggest that these compounds may function
as neurotransmitters or modulators of synaptic function in the central nervous system.    Recent interest has focused upon the functions
of taurine because of possible association with epilepsy, with cardiac function, and with retinal function.    In addition, in patients
with homocystinuria due to cystathionine synthase deficiency, the
inability to synthesize cystathionine has been related to brain
dysfunction.    These sulfur containing amino acids are the products
of a metabolic pathway of which methionine is the original precursor
(Figure 1).    This metabolic pathway also is involved with methylation
functions and folate.    This review is an attempt to correlate recent
information concerning the function of the sulfur-containing amino
acids in the central nervous system with particular emphasis upon the
possible roles of taurine.

The transmission of nervous impulses across the synaptic cleft
at neuronal junctions in the central nervous system is probably
accomplished by the release of one of a number of naturally occurring
compounds from the presynaptic portion of the synapse, followed by
interaction with receptors at the postsynaptic membrane.    The sulfur-
containing amino acids contain many of the structural characteristics
ascribed to amino acid neurotransmitters and may be defined as

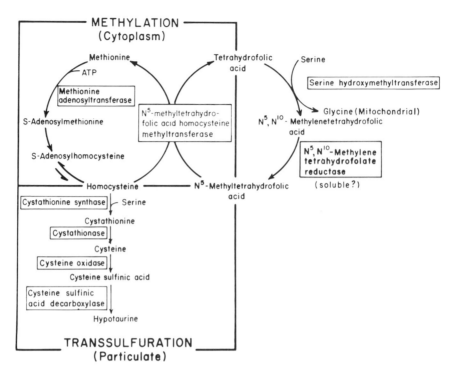

FIGURE 1.  The pathway of metabolism of methionine illustrating the
compartmentation of the enzymes.  Taurine is an oxidation product of
hypotaurine, the mechanism of this oxidation has not been fully
characterized.


neurotransmitters if they satisfy the following criteria:  presence,
collectability, identity of action and mechanism of inactivation
(Werman, 1966; Dudel, 1968; Phillis, 1970).

     We have attempted to establish an overall biochemical relation-
ship between the enzymes of the sulfur amino acid pathway and the
subcellular organelles of the brain as an indication of a possible
functional relationship.  A pattern of subcellular localization of
the enzymes in brain involved in the metabolism of methionine to
taurine exists which is compatible with compartmentation of the
methylation functions (soluble) and neurotransmitter functions
(synaptosomal) of the sulfur containing amino acids (Figure 1)
(Rassin and Gaull, 1975).  The enzymes methionine adenosyltransferase
and N5-methyltetrahydrofolate-homocysteine methyltransferase were
found in the soluble pool of rat brain; cystathionine synthase,
cysteine dioxygenase and cysteinesulfinic acid decarboxylase were

located in the synaptosomal pool; serine hydroxymethyltransferase
was associated with the mitochondria; and cystathionase was associated with a general particulate fraction of the brain which could
not be more closely defined because of the low amount of activity of
this enzyme in the brain (Rassin and Gaull, 1975). These findings
either agree with those of previous investigators, or have been confirmed by later investigators, who have examined, in most instances,
only one enzymatic step in the pathway.

Cystathionine β-synthase has been associated with a mitochondrial fraction (Kashiwamata 1971a, 1971b), although it has been
stated that this enzyme is found entirely in the soluble fraction
after brain homogenization and centrifugation (Volpe and Laster,
1972). Cysteine dioxygenase was found by some investigators to be
associated with microsomal particles (Misra and Olney, 1975) but
reexamination by these workers (Misra et al., 1977) and others
(Pasantes-Morales et al., 1977; Byrne and Salganicoff, 1977) has
confirmed the synaptosomal localization of this enzyme demonstrated
earlier (Rassin and Gaull, 1975). Cysteinesulfinic acid decarboxylase has been found to be occuluded within synaptosomal particles
(Agrawal et al., 1971; Pasantes-Morales et al., 1976). Serine
hydroxymethyltransferase has been associated with mitochondrial and
cytoplasmic fractions of the central nervous system (Davies and
Johnston, 1973; Daly and Aprison, 1974; Burton and Sallach, 1975).
Methyltetrahydrofolate-homocysteine methyltransferase has been found
to be associated with the soluble fraction of rat brain (Burton and
Sallach, 1975), and, as would be expected if our hypothesis concerning the soluble nature of the methylation cycle was correct (Rassin
and Gaull, 1975), methylenetetrahydrofolate reductase is localized
in the soluble fraction of rat brain (Burton and Sallach, 1975).
So, in general, there is good agreement between these individual
assessments of enzyme localization and our own overall study of the
enzymes of sulfur amino acid metabolism.

Present evidence does not support the hypothesis that storage
of the amino acids in synaptic vesicles may account for the separation of the neurotransmitter pool of these compounds in a manner
analogous to that of acetylcholine (Neal and Iversen, 1969; Rassin,
1972; DeBelleroche and Bradford, 1973). Although taurine (De-
Belleroche and Bradford, 1973; Rassin et al., 1977e) and glutamate
(DeBelleroche and Bradford, 1973) may be exceptions since very small
amounts of these compounds have been found to be bound to synaptic
vesicles isolated from rat brain. Thus, compartmentation of the
enzymes may help to explain how the putative neurotransmitter sulfur
containing amino acids are separated from the general metabolic pool
of amino acids so that they can function at the synapse. These
biochemical and morphological relationships provide a basis for
discussing the functional properties of the various precursors and
products of the sulfur amino acid metabolic pathway.

## THE FUNCTION OF TAURINE IN THE CENTRAL NERVOUS SYSTEM

Taurine, the decarboxylation product of cysteinesulfinic acid via hypotaurine or by direct decarboxylation of cysteic acid, has been associated with a variety of physiological functions (Jacobsen and Smith, 1968; Barbeau et al., 1976; Huxtable and Barbeau, 1976). It has been suggested as a transmitter, since it satisfies the criteria of presence, collectibility, inactivation and pharmacologic identity (Davison and Kaczmarek, 1971; Oja and Lahdesmaki, 1974; Mandel and Pasantes-Morales, 1976). Both the compound and its synthesizing enzyme have been identified in nerve ending particles (Agrawal et al., 1971; Rassin and Gaull, 1975; Rassin et al., 1977e). Uptake mechanisms capable of inactivating taurine have been described (Davison and Kaczmarek, 1971; Kaczmarek and Davison, 1972) and are necessary because of the slow catabolism of taurine to isethionic acid (Peck and Awapara, 1967). In fact, taurine may not be metabolized to isethionic acid (Applegarth et al., 1976; Fellman et al., 1977; Hoskin and Kordik, 1977). Release of taurine after electrical stimulation in a manner analogous to presynaptic excitation has been observed (Hammerstad et al., 1971; Davison and Kaczmarek, 1971; Kaczmarek and Davison, 1972). An unexplained, electrically-stimulated influx of taurine in brain slices has been observed (Lahdesmaki and Oja, 1972). Also, electrical stimulation apparently increases the rate at which taurine is synthesized by the decarboxylation of cysteinesulfinic acid (Oja et al., 1973).

Taurine reuptake and metabolism in the central nervous system may be regulated by mechanisms in the glial cells rather than in the neuronal cells. Taurine has been shown to have special transport systems in glial cells (Henn, 1976a; Borg et al., 1976). The uptake of taurine, and other putative amino acid transmitters, has been described in cultured glial cells (Schrier and Thompson, 1974). Indeed, glial cells may be important in the regulation of the availability of neurotransmitters at the synapse (Henn, 1976b).

The depressant actions of taurine on spinal neurones, brain stem neurones, and cortical neurones have been observed, and pharmacological interactions with strychnine and bicuculline have been examined in order to find a specific antagonist. In brain stem neurones, strychnine blocks the depressant effect of taurine and of glycine but not of GABA (Haas and Hosli, 1973; Hosli et al., 1973). The antagonism of glycine by strychnine in spinal neurones, while the action of GABA continues unaffected, has led to the classification of those inhibitory neurotransmitters as "glycine-like" or "GABA-like" (Curtis et al., 1967). The failure of bicuculline to antagonize taurine, while it antagonizes GABA, and the antagonistic effect of strychnine on glycine and on taurine but not on GABA in the brain stem neurones has led to classification of taurine as a "glycine-like" amino acid (Haas and Hosli, 1973). In addition, taurine produces a depressant effect on the direct cortical response that is identical to that of GABA (Kaczmarek and Adey, 1975). These pharmacological interactions are positive evidence for specific taurine post-synaptic receptor sites and favor a role as a possible neurotransmitter.

The considerable evidence for the function of taurine as a neurotransmitter in the retina has recently been reviewed (Mandel et al., 1976). Taurine is found in particularly high concentrations in the retina (Pasantes-Morales et al., 1972a), in which it appears to be localized within the photoreceptor cells (Cohen et al., 1973; Kennedy and Voaden, 1974). Although all the layers contain considerable amounts of taurine, in a study of five different species, the greatest amount consistently has been found in the outer nuclear layer (Orr et al., 1976b). Taurine has been implicated in retinal function because of its depressant activity there (Pasantes-Morales et al., 1972b). Also, light-stimulation was found to cause release of taurine from the retina of dark-adapted chickens (Pasantes-Morales et al., 1973). Studies of taurine transport and metabolism in rat retina failed to reveal a mechanism which was sufficiently finely-tuned to explain how taurine could be inactivated after release (Starr and Voaden, 1972), although specific transport systems appear to exist for taurine and for GABA (Starr, 1973; Kennedy and Voaden, 1976). It has been suggested that although taurine may not be a transmitter in the retina, it is quite possible that taurine may be a modulator of synaptic function in this neural tissue (Starr and Voaden, 1972).

Low concentrations of taurine have been observed in rats with retinitis pigmentosa (Brotherton, 1962). The retinas of dystrophic mice fail to develop increasing taurine concentrations in the same way that normal mice do (Orr et al., 1976a).

Further evidence for the importance of taurine in the retina is the degeneration of the retinal photoreceptor cells in cats fed a diet of purified casein which lacks taurine (Hayes et al., 1975a, b; Schmidt et al., 1976; Berson et al., 1976). Progressive retinal degeneration which eventually results in blindness occurs, which can be prevented or reversed by feeding supplemental taurine, but not by feeding methionine, cysteine or inorganic sulfate (Hayes et al., 1975a,b; Schmidt et al., 1975, 1977; Berson et al., 1976; Knopf et al., 1977). The cat converts only a limited amount of cysteine to taurine, apparently because the enzyme which synthesizes it, cysteinesulfinic acid decarboxylase, is limiting (Gaull et al., 1977; Knopf et al., 1977; Hardison et al., 1977).

The dietary restriction of taurine in the cat produces large decreases in the taurine concentration of various tissues of the cat (Rabin et al., 1976; Knopf et al., 1977; Sturman et al., 1977e).

Bile and retina, however, conserve taurine in the face of the general depletion observed in other organs and body fluids of the taurine deficient cat (Sturman et al., 1977e). These two instances of relative conservation occur in areas which are dependent upon adequate taurine for proper function, the bile for bile salt conjugation and the retina to maintain its structure. Unlike these instances of taurine conservation in anatomical regions where taurine is important to function, taurine does not appear to be especially conserved by the synaptosomes isolated from occipital lobe of this taurine-deficient kitten (Rassin et al., 1977f). It is interesting to note that the only other tissue that conserves taurine in the manner is the olfactory bulb (Sturman et al., 1977e). Although no relationship of taurine to olfaction has been described as yet, there is a report of a high taurine concentration in the olfactory bulb of mice (Margolis, 1974; Neidle and Kandera, 1974), and it is possible that taurine is axonally transported from the nasal epithelium to the olfactory bulb (Margolis, F.L., personal communication). Taurine is transported down the axon of the goldfish optic tract unlike any other amino acids, including gamma-aminobutyric acid and the taurine precursors (Ingoglia et al., 1976). In addition, taurine has been associated with the molecular layer of the cerebellum suggesting it may be the neurotransmitter in the stellate cells in this layer (McBride et al., 1977).

Study of the amino acid content in brain tissue from patients undergoing neurosurgery for the treatment of focal epilepsy has revealed that cortex from the region of the epileptic focus compared with directly adjacent cortex has low concentrations of taurine and glutamic acid and a high concentration of glycine, accompanied by a decrease in cortical concentrations of GABA and aspartic acid (Van Gelder et al., 1972). These differences could not be detected, however, when brain tissue from patients with epilepsy was contrasted to that acquired from other sources (Perry et al., 1975b). Decreased taurine concentrations have been found in the focal region of cats made epileptic by application of cobalt and penicillin to the cortex (Van Gelder and Courtois, 1972; Mutani et al., 1977). Taurine treatment of cats and mice made epileptic by topical application of cobalt reduced the seizure activity and also restored the concentrations of the affected amino acids to normal (Van Gelder, 1972). Intraventricular ouabain injections have been used as a model of epilepsy in animals, and the resultant seizures may be decreased more efficiently by taurine than by GABA (Izumi et al., 1973). Also, taurine may have a protective effect against photically stimulated seizures in the "photo-sensitive" baboon (Derouaux et al., 1973), but not in other species (Wada et al., 1975). It has been suggested that taurine may function to stabilize excitable membranes in the CNS, and it is this action that gives it anticonvulsant properties rather than any action as a neurotransmitter (Barbeau and Donaldson, 1974).

Taurine has been reported to have an anti-convulsant effect in man (Barbeau and Donaldson, 1973, 1974) and to be increased in concentration in plasma from patients with epilepsy (Monaco et al., 1975; Van Gelder et al., 1975; Mutani et al., 1975). Intravenously administered taurine has been reported to be efficacious in treating patients with highly refractory epilepsy (Bergamini et al., 1974). Low doses are said to work better than high doses and the schedule of administration is thought to be crucial (Van Gelder et al., 1975).

Taurine has been associated with other diseases that involve brain dysfunction. Decreased taurine excretion has been reported in patients with mongolism (Goodman et al., 1964) although this may be due to a vitamin $B_6$ deficiency (Barbeau et al., 1975). An association of taurinuria in patients with camptodactyly and mental deficiency has been reported (Nevin et al., 1965). The content of taurine was reduced in most regions of brain in a patient with an inherited form of mental depression and characteristics of Parkinsonism (Perry et al., 1975a). Two patients who died with an inherited olivopontocerebellar atrophy were found to have increased taurine concentrations in the cerebellar cortex and dentate nucleus (Perry et al., 1977).

Intracisternal injections of taurine in the rat have been found to cause slow recovery of the righting reflex, a drop and slow recovery of colonic temperature, and a fall in arterial blood pressure. These effects were similar to but more dramatic than those of the inhibitory transmitters GABA and glycine when they were administered in the same way (Sgaragli and Pavan, 1972). Inhibition of the hypothermic effect of taurine by p-chlorophenylalanine and the failure of taurine to modify the thermal response of rats to α-methyltyrosine has suggested to these authors that taurine responses may be mediated by a serotonergic mechanism (Sgaragli et al., 1975). Taurine administration during development can weakly influence adult inhibitory behavior (Persinger et al., 1976a). This influence is best expressed during periods of adjustment but does not influence well-learned or well-established responses (Persinger et al., 1976b). Rats injected, between 4 and 20 days, with 62.5 or 125 µg taurine per gm body weight on every other day subsequently ran less in a spinning wheel test and had lower response/reinforcement ratios than did saline injected controls (Persinger et al., 1976a). Intraventricular and intraperitoneal administration of taurine depress psychomotor activity in rats (Baskin et al., 1974).

Taurine and its metabolite isethionic acid have been shown to influence the excitable tissue of the heart, through direct and indirect effects upon calcium and potassium flux during arrhythmias associated with large doses of cardiac glycosides (Read and Welty, 1963, 1965; Welty and Read, 1964). Taurine has been shown to potentiate the positive inotropic effect of strophanthin-K on

guinea-pig auricles (Guidotti et al., 1971) and to exert negative
inotropic effects in rat heart and positive inotropic effects in
guinea-pig heart similar to those of ouabain (Dietrich and Diacono,
1971). A number of relationships have been observed between heart
function or pathology and taurine but no true cause and effect relationships have been defined as yet (Grosso and Bressler, 1976).
The function of taurine in muscle may be as a membrane stabilizer
rather than as a transmitter (Huxtable and Bressler, 1973) a
mechanism that has also been suggested for the brain (Barbeau and
Donaldson, 1974). Failure of this mechanism in muscle may be a
part of the biochemical basis of muscular dystrophy (Banks et al.,
1971; Baskin and Dagirmanjian, 1973).

We have been particularly interested in the special pattern of
taurine concentration in brain during development and have reviewed
this relationship recently (Sturman et al., 1977c,d). In brief,
taurine is present in high concentrations during development, at
which time it is generally the free amino acid present in the
greatest concentration. The decrease in concentration in brain
from birth to maturity is gradual and seems to be complete approximately by weaning (Sturman and Gaull, 1975b). The most well documented instance of this pattern of development is the rat but it is
true for many other species (cf. Sturman et al., 1977c). This pattern of development is common to most species despite a fairly wide
variation in the taurine concentration among species (Sturman et al.,
1977c,d). Taurine is certainly present in greater concentrations in
the brain than putative neurophysiological functions would require,
if our present understanding of such functions is correct.

We have recalculated the decrease in concentration of taurine
during development and found that there is actually an increase in
the taurine pool when it is represented as μmoles/brain rather than
μmoles/gram of brain tissue (Sturman et al., 1977b). Thus, during
early development it appears that taurine is important for some cell
types but not for others. The latter types dilute the overall brain
taurine to cause an apparent decrease in concentration. At the same
time there is a relative enrichment of the taurine stored within
synaptosomes isolated from rat brain (Rassin et al., 1977e) indicating that a possible neurotransmitter pool of taurine is being protected or is developing.

During development a major source of taurine is the milk. This
is true for man (Rassin et al., 1977a; Gaull et al., 1977), the cat
(Rassin et al., 1977d) and a number of other species (Rassin et al.,
1977c,d). Even the rat, which can synthesize more taurine than any
other species studied (Gaull et al., 1977), derives a significant
proportion of its brain taurine from the milk of the mother (Sturman
et al., 1977a). Thus, there is a unique pattern of development of
taurine in the brain of most species and a number of species supply

their young with taurine rich milk during this important period of
brain growth, further suggesting the importance of this compound to
normal brain development.

Speculation concerning the true function or functions of taurine
in brain must rely on the information that we have at hand.  So far
there is a growing volume of information that implies that taurine is
an inhibitory neurotransmitter, however, this evidence is not yet
conclusive.  Taurine appears to be important during development so
it may be required also for some biochemical or structural changes
that occur during early brain growth.  Finally, and based on the
least evidence, it is possible that taurine is important to structures which function via some mechanism of membrane disruption.
High concentrations of taurine have been reported in platelets
(Ahtee et al., 1974); in mast cells (Green et al., 1962); in adrenal
medullary granules, which may be stabilized by taurine (Nakagawa and
Kuriyama, 1975); and some taurine is apparently stored within synaptic vesicles isolated from rat brain (DeBelleroche and Bradford,
1973; Rassin et al., 1977e).  In addition, taurine has been reported
to be related to the assembly mechanism of microtubules isolated
from brain (MacIntosh, R. and Meyers, C., personal communication).
These are all instances in which taurine could play an important role
in the regulation of function by controlling the stability and/or
breakdown of membranes and structures designed to function via such
changes.

## THE METHYLATION CYCLE OF THE SULFUR CONTAINING AMINO ACIDS

Ingestion of large amounts of methionine has been related to
inhibition of growth and to tissue damage in animals (Harper et al.,
1970; Benevenga, 1974).  Methionine has also been shown to have behavioral effects in rats and mice (Taylor, 1976; Beaton et al., 1975).
These effects of methionine may be mediated through the metabolites
S-adenosylmethionine or possibly homocysteine.  S-Adenosylmethionine
(SAM) and N5-methyltetrahydrofolate (MTHF) are both methyl donors.
SAM is of particular importance to the metabolism of the catecholamines and histamine in brain.  Evidence has been presented that MTHF
might be a methyl donor for serotonin, tyramine (Banerjee and
Snyder, 1973) and dopamine (Laduron et al., 1974).  However, the
importance of MTHF to these particular methylation functions has been
questioned as the products involved are not those that are usually
observed in vivo (Meller et al., 1975; Fuller, 1976).  Both SAM and
MTHF are involved in the cycle of demethylation and methylation reactions that takes methionine to homocysteine and homocysteine back
to methionine.

SAM has been shown to be related to L-dihydroxyphenylalanine
(L-DOPA) metabolism.  L-DOPA is methylated to 3-0-methyldihydroxy-
phenylalanine rapidly after intraperitoneal injection in rats, with

an accompanying decrease in brain SAM concentrations (Wurtman et al., 1970). This reduction in rat brain SAM concentration, as well as a reduced concentration of rat blood SAM (Matthysse et al., 1971), has been reported to be accompanied by increased (Liu et al., 1972), unchanged (Ordonez and Wurtman, 1973) or decreased (Cotzias et al., 1971) rat brain methionine concentrations after a single intraperitoneal injection of L-DOPA. Repeated intraperitoneal administration of L-DOPA did cause the methionine concentration in brain to decrease to 69% of control values (Ordonez and Wurtman, 1973). Single intraperitoneal injections of L-DOPA caused significant decreases in brain methionine concentrations in folic acid deficient rats, implying that maintenance of methionine brain concentrations is dependent upon remethylation of homocysteine by the folate cycle (Ordonez and Wurtman, 1974). It is of interest, in this regard, that the activity of methyltetrahydrofolate-homocysteine methyltransferase was found to be high in brain throughout development (Gaull et al., 1973b). Intraperitoneal injections of L-DOPA given every 24 hours for 7 days to rats have been reported to result in increased concentrations of cystathionine in brain and kidney (Brown and DeFoor, 1974). The effectiveness of L-DOPA in treating patients with Parkinson's disease may be decreased by supplementation with methionine but restriction of methionine does not appreciably increase the ability of L-DOPA to ameliorate the symptoms of this disease (Pearce and Waterbury, 1974).

L-DOPA also inhibits the uptake of methionine by synaptosomal particles in vitro (Baldessarini and Karobath, 1972). In the converse situation of high methionine concentrations, dopamine and its metabolites might be affected since methylation reactions may be increased. Worsened behavior has been observed in schizophrenic patients given methionine or cysteine loads with a monoamine oxidase inhibitor (Spaide et al., 1971). L-Methionine has been reported to induce behavioral and sleep-cycle disturbances in rats and mice which could be removed by the simultaneous administration of L-serine, suggesting to these workers that the worsening effect of methionine in szhizophrenia may result from homocysteine formation rather than from formation of methylated derivatives of S-adenosyl-methionine (Beaton et al., 1975). An alternative interpretation of these data is that the serine is used to facilitate the replenishment of SAM as the β-carbon of serine is used for the remethylation of folate to MTHF in brain (see Fig. 1). Cysteine loading together with administration of tranylcypromine caused worsened behavior accompanied by excretion of the psychotomimetic methylated tryptamines (N-dimethyltryptamine, 5-hydroxy-N-dimethyltryptamine and 5-methoxy-N-dimethyltryptamine) (Narasimhachari et al., 1970). The increased excretion of these methylated derivatives may be a reflection of the methionine-sparing effects of cysteine and a favoring of the use of methionine for methylation and protein synthesis as opposed to its metabolism by the transsulfuration pathway to sulfate

(Finkelstein and Mudd, 1967).

S-Adenosylmethionine has been implicated in the mechanism of action of antidepressant drugs such as imipramine (Taylor and Randall, 1975). Imipramine, pargyline, L-DOPA, amphetamine, cyclo-leucine (Taylor and Randall, 1975) and α-methyldopa (Lo et al., 1976) all caused decreased brain S-adenosylmethionine concentrations. The possibility that depressed patients might have too little SAM has been studied also and administration of SAM was associated with some improvement, although in some patients with a severe anxiety state worsening of the symptoms was observed (Agnoli et al., 1976).

Homocysteine and folic acid also have been found to have some CNS effects. Homocysteine given in large concentrations in rats by intraperitoneal injection has been shown to have a convulsant action. These concentrations are admittedly excessive from either a physio-logical or pharmacological viewpoint but other metabolites of the pathway (methionine, cystine, serine, homoserine, cysteine) did not have such an effect in similar doses. The convulsant effect could be eliminated by prior administration of homoserine, serine, betaine, glycine or glucose (Sprince et al., 1969b). Folate and folinate have been shown to facilitate the excitatory effects of glutamate on single neurones of cat cerebral cortex and have weak excitatory effects of their own when applied to quiescent neurones (Davies and Watkins, 1973). Recently a number of neurological syndromes have been rela-ted to folate deficiencies (reviewed by Turner, 1977). The enzyme serine hydroxymethyltransferase, a crucial step in the remethylation of tetrahydrofolic acid, catalyzes the synthesis of glycine, an amino acid for which there is considerable evidence suggesting a neurotransmitter function (Aprison et al., 1968, Werman, 1972). This enzyme appears to be associated with mitochondria perhaps originating from glial cells (Rassin and Gaull, 1975). The locali-zation is compatible with the hypothesis that glial cells function in the regulation of synaptic transmission (Schrier and Thompson, 1974; Henn, 1977b). Serine, a substrate for this enzyme, also func-tions as a cosubstrate in the first step in the transsulfuration pathway from homocysteine to cysteine.

Another group of compounds, the polyamines, are products of the metabolism of S-adenosylmethionine. Two of these compounds, spermi-dine and spermine, have been found to have behavioral effects in the CNS. Intraventricular administration of these polyamines initially caused sedation and hypothermia but after some hours hyperexcit-ability and convulsions were observed (Anderson et al., 1975). These convulsions were sometimes lethal and were associated with severe pyramidal tract lesions. In addition, electroshock induced aggression in mice has been correlated with increased brain sper-mine concentrations but no changes in norepinephrine, dopamine, serotonin or spermidine were observed (Tadano et al., 1974).

Isolation induced aggression in mice was associated with increased spermidine concentrations that were reduced when the isolates were returned to the group (Tadano, 1974). Spermine and spermidine also have a general depressant effect on the spontaneous activity of brain stem neurons in the cat and the rat when applied by microiontophoresis (Wedgewood and Wolstencroft, 1977).

The function of spermidine, other than as some sort of mediator of rapid growth, also may be suggested by the pattern of development of this compound in brain. The concentration of putrescine and the specific activity of ornithine decarboxylase, which catalyzes its synthesis, increase during the middle of gestation at the time of rapid growth in the rhesus monkey (Sturman and Gaull, 1975a). The concentration of spermidine and spermine and the specific activities of the enzymes S-adenosylmethionine decarboxylase and spermidine synthase, however, increase slowly after birth and take several months to reach values observed in the adult (Sturman and Gaull, 1975a). Thus, spermidine apparently is not important just during the prenatal period of rapid brain growth.

## THE FUNCTION OF CYSTATHIONINE, CYSTEINE, CYSTEIC ACID AND CYSTEINE-SULFINIC ACID IN THE CENTRAL NERVOUS SYSTEM

The remaining sulfur-containing amino acids have not been studied as intensely as taurine and S-adenosylmethionine, but there is evidence for their importance in CNS function and some of them appear to be possible neurotransmitters or neuromodulators. Cystathionine and hypotaurine have been shown to have inhibitory properties (Werman et al., 1966; Curtis and Watkins, 1960) and cysteic acid and cysteinesulfinic acid have been shown to have excitatory properties (Curtis and Watkins, 1960).

The first metabolite formed in the transsulfuration route away from the methylation cycle is cystathionine, a compound found in relatively high concentrations in human brain (Tallan et al., 1958; Brenton et al., 1965; Gerritsen and Waisman, 1964; Sturman et al., 1970b). Cystathionine also has been found in spinal cord, where it has been implicated as a neurotransmitter because of its depressant actions on neurons after application by microiontophoresis (Werman et al., 1966). After intracerebral injection of [$^{35}$S]cystathionine into rats, something less than 4 percent of the total radioactivity in the brain was associated with synaptosomes so some cystathionine is present at the nerve ending (Griffiths and Tudball, 1976). The importance of cystathionine as a putative transmitter has been questioned because of the nature of its distribution in spinal cord: the spinal gray matter does not appear to have significantly higher concentrations than the spinal white matter (Johnston, 1968), as has been found for glycine (Aprison et al., 1968).

Cat electrocorticogram patterns may be affected by cystathionine and by cysteine, one of the cleavage products of cystathionine.
Cystathionine caused increased synchrony and reduced blood pressure
in an encephalé isolé preparation (the spinal cord was sectioned at
the $C_1$ level) of cats with permanently implanted ventricular cannulae.
Cysteine caused desynchrony of the electrocorticogram and raised
blood pressure in this type of preparation. Cystathionine (2 mg
intraventricularly) given two minutes before cysteine (1 mg intraventricularly) abolished the usual desynchronous effect of the latter
compound, although if cysteine were given eleven minutes after the
cystathionine the characteristic desynchronous response was observed
(Key and White, 1970). Cats with chronically implanted ventricular
cannulae but no spinal transection in whom cysteine was injected
showed hyperactivity, increased time before onset of sleep and desynchrony of the electrocorticogram. The only effect of injected
cystathionine in this group of animals was to shorten the time until
the onset of sleep (Key and White, 1970). These effects are compatible with the suggested inhibitory transmitter properties of
cystathionine (Werman et al., 1966) and the possible excitatory
properties of cysteine or its metabolites (Olney et al., 1971).

The interactions of cystathionine and cysteine may be important during the development of the human fetus. The cystathionine
concentration in human fetal brain is lower than that of the mature
human brain: Furthermore, cystathionase, the enzyme that cleaves
cystathionine to cysteine, is virtually absent in fetal human brain
(Gaull et al., 1972). Cystine may be an essential amino acid for
immature man (Sturman et al., 1970a), but cystine is the only plasma
free amino acid found in concentrations equal to or lower than that
of the maternal plasma (Gaull et al., 1973a). L-Methionine, L-
leucine and L-ornithine are rapidly transferred to the fetus by the
placenta against concentration gradients, but cystine appears slowly
in the fetus after L-cysteine or L-cystine loads, suggesting that
the fetus may be protected from excessive quantities of this
metabolite (Gaull et al., 1973a). Cystine concentrations may be
regulated in this unique way by the placenta to ensure the correct
balance between cystine and cystathionine, for cysteine (or its
metabolites) may be neurotoxic (Olney et al., 1971), expecially in
the presence of low concentrations of cystathionine. It is interesting in this regard that cysteine has been shown to be cytotoxic
in two separate laboratories studying cell culture systems (Nishiuch
et al., 1976; Ham et al., 1977). Cysteine has also been reported to
be an irreversible inhibitor of dopamine β-hydroxylase, the enzyme
responsible for the synthesis of the neurotransmitter norepinephrine
(Izumi et al., 1976).

The reduced concentrations of cystathionine in the absence of
its cleavage enzyme, cystathionase, may be explained by the high
specific activities of $N^5$-methyltetrahydrofolic acid-homocysteine

methyltransferase and serine hydroxymethyltransferase found in
human fetal brain during the period of neuroblast proliferation
(Gaull et al., 1973b). The $N^5$-methyltetrahydrofolic acid homocys-
teine methyltransferase also has a higher affinity for homocysteine
(Km = $10^{-5}$M) than does cystathionine β-synthase (Km = $10^{-3}$M)
(Finkelstein, 1971) or S-adenosylhomocysteine hydrolase (Km = $10^{-3}$M)
(J. Duerre, personal communication) two other enzymes for which
homocysteine is a substrate.

        Cysteinesulfinic acid and cysteic acid are two oxidation prod-
ucts of cysteine to which excitatory activity has been attributed
(Curtis and Watkins, 1960). These compounds also may be responsible
for the apparently excitatory neurotoxic effects observed after subcutaneous injection of L-cysteine because of in vivo conversion of
its sulfhydryl group to the sulfinic or sulfonic groups (Olney
et al., 1971). Cysteic acid and cysteinesulfinic acid are the most
potent competitive inhibitors of the high affinity transport system
that has been suggested as the mechanism by which glutamic acid may
be removed from receptor sites at the synapse (Balcar and Johnston,
1972a,b). The inhibition may reflect a mechanism by which cysteic
acid and cysteinesulfinic acid modulate the excitatory effects of
glutamic acid. Alternatively this high affinity transport system
may be a general reuptake mechanism for amino acids that function
as excitatory neurotransmitters. Rat brain is the only tissue in
which cysteinesulfinic acid has been detected without artifically
raising concentrations of this metabolite by preloading (Bergeret
and Chatagner, 1954). Rat brain has the capacity to synthesize
cysteinesulfinic acid from cysteine (Yamaguchi et al., 1973;
Rassin and Gaull, 1975).

        The evidence cited neither establishes these sulfur containing
compounds as neurotransmitters nor does it establish any other
specific CNS function. These metabolites do seem to be important
to the CNS, however, and eventually they may be defined as transmitters or modulators of synaptic function when enough evidence has
been accumulated.

        It is also germane that inborn errors of metabolism involving the
pathway of metabolism of sulfur amino acids have been reported. These
diseases are sometimes associated with mental retardation, implying
that normal CNS function is dependent upon normal sulfur amino acid
metabolism. Some of the findings related to these disorders are relevant to this discussion of sulfur amino acids and CNS function. Homocystinuria associated with deficient activity of cystathionine
β-synthase is the most common of these disorders (Mudd et al., 1964,
1965). This defect prevents the metabolism of homocysteine to cys-
thathionine, causing increased plasma concentrations of methionine
and homocystine and decreased concentrations or absence of plasma
cystine. No detectable homocystine and normal concentrations of

cystine are found in the liver of patients with homocystinuria despite the abnormal amounts of these metabolites in the blood and urine (Rassin et al., 1977b). Post-mortem studies of the brains of affected individuals have demonstrated an absence of cystathionine (Brenton et al., 1964, 1965; Gerritsen and Waisman, 1964) in contrast to the relatively high concentrations reported in normal brain (Tallan et al., 1958). A tentative conclusion is that an inability to synthesize cystathionine in brain may be associated with CNS dysfunction.

Homocystinuria also may be associated with enzymatic defects of $N^5$-methyltetrahydrofolic acid-homocysteine methyltransferase and $N^{5,10}$-methylenetetrahydrofolate reductase. Since remethylation is impaired, these defects are accompanied by high plasma homocystine concentrations but normal or low methionine concentrations. The methyltransferase deficiency was also accompanied by a cystathioni-nemia (Mudd et al., 1972). The clinical picture in the last two types of homocystinuria is not clear, because so few cases have been identified. It is likely, however, that some have been associated with brain dysfunction (Mudd et al., 1972).

A defect in the conversion of cystathionine to cysteine asso-ciated with cystathioninuria (Harris et al., 1959) has been found to result from a deficiency of the enzyme cystathionase (Frimpter, 1965). A number of cases of this disease have no mental retardation (Perry et al., 1968) and even within a single family both retarded and men-tally normal individuals have been observed (Hooft and Carton, 1968). Thus, there is reason to question the association of this disease with mental retardation and its relevance to CNS function remains unclear (Gaull, 1972).

## CONCLUSION

There is considerable evidence for the importance of taurine and its metabolic precursors to the central nervous sytem. Cysta-thionine, cysteine, cysteinesulfinic acid and hypotaurine may even-tually satisfy all the criteria necessary to define them as neuro-transmitters. Methionine, S-adenosylmethionine and homocysteine are intermediates in the supply of methyl groups to the central nervous system necessary for normal metabolism. Taurine may well be an in-hibitory neurotransmitter in the central nervous system, and, in addition, is important to the brain during development. Finally, taurine is associated with many organelles which function via vari-ous forms of membrane disruption and may be important in controlling the stability of these structures. The biochemical, electrophysio-logical and behavioral properties of the sulfur-containing amino acids suggest their importance to the function of the central nervous system and provide a basis for further study of the role of these compounds in the brain.

## REFERENCES

Agnoli, A., Andreoli, V., Casacchia, M., and Cerbo, R., 1976, Effect of S-adenosyl-L-methionine (SAMe) upon depressive symptoms, J. Psychiatr. Res. 13:43-54.

Agrawal, H. C., Davison, A. N., and Kaczmarek, L. K., 1971, Subcellular distribution of taurine and cysteinesulphinate decarboxylase in developing rat brain, Biochem. J. 122:759-763.

Ahtee, L., Boullin, D. J., and Paasonen, M. K., 1974, Transport of taurine by normal human blood platelets, Br. J. Pharmac. 52: 245-251.

Anderson, D. J., Crossland, J., and Shaw, G. G., 1975, The actions of spermidine and spermine on the central nervous system, Neuropharmacol. 14:571-577.

Aprison, M. H., Shank, R. P., Davidoff, R. A., and Werman, R., 1968, The distribution of glycine, a neurotransmitter suspect in the central nervous system of several vertebrate species, Life Sci. 7;583-590.

Applegarth, D. A., Remtulla, M., and Williams, I. H., 1976, Does isethionic acid occur in heart and brain tissue. Clin. Res. XXIV:646A.

Balcar, V. J., and Johnston, G. A. R., 1972a, The structural specificity of the high affinity uptake of L-glutamate and L-aspartate by rat brain slices, J. Neurochem. 19:2657-2666.

Balcar, V. J., and Johnston, G. A. R., 1972b, Glutamate uptake by brain slices and its relation to the depolarization of neurones by acidic amino acids, J. Neurobiol. 3:295-301.

Baldessarini, R. J., and Karobath, M., 1972, Effects of L-DOPA and L-3-0-methyl-DOPA on uptake of $^3$H L-methionine by synaptosomes, Neuropharmacol. 11:715-720.

Banerjee, S. P., and Snyder, S. H., 1973, Methyltetrahydrofolic acid mediates N-and O-methylation of biogenic amines, Science 182: 74-75.

Banks, W. J., Rowland, L. P., and Ipsen, J., 1971, Amino acids of plasma and urine in diseases of muscle, Arch. Neurol. 24: 176-186.

Barbeau, A., and Donaldson, J., 1973, Taurine in epilepsy, Lancet, 2:387.

Barbeau, A., and Donaldson, J., 1974, Zinc, taurine and epilepsy, Arch. Neurol. 30:52-58.

Barbeau, A., Inoue, N., Tsukada, Y., and Butterworth, R. F., 1975, The neuropharmacology of taurine. Life Sci. 17:669-678.

Baskin, S. I., and Dagirmanjian, R., 1973, Possible involvement of taurine in the genesis of muscular dystrophy, Nature 245: 464-465.

Baskin, S. I., and Hinkamp, D. L., Marquis, W. J., and Tilson, H. A., 1974, Effects of taurine on psychomotor activity in the rat. Neuropharmacol. 13:591-594.

Beaton, J. M., Smythies, J. R., and Bradley, R. J., 1975, The be-
    havioral effects of L-methionine and related compounds in rats
    and mice. Biolog. Psychiatr. 10:45-52.

Benevenga, N. J., 1974, Toxicities of methionine and other amino
    acids, Agric. and Food Chem. 22:2-9.

Bergamini, L., Mutani, R., Delsedime, M., and Durelli, L., 1974,
    First clinical experience on the antiepileptic action of
    taurine, Europ. Neurol. 11:261-269.

Bergeret, B., and Chatagner, F., 1954, Sur la présence d'acide
    cystéinesulfinique dans le cerveau du rat normal, Biochim.
    Biophys. Acta 14:297.

Berson, E. L., Hayes, K. C., Rabin, A. R., Schmidt, S. Y., and
    Watson, G., 1976, Retinal degeneration in cats fed casein.
    2.  Supplementation with methionine, cysteine or taurine,
    Invest. Ophthalmol. 15:52-58.

Borg, J., Balcar, V. J., and Mandel, P., 1976, High affinity uptake
    of taurine in neuronal and glial cells, Brain Res. 118:514-516.

Brenton, D. P., Cusworth, D. C., and Gaull, G. E., 1964, Homocys-
    tinuria:  Some biochemical studies, Proc. Int. Copenhagen,
    Congr. on the Scient. Study of Mental Retardation, p.79.

Brenton, D. P., Cusworth, D. C., and Gaull, G. E., 1965, Homocys-
    tinuria:  Biochemical studies of tissues including a compari-
    son with cystathioninuria, Pediatr. 35:50-56.

Brotherton, J., 1962, Studies on the metabolism of the rat retina
    with special reference to retinitis pigmentosa.  2.  Amino
    acid content as shown by chromatography, Exptl. Eye Res. 3:
    246-252.

Brown, F. C., and DeFoor, M., 1974, Trans-sulfuration in rat brain -
    Effects of 3,4 - dihydroxyphenylalanine (L-Dopa), Biochem.
    Pharmacol. 23:1135-1137.

Burton, E. G., and Sallach, H. J., 1975, Methylenetetrahydrofolate
    reductase in the rat central nervous system:  Intracellular and
    regional distribution. Arch. Biochem. Biophys. 166:483-493.

Byrne, M. C., and Salganicoff, L., 1977, Stimulation of cysteine
    oxidase activity of catecholamines.  Fed. Proc. 36:1007.

Cohen, A. I., McDaniel, M., and Orr, H., 1973, Absolute levels of
    some free amino acids in normal and biologically fractionated
    retinas.  Invest. Ophthalm. 12:686-693.

Cotzias, G. C., Papavasiliou, P. S., Steck, A., and Duby, S., 1971,
    Parkinsonism and levodopa, Clin. Pharmac. Ther. 12:319-322.

Curtis, D. R., and Watkins, J. C., 1960, The excitation and de-
    pression of spinal neurones by structurally related amino acids,
    J. Neurochem. 6:117-141.

Curtis, D. R., Hosli, L., and Johnston, G. A. R., 1967, Inhibition
    of spinal neurones by glycine, Nature 215:1502-1503.

Daly, E. C., and Aprison, M. H., 1974, Distribution of serine hy-
    droxymethyltransferase and glycine transaminase in several
    areas of the central nervous system of the rat.  J. Neurochem.
    22:877-885.

Davies, J., and Watkins, J. C., 1973, Facilitatory and direct ex-
    citatory effects of folate and folinate on single neurones of
    cat cerebral cortex. Biochem. Pharmacol. 22:1667-1668.
Davies, L. P., and Johnston, G. A. R., 1973, Serine hydroxymethyl-
    transferase in the central nervous system: Regional and sub-
    cellular distribution studies. Brain Res. 54:149-156.
Davison, A. N., and Kaczmarek, L. K., 1971, Taurine - a possible
    neurotransmitter? Nature 234:107-108.
DeBelleroche, J. S., and Bradford, H. F., 1973, Amino acids in
    synaptic vesicles from mammalian cerebral cortex: a re-
    appraisal, J. Neurochem. 21:441-451.
Derouaux, M., Puil, E., and Naquet, R., 1973, Antiepileptic effect
    of taurine in photosensitive epilepsy. Electroenceph. Clin.
    Neurophysiol. 34:770.
Dietrich, J., and Diacono, J., 1971, Comparison between ouabain and
    taurine effects on isolated rat and guinea-pig hearts in low
    calcium medium, Life Sci. 10:499-507.
Dudel, J., 1968, Criteria for identification of transmitter sub-
    stances, in "Structure and Function of Inhibitory Neuronal
    Mechanisms," (C. von Euler, S. Skoglund, and V. Soderburg, eds.),
    pp. 523-525, Pergamon Press, Oxford.
Fellman, J. H., Roth, E. S., and Fujita, T. S., 1977, Is taurine
    metabolized to isethionic acid in mammalian tissue? Trans. Am.
    Soc. Neurochem. 8:90.
Finkelstein, J. D., 1971, Methionine metabolism in mammals, in
    "Inherited Disorders of Sulphur Metabolism," (N. A. J. Carson
    and D. N. Raine, eds.), pp. 1-13, London.
Finkelstein, J. D., and Mudd, S. H., 1967, Trans-sulfuration in
    mammals: The methionine sparing effect of cystine, J. Biol.
    Chem. 242:873-880.
Frimpter, G. W., 1965, Cystathioninuria: Nature of the defect,
    Science 149:1095-1096.
Fuller, R. W., 1976, The rise and fall of MTHF as a methyl donor in
    biogenic amine metabolism, Life Sci. 19:625-628.
Gaull, G. E., 1972, Abnormal metabolism of sulfur-containing amino
    acids associated with brain dysfunction, in "Handbook of Neuro-
    chemistry," V. 7, (A. Lajtha, ed.) pp. 169-190, Plenum Press,
    New York.
Gaull, G. E., Sturman, J. A., and Raiha, N. C. R., 1972, Development
    of mammalian sulfur metabolism: Absence of cystathionase in
    human fetal tissues. Pediatr. Res. 6:538-547.
Gaull, G. E., Raiha, N. C. R., Saarikoski, S., and Sturman, J. A.,
    1973a, Transfer of cyst(e)ine and methionine across the human
    placenta, Pediat. Res. 7:908-913.
Gaull, G. E., vonBerg, W., Raiha, N. C. R., and Sturman, J. A.,
    1973b, Development of methyltransferase activities of human
    fetal tissues, Pediat. Res. 7:527-533.
Gaull, G. E., Rassin, D. K., Raiha, N. C. R., and Heinonen, K.,
    1977, Milk protein quantity and quality in low-birth-weight

infants.  3. Effects on sulfur amino acids in plasma and
    urine.  J. Pediatr. 90:348-355.
Gerritsen, T., and Waisman, H. A., 1964, Homocystinuria:  Absence
    of cystathionine in the brain, Science 145:588.
Goodman, H. O., King, J. S., and Thomas, J. J., 1964, Urinary ex-
    cretion of beta-aminobutyric acid and taurine in mongolism,
    Nature 204:650-652.
Green, J. P., Day, M., and Robinson, J. D., 1962, Some acidic sub-
    stances in neoplastic mast cells and in the pineal body,
    Biochem. Pharmacol. 11:957-960.
Griffiths, R., and Tudball, N., 1976, Observations on the fate of
    cystathionine in rat brain, Life Sci. 19:1217-1224.
Grosso, D. A., and Bressler, R., 1976, Taurine and cardiac physi-
    ology, Biochem. Pharmacol. 25:2227-2232.
Guidotti, A., Badiani, G., and Giotti, A., 1971, Potentiation by
    taurine of inotropic effect of strophanthin-K on guinea pig
    isolated auricles, Pharmacol. Res. Comm. 3:29-38.
Haas, H. L., and Hosli, L., 1973, The depression of brain stem
    neurones by taurine and its interaction with strychnine and
    bicuculline, Brain Res. 52:399-402.
Ham, R. G., Hammond, S. L., and Miller, L. L., 1977, Critical
    adjustment of cysteine and glutamine concentrations for im-
    proved clonal growth of WI-38 cells, in vitro 13:1-10.
Hammerstad, J. P., Murray, J. E., and Cutler, R. W. P., 1971,
    Efflux of amino acid neurotransmitters from rat spinal cord
    slices.  II. Factors influencing the electrically induced
    efflux of $^{14}C$ glycine and $^3H$-GABA, Brain Res. 35:357-367.
Hardison, W. G. M., Wood, C. A., and Proffitt, H. J., 1977, Quanti-
    fication of taurine biosynthesis in the intact rat and cat
    liver, Proc. Soc. Exp. Biol. Med. 155:55-58.
Harper, A. E., Benevenga, N. J., and Wohlhueter, R. M., 1970,
    Effects of ingestion of disproportionate amounts of amino
    acids, Physiol. Rev. 50:428-558.
Harris, H., Penrose, L. S., and Thomas, D. H. H., 1959, Cysta-
    thioninuria, Ann. Hum. Genet. 23:442-453.
Hayes, K. C., Carey, R. E., and Schmidt, S. Y., 1975a, Retinal de-
    generation associated with taurine deficiency in the cat,
    Science 188:949-951.
Hayes, K. C., Rabin, A. R., and Berson, E. L., 1975b, An ultrastruc-
    tural study of nutritionally induced and reversed retinal de-
    generation in cats, Am. J. Pathol. 78:505-524.
Henn, F. A., 1976a, Glial transport of amino acid neurotransmitter
    candidates, in "Metabolic Compartmentation and Neurotrans-
    mission.  Relation to Brain Structure and Function," (S. Berl,
    D. D. Clarke, and D. Schneider, eds.), pp. 91-97, Plenum
    Press, New York.
Henn, F. A., 1976b, Neurotransmission and glial cells:  A functional
    relationship?, J. Neurosci. Res. 2:271-282.

Hooft, C., and Carton, D., 1968, Cystathioninemia in three siblings, Abstr. Soc. for Study Inborn Errors of Metab. Zurich.

Hoskin, F. C. G., and Kordik, E. R., 1977, Hydrogen sulfide as a precursor for the synthesis of isethionate in the squid giant axon, Arch. Biochem. Biophys. 180:583-586.

Hosli, L., Haas, H. L., and Hosli, E., 1973, Taurine - a possible transmitter in the mammalian central nervous system, Experientia 29:743-744.

Huxtable, R., and Barbeau, A. (eds.), 1973, "Taurine," Raven Press, New York.

Huxtable, R., and Bressler, R., 1973, Effect of taurine on a muscle intracellular membrane, Biochim. Biophys. Acta 323:573-583.

Ingoglia, N. A., Sturman, J. A., Lindquist, T. D., and Gaull, G. E., 1976, Axonal migration of taurine in the goldfish visual system, Brain Res. 115:535-539.

Izumi, K., Donaldson, J., Minnich, J. L., and Barbeau, A., 1973, Ouabain-induced seizures in rats: Suppressive effects of taurine and γ-aminobutyric acid, Can. J. Physiol. Pharmacol. 51:885-889.

Izumi, H., Oyama, H., Hayakari, M., and Ozawa, H., 1976, Irreversible inhibition of dopamine-β-hydroxylase by cysteine, Biochem. Pharmacol. 25:488-489.

Jacobsen, J. G., and Smith, L. H., Jr., 1968, Biochemistry and physiology of taurine and taurine derivatives, Physiol. Rev. 48:424-511.

Johnston, G. A. R., 1968, The intraspinal distribution of some depressant amino acids, J. Neurochem. 15:1013-1017.

Kaczmarek, L. K., and Adey, W. R., 1975, Modification of the direct cortical response by taurine, Electroencephalog, Clin. Neurophysiol. 39:292-294.

Kaczmarek, L. K., and Davison, A. N., 1972, Uptake and release of taurine from rat brain slices, J. Neurochem. 19:2355-2362.

Kashiwamata, S., 1971a, Brain cystathionine synthase: vitamin-$B_6$ requirement for its enzymic reaction and changes in enzymic activity during early development of rats, Brain Res. 30: 185-192.

Kashiwamata, S., 1971b, Subcellular localization of cystathionine synthase in rat brain, FEBS Lett. 19:69-71.

Kennedy, A. S., and Voaden, M. J., 1974, Free amino acids in the photoreceptor cells of the frog retina, J. Neurochem. 23: 1093-1095.

Kennedy, A. S., and Voaden, M. J., 1976, Studies on the uptake and release of radioactive taurine by the frog retina, J. Neurochem. 27:131-137.

Key, B. J., and White, R. P., 1970, Neuropharmacological comparison of cystathionine, cysteine, homoserine and alpha-ketobutyric acid in cats, Neuropharmac. 9:349-357.

Knopf, K., Sturman, J. A., Armstrong, M., and Hayes, K. C., 1977, Taurine: An essential nutrient for the cat, J. Nutr. (in press).

Laduron, P. M., Gommeren, W. R., and Leysen, J. E., 1974, N-
    Methylation of biogenic amines. I. Characterization and
    properties of N-methyltransferase in rat brain using 5-
    methyltetrahydrofolic acid as a methyl donor, Biochem.
    Pharmacol. 23:1599-1608.
Lahdesmaki, P., and Oja, S. S., 1972, Effect of electrical stimula-
    tion on the influx and efflux of taurine in brain slices of
    newborn and adult rats, Exp. Brain Res. 15:430-438.
Liu, Y. P., Ambani, L. M., and VanWoert, M. H., 1972, L-Dihydroxy-
    phenylalanine: Effect on levels of amino acids in rat brain.
    J. Neurochem. 19:2237-2239.
Lo, C.-M., Kwok, M.-L., and Wurtman, R. J., 1976, O-Methylation and
    decarboxylation of α-methyldopa in brain and spinal cord:
    Depletion of S-adenosylmethionine and accumulation of metabo-
    lites in catecholaminergic neurons, Neuropharmacol. 15:395-402.
McBride, W. J., Nadi, N. S., Neuss, M., and Frederickson, R. C. A.,
    1977, Association of taurine with stellate cells in the cere-
    bellum of the rat, Trans. Am. Soc. Neurochem. 8:91.
Mandel, P., and Pasantes-Morales, H., 1976, Taurine: A putative
    neurotransmitter, Adv. in Biochem. Psychopharmacol. 15:141-151.
Mandel, P., Pasantes-Morales, H., and Urban, P. F., 1976, Taurine,
    a putative transmitter in retina, in "Transmitters in the
    Visual Process," (S. L. Bonting, ed.) pp. 89-104, Pergamon
    Press, N. Y.
Matthysse, S., Lipinski, J., and Shih, V., 1971, L-Dopa and S-
    adenosylmethionine, Clin. Chim. Acta 35:253-254.
Meller, E., Rosengarten, H., Friedhoff, A. J., Stebbins, R. D., and
    Sibler, R., 1975, 5-Methyltetrahydrofolic acid is not a methyl
    donor for biogenic amines: Enzymatic formation of formaldehyde,
    Science 187:171-173.
Misra, C. H., and Olney, J. W., 1975, Cysteine oxidase in brain,
    Brain Res. 97:117-126.
Misra, C. H., Mena, E. E., Rhee, V., and Olney, J. W., 1977, Intra-
    cellular distribution of cysteine oxidase in the rat central
    nervous system, Fed. Proc. 36:751.
Monaco, F., Mutani, R., Durelli, L., and Delsedime, M., 1975, Free
    amino acids in serum of patients with epilepsy: Significant
    increase in taurine, Epilepsia 16:245-249.
Mudd, S. H., Finkelstein, J. D., Irreverre, F., and Laster, L.,
    1964, Homocystinuria: An enzymatic defect, Science 143:1443-
    1445.
Mudd, S. H., Finkelstein, J. D., Irreverre, F., and Laster, L.,
    1965, Transsulfuration in mammals: Microassays and tissue
    distributions of three enzymes of the pathway, J. Biol. Chem.
    240:4382-4392.
Mudd, S. H., Levy, H. L., and Morrow, G., 1970, Deranged $B_{12}$ metabo-
    lism: Effects on sulfur amino acid metabolism, Biochem. Med.
    4:193-213.

Mudd, S. H., Uhlendorf, B. W., Freeman, J. M., Finkelstein, J. D., and Shih, V. E., 1972, Homocystinuria associated with decreased methyltetrahydrofolate reductase activity, Biochem. Biophys. Res. Commun. 46:905-912.

Mutani, R., Monaco, F., Durelli, L., and Delsedime, M., 1975, Levels of free amino acids in serum and cerebrospinal fluid after administration of taurine to epileptic and normal subjects, Epilepsia 16:765-769.

Mutani, R., Durelli, L., Mazzarino, M., Valentini, C., Monaco, F., Fumero, S., and Mandino, A., 1977, Longitudinal changes of brain amino acid content before, during and after epileptic activity, Brain Res. 122:513-521.

Nakagawa, K., Kuriyama, K., 1975, Effect of taurine on alteration in adrenal functions induced by stress, Japan, J. Pharmacol. 25: 737-746.

Narasimhachari, N., Heller, B., Spaide, J., Haskovec, L., Fujimori, M., Tabushi, K., and Himwich, H. E., 1970, Comparative behavioral and biochemical effects on tranylcypromine and cysteine on normal controls and schizophrenia patients, Life Sci. 9:1021-1032

Neal, M. J., and Iversen, L. L., 1969, Subcellular distribution of endogenous and 3H γ-aminobutyric acid in rat cerebral cortex, J. Neurochem. 16:1245-1252.

Neidle, A., and Kandera, J., 1974, Carnosine - an olfactory bulb peptide, Brain Res. 80:359-364.

Nevin, N. C., Hurwitz, L. J., and Neill, D. W., 1966, Familial camptodactyly with taurinuria, J. Med. Genet. 3:265-268.

Nishiuch, Y., Sasaki, M., Nakayasu, M., and Oikawa, A., 1976, Cytotoxicity of cysteine in culture media, in vitro 12:635-638.

Oja, S. S., Karvonen, M.-L, and Lahdesmaki, P., 1973, Biosynthesis of taurine and enhancement of decarboxylation of cysteine sulphinate and glutamate by the electrical stimulation of rat brain slices, Brain Res. 55:173-178.

Oja, S. S., and Lahdesmaki, P., 1974, Is taurine an inhibitory neurotransmitter? Med. Biol. 52:138-143.

Olney, J. W., Ho, O. L., and Rhee, V., 1971, Cytotoxic effects of acidic and sulphur containing amino acids on the infant mouse central nervous system. Exp. Brain Res. 14:61-76.

Ordonez, L. A., and Wurtman, R. J., 1973, Methylation of exogenous 3,4-dihydroxyphenylalanine (L-Dopa)-Effects on methyl group metabolism, Biochem. Pharmacol. 22:134-137.

Ordonez, L. A., and Wurtman, R. J., 1974, Folic acid deficiency and methyl group metabolism in rat brain: Effects of L-Dopa, Arch. Biochem. Biophys. 160:372-376.

Orr, H. T., Cohen, A. I., and Carter, J. A., 1976, The levels of free taurine, glutamate, glycine and γ-aminobutyric acid during the postnatal development of the normal and dystrophic retina of the mouse, Exptl. Eye Res. 23:377-384.

Orr, H. T., Cohen, A. I., and Lowry, O. H., 1976, The distribution of taurine in the vertebrate retina, J. Neurochem. 26:609-611.

Pasantes-Morales, H., Klethi, J., Ledig, M., and Mandel, P., 1972a, Free amino acids of chicken and rat retina, Brain Res. 41: 494-497.

Pasantes-Morales, H., Klethi, J., Urban, P. F., and Mandel, P., 1972b, The physiological role of taurine in retina: uptake and effect on electroretinogram (ERG), Physiol. Chem. and Phys. 4:339-348.

Pasantes-Morales, H., Urban, P. F., Klethi, J., and Mandel, P., 1973, Light stimulated release of $^{35}$S taurine from chicken retina, Brain Res. 51:375-378.

Pasantes-Morales, H., Mapes, C., Tapia, R., and Mandel, P., 1976, Properties of soluble and particulate cysteine sulfinate decarboxylase of the adult and developing rat brain, Brain Res. 107:575-589.

Pasantes-Morales, H., Loriette, C., and Chatagner, F., 1977, Regional and subcellular distribution of taurine synthesizing enzymes in rat brain, in "Taurine in Neurological Disease," (R. Huxtable and A. Barbeau, eds.) Raven Press, N. Y. (in press).

Pearce, L. A., and Waterbury, L. D., 1974, L-Methionine: A possible levodopa antagonist, Neurol. 24:640-611.

Peck, E. J., Jr., and Awapara, J., 1967, Formation of taurine and isethionic acid in rat brain, Biochim. Biophys. Acta 141:499-506.

Perry, T. L., Hardwick, D. F., Hansen, S., Love, D. L., and Israels, S., 1968, Cystathioninuria in two healthy siblings, New Engl. J. Med. 278:590-592.

Perry, T. L., Bratty, P. J. A., Hansen, S., Kennedy, J., Urquhart, N., and Dolman, C. L., 1975a, Hereditary mental depression and Parkinsonism with taurine deficiency, Arch. Neurol. 32:108-113.

Perry, T. L., Hansen, S., Kennedy, J., Wada, J. A., and Thompson, G. B., 1975b, Amino acids in human epileptogenic foci, Arch. Neurol. 32:752-754.

Perry, T. L., Currier, R. D., Hansen, S., and MacLean, J., 1977, Aspartate-taurine imbalance in dominantly inherited olivopontocerebellar atrophy, Neurol. 27:257-261.

Persinger, M. A., Lafreniere, G. F., and Falter, H., 1976a, Oral taurine effects on inhibitory behavior: Response transients to step-like schedule changes, Psychopharmacol. 49:249-252.

Persinger, M. A., Valliant, P. M., and Falter, H., 1976b, Weak inhibitory behavioral effects of postnatal/preweaning taurine injection in rats, Develop. Psychobiol. 9:131-136.

Phillis, J. W., 1970, "The Pharmacology of Synapses," pp. 6-7, Pergamon Press, Oxford.

Rabin, B., Nicolosi, R. J., and Hayes, K. C., 1976, Dietary influence on bile acid conjugation in the cat, J. Nutr. 106:1241-1246.

Rassin, D. K., 1972, Amino acids as putative transmitters: failure to bind to synaptic vesicles of guinea pig cerebral cortex.

J. Neurochem. 19:139-148.

Rassin, D. K., and Gaull, G. E., 1975, Subcellular distribution of enzymes of transmethylation and transsulphuration in rat brain, J. Neurochem. 24:969-978.

Rassin, D. K., Gaull, G. E., Heinonen, K., and Raiha, N. C. R., 1977a, Milk protein quantity and quality in low-birth-weight infants. 2. Effects on selected aliphatic amino acids in plasma and urine, Pediatr. 59:407-422.

Rassin, D. K., Longhi, R. C., and Gaull, G. E., 1977b, Free amino acids in liver of patients with homocystinuria due to cystathionine synthase deficiency: Effects of vitamin $B_6$, J. Pediatr. (in press).

Rassin, D. K., Sturman, J. A., and Gaull, G. E., 1977c, Taurine and other free amino acids in milk of man and other mammals, Early Human Develop. (submitted).

Rassin, D. K., Sturman, J. A., and Gaull, G. E., 1977d, Taurine in milk: Species variation, Pediatr. Res. 11:449.

Rassin, D. K., Sturman, J. A., and Gaull, G. E., 1977e, Taurine in developing rat brain: Subcellular distribution and association with synaptic vesicles of [$^{35}$S]taurine in maternal, fetal and neonatal rat brain, J. Neurochem. 28:41-50.

Rassin, D. K., Sturman, J. A., Hayes, K. C., and Gaull, G. E., 1977f, Taurine deficiency in the kitten: Subcellular distribution of taurine and [$^{35}$S]taurine, Neurochem. Res. (submitted).

Read, W. O., and Welty, J. D., 1963, Effect of taurine on epinephrine and digoxin induced irregularities of the dog heart, J. Pharmacol. 139:283-289.

Read, W. O., and Welty, J. D., 1965, Taurine as a regulator of cell potassium in the heart, in "Electrolytes and Cardiovascular Disease," v. 1, (E. Bajusz, ed.) pp. 70-85, S. Karger, Basal/New York.

Schmidt, S. Y., Berson, E. L., and Hayes, K. C., 1976, Retinal degeneration in cats fed casein. I. Taurine deficiency, Invest. Ophthalmol. 15:47-52.

Schmidt, S. Y., Berson, E. L., Watson, G., and Juang, C., 1977, Retinal degeneration in cats fed casein. 3. Taurine deficiency and ERG amplitudes, Invest. Ophthalmol. (in press).

Schrier, B. K., and Thompson, E. J., 1974, On the role of glial cells in the mammalian nervous system. Uptake, excretion and metabolism of putative neurotransmitters by cultured glial tumor cells, J. Biol. Chem. 249:1769-1780.

Sgaragli, G., and Pavan, F., 1972, Effects of amino acid compounds injected into cerebrospinal fluid spaces, on colonic temperature, arterial blood pressure and behavior of the rat, Neuropharmac. 11:45-56.

Sgaragli, G. P., Pavan, F., and Galli, A., 1975, Is taurine induced hypothermia in the rat mediated by 5-HT, Nauyn-Schmied. Arch. Pharmacol. 288:179-184.

Spaide, J. K., Davis, J. M., and Himwich, H. E., 1971, Plasma amino
     acids in schizophrenic patients with methionine or cysteine
     loading and a monoamine oxidase inhibitor, Am. J. Clin. Nutr.
     24:1053-1059.
Sprince, H., Parker, C. M., and Josephs, J. A., Jr., 1969a, Homo-
     cysteine-induced convulsions in the rat:  Protection by homo-
     serine, betaine, glycine and glucose, Agents and Actions 1:
     9-13.
Sprince, H., Parker, C. M., Josephs, J. A., Jr., and Magazino, J.,
     1969b, Convulsant activity of homocysteine and other short-
     chain mercaptoacids:  Protection therefrom. Ann. N. Y. Acad.
     Sci. 166:323-325.
Starr, M. S., 1973, Effects of changes in the ionic composition of
     the incubation medium on the accumulation and metabolism of
     $^{3}$H-$\gamma$-aminobutyric acid and $^{14}$C-taurine in isolated rat retina,
     Biochem. Pharmacol. 22:1693-1700.
Starr, M. S., and Voaden, M. J., 1972, The uptake, metabolism and
     release of $^{14}$C-taurine by rat retina in vitro, Vision Res. 12:
     1261-1269.
Sturman, J. A., Gaull, G., and Raiha, N. C. R., 1970a, Absence of
     cystathionase in human fetal liver:  Is cystine essential?
     Science 169:74-76.
Sturman, J. A., Rassin, D. K., and Gaull, G. E., 1970b, Relation of
     three enzymes of transsulphuration to the concentration of
     cystathionine in various regions of monkey brain. J. Neurochem.
     17:1117-1119.
Sturman, J. A., and Gaull, G. E., 1975a, Polyamine metabolism in the
     brain and liver of the developing monkey. J. Neurochem. 25:
     267-272.
Sturman, J. A., and Gaull, G. E., 1975b, Taurine in the brain and
     liver of the developing human and monkey, J. Neurochem. 25:
     831-835.
Sturman, J. A., Rassin, D. K., and Gaull, G. E., 1977a, Taurine in
     developing rat brain:  Transfer of [$^{35}$S]taurine to pups via
     the milk, Pediatr. Res. 11:28-33.
Sturman, J. A., Rassin, D. K., and Gaull, G. E., 1977b, Taurine in
     rat brain:  Maternal-fetal transfer of [$^{35}$S]taurine and its
     fate in the neonate, J. Neurochem. 28:31-39.
Sturman, J. A., Rassin, D. K., and Gaull, G. E., 1977c, Taurine in
     development, Life Sci. 21:1-22.
Sturman, J. A., Rassin, D. K., and Gaull, G. E., 1977d, Taurine in
     development of the central nervous system, in "Taurine in
     Neurological Disease," (R. Huxtable, and A. Barbeau, eds.),
     Raven Press, New York (in press).
Sturman, J. A., Rassin, D. K., and Gaull, G. E., 1977e, Taurine de-
     ficiency in the kitten:  Uptake and turnover of [$^{35}$S]taurine
     in brain, retina and other tissues, Neurochem. Res. (submitted).
Tadano, T., 1974, Behavioral pharmacological study of alkali metals
     (Report 3).  Changes in brain polyamines and emotional behavior

in mice when aggressive mice induced by isolation were moved to
    grouped circumstances, Folia Pharmacol. Japan. 70:457-464.

Tadano, T., Onoki, M., and Kisara, K., 1974, Behavioral pharma-
    cological study of alkali metals (Report 2). Changes of brain
    polyamine in aggressive mice induced by electro-shock and iso-
    lation, and effects of LiCl on behavior in aggressive mice,
    Folia Pharmacol. Japan. 70:9-18.

Tallan, H. H., Moore, S., and Stein, W. H., 1958, L-Cystathionine
    in human brain, J. Biol. Chem. 230:707-716.

Taylor, M., 1976, Effects of L-tryptophan and L-methionine on
    activity in the rat. Br. J. Pharmac. 58:117-119.

Taylor, K. M., and Randall, P. K., 1975, Depletion of S-adenosyl-L-
    methionine in mouse brain by antidepressive drugs, J. Pharmacol.
    Exp. Ther. 194:303-310.

Turner, A. J., 1977, The roles of folate and pteridine derivatives
    in neurotransmitter metabolism, Biochem. Pharmacol. 26:1009-
    1014.

Van Gelder, N. M., 1972, Antagonism by taurine of cobalt induced
    epilepsy in cat and mouse, Brain Res. 47:157-165.

Van Gelder, N. M., and Courtois, A., 1972, Close correlation between
    changing content of specific amino acids in epileptogenic cor-
    tex of cats and severity of epilepsy, Brain Res. 43:477-484.

Van Gelder, N. M., Sherwin, A. L., and Rasmussen, T., 1972, Amino
    acid content of epileptogenic human brain: focal versus sur-
    rounding regions, Brain Res. 40:385-393.

Van Gelder, N. M., Sherwin, A. L., Sacks, C., and Andermann, F.,
    1975, Biochemical observations following administration of
    taurine to patients with epilepsy, Brain Res. 94:297-306.

Volpe, J. J., and Laster, L., 1972, Transsulfuration in fetal and
    postnatal mammalian liver and brain, Biol. Neonate 20:385-403.

Wada, J. A., Osawa, T., Wake, A., and Corcoran, M. E., 1975, Effects
    of taurine on kindled amygdaloid seizures in rats, cats and
    photosensitive baboons, Epilepsia 16:229-234.

Wedgewood, M. A., and Wolstencroft, J. H., 1977, Effects of spermine
    and spermidine on single brainstem neurones, Neuropharmacol.
    16:445-446.

Welty, J. D., and Read, W. O., 1964, Studies on some cardiac effects
    of taurine, J. Pharmacol. 144:110-115.

Werman, R., 1966, A Review - Criteria for identification of a cen-
    tral nervous system transmitter, Comp. Biochem. Physiol. 18:
    745-766.

Werman, R., 1972, Amino acids as central neurotransmitters, in
    "Neurotransmitters" (I. J. Kopin, ed.), pp. 147-180, v. 50,
    The association for research in nervous and mental disease,
    Williams and Wilkins Co., Baltimore.

Werman, R., Davidoff, R. A., and Aprison, M. H., 1966, The inhibi-
    tory action of cystathionine, Life Sci. 5:1431-1440.

Wurtman, R. J., Rose, C. M., Matthysse, S., Stephenson, J., and
    Baldessarini, R., 1970, L-Dihydroxyphenylalanine: Effect on

S-adenosylmethionine in brain, Science 169:395-397.

Yamaguchi, K., Sakakibara, S., Asamizu, J., and Ueda, I., 1973, Induction and activation of cysteine oxidase of rat liver. II. The measurement of cysteine metabolism in vivo and the activation of in vivo activity of cysteine oxidase, Biochim. Biophys. Acta 297:48-59.

A FUNCTIONAL ROLE FOR AMINO ACIDS IN THE ADAPTATION OF TISSUES

FROM THE NERVOUS SYSTEM TO ALTERATIONS IN ENVIRONMENTAL OSMOLALITY

Claude F. Baxter and Roger A. Baldwin

Neurochem. Labs., V.A. Hosp., Sepulveda, CA 91343 and

Dept. Psychiatry, UCLA Sch. Med., Los Angeles, CA 90024

## INTRODUCTION

The cellular volume and water content of the healthy vertebrate brain are maintained within very narrow limits by mechanisms which help to adapt the intracellular osmolality of brain tissue to that of surrounding fluids. Adaptation to a hyperosmotic condition in these fluids elicits an accumulation of additional, osmotically-active solutes in brain tissues whereas adaptation to a hypoosmotic condition elicits the opposite effect.

Under conditions of salt retention, hyperglycemia, acute renal failure, renal tubular damage, premenstrual tension, dehydration and a variety of pharmacological and clinical conditions, plasma osmolality is elevated. Alternately, under conditions of hyponatremia due to water intoxication, dialysis disequilibrium, inappropriate secretion of antidiuretic hormone (ADH) or an excess administration of barbiturates or certain other drugs, plasma osmolality is depressed. All of the aforementioned conditions involve the osmotic adjustment of brain tissue and are usually accompanied by changes in mood, mentation and/or neurological function.

Osmotic alterations and the regulation of body fluids have been correlated with changes in mood and the exacerbation of symptoms of psychiatric illness in man (Coppen, 1969; Hullin et al., 1967; Coppen et al., 1966); also, with the activation of epileptogenic foci (Vastola et al., 1967), the susceptibility to epileptic seizures (Benga and Morariu, 1977), restlessness and irritability (Sotos et al., 1960), the neurological symptoms of the dialysis disequilibrium syndrome (Rodrigo et al., 1977) and even with the incidence of crimes committed by women during periods of premenstrual tension (Dalton, 1961).

In most of the studies conducted over the past 25 years, intracellular osmotic regulation in brain tissue has been examined as a phenomenon involving primarily, if not exclusively, inorganic ions (Katzman and Pappius, 1973). Although it was recognized more than 20 years ago that inorganic ions alone could not account for increases in osmolality in brain tissue in response to a hyperosmotic plasma condition, the involvement of organic molecules in osmotic regulation received scant notice. The term "idiogenic osmoles" was used to describe osmoles of unknown origin, not identifiable as inorganic ions, that appeared in brain tissues in response to an increased plasma osmolality (McDowell et al., 1955). It was suggested that solutes were being generated in the brain and other organs to achieve osmotic balance (Finberg et al., 1959; Sotos et al., 1960; Olmstead, 1964; Holliday et al., 1968). Recently, a number of laboratories have begun to identify systematically the nature of the compounds that contribute to the idiogenic osmoles of nervous system tissues. The work of a Belgian group using invertebrate nerve axons (Gerard and Gilles, 1972; Gilles and Schoffeniels, 1969), the studies in our laboratory of toad brain (Baxter and Ortiz, 1966; Baxter, 1968; Shank and Baxter, 1973, 1975), the work of two groups in San Francisco with rabbit brain (Arieff et al., 1972; Arieff and Guisado, 1976) and rat brain (Rymer and Fishman, 1973; Fishman et al., 1977) and the in vivo studies in St. Louis of mouse brain (Holowach-Thurston et al., 1975) leave little doubt that in the species studied, the "idiogenic osmoles" in brain tissues are composed primarily of amino acids, ammonia, urea and some related compounds.

Some of the largest changes observed in brain as an adaptive response to hyperosmolality in the blood plasma involve amino acids that are putative neurotransmitters or their precursors. It is quite possible, therefore, that the etiology of neurological and behavioral symptomatology associated with osmotic change is the result of changes in one or more of these amino acids or their derivatives. Such a hypothesis is made even more attractive by the findings of Arieff et al. (1973) and Arieff and Guisado (1976) that in mammals, the "idiogenic osmoles" appear to be the major variable that regulates the osmolality of brain tissues under conditions of changing plasma osmolality.


THE EXPERIMENTAL MODEL


Our studies of the "idiogenic osmoles" in tissues of the nervous system were started some years ago with a fourfold objective: (1) to identify those "idiogenic osmoles" which are affected most by changes in plasma osmolality; (2) to study the underlying mechanisms that connect the osmotic changes in blood plasma with biochemical changes in brain tissues; (3) to find the metabolic origin of the newly formed "idiogenic osmoles" in the brains of hyperosmotic or hypernatremic subjects; and, finally (4) to determine which of these biochemical changes can be linked most appropriately to behavioral changes and neurological diseases.

To accomplish the first three objectives, an animal model was required in which plasma osmolality could be altered over a wide range under normal "physiological" conditions (if possible). It was assumed that the biochemical changes in brain tissues in such an animal model would be proportional to the changes in plasma osmolality. A large biochemical change would simplify the identification of key biochemical reactions and control points that could be altered by changes in plasma osmolality.

For the initial studies a mammalian model seemed inappropriate because the induction of large changes in plasma osmolality hardly could be considered a normal physiological condition.

After some trial and error, the toad Bufo boreas was found to be a most appropriate model. These amphibians are osmoconformers so that their internal environment adjusts to parallel a hyperosmolal external environment (Gordon, 1965). Their natural California habitat is near both fresh and brackish water where they are exposed to conditions of differing environmental salinity. Fairly large fluctuations in the osmolality of their internal environment should be a normal physiological occurrence. Amphibian skin is quite permeable to some ions; thus, live toads can be treated in the laboratory like pieces of mammalian tissue. They can be placed into environments of differing salinities and will adapt by reaching osmotic equilibrium with the environment in a reasonably short period of time.

Bufo boreas toads in a fresh water environment have an apparent blood plasma pH of around 7.7 and a serum osmolality ranging from 220 to 270 milliosmoles (mOs). The exact pH and serum osmolality appears to depend, to some extent, upon the season and the nutritional state of each animal. In the laboratory these toads will adapt to an environmental salinity of 420 mOs without difficulty within 24 to 36 h. At the time of full adaptation, their serum osmolality is around 450 mOs, and their blood pH may have dropped by as much as 0.2 pH units. Bufo boreas cannot adapt to osmolalities much above 440 mOs, even if preadapted first to a lower salinity.

All experiments described, below, were performed with toads ranging in body weight from 35 to 80 g. Animals were conditioned first to the laboratory environment (20°C; light cycle: 12 h light, 12 h dark; tilted aquaria with optional access to the aqueous environment) for one month before experimentation. The procedures used for the preparation of control toads adapted to fresh water (FWA) and experimental toads adapted to a hyperosmotic environment (HOA) have been described in detail (Baxter, 1968; Shank and Baxter, 1973). The preparation of toads adapted to a hypoosmotic internal environment (HOOA) has been a fairly recent innovation. The intraperitoneal perfusion technique used to produce such animals was modeled after the one described by Elkinton et al. (1946). Toads were weighed and a volume of 20 mOs saline, equivalent to 25% of

body weight, was infused slowly through a fixed, plastic cannula
into the pleural-intraperitoneal cavity (Figure 1). An equal volume was withdrawn about 20 min later. This same procedure was repeated five times during the following 46 h. All toads treated in
this manner were allowed to adapt for another 2 h. During the
adaptation period, they had access to distilled water. The toads
reached a hypoosmotic steady state about 48 h after initiating this
procedure. Their serum osmolality had dropped to a level ranging
from 125 to 170 mOs but their plasma pH was the same as in untreated
animals. Animals with serum osmolalities much below 125 mOs
appeared sick and usually died within 24 h. No such animals were
used in any studies.

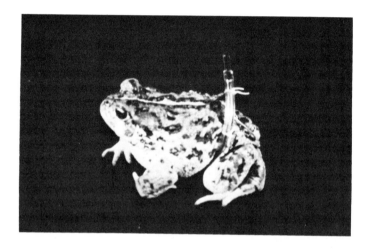

FIGURE 1. Implanted cannula for use in hypoosmotic adaptation of
the toad Bufo boreas. The cannula is fashioned from a 7-cm length
of Tygon tubing (6.4mm OD; 3.2mm ID). One end of this tubing is
sealed by the application of heat and pressure. Holes are then
punched randomly into the side of the tubing for about 1-1/2 cm
from the sealed end. The open end of the tubing is fitted with a
glass plug. This completes construction of the cannula. The per-
forated end of the cannula is inserted into the intraperitoneal
cavity of the toad through a small transverse incision made to the
left of the anterior abdominal vein about half way between fore and
hind legs. The cannula is secured in place by sutures around the
edges of the incision and by two loops of surgical thread attached
to the cannula and sewn into the skin on the back of the toad.

SOME METABOLIC CHANGES IN THE BRAINS OF HYPEROSMOTICALLY-
ADAPTED (HOA) AND HYPOOSMOTICALLY-ADAPTED (HOOA) TOADS

The relationship between different salinities in the environment and changes in the content of some representative small nitrogenous compounds in the brains of toads adapted to these salinities
is shown in Figure 2.  Whereas urea levels in brain tissue increase
to an extent that is proportional to the elevation of serum osmolality (about 80% at 420 mOs), levels of glutamic acid and aspartic
acid, in particular, are elevated to a considerably greater extent.
The drop in the level of aspartate and urea in animals adapting to
an even higher osmolality is a reflection of the breakdown of the
adaptive system.

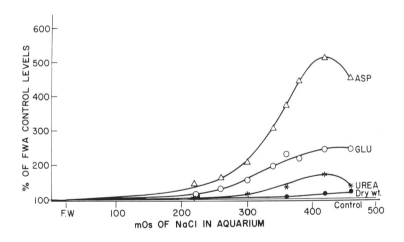

FIGURE 2. Effect of environmental osmolality upon the concentrations of two amino acids and urea in brain tissues of toad Bufo
boreas.  Toads were exposed to environments containing saline
solutions of differing osmolalities.  Exposure was for a period
of 48 h.  During this time period toads had a choice of habita-
ting in the dry, elevated portion of the aquarium or in the
saline solution in the lower part of the aquarium.  All toads
spent time in both environments.  The F.W on X axis denotes
fresh tap water (20 mOs); ASP = aspartate and GLU = glutamate.

A comparison is made in Table I between a select group of amino acids in the brain tissues of FWA, HOA and HOOA toads. In order to distinguish between significant and insignificant changes, alterations in water content, dry mass and serum osmolality are recorded. It should be noted that although the water content of HOA toads decreased by only about 3%, this corresponds to an increase in dry wt. of 22%. Thus, any amino acid increase of less than 22% in the brains of HOA toads (expressed as μmol/g tissue wet wt.) should be attributed to dehydration and not to any metabolic change.

## CHANGES IN "NON-ESSENTIAL" AMINO ACIDS (TABLE IA)

As shown in Table IA, all amino acids related metabolically to the tricarboxylic acid cycle are elevated significantly in the brains of HOA toads, with aspartate, glutamate and glutamine being quantitatively the most important. In HOOA toads, these same amino acids are all decreased. Glutamine, asparagine and GABA behave in a manner that mirrors their amino acid precursors.

Of the "non-essential" amino acids, the behavior of tyrosine is noteworthy. In the brains both of HOA and HOOA toads, the level of this amino acid is significantly depressed, and experiments with HOA toads revealed that this decrease in brain is correlated with a large adaptive increase in tyrosine aminotransferase activity in the liver tissues of these toads (C. Baxter and A. Yuwiler, unpublished). Levels of this enzyme in brain were not significantly affected. These observations support the claim that the enzymes in brain and liver are regulated by different mechanisms and that the changes in the tyrosine levels in brain tissues can be correlated inversely with the activity of tyrosine aminotransferase in the liver (Fuller, 1970). Changes in the activity of the liver enzyme are inducible by a large variety of stimuli including some putative neurotransmitters, environmental factors and stress (Black and Axelrod, 1968; Geller et al., 1969). It is possible, therefore, that the depression of tyrosine levels in the brains both of HOA and HOOA toads is the result of a generalized stress rather than a specific response to changes in plasma osmolality. It is equally possible, however, that the low tyrosine levels represent a true adaptive change in response to an altered plasma osmolality. In this connection it is of interest to note that abnormally low tyrosine levels have been observed in patients suffering from endogenous depression (Birkmayer et al., 1969) and could be the consequence of an altered plasma osmolality.

## CHANGES IN "ESSENTIAL" AMINO ACIDS (TABLE IB)

In the brains of HOA toads, all but the most basic of the "essential" amino acids are significantly elevated; this includes phenylalanine. In the case of lysine, histidine and arginine (the last-named not shown in Table I), there is a significant depression.

TABLE 1A. "NON-ESSENTIAL" AMINO ACID LEVELS IN BRAIN TISSUES OF NORMAL CONTROL AND HYPEROSMOTIC AND HYPOOSMOTIC TOADS[a]

| | | FWA (control) | HOA (hyperosmotic) | HOOA (hypoosmotic) | HOA % of control[b] | HOOA % of control[b] |
|---|---|---|---|---|---|---|
| blood serum | (mOs) | 248 ± 12 | 450 ± 6 | 152 ± 26 | 181[d] | 61[c] |
| brain H2O content | (%) | 85.5 | 82.4 | 86.0 | 96 | 101 |
| brain dry wt. | (%) | 14.5 | 17.6 | 14.0 | 122 | 97 |
| (μmol/g tissue wet wt. ± SD) | | | | | | |
| ALANINE | | 0.33 ± .04 | 1.43 ± .18 | 0.27 ± .006 | 440[d] | 83[c] |
| ASPARTATE | | 1.63 ± .16 | 5.32 ± .32 | 1.16 ± .25 | 327[d] | 71[c] |
| GLUTAMATE | | 6.30 ± .30 | 13.69 ± 1.16 | 4.93 ± .71 | 217[d] | 78[c] |
| GABA | | 2.20 ± .18 | 4.87 ± .50 | 1.78 ± .26 | 221[d] | 81 |
| SERINE | | 0.33 ± .04 | 0.82 ± .11 | 0.21 ± .05 | 250[d] | 65[c] |
| GLYCINE | | 0.44 ± .06 | 1.04 ± .24 | 0.28 ± .06 | 239[d] | 64[c] |
| ASPARAGINE | | 0.16 ± .02 | 0.40 ± .03 | 0.09 ± .02 | 252[d] | 54[d] |
| GLUTAMINE | | 4.55 ± .49 | 8.45 ± .72 | 3.19 ± .21 | 186[d] | 70[d] |
| TYROSINE | | 0.17 ± .04 | 0.12 ± .015 | .062 ± .001 | 72[c] | 37[d] |

TABLE 1B.　"ESSENTIAL" AMINO ACID LEVELS IN BRAIN TISSUES OF NORMAL CONTROL AND HYPEROSMOTIC AND HYPOOSMOTIC TOADS[a]

| | FWA | HOA | HOOA | HOA | HOOA[b] |
|---|---|---|---|---|---|
| | (control) | (hyperosmotic) | (hypoosmotic) | % of control | |
| | ($\mu$mol/g tissue wet wt. ± SD) | | | | |
| THREONINE | 0.23 ± .09 | 0.55 ± .12 | 0.15 ± .03 | 235[c] | 64 |
| VALINE | 0.07 ± .01 | 0.15 ± .02 | 0.06 ± .01 | 227[d] | 91 |
| METHIONINE | 0.036 ± .005 | 0.064 ± .014 | 0.078 ± .027 | 178[c] | 217[c] |
| ISOLEUCINE | 0.026 ± .002 | 0.076 ± .01 | 0.036 ± .004 | 292[d] | 138[d] |
| LEUCINE | 0.066 ± .006 | 0.18 ± .02 | 0.094 ± .02 | 271[d] | 142[c] |
| PHENYLALANINE | 0.05 ± .01 | 0.12 ± .04 | 0.08 ± .02 | 232[c] | 164[c] |
| LYSINE | 0.140 ± .04 | 0.10 ± .02 | 0.17 ± .04 | 67[c] | 120 |
| HISTIDINE | 0.086 ± .02 | 0.063 ± .01 | 0.092 ± .02 | 73[c] | 107 |

[a]Five toads per experimental group, each brain analyzed separately. Results are average ± SD. Extracts were prepared from frozen brains using 5-sulfosalicylic acid as a deproteinizing agent (Hamilton, 1962) and norleucine as an internal standard. Amino acids in 5 mg tissue equivalent of extract were separated using a high-pressure, narrow-bone Durrum column (30 cm), filled with DC-4A resin in the Li+ form. Amino acids were eluted using the Durrum-Pico Buffer System IV (Li+) program (Benson, 1974) with minor modifications. Amino acids and related compounds were detected and measured in the effluent as the fluorescent addition product with O-phthalaldehyde (Roth and Hampai, 1973; Benson and Hare, 1975), using an Aminco Model 4-7461 fluoro-monitor.
[b]The biochemical significance of the difference in values from experimental brains compared to control brains was calculated in a way that discounted any apparent changes caused by alterations in the dry wt. content of brains from experimental animals. [c]P<0.05. [d]P≤ 0.01.

Also, in the HOOA toads, some "essential" amino acid levels in brain tissue appear elevated.  As in the case of tyrosine, these changes could be the result of some phenomenon that is common both to HOA and HOOA toads but unrelated to osmotic conditions.  Any interpretation of these data must take into consideration also that "essential" amino acids for amphibians have not been established.

## Changes in Other Parts of Nervous System

The large <u>percentage</u> increase of aspartate and alanine, in brain tissues of HOA toads, is not confined to the central nervous system.  Gilles and Schoffeniels (1969) have reported a similar increase in the peripheral nerve of <u>Eriocheir</u> <u>sinensis</u> when this species adapted to a hyperosmotic environment.  In their studies, a large change in proline levels also was reported.  In the toad, the most dramatic changes were found in retinal tissue.  The normal levels of amino acids in toad retina are considerably lower than in brain but the response to osmotic adaptation is greater - and, in the case of aspartate, very much greater - than in brain tissues (Table II).  The nine- to ten-fold increase in aspartate content of the HOA retina represents the largest adaptive response to an altered osmolality that has been recorded for any organic compound in any tissue of the toad.

TABLE II.   SOME AMINO ACID LEVELS IN BRAIN AND RETINA OF TOADS ADAPTED TO EITHER A FRESH WATER OR A HYPEROSMOTIC NaCl ENVIRONMENT (400 to 420 mOs)[a]

|  | FWA Toad | | HOA Toad | |
|---|---|---|---|---|
|  | Brain | Retina | Brain | Retina |
|  | μmol/g wet wt. | | % of FWA levels | |
| Aspartate | 1.3 | 0.3 | 385 | 1060[b] |
| Alanine | 0.7 | 0.2 | 241 | 300 |
| Glutamate | 6.6 | 1.9 | 192 | 251 |
| GABA | 2.7 | 1.5 | 194 | 172 |
| Urea | 19.3 | 21.0 | 197 | 200 |

[a]Three retinal samples and six brain samples were used for each group of data in the Table.  Variability between samples was within the range of ± 12%.

[b]We are indebted to Dr. Paul B. Hamilton of the Alfred I. Du Pont Institute for making an independent analysis and verifying this surprisingly large change.

ADAPTIVE MECHANISMS REGULATING AMINO ACID LEVELS IN TOAD BRAIN

The mechanisms regulating amino acid levels and metabolism in brain tissues during osmotic adaptation are not fully understood. Regulation in the brain appears to differ from regulation in liver tissues (Benuck and Lajtha, 1974), and regulatory mechanisms appear to differ for different amino acids. This is suggested in toad brain by the pattern of amino acid changes during early stages of adaptation to a hyperosmotic environment. Partial results of such a study are shown in Figure 3. Plasma osmolality was elevated rapidly in these studies by injecting concentrated hyperosmotic solutions directly into the bloodstream or into the intraperitoneal cavity, thereby bypassing any barriers to the hyperosmotic solutes in the skin of the toad. For some details of the in vivo procedure, the legend for Figure 3 and an earlier description (Baxter, 1968) should be consulted.

## Differences Between Alanine and Aspartic Acid

As noted earlier, aspartate and alanine both increase substantially in the brain of the HOA toad. Yet, it is apparent that whereas the mechanism responsible for the elevation of alanine is very rapid initially, the mechanism for the accumulation of aspartate is preceded by a considerable delay period during which aspartate levels actually decrease (Figure 3). A similar delay has been noted for aspartate when the HOA toad is readapted to a fresh water environment (C. Baxter and B. Chang, unpublished). When the metabolism of $[U-^{14}C]$-glucose by toad brain was studied (Shank and Baxter, 1973), the rate of alanine biosynthesis from pyruvate appeared to increase with hyperosmotic adaptation but an increase in the rate of aspartate biosynthesis could not be demonstrated.

Alanine and aspartate also behave differently during in vitro incubations of toad brain. Although it was possible to demonstrate a sizable increase in the content of alanine in toad brain tissues incubating in a hyperosmotic, aerated Ringer-type medium in vitro, this was not the case for aspartic acid (Whiten and Baxter, 1973). All of these results suggest that the mechanism responsible for the adaptive increase of alanine in brain tissue is intrinsic but that the increase in aspartate requires the "turning on" of some mechanism located outside the brain.

## The Role of Urea, Ammonia and Taurine in the Osmotic Regulation of Nervous Tissue

Urea is metabolically related to amino acids and appears to play an important role in the osmotic adaptation of many aquatic animals (McBean and Goldstein, 1967; Jungreis, 1976). It is present

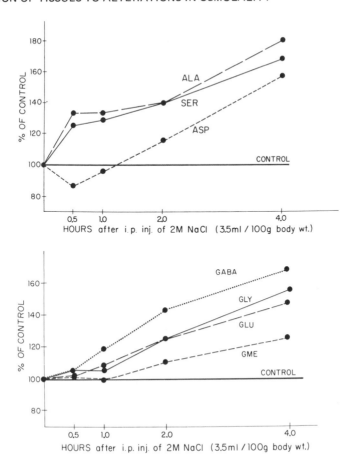

FIGURE 3. Early amino acid changes in toad brain tissues in response to injection of hyperosmotic NaCl.  Saline solutions were
injected into the externalized toad heart (2 M NaCl, 3.5 ml/100 g
body wt.).  The experimental design and analytical methods have
been described (Baxter, 1968; Shank and Aprison, 1970; Shank and
Baxter, 1973).  With proper precautions, toads with externalized
hearts survive in the laboratory for weeks without apparent dis-
comfort.  They eat, mate and behave like normal toads with inter-
nalized hearts.  After injection, these toads were placed into
aquaria containing 400 mOs saline solution.  At time periods after
injection (as indicated on the X axis), amino acid levels were
measured in the brain tissues of these animals.  Each experimental
point shown represents the average amino acid level in the brains
of 6 to 10 toads.  Zero time control toads with externalized hearts
and injected with isoosmotic saline solution showed no difference
from normal (FWA) untreated controls.  ALA = alanine; SER = serine;
ASP = aspartate; GABA = γ-aminobutyric acid; GLY = glycine; GLU =
glutamate; GME = glutamine.

in large quantities in the tissues of amphibians including brain and retina (Table II). Its distribution appears to be quite uniform, and levels in brain, retina and plasma are almost identical at most times. The concentration of urea in brain and plasma both under hypo- and hyper-osmotic conditions appears to be correlated linearly with serum osmolality. A somewhat similar observation has been made with dogfish (Alexander et al., 1968). Elevated urea levels in the hyperosmotically-adapting toad could increase the transport and metabolism of amino acids entering the brain (Amos and Harvey, 1969; Rapoport, 1976; Pickard et al., 1977). However, when the levels of urea in the hyperosmotically-adapting toad were prevented from rising and levels actually decreased in blood and brain, the levels of amino acids in brain tissue continued to rise (Baxter and Shank, 1973). On the basis of these experiments, it seems unlikely that there is a decisive interaction of urea with the mechanisms regulating amino acid levels in brain during hyperosmotic adaptation.

Ammonia production in brain slices incubated in a hyperosmotic medium increases fourfold (Fishman et al., 1977), and glutamine levels are increased tenfold in the brains of fish exposed to an ammonia-containing environment (Levi et al., 1974). Thus, in brain tissues of animals adapting to a hyperosmotic environment, ammonia is assumed to play an important role as a nitrogen donor in the synthesis of amino acids and amines. However, the actual levels of ammonia in the brains both of HOA and HOOA toads remain essentially unchanged from the levels found in the brains of FWA toads. Therefore, despite its metabolic importance, ammonia is unimportant as a component of the "idiogenic osmoles."

Taurine is present in the brain of most species at very high concentrations (Jacobsen and Smith, 1968) and at even higher concentrations in the retina (Orr et al., 1976a,b). In the toad, where taurine is present at somewhat lower levels, this amino acid does not appear to participate in the regulation of brain tissue osmolality. Some authors have found evidence to suggest that taurine participates as an osmoregulator in muscle tissue (Lynch and Wood, 1966; Vincent-Marique and Gilles, 1970; Lasserre and Gilles, 1971; Colley et al., 1974). However, the most recent evidence casts taurine in the role of a non-participant during osmoregulation of muscle tissue - at least in teleosts (Ahokas and Sorg, 1977).


ARE IONIC OR OSMOTIC MECHANISMS INVOLVED IN THE INDUCTION OF THE BIOCHEMICAL CHANGES OBSERVED IN THE HOA TOAD BRAIN?

The publications of various investigators leave little doubt of their belief that inorganic ionic mechanisms (predominantly $Na^+$ and $Cl^-$) are acting directly upon specific enzyme systems to regulate amino acid metabolism (Gilles, 1969, 1974; Wickes and Morgan, 1976), urea cycle enzymes (McBean and Goldstein, 1967; Sharma, 1969;

Balinsky et al., 1972a), and Krebs cycle enzymes (Ramamurthi, 1966;
Sarkissian and Boatwright, 1974) during periods of osmotic adaptation.  Other authors investigating the effect of salt concentrations
upon enzymes of the urea cycle and energy metabolism have been more
cautious by referring to the effects as osmotically- rather than
ionically-induced (Watts and Watts, 1966; Atsmon and Davis, 1967;
Gilles and Jöbsis, 1972; Colley et al., 1972).

An attempt was made to determine whether ionic or osmotic
mechanisms initiate the biochemical changes seen in the brain tissues
of toads adapting to a hyperosmotic environment (Baxter and Baldwin,
1975).  In short-term studies (4 h), toads were injected intraperitoneally with hypertonic solutions of either NaCl (ionic) or mannitol
(non-ionic).  Results are shown in Table III, and experimental details are recorded in the Table footnote and in the legend for
Figure 3.

Identical, elevated serum osmolalities were found in both
groups of experimental toads.  The $Na^+$ levels in brain and blood
were elevated substantially in the NaCl-treated toads but were unchanged or slightly below normal in the mannitol-treated toads.  Yet,
despite the lack of an increase in $Na^+$ ion in the brain or plasma of
the mannitol-injected toads, the changes in amino acid patterns are
very similar to the changes observed in the NaCl-injected toads.

The experiment suggests but does not prove conclusively that
the adaptive regulation of amino acid levels in the brains of HOA
toads is primarily dependent upon osmotically-activated mechanisms.

### Hormones, Putative Neurotransmitters and
### Second Messengers in Osmoregulatory Processes

The role of neurohypophyseal, antidiuretic hormones in the regulation of water metabolism both in mammals and amphibians is well
established (Sawyer, 1964).  A role for these hormones in the adaptation of amphibians and mammals to high environmental salinities
has been suggested (Katz and Weisberg, 1971; Pavel and Coculescu,
1972).  There are delicate interrelationships between neurohypophyseal hormones, putative neurotransmitters and cyclic nucleotides
(Eggena et al., 1970).  Specific effects of these hormones on the
nervous system have been reviewed (Severs and Daniels-Severs, 1973),
and relationships between a hypertonic internal environment and
these hormones also have been documented (Andersson and Westbye,
1970; George, 1976).  In addition, corticosteroids may contribute to
osmoregulation (Jungreis et al., 1970).  It is quite possible that
some of these hormones are involved directly or indirectly in the
metabolic changes seen in brain tissues during osmotic adaptation.
It is known, for example, that the injection of vasotocin into the
amphibian Bufo bufo mobilizes blood glucose in a way that is identical to the injection of a solution of hypertonic saline (Bentley,
1965).  The delays in the onset of some metabolic changes (Figure 3)

also suggest such a possibility.  A full discussion of this topic
is outside of the scope of this chapter.

TABLE III.   EARLY (4 h)ADAPTIVE RESPONSE OF AMINO ACID
             LEVELS IN TOAD BRAIN TO SUDDEN IONIC AND NON-
             IONIC HYPEROSMOTIC CHANGE IN BLOOD PLASMA IN VIVO[a]

| | Adapting to hyperosmotic | |
| | NaCl | Mannitol |
| | % of control (FWA) values[b] | |
| Serum osmolality[b] | 171 | 169 |
| Brain Na$^+$ [b] | 139 | 91 |
| Serum Na$^+$ [b] | 126 | 74 |
| Alanine | 180 | 165 |
| Aspartate | 157 | 142 |
| Glutamate | 147 | 132 |
| GABA | 162 | 122 |
| Glutamine | 123 | 100 |
| Serine | 167 | 173 |
| Glycine | 154 | 148 |

[a]Four identical groups of experimental toads were used.  One
group was injected i.p. with 2 M NaCl (3.5 ml/100 g body
wt.) and a second group with 0.9 M mannitol (15.6 ml/100g
body wt.).  Of the two control groups, one was injected
with 0.25 M mannitol (15.6 ml/100 g body wt.) and the other
remained uninjected.  Since the results from both control
groups were identical, they are treated as one group.  In
subsequent experiments, i.v. and intracardiac injections
(see Figure 3) produced identical results.  At the end of
the 4-h adaptation period, toads were decapitated and the
brains excised and hemisected in the cold.  One-half of
each brain was analyzed for amino acids as previously described (Shank and Baxter, 1973).  The other half was homogenized in 5% TCA and the extract analyzed for Na$^+$ and K$^+$
using flame photometry.
[b]All results are expressed in terms of the levels found in
the fresh water adapted control groups.  Actual levels of
amino acids in FWA toad brain are shown in Table I.  The
osmolality of the serum in untreated FWA toads was 233 mOs
with a corresponding Na$^+$ concentration of 119 mequiv/kg.
The Na$^+$ concentration in the brain of untreated toads averaged 58 mequiv/kg.

## WHAT ARE THE ORIGINS OF THE CARBON ATOMS COMPRISING THE NEW AMINO ACIDS ACCUMULATING IN NERVOUS TISSUES DURING HYPEROSMOTIC ADAPTATION?

### Transport Into Nervous Tissues

The exact origin of the carbon skeleton for amino acids accumulating in brain tissues of the toad adapting to a hyperosmotic environment is not known. Such carbon atoms could originate from outside the brain and be transported into the brain tissue at a faster rate (or carried out at a slower rate) during periods of hyperosmotic adaptation. Since it is generally believed that mechanisms for the

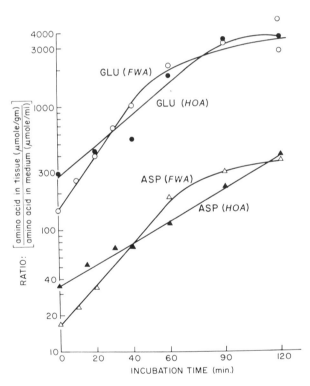

FIGURE 4. Uptake in vitro of glutamate and aspartate by brains from FWA and HOA toads: Establishment of concentration gradient in vitro. For some experimental details, see footnote of Table IV. There was no preincubation in these experiments which were conducted as previously described (Shank et al., 1973) but for different periods of incubation.

transport of amino acids in and out of the brain are primary deter-
minants of amino acid levels within the brain (Lajtha, 1974), the
rates of amino acid uptake into the brain tissues of the toad Bufo
boreas were studied (Shank et al., 1973). A comparison of glutamate
uptake in vitro into hemisected brains of HOA and FWA toads has been
reported also (Shank and Baxter, 1975). When the HOA toad brain was
incubated in a medium that simulated the extracellular fluid both
in ionic and osmotic composition, the transport of glutamate was
not enhanced. Uptake was tested also for a variety of other amino
acids.

High- and low-affinity uptake could be distinguished in 5-min
uptake studies at 25°C. The methods used in this study with $[^{14}C]$-
labeled amino acids are those described by Logan and Snyder (1972)
and Balcar and Johnston (1972) as well as other investigators. The
ability to concentrate glutamate and aspartate against unusually
large concentration gradients is the same both in FWA and HOA toad
brains (Figure 4). A summary of Km and Vmax for both high- and low-
affinity uptake of four amino acids (as calculated from the experimental data) is shown in Table IV. The Km and Vmax for the high-
affinity uptake are similar for FWA and HOA toad brains. The Km
and Vmax for the low-affinity uptake of glutamate, GABA and leucine
are significantly altered in the HOA brains. Low-affinity uptake
has been equated with exchange diffusion (Benjamin and Quastel,
1976). According to such an interpretation, the altered low-
affinity Km and Vmax are the result of the very much higher tissue
levels of these amino acids in the HOA toad brains, rather than a
function of altered membrane transport parameters.

The results have no bearing upon possible regulatory changes
in the transport of amino acids across the blood-brain barrier. The
movement of a variety of substances across the blood-brain barrier
can be altered in vivo by changes in environmental osmolality
(Gerard and Gilles, 1972b; Rapoport and Thompson, 1973; Sterrett et
al., 1974; Treherne et al., 1977; Pickard et al., 1977). The possible alteration of this barrier in the toad adapting to a hyperosmotic environment is a distinct possibility. It is presently under
investigation.


## Source of Essential Amino Acids in Brain Tissues

In the normal mammalian brain, essential amino acids appear to
be taken up more effectively than other amino acids (Oldendorf,
1971). Results from experiments conducted with crustacean nerve in
vitro have been interpreted to indicate that during osmotic adaptation, the levels of essential amino acids in brain tissue are regulated by changes in membrane permeability (Gilles and Schoffeniels,
1969; Gilles and Gerard, 1974). In studies with leucine, this
effect was not observed at the tissue membrane level of the toad
brain (Table IV). It remains to be seen whether such regulation
takes place at the level of the blood-brain barrier.

TABLE IV.  THE HIGH-AND LOW-AFFINITY UPTAKE OF AMINO ACIDS
INTO TISSUES OF HEMISECTED BRAIN IN VITRO OF TOADS
ADAPTED IN VIVO TO EITHER A FRESH WATER (FWA) OR A
400 mOs SALINE (HOA) ENVIRONMENT[a]

| Amino Acid | Toad Condition | Apparent $K_m$ $\mu M$ | | Apparent $V_{max}$ $\mu mol/g/min$ | |
|---|---|---|---|---|---|
| | | HIGH | LOW | HIGH | LOW |
| Glutamate | FWA | 167 | 1100 | 0.36 | 1.25 |
| | HOA | 143 | 500 | 0.27 | 0.77 |
| Aspartate | FWA | 23 | 200 | 0.06 | 0.33 |
| | HOA | 22 | 333 | 0.05 | 0.33 |
| GABA | FWA | 104 | 1000 | 0.12 | 0.50 |
| | HOA | 111 | 714 | 0.12 | 0.42 |
| Leucine | FWA | 200 | 2000 | 0.10 | 0.50 |
| | HOA | 222 | 588 | 0.11 | 0.25 |

[a]The preparation of the hemisected brains, the viability of
this system and the details of the incubation conditions
have been described elsewhere (Shank et al., 1973, 1975;
Shank and Baxter, 1975).  The uptake studies were conducted
essentially as described by Logan and Snyder (1972) and
Balcar and Johnston (1972).  Brain tissues were preincubated without labeled amino acid for 5 min at 25°C.  The
labeled amino acid and amino acid carrier were added so
that the final amino acid concentration in incubation tubes
ranged from 10 to 1000$\mu$M. Uptake was measured during a 5-
min incubation period at 25°C.  Uptake was stopped and tissues analyzed as already described (Shank and Baxter, 1975).

The higher concentration of "free," essential amino acids in
brain tissues of HOA toads indicates that either inside or outside
of their brain tissues, some essential amino acids are becoming
available more rapidly or are utilized more slowly.  Since a more
plentiful dietary supply of these amino acids in the HOA toad seems
to be excluded by the postabsorptive condition of the experimental
animals, the most likely source appeared to be from an enhanced degradation of proteins and peptides.  This hypothesis was tested by
measuring the effect of hyperosmotic adaptation on some proteolytic
activities in brain and liver of the toad Bufo boreas.  A summary of
the most pertinent results is shown in Table V.  Neither the protein

TABLE V.  PROTEOLYTIC AND AMINOPEPTIDASE ACTIVITY IN BRAIN AND LIVER TISSUES OF NORMAL (FWA) AND HYPEROSMOTICALLY-ADAPTED (HOA) TOADS[a]

| | Brain | | Liver | |
|---|---|---|---|---|
| | FWA | HOA | FWA | HOA |
| Total tissue wet wt. per organ | 62 mg (± 6) | 57 mg (± 7) | 1.44 g (± 0.2) | 0.65 (± 0.07) |
| Protein content mg/g tissue | 105 | 122 | 164 | 228 |
| $\mu$mol/g tissue protein/h | | | | |
| Acid proteolysis[b] pH 3.2 | 122 (± 12) | 90 (± 13) | 377 (± 72) | 477 (± 78) |
| Neutral proteolysis[c] pH 7.6 | 252 (± 70) | 211 (± 114) | 116 (± 30) | 140 (± 33) |
| Aminopeptidase[c] pH 7.6 | 2032 (± 161) | 2240 (± 176) | 4760 (± 1074) | 6442 (± 764) |

[a]Brains and livers used for these analyses were removed immediately after decapitation. They were homogenized in 9 volumes of 10 mM potassium phosphate buffer, pH 7.6, containing 0.2% Triton X100. The data in this Table are based upon experiments with eight toads.

[b]Acidic proteolytic activity was measured in citrate buffer, pH 3.2, with denatured hemoglobin as substrate by the method of Serra et al. (1972) as modified by Marks et al. (1975). Results are expressed as $\mu$mol of tyrosine equivalent formed/g tissue protein/h (± SD).

[c]Neutral proteolytic activity as well as aminopeptidase activity were measured according to the methods of Marks and Lajtha (1970) and Boehme et al. (1974) using denatured hemoglobin and leucylglycylglycine as substrates. Results are expressed as  mol of glycine equivalent formed/g of tissue protein/h (± SD).

content per brain nor the proteolytic activities measured in brain
tissues are significantly different in FWA as compared to HOA toads.
Even the increased activity (per unit of liver protein) in HOA toads
is small when compared to the loss of water from their livers.   Calculations from the data provided in Table V indicate that in HOA
toads, the proteolytic capacity per whole liver was less than in the
FWA control animals.   Thus, the methods employed did not reveal any
evidence to support the belief that an altered proteolytic activity
in brain or liver contributed to the elevated levels of essential
amino acids in the nervous tissues of the HOA toads.

The observation that the protein content of brain tissues
appears to be unaffected by hyperosmotic adaptation is in agreement
with a preliminary result obtained by different methods (Shank and
Baxter, 1973).   Recent studies with crustaceans adapting to a hyperosmotic environment suggest that the additional essential amino acids
are generated by a more rapid breakdown of blood proteins (Gilles,
1977).   This possibility remains untested in the toad.

## Sources of Non-Essential Amino Acids:
## Glycolysis and Related Reactions

There are a variety of ways in which carbon skeletons for additional amino acids in the HOA toad brain could become available.
Initially, an increased rate of glycogen breakdown could provide the
carbon atoms.   Subsequently, a decreased rate of glucose utilization
for energy metabolism and possibly an enhanced rate of $CO_2$ fixation
might assure the maintenance of the higher levels of amino acids
(providing, of course, that there is an ample source of amino
groups).   Studies have been conducted on a variety of enzymes leading from glycogen to amino acids to show that ionic or osmotic concentrations can regulate key enzymes along this pathway.   The levels
of glucose, lactate pyruvate and α-ketoglutarate in brain and the
levels of glycogen in liver and brain are shown for the FWA and HOA
toad (Table VI).   Although the glycogen content of amphibian brain is
much higher than that found in mammals (Passonneau and Lauderdale,
1974), there is no significant alteration in the glycogen content of
the HOA toad brain.   By contrast, the glycogen content in the livers
of HOA toads was drastically reduced.   (Since the wet wt. of the
livers in HOA toads is usually less than one-half that of livers in
FWA toads, the glycogen mobilization is even greater than it would
appear at first sight.)   The increased glycogenolysis in the liver
but not in brain of HOA toads follows the pattern (mentioned
earlier) for tyrosine aminotransferase which is activated also in
liver but not in brain.   It represents a much greater adaptability
(plasticity) of enzymes of liver tissue when compared with the same
enzymes in brain.   This same observation has been made by other investigators who have compared circadian rhythms and nutritional responses of brain and liver enzymes (Fuller, 1970; Benuck and Lajtha,
1974).   In HOA toads, the precipitous drop in liver glycogen is not

related to nutrition. The FWA and HOA toads both were postabsorptive during the period of hyperosmotic adaptation. Glucose levels
in the brain tissues of the HOA toad were elevated, thereby contributing to the osmolality of the HOA brain tissue. These observations
confirm similar studies from another laboratory (Jurss and Schlisio,
1975).

The levels of lactate and pyruvate in the HOA toad brains were
essentially the same as those found in FWA toad brains; the levels
of α-ketoglutarate were only marginally different in the HOA toad
brain as compared with the FWA toad brain. Such results agree with
the findings of other investigators: that key enzymes such as
citrate synthetase and pyruvate kinase (Sarkissian and Boatwright,
1975; Wickes and Morgan, 1976) remain unchanged in osmoconformers
adapting to hyperosmotic conditions. However, this lack of response does not apply to at least one of these enzymes in aquatic
osmoregulators (Sarkissian and Boatwright, 1974) and may not reflect the behavior of these enzymes in mammalian brain.

TABLE VI.   LEVELS OF GLYCOGEN, GLUCOSE AND SOME METABOLIC
            PRODUCTS IN FWA AND HOA TOADS

| Substance | Organ | Toads | | Adaptation |
| | | FWA | HOA | |
| | | μmol/g wet wt. | | Δ% |
| Glycogen[a] | Brain | 12.1 | 11.8 | NS[c] |
| Glycogen[a] | Liver | 284[b] | 166[b] | -42 |
| Glucose | Brain | 1.14 | 2.84 | +149 |
| Lactate | ↓ | 1.21 | 1.12 | NS |
| Pyruvate | | 0.078 | 0.086 | NS |
| α-ketoglutarate | | 0.073 | 0.057 | -22 |

[a]The measurement of glycogen in brain and liver tissues of
amphibians is complicated by a soluble glycogen fraction
(McDougal et al., 1963) which requires a modified analysis.
The values given are for total glycogen, including both
soluble and insoluble fractions. Although there were large
seasonal variations in the glycogen content of toad liver,
the differences in glycogen content between FWA and HOA
toads could be demonstrated at all times, but not always to
the same extent.
[b]Expressed as glucose equivalents.
[c]NS = not significant (P > 0.1).

The effect of osmotic adaptation upon overall energy metabolism is not clear. Experiments with a large variety of osmoconformers have saturated the literature with inconsistent results. Whether this reflects the nutritional state of the different invertebrate species at the time of testing or some other unknown variable, or represents a basic difference in the different osmoconformers is not known. Based upon rather limited data, hyperosmotic adaptation in the toad Bufo boreas appears to be accompanied by a downward shift in nervous tissues of NAD/NADP ratios, ATP levels and phosphocreatine content. However, this shift is extremely small when compared to the shifts observed under anoxic conditions in brain tissues (Norberg and Siesjö, 1975), and glucose utilization by brain tissues of FWA and HOA toads did not appear to be significantly different (Shank and Baxter, 1973).

### Changes in Urea Cycle Enzymes and Products as a Consequence of Hyper- and Hypo-Osmotic Adaptation

The accumulation of urea in amphibians adapting to a hyperosmotic environment is well documented. Whereas a variety of mechanisms appear to be responsible for the initial urea elevation (Colley et al., 1972; Balinsky et al., 1972a,b), the effect of long-term adaptation to salinity appears to be correlated in the liver with an elevation of a select group of enzyme activities (Balinsky et al., 1972b; McBean and Goldstein, 1967; Watts and Watts, 1966; Janssens and Cohen, 1968). In brain tissues of the HOA toad, ornithine, citrulline and ammonia levels appear elevated while arginine levels are depressed. Since the activities of some of the urea cycle enzymes in brain are extremely low, it is likely that the metabolic alterations responsible for the altered levels of the urea-ornithine cycle intermediates occur outside the nervous system.

## SOME GENERAL COMMENTS ABOUT AMINO ACIDS AND OSMOTIC ADAPTATION

### Localization

The participation of nitrogenous and other organic molecules in the regulation of osmolality in nervous system tissues raises a variety of questions. One of the most obvious concerns the localization of the extra nitrogenous molecules that accumulate in the brains of HOA toads or that are lost from the brains of HOOA toads. Compartmentation would have to be invoked to explain the large increases of so many putative neurotransmitters (and their precursors) with little apparent affect on the behavior of HOA toads. Even in man, where hyperosmotic adaptation is accompanied by some neurological abnormalities and deficits, it is likely that most of the increased

number of putative neurotransmitter molecules are not being stored
at sites of their neuronal action.  It is tempting to suggest that
glial cells are the major sites for the storage and accumulation of
the "idiogenic osmoles," and methods are being devised which should
permit the testing of this hypothesis.  It will be necessary to
ascertain whether neurons, glia and other cell types in the nervous
system adapt to an altered osmotic environment via different regulatory and biochemical mechanisms.

### Some Alternate Methods for the Regulation of "Free" Amino Acid Levels in Brain Tissues

Throughout this chapter, emphasis has been placed upon the additional carbon and nitrogen sources that must be found to account
for the elevated "idiogenic osmoles" in the HOA toad brain.  The
possibility that this buildup is the result of decreased utilization
of these compounds for synthetic and energy metabolism has received
scant attention, although it constitutes a real possibility.  Similarly, the osmotic regulation of the efflux of amino acids from
brain tissues deserves more careful consideration, both at the tissue level and at the level of the blood-brain barrier.

Several potential sources for an extra supply of carbon and
nitrogen atoms in the hyperosmotically-adapting toad have not been
considered in this chapter.  Among others, these include the purines,
$CO_2$ fixation and short-chain fatty acids.  There are suggestions from
related experiments in the literature that these compounds and related
biochemical mechanisms could be involved in osmotic regulation.

No distinction has been made - except incidentally - between
short-term and long-term adaptation to an altered osmotic environment
(i.e. glycogen mobilization may be a short-term effect while induction of urea-ornithine cycle enzymes in the liver may be a long-term
effect).  Other authors have suggested that such a distinction should
be made.  The possibility exists also that some of the osmotically-
triggered changes in amino acid metabolism and transport are more
closely related to the slight drop in the blood pH of the HOA toad.

The toad brain has proven to be a most convenient model for
studying the identities, the origins and the regulation of "idiogenic
osmoles" in the nervous system.  Since all available evidence suggests that the amino acid constituents of the "idiogenic osmoles" in
mammalian brain are similar and are regulated by similar mechanisms,
the brain of Bufo boreas would appear to be also a most appropriate
model for this study.

### ACKNOWLEDGEMENTS

Aside from those individuals acknowledged for their contribution
by authorship in our publications, we would like to thank Dr. C. Leo
Ortiz, Dr. Arthur Yuwiler, Dr. Paul B. Hamilton, Mr. Benjamin Chang,

Mr. Ronald Burkholder, Ms. Sandra Murray, Mr. Joseph Ravida and
Mr. John Bright for their indispensable collaboration and technical
support. We gratefully acknowledge the editorial and administrative
support provided by Ms. Louise Eaton, not only in the preparation of
this manuscript but also in facilitating the overall project. Administrative support was received also from the Brain Research Institute
and the Neuropsychiatric Institute of the Center for the Health
Sciences at UCLA as well as the Division of Neurosciences, City of
Hope National Medical Center, Duarte, Calif. This research was supported in part by the Medical Research Service of the Veterans
Administration and by USPHS grant #NS03743 from the National Institute of Neurological and Communicative Disorders and Stroke.

## REFERENCES

Ahokas, R. A., and Sorg, G., 1977, The effect of salinity and
temperature on intracellular osmoregulation and muscle free
amino acids in Fundulus diaphanus, Comp. Biochem. Physiol.
56(A):101-105.

Alexander, M. D., Haselwood, E. S., Haselwood, G. A. D., Watts,
D. C., and Watts, R. L., 1968, Osmotic control and urea biosynthesis in selachians, Comp. Biochem. Physiol. 26:971-978.

Amos, H., and Harvey, M. L., 1969, Induction of glutamine synthetase
by urea, Biochem. Biophys. Res. Comm. 35:280-287.

Andersson, B., and Westbye, O., 1970, Synergistic action of sodium
and angiotensin on brain mechanisms controlling fluid balance,
Life Sci. 9:601-608.

Arieff, A. I., and Guisado, R., 1976, Effects on the central nervous
system of hyper- and hypo-natremic states, Kidney Int. 10:41-53.

Arieff, A. I., Kleeman, C. R., Keushkerian, A., and Bagdoyan, H.,
1972, Brain tissue osmolality: Method of determination and
variation in hyper- and hypo-osmolar states, J. Lab. Clin. Med.
79:334-343.

Arieff, A. I., Massry, S. G., Barrientos, A., and Kleeman, C. R.,
1973, Brain water and electrolyte metabolism in uremia: Effects
of slow and rapid hemodialysis, Kidney Int. 4:177-187.

Atsmon, A., and Davis, R. P., 1967, Mitochondrial respiration under
conditions of varying osmolarity, Biochim. Biophys. Acta 131:
221-233.

Balcar, V. J., and Johnston, G. A. R., 1972, The structural specificity of the high affinity uptake of L-glutamate and L-aspartate
by rat brain slices, J. Neurochem. 19:2657-2666.

Balinsky, J. B., Coetzer, T. L., and Mattheyse, F. J., 1972a, The
effect of thyroxine and hypertonic environment on the enzymes of
the urea cycle in Xenopus laevis, Comp. Biochem. Physiol. 43(B):
83-95.

Balinsky, J. B., Dicker, S. E., and Elliott, A. B., 1972b, The effect
of long-term adaptation to different levels of salinity on urea

synthesis and tissue amino acid concentrations in Rana cancrivora, Comp. Biochem. Physiol. 43(B):71-82.

Baxter, C. F., 1968, Intrinsic amino acid levels and the blood-brain barrier, in "Progress in Brain Research," Vol. 29 (A. Lajtha and D. H. Ford, eds.), pp. 429-444, Elsevier, Amsterdam.

Baxter, C. F., and Baldwin, R. A., 1975, Adaptation to environmental osmolality: Apparent non-ionic induction of elevated amino acid levels in the brain of the toad Bufo boreas, Trans. Am. Soc. Neurochem. 6:96.

Baxter, C. F., and Ortiz, C. L., 1966, Amino acids and the maintenance of osmotic equilibrium in brain tissue, Life Sci. 5:2321-2329.

Baxter, C. F., and Shank, R. P., 1973, Mechanisms in the regulation of amino acids and related metabolites of brain tissues in a hyperosmotic environment, Int. Soc. Neurochem. Abst. 4:349.

Benga, G., and Morariu, V. V., 1977, Membrane defect affecting water permeability in human epilepsy, Nature (London) 265:636-638.

Benjamin, A. M., and Quastel, J. H., 1976, Cerebral uptakes and exchange diffusion in vitro of L- and D-glutamates, J. Neurochem. 26:431-441.

Benson, J. R., 1974, Single-column analysis of amino acids; biological fluids analyzed in five hours, Durrum Resin Report No. 5.

Benson, J. R., and Hare, P. E., 1975, O-Phtalaldehyde: Fluorgenic detection of primary amines in the picomole range. Comparison with fluorescamine and ninhydrin, Proc. Natl. Acad. Sci. U.S.A. 72:619-622.

Bentley, P. J., 1965, Hyperglycaemic effect of vasotocin in toads, Nature (London) 206:1053-1054.

Benuck, M., and Lajtha, A., 1974, The effect of elevated amino acids on aminotransferase levels in brain and liver of the mouse, J. Neurochem. 23:553-559.

Birkmayer, W., Neumayer, E., Stöckl, W., and Weiler, C., 1969, in "Das Depressive Syndrom" (H. Hippius and H. Selbach, eds.), Urban and Schwarzberg, Munich.

Black, I. B., and Axelrod, J., 1968, Regulation of the daily rhythm in tyrosine transaminase activity by environmental factors, Proc. Natl. Acad. Sci. U.S.A. 61:1287-1291.

Boehme, D. H., Fordice, M. W., and Marks, N., 1974, Proteolytic activity in brain and spinal cord in sensitive and resistant strains of rat and mouse subjected to experimental allergic encephalomyelitis, Brain Res. 75:153-162.

Colley, L., Fox, F. R., and Huggins, A. K., 1974, The effects of changes in external salinity on the non-protein nitrogenous constituents of parietal muscle from Agonus cataphractus, Comp. Biochem. Physiol. 48(A):757-763.

Colley, L., Rowe, W. C., Huggins, A. K., Elliott, A. B., and Dicker, S. E., 1972, The effect of short-term changes in the external salinity on the levels of the non-protein nitrogenous compounds and the ornithine-urea cycle enzymes in Rana cancrivora, Comp. Biochem. Physiol. 41(B):307-322.

Coppen, A. J., 1969, Disorders of mineral metabolism on depressive
    patients, Psychiat. Neurol. Neurochir. 72:189-193.
Coppen, A. J., and Shaw, D. M., 1963, Mineral metabolism in melan-
    cholia, Br. Med. J. 5370:1439-1445.
Coppen, A. J., Shaw, D. M., Malleson, A., and Costain, R., 1966,
    Mineral metabolism in mania, Br. Med. J. 5479:71-75.
Dalton, K., 1961, Menstruation and crime, Br. Med. J. 5269:1752-1753.
Eggena, P., Schwartz, I. L., and Walter, R., 1970, Threshold and re-
    ceptor reserve in the action of neurohypophyseal peptides, J.
    Gen. Physiol. 56:250-271.
Elkinton, J. R., Danowsky, T. S., and Winkler, A. W., 1946, Hemo-
    dynamic changes in salt depletion and in dehydration, J. Clin.
    Invest. 25:120-129.
Finberg, L., Luttrell, C., and Redd, H., 1959, Pathogenesis of
    lesions in the nervous system in hypernatremic states: experi-
    mental studies of gross anatomic changes and alterations of
    chemical composition of the tissues, Pediatrics 23:46-53.
Fishman, R. A., Reiner, M., and Chan, P. H., 1977, Metabolic changes
    associated with iso-osmotic regulation in brain cortex slices,
    J. Neurochem. 28:1061-1067.
Fuller, R. W., 1970, Differences in the regulation of tyrosine amino-
    transferase in brain and liver, J. Neurochem. 17:539-543.
Geller, E., Yuwiler, A., and Schapiro, S., 1969, Tyrosine aminotrans-
    ferase: Activation or repression by a stress, Proc. Soc. Exp.
    Biol. Med. 130:458-461.
George, J. M., 1976, Vasopressin and oxytocin are depleted from rat
    hypothalamic nuclei after oral hypertonic saline, Science 193:
    146-148.
Gerard, J. F., and Gilles, R., 1972a, The free amino-acid pool in
    Callinectes sapidus (Rathbun) tissues and its role in the osmotic
    intracellular regulation, J. Exp. Mar. Biol. Ecol. 10:125-136.
Gerard, J. F., and Gilles, R., 1972b, Modification of the amino-acid
    efflux during the osmotic adjustment of isolated axons of
    Callinectes sapidus, Experientia 28:863-864.
Gilles, R., 1969, Effect of various salts on the activity of enzymes
    implicated in amino-acid metabolism, Arch. Int. Physiol. Biochem.
    77:441-464.
Gilles, R., 1974, Studies on the effect of NaCl on the activity of
    Eriocheir sinesis glutamate dehydrogenase, Int. J. Biochem. 5:
    623-628.
Gilles, R., 1977, Effects of osmotic stresses on the proteins
    concentration and pattern of Eriocheir sinesis blood, Comp.
    Biochem. Physiol. 56(A):109-114.
Gilles, R., and Gerard, J. F., 1974, Amino-acid metabolism during
    osmotic stress in isolated axons of Callinectes sapidus, Life
    Sci. 14:1221-1229.
Gilles, R., and Jóbsis, F. F., 1972, Isoosmotic intracellular regu-
    lation and redox changes in the respiratory chain components of
    Callinectes sapidus isolated muscle fibers, Life Sci. 11:877-885.
Gilles, R., and Schoffeniels, E., 1969, Isosmotic regulation in

isolated surviving nerves of Eriocheir sinensis Milne Edwards,
   Comp. Biochem. Physiol, 31;927-939.
Gordon, M.S., 1965, Intracellular osmoregulation in skeletal muscle
   during salinity adaptation in two species of toads, Biol. Bull.,
   12:218-229.
Hamilton, P.B., 1962, Ion exchange chromatography of amino acids-
   microdetermination of free amino acids in serum, Ann. N.Y. Acad.
   Sci., 102:55-57.
Holliday, M.A., Kalyci, M.N., and Harrah, J., 1968, Factors that
   limit brain volume changes in response to acute and sustained
   hyper- and hypo-natremia, J. Clin. Invest., 47:1916-1923.
Holowach-Thurston, J., Hauhart, R.E., Jones, E.M., and Ater, J.L.,
   1975, Effect of salt and water loading on carbohydrate and
   energy metabolism and levels of selected amino acids in the
   brains of young mice, J. Neurochem., 24:953-957.
Hullin, R.P., Bailey, A.D., McDonald, R., Dransfield, G.A., and
   Milne, H.B., 1967, Variations in body water during recovery
   from depression, Br. J. Psychiatry, 113:573-583.
Jacobsen, J.G., and Smith, L.H. Jr., 1968, Biochemistry and physiology of taurine and taurine derivatives, Physiol. Rev., 48:
   424-511.
Janssens, P.A., and Cohen, P.P., 1968, Biosynthesis of urea in the
   estivating African Lungfish and in Xenopus laevis under condi-
   tions of water shortage, Comp. Biochem. Physiol., 24:887-898.
Jungreis, A.M., 1976, Partition of excretory nitrogen in amphibia,
   Comp. Biochem. Physiol., 53(A):133-141.
Jungreis, A.M., Huibregtse, W.H., and Ungar, F., 1970, Corticoster-
   oid identification and corticosterone concentration in serum of
   Rana pipiens during dehydration in winter and summer, Comp.
   Biochem. Physiol., 34:683-689.
Jürss, K., and Schlisio, W., 1975. Osmo- and Ionenregulation von
   Xenopus laevis Daud. nach Adaption in verschiedenen osmotisch
   wirksamen Lösungen. IV. Veränderung der Stickstoffexcretion,
   Harnstoff- und Glycogenkonzentration der Lever sowie des Blut-
   zuckers, Zool. Jahrb. Abt. Allg. Zool. Physiol., 79:1-8.
Katz, U., and Weisberg, J., 1971, Role of skin and neurohypophyseal
   hormones in the adaptation of the toad Bufo viridis to high sa-
   linities, Nature (London), 232:344-345.
Katzman, R., and Pappius, H.M., 1973, "Brain Electrolytes and Fluid
   Metabolism", Williams & Wilkins, Baltimore.
Lajtha, A., 1974, Amino acid transport in the brain in vivo and in
   vitro, in Aromatic Amino Acids in the Brain, Ciba Found. Symp.
   22:25-49.
Lasserre, P., and Gilles, R., 1971, Modification of the amino acid
   pool in the parietal muscle of two euryhaline teleosts during
   osmotic adjustment, Experientia, 27:1434-1435.
Levi, G., Morosi, G., Coletti, A., and Catanzaro, R., 1974, Free
   amino acids in fish brain:  Normal levels and changes upon
   exposure to high ammonia concentrations in vivo, and upon

exposure to high ammonia concentrations in vivo, and upon incubation of brain slices, Comp. Biochem. Physiol., 49(A): 623-626.

Logan, W.J., and Snyder, S.H., 1972, High affinity uptake systems for glycine, glutamic and aspartic acids in synaptosomes of rat central nervous tissues, Brain Res., 42:413-431.

Lynch, M.P., and Wood, L., 1966, Effects of environmental salinity on free amino acids of Crassostrea virvinica gmelin, Comp. Biochem. Physiol., 19:783-790.

Marks, N., and Ljatha, A., 1970, Brain aminopeptidase hydrolyzing leucylglycylglycine and similar substrates, in "Methods in Enzymology", Vol. 19 (G.E. Perlman and L. Lorand, eds.), pp. 534-543, Academic Press, New York.

Marks, N., Stern, F., and Lajtha, A., 1975, Changes in proteolytic enzymes and proteins during maturation of the rat brain, Brain Res., 86:307-322.

McBean, R.L., and Goldstein, L., 1967, Ornithine-urea cycle activity in Xenopus laevis. Adaptation to saline, Science, 157:931-932.

McDougal, D.B. Jr., Holowach, J., Howe, M.C., Jones, E.M., and Thomas, C.A., 1963, The effects of anoxia upon energy sources and selected metabolic intermediates in the brains of fish, frog and turtle, J. Neurochem., 15:577-588.

McDowell, M.A., Wolf, A.V., and Steer, A., 1955, Osmotic volumes of distribution, idiogenic changes, in osmotic pressure associated with administration of hypertonic solutions, A. J. Physiol., 180:545-558.

Norberg, K., and Siesjö, B.K., 1975, Cerebral metabolism in hypoxic hypoxia. II. Citric acid cycle intermediates and associated amino acids, Brain Res., 86:45-54.

Oldendorf, W.H., 1971, Brain uptake of radiolabelled amino acids, amines and hexoses after arterial injection, Am. J. Physiol., 221:1629-1639.

Olmstead, E.G., 1964, Organic contribution to intracellular osmolarity in rabbits, Arch. Int. Physiol. Biochim., 72:794-798.

Orr, H.T., Cohen, A.I., and Carter, J.A., 1976a, The levels of free taurine, glutamate, glycine and γ-amino butyric acid during the postnatal development of the normal and dystrophic retina of the mouse, Exp. Eye Res., 23:377-384.

Orr, H.T., Cohen, A.I., and Lowry, O.H., 1976b, The distribution of taurine in the vertebrate retine, J. Neurochem., 26:609-611.

Passonneau, J.V., and Lauderdale, V.R., 1974, A comparison of three methods of glycogen measurement in tissues, Anal. Biochem., 60:405-412.

Pavel, S., and Coculescu, M., 1972, Arginine vasotocin-like activity of cerebrospinal fluid induced by injection of hypertonic saline into the third cerebral ventricle of cats, Endocrinology, 91:825-827.

Pichard, J.D., Durity, F., Welsh, F.A., Langfitt, T.W., Murray-Harper, A., and MacKenzie, E.T., 1977, Osmotic opening of the

blood-brain barrier; Value in pharmacological studies on the
    cerebral circulation, Brain Res., 122:170-176.
Ramamurthi, R., 1966, Succinic dehydrogenase activity in a fresh-
    water crab in relation to slainity stress, Comp. Biochem.
    Physiol., 19:645-648.
Rapoport, S.I., 1976, "Blood-Brain Barrier in Physiology and Medi-
    cine", Raven Press, New York.
Rapoport, S.I., and Thompson, H.K., 1973, Osmotic opening of the
    blood-brain barrier in the monkey, without associated neurolo-
    gical deficits, Science, 180:971-973.
Rodrigo, F., Shideman, J., McHugh, R., Buselmeier, T., and
    Kjellstrand, C., 1977, Osmolality changes during hemodialysis,
    Ann. Intern. Med., 86:554-561.
Roth, M., and Hampai, A., 1973, Column chromatography of amino
    acids with fluorescence detection, J. Chromatog., 83:353-356.
Rymer, M., and Fishman, R.A., 1973, Protective adaptation of brain
    to water intoxication, Arch. Neurol., 28:49-54.
Sarkissian, I.V., and Boatwright, D.T., 1974, Regulation by salt
    and by Krebs cycle metabolites of citrate synthetase from an
    osmoregulator, white shrimp Penaeus setiferus and from a non-
    osmoregulator, sea anemone, Bunedosoma cavernata, Comp. Biochem.
    Physiol., 49(B):325-333.
Sarkissian, I.V., and Boatwright, D.T., 1975, Influence of possible
    in situ ionic environment on kinetics of purified citrate syn-
    thetase from an osmoconformer sea anemone Bunedosoma cavernata,
    Enzyme, 19:110-115.
Sawyer, W.H., 1964, Vertebrate neurohypophysial principles,
    Endocrinology, 75:981-990.
Serra, S., Grynbaum, A., Lajtha, A., and Marks, N., 1972, Peptide
    hydrolases in spinal cord and brain of the rabbit, Brain Res,
    44:579-592.
Severs, W.B., and Daniels-Severs, A.E., 1973, Effects of angioten-
    sin on the central nervous system, Pharm. Rev., 25:415-449.
Shank, R.P., and Aprison, M.H., 1970, Methods of multiple analyses
    of concentration and specific radioactivity of amino acids in
    nervous tissue extracts, Anal. Biochem., 35:136-145.
Shank, R.P., and Baxter, C.F., 1973, Metabolism of glucose, amino
    acids, and some related meaabolites in the brain of toads
    (Bufo boreas) adapted to fresh water or hyperosmotic environ-
    ments, J. Neurochem., 21:301-313.
Shank, R.P., and Baxter, C.F., 1975, Uptake and metabolism of gluta-
    mate by isolated toad brains containing different levels of
    endogenous amino acids, J. Neurochem., 24:641-646.
Shank, R.P., Whiten, J.T., and Baxter, C.F., 1973, Glutamate uptake
    by the isolated toad brain, Science, 181:860-862.
Shank, R.P., Whiten, J.T., and Baxter, C.F., 1975, Viability of
    some metabolic processes in the isolated toad brain adapted to
    two osmotic environments, J. Neurobiol., 6:145-157.

Sharma, M.L., 1969, Trigger mechanism of increased urea production by the crayfish Oronectes rusticus under osmotic stress, Comp. Biochem. Physiol., 30:309-321.

Sotos, J.F., Dodge, P.R., Meara, P., and Talbot, N.B., 1960, Studies in experimental hypertonicity. I. Pathogenesis of the clinical syndrome, bichemical abnormalities and cause of death, Pediatrics, 26:925-937.

Sterrett, P.R., Thompson, A.M., Chapman, A.L., and Matzke, H.A., 1974, The effects of hyperosmorarity on the blood-brain barrier. A morphological and physiological correlation, Brain Res., 77:281-295.

Treherne, J.E., Carlson, A.D., and Skaer, H. leB., 1977, Facultative blood-brain barrier and neuronal adaptation to osmotic stress in a marine osmoconformer, Nature (London), 265:550-553.

Vastola, E.F., Maccario, A., and Homan, R., 1967, Activation of epileptogenic foci by hyperosmolality, Neurology, 17:520-526.

Vincent-Marique, C., and Gilles, R., 1970, Modification of the amino acid pool in blood and muscle of Eriocheir sinensis during osmotic stress, Comp. Biochem. Physiol., 35:479-485.

Watts, D.C., and Watts, R.L., 1966, Carbamoyl phosphate synthetase in the elasmobranchii: Osmoregulatory function and evalutionary implications, Comp. Biochem. Physiol., 17:785-798.

Whiten, J.T., and Baxter, C.F., 1973, Changes in amino acid composition of excised toad brain in response to hyperosmotic medium, Proc. Soc. Neurosci., 3:348.

Wickes, M.A., and Morgan, R.P. II, 1976, Effects of salinity on three enzymes involved in amino acid metabolism from the American oyster Crassostrea virginica, Comp. Biochem. Physiol., 53(B):339-343.

# ISOLATION AND BIOCHEMICAL CHARACTERIZATION OF MORPHOLOGICALLY

# DEFINED STRUCTURES, INCLUDING CELL TYPES, FROM THE CEREBELLUM

R. Balázs, J. Cohen, J. Garthwaite and P.L. Woodhams

MRC Developmental Neurobiology Unit
Institute of Neurology, 33 John's Mews
London WC1N 2NS

The heterogeneity of brain tissue presents major difficulties
in evaluating experimental observations on CNS metabolism from the
use of radioactive substrates. Although kinetic studies have permitted the definition of distinct metabolic compartments, the assignment of these to morphological structures rests to a great extent
on circumstantial evidence (see e.g. Berl and Clerk, 1969; Balázs et
al, 1973; Garfinkel, 1973; Cremer et al, 1975; van den Berg et al,
1975). It must be added here how gratifying it is that, with improved
technology, many recent studies of the metabolic properties of
structural components of the brain have supported major points in
the hypothesis developed by a number of workers in the field of
metabolic compartmentation of the tricarboxylic acid cycle and associated amino acids. These include differences in the localization
of the uptake and metabolism of labelled glucose compared to certain
amino acids and fatty acids and in the distribution of certain enzymes
implicated in the transfer of glutamate, GABA and glutamine between
the neuronal and glial constituents in the tissue (Quastel, 1975;
Minchin and Beart, 1975; Voaden et al, 1977; Martinez-Hernandez et
al, 1977; see also Chapter by Bradford, 1978). Nevertheless, in
order to test the hypothetical allocation of metabolic compartments
to structures it is necessary to isolate functioning structural units
from the brain in a pure form. This is evidently an outstandingly
important question in its own right. Knowledge of the biochemical
properties of specific subcellular structures of the brain, and even
more of cell types, is still limited. Our attempts to isolate various
components of the brain are the subject of this report. We have
concentrated our efforts on the 'biochemical dissection' of the
cerebellum; at first we shall consider very briefly a synaptic complex isolated in our laboratory, the cerebellar glomerulus particles,

then recent observations on the isolation of cell types will be
presented in more detail.


## I. GLOMERULUS PARTICLES

The most conspicuous complex in the granular layer of the cerebellum is the glomerulus, the core of which is the giant excitatory
mossy fibre terminal. The mossy fibre rosette is surrounded by the
dendritic digits of the granule cells, which are held together by
frequent puncta adherentia. This conveys to the glomerulus a
certain cohesion, thus facilitating the preservation of this structure when the tissue is disrupted. On the periphery of the dendrites,
the terminals of the inhibitory Golgi axons make synaptic contact.
We have recently succeeded in obtaining a preparation in which
large fragments of the cerebellar glomeruli (glomerulus particles)
accounted for over 90% of the tissue volume (Balázs et al, 1975a;
Hajós et al, 1975), and a similar preparation has been described
by Hamberger et al (1976). The important asset of the preparation
besides its purity, is that the glomerulus particles are composed,
almost exclusively, of a limited number of neuronal processes, which
can be clearly identified using electronmicroscopy (Fig. 1). We
have characterized the preparation in terms of enzyme composition
(Hajós et al, 1974; Tapia, et al, 1975; Balázs et al, 1975a) and
certain functional properties, such as glucose uptake and utilisation
(Wilson et al, 1976), so here only recent studies on the transport of
certain putative transmitter amino acids will be mentioned. Such
studies, as are also employed in mapping specific chemical pathways
in the CNS, are described in detail in Chapter by Kelly. Our investigations emphasise the need for great circumspection in interpretation
and especially for obtaining other evidence to support conclusions
drawn from uptake studies.
The glomerulus particle preparation has provided the opportunity
for testing the hypothesis that a high affinity transport system for
agents is unique to those terminals which function with those agents
as their transmitter (e.g. Logan and Snyder, 1972). Wilson et al
(1976) found that the particles contained both high and low affinity
transport systems for the putative transmitter amino acids, GABA,
glycine, glutamate and aspartate, whereas other amino acids studied
were transported only by low affinity systems. The high affinity
systems, which are $Na^+$- and energy-dependent, showed the highest
$V_{max}$ for GABA and a net accumulation of GABA and glycine in the
particles was demonstrated. The uptake of [$^3H$]GABA was competitively
inhibited by 2,4-diaminobutyric acid (DABA; the $K_I$, about 20$\mu$M, being
very near to the $K_T$ for GABA, 10$\mu$M), while it was little affected by
$\beta$-alanine. These results support the hypothesis that DABA and $\beta$-
alanine are inhibitors of the high affinity GABA uptake in neuronal
and glial structures respectively (Schon and Kelly, 1974). Furthermore electron microscopic autoradiography showed that high affinity

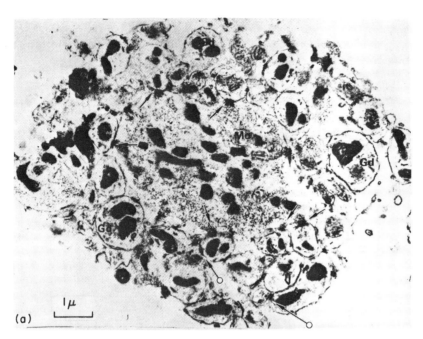

FIGURE 1. Ultrastructural appearance of glomerulus particles: the mossy fibre terminal containing numerous synaptic vesicles and mito-chondria is surrounded by the digits of the granule cell dendrites. Arrows and signed arrows respectively point at synaptic specialisa-tions and interdendritic puncta adhearentia. (From Hajós et al, 1975, by courtesy of J. Neurochem.)

$[^3H]$GABA uptake was selectively localized to the inhibitory Golgi axon terminals (Wilkin et al, 1974), which are also enriched in GAD (McLaughlin et al, 1974) and seem to function with GABA as their transmitter (e.g. Curtis, 1975).

These results indicated that GABA is not accumulated randomly in neuronal structures. However, the observations on glycine have been important to establish the limits of the selectivity of trans-mitter uptake: hitherto no evidence points to glycine as a trans-mitter in the rat cerebellum. The high affinity $[^3H]$glycine uptake in the glomerulus particles is at variance with previous reports on preparations of whole cerebellar tissue (Johnston and Iversen, 1971; Logan and Snyder, 1972), where it seems the great dilution of the relevant structures rendered this process undetectable. Recent kinetic studies by Graham Wilkin and John Wilson indicate that the carrier sites for GABA and glycine are different; they have found that glycine is a non-competetive inhibitor of $[^3H]$GABA transport with a $K_I$ of $600 \mu M$ vs its $K_T$ of $20 \mu M$ and GABA is an extremely weak inhibitor of glycine uptake (the uptake of $10 \mu M$ $[^3H]$glycine was only

inhibited by 17% by 1,5mM GABA). It seems, however, that the high
affinity [3H]glycine uptake is also localized to the Golgi axon
terminals, and preliminary electron microscopic autoradiographic
observations have suggested that [3H] GABA and [3H]glycine are accumulated by the same terminals, albeit by different carriers.


## II. SEPARATION OF CELL TYPES FROM THE DEVELOPING CEREBELLUM

### A. Isolation of Perikarya from the Cerebellum

Although methods for the separation of neuronal and glial perikarya ('cells') from the brain have been described previously (Rose,
1969; Poduslo and Norton, 1972; Sellinger and Azcurra,  1974) the
parallel preservation of both ultrastructure and metabolic activity
of the cells has presented a major obstacle (Johnston and Roots, 1970;
Hamberger and Sellström, 1975).  In collaboration with Garry Dutton
(Open University) we have succeeded in isolating from the developing
rat cerebellum, cell bodies which seem to fulfill both these criteria
(Cohen et al, 1974; Balázs et al, 1975b; Wilkin et al, 1976).  This
advance was due to a combination of factors employed in the crucial
process of tissue dissociation: low trypsin concentration (0.025%)
combined with termination with a trypsin inhibitor after a relatively
short period of tissue digestion, the use of isotonic conditions and
physiological pH throughout the procedure, and the avoidance of high
centrifugal forces.  The recovery of cells from the cerebellum of
1-15 day old rats was 26-43% depending on age.  It would appear,
however, that in comparison with these values the recovery of the
large neurones was less, whereas that of replicating cells was more.
These differences may relate to the possibility of greater damage
being inflicted during tissue dissociation upon large neurones with
many processes than on replicating cells.  Electron microscopic
studies showed good structural preservation - notably the continuity
of plasma membranes and the maintenance of mitochondrial morphology
(Fig. 2).  Regarding the Purkinje cells, for example, many characteristic features of the perikarya survived the isolation procedure,
including the perisomatic spines which are the sites of climbing
fibre synaptic contact at this age.  Viability was also indicated
by the observation that more than 80% of the cells excluded trypan
blue and that the plating efficiency in tissue culture was very high
(see below).
Metabolic integrity accompanied morphological preservation as
judged by several functional criteria, including the ability to
metabolise glucose and accumulate $K^+$ ions (Wilkin et al, 1976).
In view of the claim by Iqbal and Tellez-Nagel (1972) that the trypsinisation procedure of Norton and Poduslo (1970) induces a massive
depletion of perikaryal proteins it was very important to compare
the SDS-acrylamide gel electrophoretic pattern of whole cerebellar
homogenates with that of the total cell suspension.  After in vivo

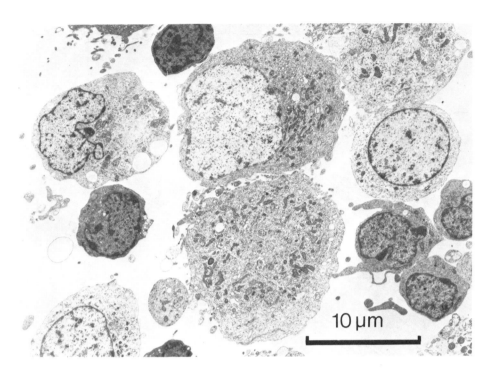

FIGURE 2. Survey electron micrograph showing the different cell types in a suspension derived from dissociated cerebellar tissue. Note the marked differences in the size of the large neurones (probably Purkinje cells) and the electron dense external granule cells.

labelling with radioactive amino acids the stained and labelled profiles of both preparations were very similar with only small quantitative differences confined to the high molecular weight region (>70 000) of the gel. Furthermore, the cell preparations incorporated labelled amino acids into protein in vitro for extended periods, and this was over 90% inhibited by cycloheximide (Fig. 3 inset). It was also found that the pattern of perikaryal protein synthesis in vitro closely resembled that in vivo (Fig. 3).

During the age period under study, cell proliferation is extensive in the rat cerebellum (Balazs et al, 1977). In the total cell suspension DNA synthesis continued since [3H] thymidine was incorporated at a linear rate (Fig. 4), and studies with appropriate inhibitors suggested that this reflected relicative DNA synthesis rather than DNA repair mechanisms (Cohen et al, 1977).

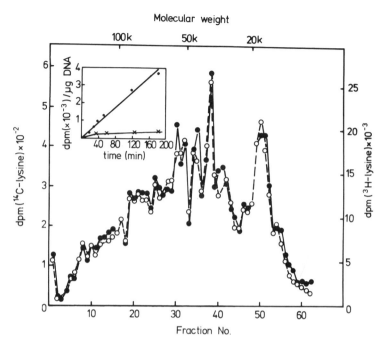

FIGURE 3. Comparison of the electrophoretic patterns of perikarya protein from 6 day old cerebella labelled 1 h in vivo with $[^{14}C]$ lysine (●——●) and with $[^3H]$ lysine for 30 min in vitro (o---o). Inset: time-course of $^{14}C$ lysine incorporation into protein of perikarya from 6 day old cerebella in the presence (X) and absence (●) of cycloheximide (50μg/ml). (From Wilkin et al, 1976).

## B. Separation of Cell Types

It would appear, therefore, that the preparation described above is suitable starting material for attempting to separate viable cell types. We have approached this by taking advantage of the marked differences in the perikaryal size of the different cell types in the cerebellum (see Fig. 2). Unit gravity sedimentation technique (Miller and Phillips, 1969) was used for this purpose. This method has been used before for the separation of perikarya from dissociated cerebellar tissue (Cohen et al, 1973; Barkley et al, 1973). Briefly, the cell suspension (maximum 150 million cells) was introduced into a conically based cylindrical sedimentation chamber (12 cm diameter), and was displaced from the bottom by a continuous gradient of 0.5 - 2% bovine serum albumin (BSA) in $Ca^{2+},Mg^{2+}$-free Krebs-Ringer medium. Sedimentation under gravity was allowed to continue in the cold for about 2.5 h when 10 ml

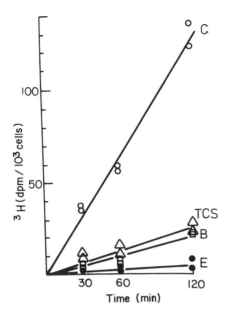

FIGURE 4. Time course of in vitro incorporation of [3H] thymidine (10 μCi/ml) in the total cell suspension (TCS) and in fractions B, C and E. (From Cohen et al, 1977).

fractions were collected (Cohen et al, 1977). The sedimentation profile of cells is shown in Fig. 5. By assigning the cells to five arbitrary size classes (Table 1) it was possible to resolve this monotonous profile into a series of well defined peaks using an electronic particle analyzer (inset in Fig. 5). Fractions that contained 50% or more of a particular size class were pooled. The following studies concentrated on these pooled fractions, which will be referred to as fractions A - E.

Electron microscopic studies indicated that the pooled fractions were, with the exception of A which contained debris, also enriched in distinct well preserved cell types. It must be emphasised here that in the separation of cell types, yield was sacrificed for purity, and only about 20% of the initial cell suspension was recovered in the peak fractions. The results are summarised in Table 1. Fraction E was remarkably enriched in large neurones accounting for about 40% of the cells vs 2% in the initial cell suspension. The structural appearance of most of these perikarya resembled Purkinje cells, but Golgi cells and neurones from the deep cerebellar nuclei must have also been present (Fi.g 6a). The structural features of the dominant cells in fraction C and B, which comprised medium sized and small perikarya respectively, were similar, and resembled those of the

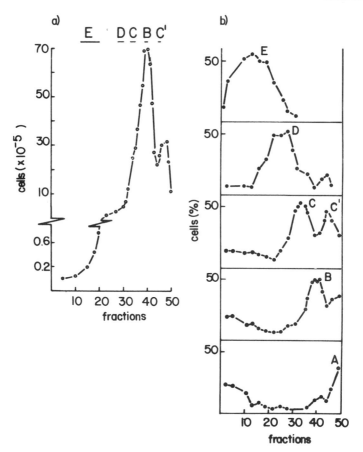

FIGURE 5. Analysis of cell numbers and cell size distributions in
fractions, collected after unit gravity sedimentation (2.5 h), of a
suspension of cerebellar cells from 6 day old rats. (a) Profile of
cell numbers. The horizontal bars denote the positions of the peaks
of enrichment in particles of the size classes defined in Table 1.
(b) Profiles of size distribution. The relative frequency of each
of the size categories A - E is expressed as a percentage of the
total cells in the separated fractions. (From Cohen et al, 1977).


external granule and differentiating internal granule cells (Fig. 6b);
these cell types represented about 70% of the total in either fraction. About 60% of the cells in fraction C' were light cells having
the appearance of astroglia (Fig. 6c). The density of these cells
must have been relatively low since, although they were of medium
size, they sedimented at a rate appropriate to cells of smaller
size. In comparison with the other fractions, the exclusion of
trypan blue by cells in this fraction was similar (over 80%), but

electron microscopy showed a higher proportion of apparently damaged cells. Fraction C' was only prominent in preparations from 6-7 day old rat cerebella.

In the absence of reference landmarks available in sections, electron microscopy has certain limitations in providing unambiguous identification of isolated cells. Supplementary information for classification, however, was obtained using certain biochemical and immunological markers for the different cell types. Replicating cells in S phase can be identified by the incorporation of labelled thymidine into DNA. Cells pulse-labelled either in vivo or in vitro exhibited the same sedimentation profile with a peak corresponding to the medium size range defined in this study (Fig. 7). Autoradiographic studies showed that over 30% of the cells in fraction C vs about 10% in the initial cell suspension became labelled after a 15 min exposure to [3H]thymidine. This fraction was also enriched in mitotic cells (3% vs 0.7% in the total cell suspension), and was thus about 4 fold enriched in a subpopulation of replicating cells mainly in the late S phase and the G2 phase of the cell cycle. Significantly it was also observed that DNA synthesis continued in the separated fractions: the rate was much higher in fraction C than in the total cell suspension (Fig. 4). However, these experiments left unanswered the question as to whether DNA synthesis simply continued in those cells which had started this process in vivo, or whether it was also initiated in vitro (see below).

Further improvements in cell separation. The notable enrichment of fraction C in replicating cells was due to the size changes which occur as multiplying cells progress through the cell cycle. However, the wide variation in size of the replicating cells also had unwanted consequences since it interferred with the resolution of differentiated cells. Further improvement in resolution was achieved by eliminating the proliferating cells in situ before cell separation using an inhibitor of cell replication (hydroxyurea). A further sophistication can be introduced here by taking into consideration the chronological sequence of the formation of the different cell types in the cerebellum. In one experimental schedule, hydroxyurea was given to rats at day 6 when the Purkinje, Golgi and a great fraction of the basket cells (Altman, 1969) and astroglia (Lewis et al, 1977), but only a small proportion of the granule and stellate cells or oligodendroglia have been formed. Confirming the observation of Ebels et al (1975), we found that two days after the administration of hydroxyurea (2mg/g), the major cerebellar germinal site, the external granular layer, has practically disappeared. Accordingly, when cerebellar cells from hydroxyurea treated rats were separated, an outstandingly pure preparation of large neurones, which constituted about 80% of the cells in fraction E, was obtained (Fig. 8). The other fraction of significance was fraction D; the dominant cells here were medium sized light cells which contained mitochondria, a rather sparce endoplasmic reticulum, numerous clusters of free ribosomes and, most notably, cytoplasmic filaments res-

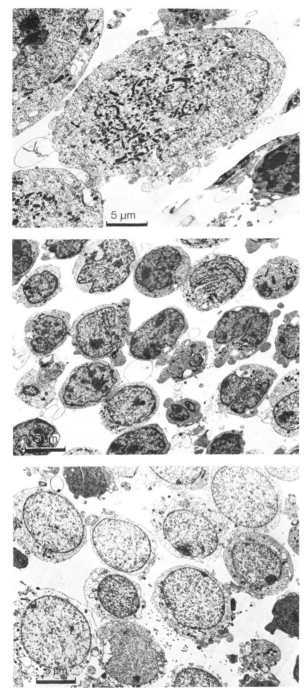

FIGURE 6. Survey electron micrograph of the peak fraction E(a),
B(b) and C'(c). (From Cohen et al, 1977).

embling those in astroglia.  However, markers other than ultrastructural appearance were required for identification.  Over the
last few years, a number of phenotypic markers for neurones and
glia, including cell type specific antigens, have been identified
(for reviews see Rajewsky and Laerum, 1977).  Initially we have
attempted to use such markers, and we are indebted for the gifts of
antisera to Drs. Claire Zomzelly-Neurath (Roche Institute of Molecular Biology, New Jersey; 14-3-2 and S-100), A. Bignami (Harvard
Medical School, Boston; glial fibrillary acidic protein, GFAP) and
J.-P. Changeux and J. Mallet (Pasteur Institute, Paris; "Purkinje
cell" antigen).

The studies now described were aimed at the identification of
cells derived from cerebella of hydroxyurea treated 8 day old rats.
At this age we were unable to demonstrate convincingly specific
staining with antisera against S-100 or 14-3-2.  However, the GFAP
antiserum showed specific staining both in situ and with the isolated
cells.  Besides the Bergmann glial fibres, numerous astrocytes could
be detected in the internal granular layer of normal cerebella, confirming previous observations (Bignami and Dahl, 1973; Ludwin et al,
1976).  Similar results were obtained from cerebella of hydroxyurea
treated rats.  In the total cell suspension of hydroxyurea treated
8 day old rats about 19% of the cells were GFAP positive vs 6% in
that derived from normal cerebella.  Fraction $D_1$ from the treated
rats was remarkably enriched in cells which were GFAP positive (46%)
and which showed ultrastructural features, including cytoplasmic
filaments, characteristic of astrocytes.  Surprisingly, fraction C'
(light cell fraction from untreated cerebella) contained very few
GFAP positive cells.

The "Purkinje cell" antiserum obtained from the Pasteur Institute
reacted always with large neurones only, but recent studies on cerebellar sections indicated that, besides the Purkinje cells, the large
nerve cells of the deep nuclei are also positive.

Thus, we have available preparations greatly enriched in two
types of neurones (large neurones, mainly Purkinje cells and external granule and primitive granule cells) and one enriched in astroglia.  This now permits the investigation of the biochemical properties of these cell types, including the testing of certain hypotheses
which, in the absence of suitable preparations, have hitherto rested
on mainly indirect evidence.

C. Properties of GABA Transport Systems in Different Cell Types

As mentioned above it has been proposed that certain compounds
can be used to distinguish between neuronal and glial uptake of
[$^3$H]GABA (Schon and Kelly, 1974).  Furthermore, autoradiographic
studies on cerebellar sections derived from animals injected with
[$^3$H]GABA have shown the labelling of glial cells and inhibitory
interneurones, but not of the GABA-ergic Purkinje cells, (Iversen

TABLE I. RESOLUTION OF TOTAL CELL SUSPENSION BY UNIT GRAVITY SEDIMENTATION[a]

| Pre-treatment | Size classes | Equivalent spherical diameter ($\mu$m) | Classification | Dominant cell types in pooled peak fractions | Purity (%) |
|---|---|---|---|---|---|
| None | A | 5.5-6.5 | (Debris) | | |
| None | C' | 8.0-10 | Light cells[b] | | 57 |
| None | B | 6.5-8.0 | External granule and primitive granule cells | | 70 |
| None | C | 8.0-10 | Replicatory cells mainly in the S and $G_2$ phase of the cell cycle | | 30-40 |
| None | D | 10-14.5 | (Mixture of large and intermediate sized cells) | | |
| None | E | 14.5 | Large neurones (Purkinje cells) | | 40 |
| HU | $D_1$ | 10 - 12 | Astroglia | | 46 |
| HU | E | 14.5 | Large neurones (Purkinje cells) | | 80 |

[a]Cells were separated from developing cerebella of either normal rats or of those pretreated with hydroxyurea (HU, 2mg/g given at day 6, animals killed at day 8) in order to delete the heterogeneously sedimenting proliferating cells (see Text).
[b]This fraction is only prominent in preparations of 6-7 day old cerebella. Very few cells in this fraction reacted with the antiserum against glial fibrillary acidic protein, although the structural features of the light cells resembled those of astrocytes.

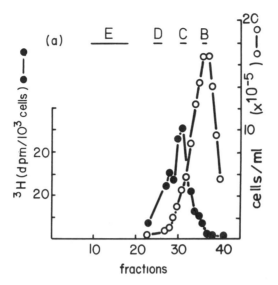

FIGURE 7.  Sedimentation profile of labelled cells separated after in
vivo incorporation of [3H]thymidine (7.5 Ci/g body wt; 2 Ci/mmole) for
30 min.  (From Cohen et al, 1977).

et al, 1975).  On the other hand, Purkinje cell labelling has been
detected in cerebellar cultures (Burry and Lascher, 1975).
     When the total cell suspension was incubated in the presence
of low concentration of GABA ($10^{-6}$M), which would favour high affinity uptake, only a relatively small proportion of the perikarya
became labelled, indicating a certain selectivity in the distribution
of the carrier.  However almost all the large cells in fraction E
were labelled, suggesting that the failure of GABA uptake by
Purkinje cells in the whole tissue is related to factors other than
the presence of specific carriers on the cell membrane.  The labelling of Purkinje cells was little affected by the presence of excess
β-alanine (1mM) in the incubation medium, but it was powerfully
inhibited by cis-1,3-aminocyclohexane carboxylic acid (ACHC, 1mM).
We are indebted to Dr. N.G. Bowery for the gift of this substance
which has been proposed to be a specific inhibitor of neuronal GABA
transport (Bowery et al, 1976).  When the experiments were performed
with the astroglial fraction D1, the results were the opposite to
those obtained with fraction E; β-alanine was a strong inhibitor of
[3H]GABA uptake, whereas ACHC was a weak inhibitor.  These observations, therefore, support the view that the GABA transport systems
in neurones and glia are different, and that β-alanine and ACHC are
selective inhibitors of the neuronal and glial high affinity uptake
respectively.

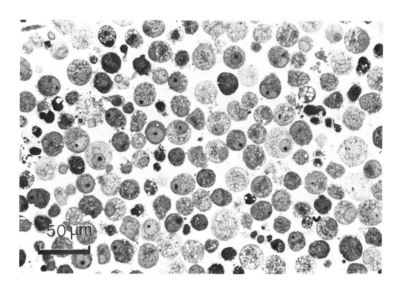

FIGURE 8.  Fraction E (large neurones) separated from cerebella of
8 day old rats which were treated with hydroxyurea (2mg/g) at day 6.


### D. Glutamate Receptor

Glutamate has been implicated recently as the transmitter of
the parallel fibres (Young et al, 1974; however see Patel and Balázs,
1975) and of the climbing fibres (Mao et al, 1974; Biggio and Guidotti,
1976; see also Chapter    ).  Glutamate action in the cerebellum is
associated with an increase in cGMP concentration and, on the basis
of circumstantial evidence, it has been suggested that this occurs
in the Purkinje cells (Mao et al, 1974; Biggio and Guidotti, 1976).
As relatively little information has been available on the effect of
glutamate on cyclic nucleotide concentrations in the immature cerebellum, this was at first investigated in slices of rat cerebellum
at different ages.  It was found that the glutamate-induced increase
in cGMP was age-related, being very small in the newborn, reaching
its maximum (over 200-fold stimulation within 3-5 min after addition
of glutamate) at days 8-14, and declining thereafter.  There was also
a rise in cAMP levels, but this was only 2-4 fold and similar from
birth to adulthood.  The increase in cGMP concentration in response
to glutamate using slices from 8 day old rats was enhanced after
hydroxyurea treatment on day 6: this is consistent with the effect
being localised to a differentiated cell type(s), such as the Purkinje cells, rather than replicating cells.
Before testing this effect of glutamate using the isolated cells,
we established that none of the steps in the cell isolation procedure

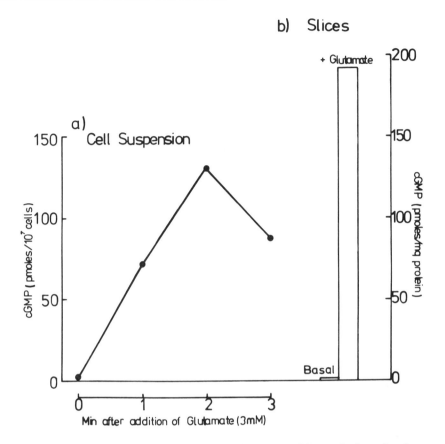

FIGURE 9.  Effect of glutamate (3mM) on cyclic GMP levels in a) cerebellar cell suspension and b) cerebellar slices, both derived from 8 day old rats treated on day 6 with hydroxyurea to deplete the tissue of replicating cells.
    The cells and slices were preincubated for 90 min in Krebs-Henseleit solution at 37º before addition of glutamate.  The suspension medium for the cells contained 1% lipid-free bovine serum albumin.  Cell concentration: 10 million cells/ml (∼1mg protein/ml).  Slices incubated at about 1 mg protein/ml.  In b), cGMP levels are shown before (= basal ) and 5 min after addition of glutamate.

prior to tissue dissociation, e.g. trypsinisation, affected the response in slices.  Accordingly, when the total cell suspension was incubated under suitable conditions, the response to glutamate was comparable to that observed using slices (Fig. 9).  These results indicate that since the isolated cells have no processes, the receptors for glutamate are located on the cell membranes.  We are currently investigating the response in the various cell fractions described above in an attempt to determine whether a specific cell type is responsible for the effect.

### III. TISSUE CULTURE

It is well documented that the enzymic digestion used for dis-
persing cells from solid tissues often causes alterations in cell
membranes, including surface receptors, and that culturing the cells
facilitates the reconstitution of the physiological state of the
membrane (Hopkins and Farquhar, 1973). Furthermore tissue culture
may assist in the study of the expression of characteristic functions
involved in cell replication, differentiation and cell to cell recognition. In collaboration with Dr. E. Thompson (Institute of
Neurology) conditions have now been established which result in remarkably high plating efficiencies, of the order of 70% or more for
the total cerebellar cell suspension. This is the most reliable
validation of the viability of the cell preparation.

Pilot studies with fractions enriched in particular cell types
(see also Currie et al, 1977 for granule cells) indicated that a
small proportion of the large neurones in fraction E undergoes marked
differentiation, usually starting after a long delay in culture.
The pattern of process formation of most cells in this fraction
resembled that of the Purkinje cells, but some looked similar to the
multipolar neurones in the deep cerebellar nuclei (Fig. 10). The
astroglial cells, which were rounded after separation, as were the
other perikarya, rapidly attached to the surface and started to
produce GFAP-positive processes (Fig. 11); by 66 h in culture they
had almost covered the whole surface. With respect to the neural
replicating cells the progressive appearance of 'flat' cells has
been a major problem (mitotic inhibitors, of course, could not be
used here). Thus hitherto, the investigations have been mainly
restricted to the first 24 h after seeding. Throughout this period
the rate of [3H]thymidine incorporation was maintained at about the
same level as was observed immediately after the isolation of cells.
Since the cell cycle time in vivo in the cerebellum is less than
20 h (Balázs et al, 1977; Lewis et al, 1977) these results suggested
that a significant proportion of the isolated cells was not only
able to continue in the S phase but also to initiate a new round of
DNA synthesis in vitro. In the rat cerebellum about 97% of the final
cell number is generated during the first 3 weeks after birth, and
the numbers of neurones and glial cells formed are similar (Balázs
et al, 1977). Thus during the early postnatal period, a high proportion of the replicating cells in the cerebellum are neuronal
precursors. Electron microscopic studies showed that many of the
isolated cells, including those in fraction C which was enriched in
S phase and mitotic cells, were similar to the external granule
cells. These considerations are therefore consistent with the view
that replicating cells - which in vivo are neuronal precursors -
were isolated from the developing cerebellum, and the present observations raise the possibility that dividing neuronal precursor
cells can be studied in vitro.

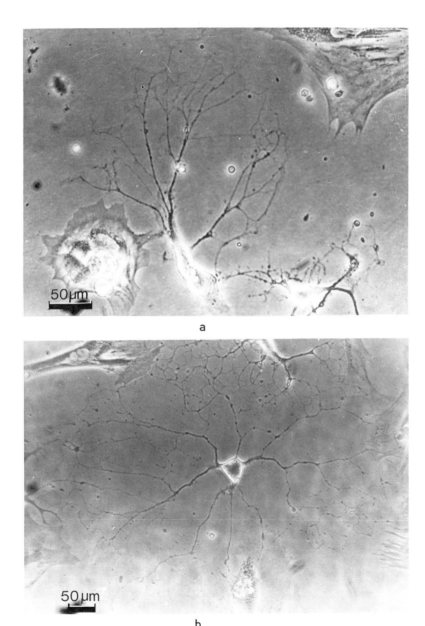

FIGURE 10. Differentiation of large neurones in tissue culture with the appearance of (a) Purkinje cells and (b) deep cerebellar neurones.

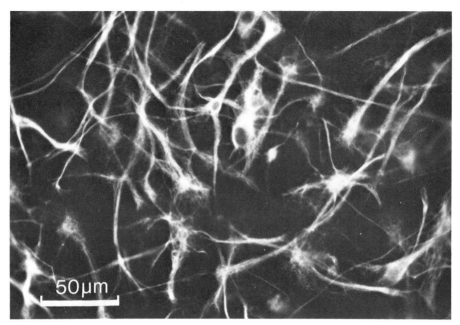

FIGURE 11. Differentiation of astroglial cells from fraction D, 18 h after plating.


IV. SUMMARY


We have concentrated on the separation of morphologically de-fined structures from the rat cerebellum: these include large frag-ments of the cerebellar glomeruli and perikarya of various cell types.

Using the glomerulus particle preparation, we explored the possible localization of high affinity transport systems for certain transmitter amino acids, such as GABA and glycine, to specific nerve terminals.

A method was developed for the isolation of perikarya from the developing cerebellum. The yield was high: with experience 40-50% of the cells in the 8 day old cerebellum were recovered, and so the preparation is fairly representative of the tissue.

The cells showed good structural preservation and were meta-bolically competent. Significantly, the pattern of protein synthesis in vitro was similar to that in vivo; cells with glutamate receptors retained their ability to respond to the amino acid stimulus with an increase in cGMP; the replicating cells continued synthesising DNA. The viability of the cells was also attested by the high plating efficiency in tissue culture (almost 70%).

The total cell suspension was fractionated by the unit gravity sedimentation technique. Further improvement in the separation of cell types was achieved by eliminating the heterogeneously sedimenting replicating cells in vivo with hydroxyurea prior to separation. By using electron microscopy, immunocytochemical as well as combined metabolic and autoradiographic criteria, we identified fractions which were enriched in the following cell types (the values in brackets give the percentage of the dominant cell type in the fractions): large neurones (about 80%); astrocytes (about 50%); late S and G2 replicating cells (about 40%); external granule and differentiating internal granule cells (about 70%).

When these fractions were cultured, cells including Purkinje cells and astrocytes, showed signs of differentiation. Furthermore, there was evidence that, at least during a limited period after seeding, a significant proportion of neural replicating cells was not only able to continue but also to initiate DNA synthesis in vitro.

## REFERENCES

Altman, J., 1969, DNA metabolism and cell proliferation, in "Handbook of Neurochemistry" Vol 2(A. Lajtha, ed.) pp. 137-182, Plenum Press, New York

Balázs, R., Patel, A.J. and Richter, D., 1973, Metabolic compartments in the brain: their properties and relation to morphological structures, in "Metabolic Compartmentation in the Brain", (R. Balázs and J.E.Cremer, eds.) pp.167-184, MacMillan,London

Balázs, R., Hajós, F., Johnson, A.L., Reynierse, G.L.A., Tapia, R. and Wilkin, G.P., 1975a, Subcellular fractionation of rat cerebellum: an electron microscopic and biochemical investigation. III. Isolation of large fragments of the cerebellar glomeruli, Brain Res. 86: 17-30

Balázs, R., Wilkin, G.P., Wilson, J.E., Cohen, J. and Dutton, G.R., 1975b, Biochemical dissection of the cerebellum. V. Isolation of perikarya from cerebellum with well preserved ultrastructure, in "Metabolic Compartmentation and Neurotransmission"(S. Berl, D.D. Clarke and D. Schneider, eds.) pp. 437-448, Plenum Press, New York

Balázs, R., Lewis, P.D. and Patel, A.J., 1977, Metabolic influences on cell proliferation, in "Biochemical Correlates of Brain Structure and Function" (A.N. Davison, ed.) pp. 43-83, Academic Press, New York

Barkley, D.S., Rakic, L.L., Chaffee, J.K. and Wong, D.L., 1973, Cell separation by velocity sedimentation of postnatal mouse cerebellum, J. Cell Physiol. 81: 271-297

Berl, S. and Clark, D.D. 1969, Compartmentation of amino acid metabolism, in "Handbook of Neurochemistry", Vol 2 (A.Lajtha, ed.) pp. 447-472, Plenum Press, New York

Biggio, G. and Guidotti, A., 1976, Climbing fibre activation and 3'-5'-cyclic guanosine monophosphate (CGMP) content in cortex and deep nuclei of cerebellum, Brain Res. 107: 365-373

Bignami, A. and Dahl, D., 1973, Differentiation of astrocytes in the cerebellar cortex and the pyramidal tract of the newborn rat. An immunofluorescence study with antibodies to a protein specific to astrocytes, Brain Res. 49: 393-402

Bowery, N.G., Jones, G.P. and Neal, M.J., 1976, Selective inhibition of neuronal GABA uptake by cis-1,3-aminocyclohexane carboxylic acid, Nature 264: 281-284

Burry, R.W. and Lascher, R.S., 1975, Uptake of GABA in dispersed cell cultures of postnatal rat cerebellum: an electron microscopic autoradiographic study, Brain Res. 88: 502-507

Cohen, J., Mares, V. and Lodin, Z., 1973, DNA content of purified preparations of mouse Purkinje neurons isolated by a velocity sedimentation technique, J. Neurochem. 20: 651-657

Cohen, J., Dutton, G.R., Wilkin, G.P., Wilson, J.E. and Balázs, R., 1974, A preparation of viable perikarya from developing rat cerebellum with preservation of a high degree of morphological integrity, J. Neurochem. 23: 879-901

Cohen, J., Balázs, R., Hajós, F., Currie, D.N. and Dutton, G.R., 1977, Separation of cell types from the developing cerebellum, Brain Res. (in press)

Cremer, J.E., Heath, D.F., Patel, A.J., Balázs, R. and Cavanagh, J.B., 1975, An experimental model of CNS changes associated with chronic liver disease: portocaval anastomosis in the rat, in "Metabolic Compartmentation and Neurotransmission" (S. Berl, D.D. Clarke and D. Schneider, eds.), pp. 461-478, Plenum Press, New York

Currie, D.N., Dutton, G.R. and Cohen, J., 1976, Primary cell cultures of separated cell fractions from developing cerebellum, Neuroscience Lett. 3: 86

Curtis, D.R., 1975, Gamma-aminobutyric and glutamic acids as mammalian central transmitters, in "Metabolic Compartmentation and Neurotransmission" (S. Berl, D.D. Clarke and D. Schneider, eds.) pp. 11-36, Plenum Press, New York

Ebels, E.J., Peters, I. and Thijs, A., 1975, Studies on ectopic granule cells in the cerebellar cortex. III. An investigation into the restoration of the external granular layer after partial destruction, Acta Neuropathol. (Berl) 31: 103-107

Garfinkel, D., 1973, Possible correlations between morphological structures in the brain and the compartmentations indicated by simulation, in "Metabolic Compartmentation in the Brain", (R. Balázs and J.E. Cremer, eds.), pp. 129-136

Hajós, F., Tapia, R., Wilkin, G., Johnson, A.L. and Balázs, R., 1974, Subcellular fractionation of rat cerebellum: and electron microscopic and biochemical investigation. I. Preservation of large fragments of the cerebellar glomeruli, Brain Res. 70: 261-279

Hajós, F., Wilkin, G., Wilson, J. and Balázs, R., 1975, A rapid procedure for obtaining a preparation of large fragments of the
cerebellar glomeruli in high purity, J. Neurochem. 24: 1273-1278

Hamberger, A. and Sellström, A., 1975, Techniques for separation of
neurons and glia and their application to metabolic studies,
in "Metabolic Compartmentation and Neurotransmission", (S. Berl,
D.D. Clarke and D. Schneider, eds.) pp. 145-166, Plenum Press,
New York

Hamberger, A., Hansson, H.A., Lazarewics, J.W., Lundh, T. and Sellström, A., 1976, The cerebellar glomerulus: isolation and metabolic properties of a purified fraction, J. Neurochem. 27:
267-272

Hopkins, C.R. and Farquhar, M.G., 1973, Hormone secretion by cells
dissociated from rat anterior pituitaries, J. Cell Biol. 59:
276-303

Iversen, L.L., Dick, F., Kelly, J.S. and Schon, F., 1975, Uptake and
localization of transmitter aminoacids in the nervous system,
in "Metabolic Compartmentation and Neurotransmission", (S. Berl,
D.D. Clarke and D. Schneider, eds.) pp. 65-89, Plenum Press,
New York

Iqbal, K. and Tellez-Nagel, I., 1972, Isolation of neurons and glial
cells from normal and pathological human brains, Brain Res.
45: 296-301

Johnston, G.A.R. and Iversen, L.L., 1971, Glycine uptake in rat central nervous system slices and homogenates: evidence for different uptake systems in spinal cord and cerebral cortex, J.
Neurochem. 18: 1951-1961

Johnston, P.V. and Roots, B.I., 1970, Neuronal and glial perikarya
preparations: an appraisal of present methods, Int. Rev. Cytol.
29: 265-280

Lewis, P.D., Fülöp, Z., Hajós, F., Balázs, R. and Woodhams, P.L.,
1977, Neuroglia in the internal granular layer of the developing rat cerebellar cortex, Neuropathol. Appl. Neurobiol. 3:
183-190

Logan, W.J. and Snyder, S.H., 1972, High affinity uptake systems
for glycine, glutamic and aspartic acids into synaptosomes
of rat central nervous tissue, Brain Res. 42: 413-431

Lugwin, S.K., Kosek, J.C. and Eng, L.F., 1976, The topographical
distribution of S-100 and GFA proteins in the adult rat brain:
an immunohistochemical study using horseradish peroxidase-
labelled antibodies, J. Comp. Neurol. 165: 197-208

Mao, C.C., Guidotti, A. and Costa, E., 1974, The regulation of cyclic
guanosine monophosphate in rat cerebellum: possible involvement
of putative amino acid neurotransmitters, Brain Res. 79: 510-514

Martinez-Hernandez, A., Bell, K.P. and Norenberg, M.D., 1977, Glutamine synthetase: glial localization in brain, Science 195:
1356-1358

McLaughlin, B.J., Wood, J.G., Saito, K., Barber, R., Vaughn, J.E., Roberts, E. and Wu, J., 1974, The fine structural localization of glutamate decarboxylase in synaptic terminals of rodent cerebellum, Brain Res. 76: 377-391

Miller, R.G. and Phillips, R.A., 1969, Separation of cells by velocity sedimentation, J. Cell Physiol. 73: 191-201

Minchin, M.C.W. and Beart, P.M., 1975, Compartmentation of amino acid metabolism in the rat dorsal root ganglion: a metabolic and autoradiographic study, Brain Res. 83: 437-449

Norton, W.T. and Poduslo, S.E., 1970, Neuronal soma and whole neuroglia of rat brain: a new isolation technique. Science 167: 1144-1146

Patel, A.J. and Balázs, R., 1975, Effect of X-irradiation on the biochemical maturation of rat cerebellum: metabolism of $[^{14}C]$ glucose and $[^{14}C]$ acetate, Radiol. Res. 62: 456-469

Poduslo, S.E. and Norton, W.T., 1972, The bulk separation of neuroglia and neuronal perikarya, in "Research Methods in Neurochemistry", (N. Marks and R. Rodnight, eds.), Vol. 1, pp. 19-32, Plenum Press, New York

Quastel, J.H., 1975, Metabolic compartmentation in the brain and effects of metabolic inhibitors, in "Metabolic Compartmentation and Neurotransmission", (S. Berl, D.D. Clarke and D. Schneider, eds.), pp. 337-361, Plenum Press, New York

Rajewsky, M.F. and Laerum, O.D., 1977, Neurobiology of Brain Tumours, U.I.C.C. Workshop, Geneva

Rose, S.P.R., 1969, Neurons and glia: separation techniques and biochemical inter-relationships, in "Handbook of Neurochemistry" (A. Lajtha, ed.), Vol. 2, pp. 183-193, Plenum Press, New York

Schon, F. and Kelly, J.S., 1974, The characterization of $[^3H]$GABA uptake into the satellite glial cells of rat sensory ganglia, Brain Res. 66: 289-300

Sellinger, O.Z. and Azcurra, J.M. 1974, Bulk separation of neuronal cell bodies and glial cells in the absence of added digestive enzymes, in "Research Methods in Neurochemistry", (N. Marks and R. Rodnight, ed.), Vol. 2, pp. 3-38, Plenum Press, New York

Tapia, R., Hajós, F., Wilkin, G., Johnson, A.L. and Balázs, R., 1974, Subcellular fractionation of rat cerebellum: an electron microscopic and biochemical investigation. II. Resolution of morphologically characterized fractions, Brain Res. 70: 285-299

Van den Berg, C.J., Reijnierse, G.L.A., Blockhuis, G.G.D., Kroon, M.C., Ronda, G., Glarke, D.D. and Garfinkel, D., 1975, A model of glutamate metabolism in brain: a biochemical analysis of a heterogenous structure, in "Metabolic Compartmentation and Neurotransmission", (S. Berl, D.D. Clarke and D. Schneider, eds.), pp. 515-543, Plenum Press, New York

Voaden, M.J., Lake, N. and Nathwani, B., 1977, A comparison of - aminobutyric acid metabolism in neurones versus glial cells using intact isolated retinae, J. Neurochem. 28: 457-459

Wilkin, G.P., Wilson, J.E., Balázs, R., Schon, F. and Kelly, J.,
    1974, A comparison of GABA uptake in the excitatory and in-
    hibitory and inhibitory nerve terminals of the isolated cere-
    bellar glomerulus, Nature (London), 252: 397-399
Wilkin, G.P., Balázs, R., Wilson, J.E., Cohen, J. and Dutton, G.R.,
    1976, Preparation of cell bodies from the developing cerebellum:
    structural and metabolic integrity of isolated cells, Brain Res.
    115: 181-199
Wilson, J.E., Wilkin, G.P. and Balázs, R., 1976, Metabolic properties
    of a purified preparation of large fragments of the cerebellar
    glomeruli: glucose metabolism and amino acid uptake, J. Neuro-
    chem. 26: 957-965
Young, A.B., Oster-Granite, M.L., Herndon, R.M. and Snyder, S.H.,
    1974, Glutamic acid: selective depletion by viral induced gra-
    nule cell loss in hamster cerebellum, Brain Res. 73: 1-13

# GLIAL CELLS AND AMINO ACID TRANSMITTERS

Anders Hamberger, Åke Sellström and Charles T. Weiler

Institute of Neurobiology, University of Göteborg

Fack, S-400 33 Göteborg 33, SWEDEN

## INTRODUCTION

The role of glial cells in connection with the termination of the electrophysiological action of neurotransmitter amino acids is an emerging subject of great interest. The background to this work goes back to the 1960's when Kuffler and coworkers, using the leech brain, showed that the basic membrane properties of glial cells differed from those of neurons. No action potentials are generated by glial cells, and they lack the polarized structure of a neuron. The glial cell, however, is continuously influenced by neuronal activity, e.g., its membrane potential is determined by the extracellular potassium concentration which increases with increased neuronal excitation. Subsequent removal of excess potassium from the extracellular space is thought to occur via glial cells. In addition, glial cell metabolism is stimulated by moderate elevation of extracellular potassium. The glia may be thought of, then, as essential for clearing the extracellular space of potassium.

This potassium-buffering effect cannot be considered, however, as a generalized property of all glial cells, but only of astrocytes, since the other morphological glial types are not intimately associated with the neuronal membrane anatomically and are not in a position to directly influence neuronal activity. Thus, whereas astrocytic processes envelop the perikaryon on all surfaces which are not occupied by synaptic contacts, the oligodendrocytes are either further removed from the neuronal perikaryon or separated from the axon by the myelin sheath. The microglia are relatively scarce and do not appear to be involved in directly regulating neuronal function. Other types of glial cells, such as the satellite cells in

653

the root ganglia and the Schwann cells, differ considerably in
function when compared with the previous group. Recent work now
carries glial specialization a step further; results have appeared
that suggest that astrocytes themselves are not uniform in their
properties, but probably differ from region to region, and may have
specialized functions at specific synapses.

In the following presentation we were interested in describing
some of the phenomena associated with the role of astroglia in amino
acid neurotransmission.

## REGIONAL SPECIALIZATION OF ASTROGLIA

Glycine, an inhibitory transmitter in the spinal cord (Aprison
et al., 1975) has no known transmitter function in the cerebral cortex. The biochemical correlate of transmitter function, high-affinity uptake, is present in spinal cord slices and synaptosomes, but
not in the corresponding fractions from cortex (Johnston & Iversen,
1971; Logan & Snyder, 1972). It is therefore of interest that in a
comparison of the kinetics of glycine uptake in bulk-isolated glia
from cortex and spinal cord (Henn, 1975), the uptake  into the cord-
glia shows high-affinity kinetics, whereas glia from cortex lack the
high-affinity uptake system. This clearly represents evidence for
regional specialization of glia with respect to glycine uptake.

Other studies also point to biochemical differences among glia
in different regions. In a comparison of dopamine-binding  by glial
cells from the caudate nucleus with binding by synaptosomes from the
same area, Henn et al. (1977) reported that the glial dopamine-
binding was almost four times that of the synaptosomes. In an extension of the above study, the dopamine-binding by caudate glia was
considerably greater than binding by glia isolated from cortex.

These observations on glycine uptake and dopamine binding suggest that glial cells are specialized according to particular synaptic regions in the CNS. Such specialization in the glia would presumably require a specific signal arising from a neighbouring synapse. In confirmation of this, studies in which kainic acid is injected to abolish neuronal dopamine-binding demonstrate the dependence of glia on neurons for the maintenance of this property. Kainic
acid injected in the caudate is known to destroy the dopamine neuron,
and to stimulate glial proliferation (McGeer et al., 1976). Although
the glia proliferate in the area of the lesion, the dopamine-binding
decreases. Dopamine-binding by glia would thus seem to depend on the
functional presence of the synapse.

Regional specialization of glia should be kept in mind when
approaching the problem of the relationship of the glia to trans-

mitter amino acid function. Our own approach with respect to GABA
and glutamate has been to use astroglia isolated in bulk from cerebral cortex, since these particular amino acids appear to have a
widespread transmitter function in that area of the CNS.

## GABA TRANSPORT AND METABOLISM

The first evidence that glial cells were involved in terminating the action of amino acid transmitters stemmed from observations
using GABA in three different system. Hökfelt & Ljungdahl (1970),
using autoradiography of cerebral tissue following incubation with
$^3$H-GABA, observed that not all grains were distributed over neuronal
structures. In similar types of experiments using the lobster neuromuscular junction, Orkand & Kravitz (1971) found a significant number of grains over Schwann cells. In the same year our group reported a high-affinity energy-dependent GABA uptake system to be present
in bulk-isolated astroglial cells (Henn & Hamberger, 1971). High-
affinity uptake systems in isolated glial cells have now been described for glutamate (Henn et al., 1974) and glycine (Henn, 1975)
as well.

In general it appears that the properties of the high-affinity
glial uptake system do not differ from those in nerve-terminals.
Both show an absolute dependence on sodium, and accumulation of GABA
is optimal in physiological concentration of potassium (Sellström
& Hamberger, 1975). Furthermore, using the bulk-isolated system, we
have been unable to confirm the suggested specificity (Iversen et
al., 1975) of the GABA analogues β-alanine and L-2,4-diaminobuty-
rate (DABA) for inhibition of GABA transport in glia vs. nerve-terminals, respectively (Sellström & Hamberger, 1975; Sieghart et al.,
1977). This inhibitor-specificity had been shown to hold true for
the situation in which dorsal root ganglion was used as the glial
cell model. Actually, glia from dorsal root ganglia differ from cortical glia in other respects as well; cortical glial cells are reported to undergo depolarization when they take up GABA (Krnjević
& Schwartz, 1967). Similar depolarization has not been found in the
ganglionic glia (Brown, personal communication).

All preparations so far known to take up $^3$H-GABA can also release $^3$H-GABA. Conditions for GABA release are essentially the reverse of those for uptake. Thus, increased $K^+$, decreased $Na^+$, and
metabolic inhibitors, all known to inhibit GABA uptake, will actively stimulate GABA release. We have been interested in further characterizing this release process for GABA. In this respect, it has
been shown that GABA release and uptake is coupled to the movement
of three $Na^+$ ions for each molecule of GABA, implying that GABA
transport is a direct function of changes in the membrane potential
and the sodium gradient (Sellström et al., 1977). The dependence of

GABA release upon the shift in the membrane potential, i.e., upon
depolarization, may explain why GABA release from terminals is
$Ca^{++}$-dependent. If $Ca^{++}$ added to cells, already exposed to high po-
tassium-concentrations, serves to further depolarize them, the result would be an increment in release which appears as $Ca^{++}$-depend-
ent. It has recently been shown that $Ca^{++}$ added to glial cells superfused in high $K^+$-media, causes release of previously accumulated
$^3H$-GABA (Sellström et al., 1977 b). The question as to whether glial cells actually release or accumulate GABA at the GABAnergic synapse is extensively dealt with elsewhere in this volume (cf. Henn
et al.). In general, it appears that due to the higher membrane potential of the glial cell compared to the neuron, and also because
of the high intraglial concentration of the GABA-degrading enzyme,
GABA-transaminase (GABA-T) (Sellström et al., 1975), the likely role
of the glial cell is to serve in the capacity of a perisynaptic
transport and metabolic apparatus, maintaining a low concentration
of GABA outside the neuronal membrane.

## GLUTAMATE AND GLUTAMINE TRANSPORT AND METABOLISM

Studies involving autoradiographic localization of exogeneous
amino acids within synaptosomal populations from the cerebral cortex suggest that 15% of the nerve-endings accumulate glutamate as
opposed to 30% for GABA and 5% for norepinephrine (Beart, 1976).
High-affinity uptake and receptor binding differ both pharmacologically and in their sodium requirements, the uptake process being
sodium-dependent. A sodium-dependent, high-affinity uptake of glutamate has been demonstrated in glioma clones (Faivre-Bauman et al.,
1974; Henn et al., 1974) and in nerve-terminal-free dorsal root
ganglia which have been employed as glial uptake systems (Roberts
& Keen, 1974). Autoradiography indicates exclusive uptake of glutamate by glial elements in the ganglia (Schon & Kelly, 1974).

In view of the close metabolic relationship between glutamine
and glutamate, transport characteristics for both these amino acids
were examined in bulk-isolated astrocytes and synaptosomes. High
tissue to medium ratios for glutamate were observed for synaptosomes and glia, and both fractions displayed the characteristic dual
high- and low-affinity system for glutamate uptake. Glutamine, on
the other hand, was accumulated only by a low-affinity uptake process in glia and synaptosomes (Table 1).Glutamate and glutamine uptake differed also in their sodium requirement, only glutamate uptake showing strict sodium dependency. High-affinity glutamate uptake in both glia and synaptosomes was strongly inhibited by aspartate, only moderately inhibited by glutamine, and unaffected by GABA.

These differences in the kinetic behavior of glutamate and
glutamine may have implications with respect to the situation in vivo.

TABLE 1.  KINETIC PARAMETERS FOR UPTAKE OF GLUTAMATE AND GLUTAMINE
IN BULK-ISOLATED GLIA ANS SYNAPTOSOMES. Vmax IS EXPRESSED IN pmols/
5 min/ mg wet wt.;  $Km_H$ AND $K_{ml}$ REFER TO HIGH- AND LOW-AFFINITY Km's
RESPECTIVELY.

| | $Km_H$ | $Vmax_1$ | $Km_L$ | $Vmax_2$ | $Km_H$ | $Vmax_1$ | $Km_L$ | $Vmax_2$ |
|---|---|---|---|---|---|---|---|---|
| | | SYNAPTOSOMES | | | | GLIA | | |
| GLUTAMATE | 10 µM | 2500 | 310 µM | 4000 | 10 µM | 300 | 710 µM | 1600 |
| GLUTAMINE | -- | -- | 240 µM | 1330 | -- | -- | 630 µM | 775 |

The extracellular glutamine concentration derived from the level in
CSF is 500 µM (Plum, 1974), whereas the glutamate level is very low,
about 10 µM. It can be seen (Table 1) that these concentrations
lie in the range at which the relevant transport systems for the
two amino acids operate at half-maximum velocity, so that transport
processes may actually determine or set the extracellular levels.
Since glutamate is neuroexcitatory, whereas glutamine has no electrophysiological effect on the neuronal membrane, the transport of
these amino acids into both nerve-terminals and glia  may function
to regulate neuronal excitability.

These observations concerning transport led us to investigate
the metabolic interrelationships between glutamine and glutamate
by studying  two relevant enzymes, glutaminase and glutamine synthetase. The degradation and biosynthesis of glutamine are thought
to take place in different compartments of the nervous system. Glutamine is a major metabolic substrate for nerve-endings, presumably
furnishing a transmitter pool of glutamate (Bradford & Ward, 1976),
whereas the biosynthesis of glutamine is thought to take place in
glial cells (Van den Berg, 1973;  Benjamin & Quastel, 1972), or in
post-synaptic elements. In this connection, the glia are thought
to be involved in a recycling process whereby transmitter glutamate,
following uptake by glia, is there converted to glutamine, from which
it diffuses back to the nerve-terminal to refurnish a transmitter-
precursor supply of glutamine. Glutamate in the extracellular space
may also be taken up by post-synaptic neuronal elements, converted
to glutamine in the neuronal cell body, and secreted or transported
down the axon to furnish a nerve-terminal supply of glutamine.

When we compared the glutaminase activity in isolated glia,
neuronal perikarya and nerve-terminals, we found that by far the
highest activity resided in the synaptosomes. Compared to this,

glial cells contained 25-30% of the activity, and neuronal perikarya 10%, which confirmed that nerve-terminals appeared to be the major site of degradation of glutamine. It was considered appropriate in these studies to express the glutaminase activities in the various fractions on a protein basis, since glutaminase is a particulate (mitochondrial) enzyme (Salganicoff & DeRobertis, 1965). In the case of glutamine synthetase, however, we related the activity to the soluble marker lactate dehydrogenase (LDH), in view of the largely cytoplasmic localization of this enzyme (Sellinger & De Balbian Verster, 1962). In relation to LDH content, glutamine synthetase was lowest in the synaptosomes. Glia contained about twice as much activity, and neuronal perikarya five times as much as synaptosomes. It appeared, then, that the major sites of glutamine biosynthesis were the neuronal cell bodies and the glia. Combined with the glutaminase data, this was consistent with either of the previously mentioned mechanisms for the compartmentation of glutamate/glutamine metabolism. The localization of glutamine synthetase has recently been studied by immunohistochemical methods (Martinez-Hernandez et al., 1977). By this means, an exclusively glial localization for this enzyme was found, with apparently no activity associated with neurons.

Consistent with the proposal that glutamine, synthesized by the glia, is cycled back into the nerve-ending where it is largely degraded into a transmitter supply of glutamate, we found that there existed a quantitative correspondence between the rate of uptake of glutamine into the nerve-terminal and its rate of catabolism, such that most of the glutamine taken up was quickly broken down to glutamate; i.e., in following the kinetics of glutamine uptake into synaptosomes, the Vmax for this low-affinity transport process lay in the same range as the measured synaptosomal glutaminase activity.

We also found that the glutaminase activity in both synaptosomes and glia could be influenced by additions of phosphate or ammonium ion. Phosphate alone at 5 mM stimulated the activity 2-3 fold whereas further addition of $NH_4Cl$ at 2 mM abolished the phosphate stimulation, reducing the activity to 50% below basal levels. A phosphate-dependent glutaminase has been purified from brain (Svenneby, 1970). The inhibitory effect of ammonium ion on glutamine degradation may be important physiologically; i.e., ammonium could exert its long-term depressant effect on neuronal excitability by suppressing synthesis of the excitatory transmitter pool of glutamate from glutamine.

## CONCLUSIONS

We have been concerned in the present review with characterizing the functions of astroglial cells in amino acid transmission. Evidence has been presented which suggests that there exist specialized populations of astroglia whose function depends on their association with particular synaptic regions of the CNS. With respect to the GABAnergic synapse, the glial cell serves as an efficient transmitter sink, due both to its uptake properties associated with its high membrane potential as well as its capacity to readily metabolize GABA via GABA-transaminase. With respect to the glutaminergic synapse, bulk-isolated glia possess a high-affinity uptake system for glutamate, whereas the transmitter-precursor glutamine is taken up by glia and synaptosomes by a low-affinity transport process, consistent with the maintenance of a high glutamine/glutamate ratio in the extracellular space. Glutaminase activity was considerably higher in synaptosomes than in glia or neuronal perikarya, whereas glutamine synthetase activity was highest in the neurons and glia. Presumably, glutamate released from nerve-terminals undergoes either re-uptake into the terminal, or uptake into the adjacent astroglia or post-synaptic elements where it is converted to glutamine. The terminal is then resupplied with its pool of transmitter-precursor either from the neuronal perikaryon or by diffusion from the glia. In the case of glutamate, then, glia not only serve to inactivate released transmitter (as with GABA), but also to furnish the terminal with a supply of glutamine for transmitter synthesis.

## ACKNOWLEDGEMENTS

This work was supported by a grant from the Swedish Medical Research Council (B77-12X-00164-13A). C.T.W. has been supported by a National Institutes of Health grant ((number 1 F 32 NS 5161-02). Part of the investigation was carried out by Å.S. as a visiting Fellow in collaboration with Dr. F.A.Henn at the University of Iowa.

REFERENCES

Aprison, M.H., Daly, E.C., Shank, R.P. and McBride, W.J. Neurobiochemical evidence for glycine as a transmitter and a model for its intrasynaptosomal compartmentation. Im: "Metabolic Compartmentation and Neurotransmission". Ed. S. Berl, D.D. Clarke and D. Schneider, Plenum Press, 1975, pp. 37-63.

Beart, P.M. (1976) The autoradiographic localization of L-($^3$H)-glutamate in synaptosomal preparations. Brain Research 103, 350-355.

Benjamin, A.M. and Quastel, J.H. (1972) Localizations of amino acids in brain slices from rat. Biochem J.128, 631-646.

Bradford, H. and Ward, H.K. (1976) On glutaminase activity in mammalian synaptosomes, Brain Research 110, 115-125.

Faivre-Bauman, A. Rossier, J. and Benda, P. (1974) Glutamate accumulation by a clone of glial cells. Brain Research 76, 371-375.

Henn, F.A. Glial transport of amino acid neurotransmitter candidates. In: "Metabolic Compartmentation and Neurotransmission". Ed. S. Berl, D.D. Clarke and D. Schneider, Plenum Press, 1975, pp. 91-97.

Henn, F.A. and Hamberger, A. (1971) Glial cell function: Uptake of transmitter substances. Proc. Natl. Acad. Sci., USA 68, 2686-2690.

Henn, F.A., Goldstein, M.N. and Hamberger, A. (1974) Uptake of the neurotransmitter candidate glutamate by glia. Nature 249, 663-664.

Henn, F.A., Anderson, D.J. and Sellström, Å. (1977) Possible relationship between glial cells, dopamine and the effects of antipsychotic drugs. Nature 266, 637-638.

Hökfelt, T. and Ljungdahl, Å. (1970) Cellular localization of labeled gammaaminobutyric acid ($^3$H-GABA) in rat cerebellar cortex: an autoradiographic study. Brain Research 22, 391-396.

Iverson, L.L., Dick, F., Kelly, J.S. and Schon, F. Uptake and localization of transmitter amino acids in the nervous system. In: "Metabolic Compartmentation and Neurotransmission". Ed. S. Berl, D.D. Clarke and D. Schneider, Plenum Press, 1975, pp. 65-89.

Johnston, G.A.R. and Iverson, L.L. (1971) Glycine uptake in rat central nervous system slices and homogenates: Evidence for different uptake systems in spinal cord and cerebral cortex. J. Neurochem. 18, 1951-1961.

Krnjević, K. and Schwartz, S. (1967) Some properties of unresponsive cells in the cerevral cortex. Exp. Brain Res. 3, 320-336.

Logan, W.I. and Snyder, S.H. (1972) High affinity uptake systems for glycine, glutamic and aspartic acids in synaptosomes of rat central nervous tissues. Brain Research 42, 413-431.

Martinez-Hernandez, A., Bell, K.P. and Norenberg, M.D. (1977) Glutamine synthetase: glial localization in brain. Science 195, 1356-1358.

McGeer, E.G., Innanen, V.T. and McGeer, P.L. (1976) Evidence on the cellular localization a adenyl cyclase in the neostriatum. Brain Research 118, 356-358.

Orkand, P.M. and Kravitz, E.A. (1971) Localization of the sites of γ-aminobutyric acid (GABA) uptake in lobster nerve-muscle preparations. J. Cell Biol. 49, 75-89.

Plum, C.M. (1974) Free amino acid levels in the cerebrospinal fluid of normal humans and their variation in cases of epilepsy. J. Neurochem. 23, 595-600.

Roberts, P.I. and Keen, P. (1974) [14]C-glutamate uptake and compartmentation in glia of rat dorsal sensory ganglion. J. Neurochem. 23, 201-209.

Salganicoff, L. and DeRobertis, E. (1965) Subcellular distribution of the enzymes of the glutamic acid, glutamine and γ-aminobutyric acid cycles in rat brain. J. Neurochem. 12, 287-309.

Schon, F. and Kelly, I.S. (1974) Autoradiographic localization of ([3]H)-GABA and ([3]H)-glutamate over satellite glial cells. Brain Research 66, 257-288.

Sellinger, O.Z. and De Balbian Verster, F. (1962) Glutamine synthetase of rat cerebral cortex: intracellular distribution and structural latency. J. Biol. Chem. 237, 2836-2844.

Sellström, Å. and Hamberger, A. (1975) Neuronal and glial cell systems for γ-aminobutyric acid transport. J. Neurochem. 24, 847-852.

Sellström, Å., Sjöberg, L.B. and Hamberger, A. (1975) Neuronal and glial systems for γ-aminobutyric acid metabolism. J. Neurochem. 25, 393-398.

Sellström, Å., Venema, R. and Henn, F.A. (1977a) Energetics for γ-aminobutyric acid transport, uptake. (Submitted for publication).

Sellström, Å., Venema, R. and Henn, F.A. (1977b) Energetics for γ-aminobutyric acid transport, release. (Submitted for publication).

Sieghart, W., Sellström, Å., and Henn, F.A. (1977) γ-aminobutyric transport in bulk-isolated glia, C-6 glioma and ganglional glial cells. A comparison. (Submitted for publication).

Svenneby, G. (1970) Pig brain glutaminase: Purification and identification of different enzyme forms. J. Neurochem. 17, 1591-1599.

Van Den Berg, C.J. A model of compartmentation in mouse brain based on glucose and acetate metabolism. In: "Metabolic Compartmentation on the Brain". Ed. R. Balazs and J. Cremer, Macmillan 1973, pp. 137-166.

# INTERACTIONS BETWEEN NEUROTRANSMITTERS AND ASTROGLIAL CELLS

Fritz A. Henn, Rick Venema and Åke Sellström

Department of Psychiatry, University of Iowa

Iowa City, Iowa 52242

## AMINO ACID TRANSPORT

Beginning with our studies of GABA transport by bulk-isolated glial cells (Henn and Hamberger, 1971) we have been interested in defining the interactions between neurotransmitter candidates, ionic transport and glial cells. We have demonstrated,using both bulk-isolated glial cells and cultured glial cells,that electrically active amino acids are transported by astroglia with transport systems having Km's in the range of $10^{-5}$ M or less. In addition, we suggested that the glial ATPase is uniquely sensitive to $K^+$ stimulation and is involved in controlling extracellular $K^+$ (Henn, Haljamae and Hamberger, 1972). This has been confirmed and extended by others (Hertz, 1973). Recently we have been concerned with the conditions necessary for amino acid uptake or release by astroglial cells. Following the demonstration that glia exhibit $K^+$ stimulated release of GABA, we undertook to examine the parameters which define the direction of amino acid transport by glial cells.

Our results suggest that three $Na^+$ ions are co-transported with GABA and one $K^+$ ion is counter-transported in the process (Sellström et al., 1977. This is in agreement with the results of Martin (1976). The energy in the electrochemical gradient across the astroglial membrane appears to be sufficient to account for GABA transport by glia (Sellström et al., 1977). This fact emerged from an investigation into the role of homoexchange in defining the amino acid transport properties of glia. Following the demonstration by Levi and Raiteri (1974) that the exchange of unlabeled endogenous amino acid for labeled tracer amino acid may constitute the major portion of the transport of these compounds measured isotopically in synaptosomes, we examined exchange reactions. We found that for both

663

astroglial cells and synaptosomal preparations net GABA uptake was
described by the following equation (Sellström, Venema and Henn,
1976)

$$[GABA]_i \big/ [GABA]_o = \left( \frac{[Na^+]_o}{[Na^+]_i} \right)^3 \left( \frac{[K^+]_i}{[K^+]_o} \right) e^{-2\Delta VF/RT} \qquad \underline{eq.1}$$

in which the subscript i refers to internal concentration, o to external concentration and V the membrane potential, F the Faraday
constant, T the absolute temperature and R the gas constant. This
describes the equilibrium point for GABA transport across a cell
membrane. Analysis of this equation showed that the ability to
concentrate GABA was critically dependent on the membrane potential.
Experimental tests confirmed the validity of the equation at varying
membrane potentials and calculations demonstrate that at a normal
glial membrane potential of -90 mv the glia can concentrate GABA
well over 100,000 fold. This applies to synaptosomes as well and
explains why preparations with damaged membranes and resulting low
membrane potentials do not exhibit net GABA uptake while slice or
cultured cell preparations do.

The critical question in evaluating GABA transport by glia is
what role it plays under in vivo conditions. In vitro demonstra-
tions of active GABA uptake and $K^+$ stimulated GABA release have
been reported in numerous laboratories. Glia clearly have the capacity for bidirectional GABA transport. This could be part of a system which regulates the level of GABA extracellulary and thereby
modulates neuronal activity, or the release of GABA could be an
artifact of in vitro experimental conditions. In an attempt to answer this question we utilized a three compartment model: 1) presynaptic compartment, 2) glial compartment and 3) the extracellular
space. Utilizing equation 2 we derived the following expression for
the equilibrium concentration of GABA inside the glial cell

$$[GABA]_{ig} = [GABA]_{is} \left( \frac{[Na^+]_{is}}{[Na^+]_{ig}} \right)^3 e^{-(3F(V_g-V_s)/RT)} \qquad \underline{eq.2}$$

where the subscript i refers to internal concentration, g refers to
glial and s to synaptosomal. The membrane potential across the glial
cell is given by $V_g$, and that across the synaptic membrane by $V_s$.
Using the synaptosomal concentration of GABA at a GABA synapse determined by Fonnum and Walberg (1973) we calculated that at rest the
glia would have an equilibrium concentration approaching 4 molar
GABA. Since this is many orders of magnitude greater than the possible glial GABA, it suggests that there is always a strong driving
force for GABA uptake across the glial membrane. During stimulation
cells lose $K^+$ and their membrane potentials decrease, so we examined

the case of stimulation to tetany in which the glial cell is maximally depolarized. This would provide the most likely situation for
glial release of GABA. The calculated intraglial equilibrium concentration of GABA is 150 mM under these conditions. In order to
determine direction of GABA transport, it is necessary to know what
the concentration of GABA is inside a glial cell. It is unlikely
to be high since the degradative enzyme for GABA, GABA transaminase
(EC 2.6.1.19), is widely distributed and found in glia, while the
synthesis of GABA, predominantly through L-glutamate decarboxylase
(EC 4.1.1.15), occurs  mainly in neurons. A quantitative estimate
of glial GABA was made from the data of Fonnum and Walberg (1973)
on the Deiter's nucleus. Assuming that all the GABA, which is not
localized synaptically, is in glial cells and that these cells
account for 25% of the volume of the nucleus, the GABA concentration
would be in the range of 5 mM inside glia. This is almost certainly
an overestimate and indicates the driving force, even at tetany, is
very much toward uptake rather than release.

Our studies on amino acid transport by glial cells suggest that
electrically active amino acids are transported into glia with high
affinity transport systems. The inward transport is driven by the
electrochemical potential across the glial cell membrane and release
of amino acids is unlikely to occur under in vivo conditions.

## NEUROLEPTIC DRUGS, DOPAMINE AND GLIA

An area which we recently began investigating involves the localization of drug receptors in the central nervous system (CNS). Of
particular interest to our laboratory is the mechanism of action of
psychiatric drugs. Our studies have focused on neuroleptic drugs,
which are effective in ameliorating the symptoms of psychosis, including delusions, hallucinations and other forms of thought disorder. In general,these drugs are equally effective in combating
these symptoms regardless of the illness which lies behind the
emergence of the symptoms. Such illnesses include mania, toxic
psychosis and schizophrenia. It is as a probe into the biochemical
basis of the latter illness, schizophrenia, that a great deal of
research has been carried out on the CNS effects of neuroleptics.
The reasons for this are,in part,a reflection of the seriousness
of schizophrenic disorders as well as a response to a number of
pharmacological observations linking neuroleptics, dopamine and
schizophrenia. These observations, which include the finding that
neuroleptics induce Parkinsonism (Hollister, 1972), that amphetamine psychosis may be mediated by excess dopaminergic activity
(Randrup and Munkvad,1966;  Snyder, 1972) and that neuroleptics
appear to interfere with dopaminergic transmission (Van Rossen, 1966;
Matthysse, 1973;  Snyder et al., 1974),led to the dopamine hypothesis
of schizophrenia which states that a functional excess of dopamine
underlies many of the abnormalities seen in schizophrenia. This
hypothesis, which appears somewhat simplistic to us in view of the

complexities in CNS function and schizophrenic symptomatology,has nonetheless served as a useful model. It recently resulted in the powerful correlation between clinical efficacy of the four chemical classes of neuroleptic drugs and their in vitro ability to block what is thought to be the dopamine antagonist receptor site ( Creese and Snyder, 1975; Seeman et al., 1975; Creese and Snyder, 1976; Seeman et al., 1976). Haloperidol, a buterophenone, is felt to bind the antagonistic state of the dopamine receptor (Creese and Snyder, 1975) and as such inhibition of its binding serves as a measure of dopamine antagonism by a neuroleptic drug. These experiments define specific binding in terms of the binding in the presence of an excess of an inactive stereoisomer of the neuroleptic butaclamol minus the binding in the presence of an excess of the active configuration. The difference is taken to be the specific binding, and exhibits saturability, high affinity (nM range) and regional localization. One problem with these results is that dopamine-sensitive adenylate cyclase is thought to be associated with postsynaptic receptors (Kebabian, Petzold and Greengard, 1972) and the ability of buterophenones to inhibit this enzyme does not correlate with their clinical potency.

The scheme for cAMP involvement in some synaptic activity suggested by Greengard and his colleagues (see Beam and Greengard, 1975) involves neurotransmitter stimulation of adenylate cyclase. Cyclic AMP is generated and activates a cAMP-dependent protein kinase. This results in the phosphorylation of specific proteins which alter the postsynaptic membrane potential. Dopamine synapses are thought to operate via this scheme and so the fact that neuroleptic inhibition of the dopamine-sensitive adenylate cyclase does not correlate with either receptor binding or clinical activity presents a problem. This fact, coupled with our observation that the specific haloperidol binding activity was similar, not increased, in a synaptosomal preparation compared to a brain membrane preparation, induced us to look for other dopamine or haloperidol receptors. Using the conditions of other workers we found the binding of haloperidol to be over fourfold greater per mg protein in a glial cell preparation from bovine caudate than in a synaptosomal preparation from this region. This led us to the conclusion that there might be a variety of dopamine receptors,rather than a single receptor with varying antagonistic and agonistic states. Our suggestion is that there exists a specific glial receptor with the properties of the antagonistic dopamine receptor.

For this receptor to be involved in the action of neuroleptics it is necessary that it be the principal binding site for the drug and cause some alteration in neuronal function. Our results with haloperidol binding demonstrate that the astroglial membrane binds more drug than the synaptic membrane. Subsequent studies on dopamine-sensitive adenylate cyclase activity showed it was enriched

3.8 fold in the glial cell fraction, or an equivalent enrichment to that found for the binding site. Studies on five different glial cell preparations indicated a greater degree of dopamine stimulation of the enzyme than found in synaptosomal preparations. If the glial receptor is associated with a specific adenylate cyclase, we might expect that activation of a phosphokinase and subsequent protein phosphorylation might be involved in the translation of receptor activation into metabolic alterations.

To examine this possibility we investigated the ability of bulk-isolated glial cells from bovine caudate to phosphorylate proteins in response to cyclic AMP. The comparative ability of synaptic plasma membrane (SPM), glial plasma membrane (GPM) and glial cells to phosphorylate specific proteins was assessed using the assay of Ueda et al. (1973). Membrane fractions were incubated for 30 sec at 25⁰ C in the presence or absence of cAMP, while glial cells were incubated in the presence of dibutyrl cAMP. The specific proteins phosphorylated were determined via SDS polyacrylamide disc gel electrophoresis and the labeling of specific proteins is increased 40 to 50% for the membrane preparations and 75% for the glial cell fraction. These results demonstrate that both membranes possess the ability to phosphorylate specific proteins and that this phosphorylation is enhanced when intact glial cells are used. As a further check on this we assayed the intrinsic protein kinase activity in synaptosomal and glial cell preparations. This was measured using the method of Weller and Morgan (1976) and the results show enzyme activity in both preparations stimulated by cAMP. The glial cell preparation proved to have a more active cAMP-sensitive protein kinase than synaptosomal preparations.

Our investigations,to date,suggest that the neuroleptic drug receptor may be localized in specific astroglial cells. This receptor is associated with an adenylate cyclase which, when activated, activates a protein kinase via cAMP production. The protein kinase appears to phosphorylate specific proteins which in turn may alter a variety of glial cell functions. For this system to play an important role in neuroleptic drug activity it would appear necessary that it result in the alteration of neuronal information processing. This might be accomplished by altered metabolism or transport properties of glia. Examples of the involvement of cAMP in such changes include increased glycogen breakdown as seen in skeletal muscle (Mayer and Stull, 1971) or membrane permeability changes found in smooth muscle (Andersson et al., 1972). The existence of such an intercellular feedback loop,with neuronal activity triggering an astroglial response which modifies neuronal output,is an intriguing possibility. Neuroleptic drugs may provide the initial clue which will lead to the elucidation of such systems in the CNS.

REFERENCES

ANDERSSON, R., LUNDHOLM, L., MOHNE-LUNDHOLM, E. & NILSSON, K. (1972) in Adv. Cyclic Nucleotide Res. (GREENGARD, P. & ROBINSON, R., eds.) Raven Press, New York.

BEAM, K. & GREENGARD, P. (1976) Cold Spring Harbor Symposium 40, 157-168.

CREESE, I., BURT, D., & SNYDER, S. H. (1975) Life Sci. 17, 993-1001.

CREESE, I., BURT, D., & SNYDER, S. H. (1976) Science 192, 481-482.

FONNUM, F. & WALBERG, F. (1973) Brain Research 54, 115-127.

HENN, F. A., HALJAME, H. & HAMBERGER, A. (1972) Brain Research 43, 437-443.

HENN, F.A. & HAMBERGER, A. (1971) Proc. Nat. Acad. Sci. (U.S.A.) 71, 2686-2690.

HERTZ, L. (1973) Biochemical Society Trans. 1, 115-118.

HOLLISTER, L. E. (1972) Clinical Use of Psychotherapeutic Drugs, C. Thomas, Springfield, Illinois.

KEBABIAN, J. W., PETZOLD, G. & GREENGARD, P. (1972) Proc. Nat. Acad. Sci. (U.S.A.) 71, 2145-2149.

LEVI, G. & RAITERI, M. (1974) Nature 250, 735-737.

MAYER, S. W. & STULL, J. T. (1971) Ann. N. Y. Acad. Sci. 185, 433-443.

MATTHYSSE, S. (1973) Fedn. Proc. 32, 200-204.

RANDRUP, A. & MUNKVAD, I. (1972) Orthomol. Psych. 1, 2-7.

SEEMAN, P., CHAU-WONG, M., TEDESCO, J. & WONG, K. (1975) Proc. Nat. Acad. Sci. (U.S.A.) 72, 4376-4380.

SEEMAN, P.,LEE, T., CHAU-WONG, M. & WONG, K. (1976) Nature 261, 717-718.

SELLSTRÖM, A., VENEMA, R. & HENN, F.A. (1976) Nature 264, 652-653.

SELLSTRÖM, A., VENEMA, R. & HENN, F.A. (1977) J. Neurochem., in press.

SNYDER, S. H. (1972) Arch. Gen. Psych. 27, 169-179.

SNYDER, S. H., BANERJEE, S. P., YAMAMURA, H. I. & GREENBERG, D. (1974) Science 184, 1243-1245.

UEDA, T., MAENO, H. & GREENGARD, P. (1973) J. Biol. Chem. 248, 8295-8301.

VAN ROSSEN, J. M. (1966) Arch. Int. Pharm. Ther. 160, 492-494.

AMINO ACID PRECURSORS:   THEIR TRANSPORT INTO BRAIN AND

INITIAL METABOLISM

Jill E. Cremer, G. S. Sarna[*], Hazel M. Teal
and V. J. Cunningham

MRC Toxicology Unit, MRC Laboratories
Woodmansterne Road, Carshalton, Surrey
*Department of Physiology, King's College
London

In the introduction to an earlier book in this series (Berl, et al., 1975) the editors expressed their view that concepts of metabolic compartmentation may contribute significantly to an understanding of transmitter pools – their storage, release, uptake and metabolism.   Included among the putative transmitter  substances were the amino acids glutamic acid, aspartic acid, GABA and glycine and these are the compounds presently under consideration.

Our own view coincides with that just expressed and we have continued to investigate aspects of metabolic compartmentation in the intact brain.   The theme of the present Chapter is to first consider the evidence that the putative transmitter amino acids do not per se enter the brain from plasma but are synthesized within nervous tissue from various precursors.   Secondly, to describe the metabolic fate of different amino acid precursors at very short times after their entry into the brain.   Thirdly, to discuss some quantitative aspects of brain metabolism with particular reference to GABA and the anticonvulsant di-n-propylacetate.


I   TRANSPORT PROCESSES BETWEEN BLOOD AND BRAIN

Several laboratories have developed procedures for measuring the transport of amino acids between the blood and brain (Lajtha et al., 1963;   Oldendorf 1971;   Yudilevich et al.,1972; Baños et al., 1973;   Betz et al., 1975).   There is general agreement that the influx of many amino acids across brain

669

capillary endothelial cells is via facilitated diffusion processes that show saturation kinetics and are uninfluenced by
sodium.

The comprehensive lists of amino acids studied for self-
saturation and cross-competition have shown the presence of
carriers with selective affinities for groups of amino acids.
There appears to be a common carrier system for the transport
of neutral amino acids.  The specificity is broad but two
notable exclusions are GABA and glycine, both of which show
negligible rates of influx from plasma to brain (Oldendorf, 1971;
Yudilevich et al., 1972).  For the two acidic amino acids,
glutamic and aspartic, there is some evidence for a specific,
saturable carrier system (Oldendorf and Szabo, 1976) but the
estimated maximal rates of influx are extremely small and at
normal plasma levels the system would be fully saturated.
Other work has shown negligible uptake for these two amino
acids (Yudilevich et al., 1972).

Among the amino acids showing the highest transport capacities are the precursors of monoamine neurotransmitters,
namely phenylalanine, tyrosine and tryptophan (Oldendorf, 1971;
Yudilevich et al., 1972).  Glutamine could be considered a
precursor of glutamate and GABA, and there has been some mis-
conception in the past that it passes fairly readily across
the blood-brain barrier.  However, in the more definitive
experiments on transport processes the passage of glutamine
has been found to be very low (Yudilevich et al., 1972;
Oldendorf and Szabo, 1976).

Based on available data there is a growing opinion that
chemical neurotransmitters have restricted rates of transport
between blood and brain.  So, by this argument the demonstration that the flux rates for GABA, glycine, glutamic and aspartic acids are extremely low adds to other evidence that these
amino acids play a direct role in neurotransmission.

From the same reasoning it would be expected that selective permeability to the different amino acids would occur
early in maturation.  That this is indeed the case is shown
in recent studies on rats of different ages (Table I).  Even
in the newborn rat there are differences in the uptake index
for different groups of amino acids.  The uptake of essential
amino acids, such as valine, is several times greater than that
of the putative neurotransmitter amino acids (Sershen and
Lajtha, 1976).  By 3 weeks of age the properties of the amino
acid carriers seem to be the same as those in young adults
(Cremer et al., 1976, and Table I).

The experimental data referred to has all been from living animals and, although not proven, the site of transport in

TABLE I. BRAIN UPTAKE INDEX FOR AMINO ACIDS DURING POST-
NATAL DEVELOPMENT

| | Newborn a | 19-23 Day-old b | Adult a | c |
|---|---|---|---|---|
| Valine | 60 | 19 | 19 | 21 |
| Lysine | 70 | 21 | 10 | 26 |
| Glycine | 22 | 2.2 | 3.3 | 2.5 |
| GABA | 19 | 2.2 | 2.3 | 2.2 |
| Glutamate | 26 | 2.5 | 3.8 | 3.2 |

Data are taken from a Sershen and Lajtha, 1976;  b Cremer
et al., 1976 and Cremer and Teal unpublished observations;
c Oldendorf, 1971.  A trace quantity of $[^{14}C]$amino acid, with
$^3H_2O$ as a reference, was injected as a bolus in Ringer's solution into the carotid artery of rats under anaesthesia followed
by decapitation 10 to 15 sec later.  Results are expressed
as the

$$\text{Brain Uptake Index} = \frac{\text{Brain } ^{14}C/\text{Brain } ^3H}{\text{Injectate } ^{14}C/\text{Injectate } ^3H} \times 100$$

the brain is likely to be at the capillary endothelial cell
membrane (see Yudilevich and Sépulveda, 1976).  The properties
of these amino acid transport systems are different from those
observed in vitro using other types of nervous system preparations.  In capillary transport there is no evidence for both
'high' and 'low' affinity carriers for a particular amino acid
nor do cations appear to have an influence.

Although the putative neurotransmitter amino acids enter
the brain from the blood only slowly, there is evidence that
when injected intracisternally, thus bypassing the blood-brain
barrier, they are rapidly metabolized within the brain (Data
for glutamic acid and glycine have been reviewed by Berl, 1973,
and Aprison et al., 1975, respectively).  Also, these amino
acids are rapidly labelled from non-amino acid precursors that
enter the brain from the blood.  There is no doubt, therefore,
of the dynamic state of the amino acids in nervous tissue and
since the quantities present are large, ranging between 1 to
12 μmoles/g wet wt of tissue, flux rates will be high.  Some
values are given in Table II.

For comparative purposes some quantitative aspects of
non-amino acid neurotransmitters and their precursors are

TABLE II. QUANTITIES AND TURNOVER RATES OF SOME AMINO ACIDS
IN RAT BRAIN

|  | Brain concn. μmol/g | Turnover μmol/g min |
|---|---|---|
| Glycine | 1.1 | 0.04 a |
| GABA | 1.5 | 0.12 b |
| Glutamate | 12.0 |  |
| Aspartate | 2.5 |  |

Data are taken from a Shank and Aprison, 1970;  b Patel et al.,
1974.

given in Table III.   Data from the literature are shown for
turnover rates of neurotransmitters and influx rates of the
precursors from the blood.   The amounts in the brain of the
various compounds are also listed.   References to data sources
are given and we realize that these are a limited selection.
What is notable is that for the non-amino acid neurotransmitters all values are in nanomol quantities or less whereas for
those amino acids that may be neurotransmitters the quantities
are many times greater.

TABLE III. QUANTITATIVE ASPECTS OF NON-AMINO ACID NEUROTRANS-
MITTERS AND THEIR PRECURSORS

|  | Precursor | | | Neurotransmitter | |
|---|---|---|---|---|---|
|  | Influx nmol/g.min | Brain concn. nmol/g |  | Brain concn. nmol/g | Turnover nmol/g.min |
| Tyrosine | 6.2 | 105 | Dopamine | 33 | ·3 |
| ditto | 6.2 | 105 | Noradrenaline | 3 | ·01 |
| Tryptophan | 4.1 | 25 | 5-HT | 5 | ·04 |
|  |  |  | Acetylcholine | 50 | 15 |

Influx rates from blood to brain are taken from Pardridge,
1977 and turnover values are from Costa and Neff, 1970, and
Costa et al., 1975.

As has been commented by others, if certain of the amino
acids do function directly as neurotransmitters then the amounts
used for this purpose are likely to be a small fraction of the
total present in brain.   The identification of such small
pools within overall metabolism is a challenging problem.

Nevertheless, a knowledge of the rates of formation and degradation of total pools of precursors and products, and changes
in these rates in response to drugs etc. might well throw
light on the neurotransmitter portion if the situation is
analagous to that of acetylcholine.   Gibson and Blass (1975;
1976) have shown that although the synthesis of acetylcholine
accounts for less than 1% of the total flux through the metabolic step of pyruvate conversion to acetyl CoA (ie pyruvate
dehydrogenase) there is a high correlation coefficient between
the degree of inhibition of the total flux and of acetylcholine
formation.

The most important precursor, quantitatively, of the amino
acids under consideration is glucose.   Following a systemic
injection of $[^{14}C]$glucose label rapidly becomes incorporated
into each of these brain amino acids, GABA, glutamate, aspartate and glycine (Cremer, 1964;   Shank and Aprison, 1970).
This must occur by metabolism of glucose within the CNS.
Glucose enters the brain from blood mainly by a stereospecific,
saturable transport process (Crone, 1965; Oldendorf, 1971);
the diffusional component is small.   At normal plasma glucose
concentrations, around 8 mM, the carrier is half saturated and
the flux rate between blood and brain of rats is about 2 µmol/
g. min (Bachelard et al., 1973; Pardridge and Oldendorf, 1975).
This is several times greater than the net rate of glucose
utilization by brain which, in conscious rats is about 0.7
µmol/g.min (Hawkins et al., 1974; Borgström et al., 1976).
The normal pool size of rat brain glucose is 1.8 µmol/g.
Consequently, following an intravenous injection of labelled
glucose the specific radioactivity of brain glucose reaches
that of plasma within two minutes (Hawkins et al., 1974 and
Figure 2).   Therefore, via glycolysis and pyruvate oxidation
label entering the brain as glucose rapidly becomes incorporated into metabolites, including the amino acids.   Some experiments of this type are discussed in section III.

In certain circumstances glucose utilization by brain is
partially replaced by the ketone-bodies, acetoacetate and 3-
hydroxybutyrate.   This occurs in starvation (Owen et al., 1967)
and, in many species including man, during the period of postnatal development (Hawkins et al., 1971;   Persson et al., 1972;
Kraus et al., 1974; Cremer and Heath, 1974).   There is evidence
that both acetoacetate and 3-hydroxybutyrate enter brain from
the blood by a facilitated transport process (Gjedde and Crone,
1975) which is distinct from the carrier mechanism for glucose
transport.   Interestingly, it has a greater capacity during
the post-natal period (Figure 1 and Cremer et al., 1976; Moore
et al., 1976) and can be induced in adults by a period of
fasting (Gjedde and Crone, 1975).

Within the CNS the ketone bodies are oxidatively metabolized via the formation of acetyl CoA.   Radioactive tracer
experiments show that carbon from either $[^{14}C]$-acetoacetate
or $[^{14}C]$-3-hydroxybutyrate becomes incorporated into amino
acids of brain in a way very similar to that found when $[^{14}C]$-
glucose is the precursor (Cremer, 1971; Van den Berg, 1973;
Cremer and Heath, 1974).

During the post-natal period it should be appreciated that
the rate of ketone-body oxidation by the brain can equal that oj
glucose so that amino acid formation is dependent on both
classes of substrate.   Experiments on CNS amino acid turnover
in which only $[^{14}C]$-glucose or only $[^{14}C]$-ketone-bodies are
used will be misleading in quantitative terms.   A compartmental analysis of glucose and ketone-body utilization in young
rat brains was presented previously (Cremer and Heath, 1975).

The carrier mechanism by which ketone-bodies are transported into the brain appears to have a fairly broad specificity for other monocarboxylic acids.   A study on young suckling rats by Cremer et al.,(1976) showed that lactate and
acetate were probably also transported by this carrier.   Not
only was there cross-competition between the acids but the
change in the brain uptake index with age was virtually identical (Figure 1).

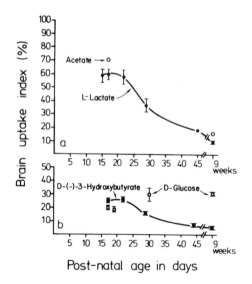

FIGURE 1.   Changes with age in the Brain Uptake Index for oxidizable
metabolites.   The definition of BUI is given in the legend to Table
I.   Data are from Cremer et al., 1976.

In terms of what is known about the labelling of amino acids in the brain from different precursors, the list of substances apparently transported across the blood-brain barrier by the same carrier process is an interesting one (Table IV). For example, it includes acetate and butyrate, two precursors that have been shown to give rise to a high labelling of glutamine in relation to glutamate, a finding which was the start of the subject of metabolic compartmentation in brain.

The following section describes some recent studies on the blood-brain barrier transport and initial cerebral metabolism of selected monocarboxylic acid precursors.

TABLE IV. THE UPTAKE OF MONOCARBOXYLIC ACIDS BY THE BRAIN OF ADULT RATS

|                   | Brain Uptake Index | Reference |
|-------------------|:------------------:|:---------:|
| Acetate           | 14                 | a         |
| Propionate        | 31                 | a         |
| Butyrate          | 46                 | a         |
| Octanoate         | 94                 | a         |
| Pyruvate          | 42                 | a         |
| Lactate           | 16                 | a         |
| Acetoacetate      | 11                 | b         |
| 3-Hydroxybutyrate | 8                  | b         |

References are a Oldendorf, 1973; b Gjedde and Crone, 1975.

II   INITIAL METABOLISM OF LABELLED PRECURSORS

One of the techniques, widely used, for measuring the influx of substances from the blood to brain is to rapidly inject a bolus of fluid, containing the test compounds, into the common carotid artery.   There is good evidence that mixing between the injectate solution and blood is minimal during the first passage through the brain and blood flow is not impeded. So, by this means for about 1 second the brain is exposed to a solution of known composition (Oldendorf, 1970; Oldendorf and Braun, 1976).   For many substances this is sufficient time for appreciable quantities to enter the brain.   We have recently used this technique for combined studies on transport processes and the initial metabolism of compounds entering the brain (Cremer et al., 1977b).   The two labelled precursors chosen for comparison were $[2-^{14}C]$pyruvate and $[1-^{14}C]$butyrate both of which can be converted to carboxyl-labelled acetyl CoA.

Earlier work by Oldendorf (1973) had indicated competition between the two substances for transport across the blood-brain barrier.   Previous studies on metabolism had shown that following an intravenous injection of $[1-^{14}C]$ butyrate the amino acids in brain become highly labelled (O'Neal and Koeppe, 1966:   Cremer et al., 1975(a) and 1975(b). The few studies with labelled pyruvate (Albers et al., 1961; O'Neal and Koeppe, 1966) were equivocal because of the rapidity with which pyruvate is converted to glucose by the liver. Bolus injections into the carotid artery circumvent peripheral influences on the labelled precursor.   Experiments were on adult rats under pentobarbital anaesthesia.   At selected times following the carotid injection the brains were removed by the "blow-freeze" technique (Veech et al., 1973) and various brain metabolites analysed for the incorporation of radioactivity. The shortest time studied was 9 seconds and with either precursor, considerable transformation to other metabolites had occurred (Table V and VI).   With $[1-^{14}C]$butyrate, at 50 sec after the injection 75 per cent of label originating as butyrate had become incorporated into the total amino acid fraction.   Glutamine had acquired 50 per cent of the label in this fraction (Table V).

The quantity of butyrate that had entered the brain was 1 nmol/g (calculated from the total radioactivity in brain at 9 sec).   There was no obvious loss of $^{14}C$ radioactivity between 9 and 50 sec, suggesting that once butyrate molecules had entered the brain they were transformed into, and mixed with, other intermediary metabolites.

When $[2-^{14}C]$pyruvate was the precursor it was notable that within 10 sec of the injection more than 40 per cent of the label was in brain lactate.   By 50 sec much of the label left lactate and was present in amino acids, mostly glutamic acid (Table VI).

The total radioactivity in the brain at 10 sec after a carotid injection of $[2-^{14}C]$pyruvate was equivalent to 3 nmol pyruvate/g.   If there was complete mixing with all brain pyruvate + lactate, present at 1.3 μmol/g, and no further metabolism then a specific radioactivity of 50,000 dpm/μmol would be expected.   The observed radioactivity of lactate was 25,700 dpm/μmol at 10 sec and dropped to 13,890 by 50 sec.   These results indicated that the initial rate of interconversion between pyruvate and lactate was very high and involved a large portion of the total lactate and pyruvate present in brain. There was also a high rate of oxidative metabolism of pyruvate via a tricarboxylate cycle from which label became incorporated into glutamate, glutamine and aspartate.

TABLE V. INCORPORATION OF LABEL INTO BRAIN METABOLITES FOLLOWING A CAROTID INJECTION OF [1-$^{14}$C]BUTYRATE

| Time after injection | BUI | Total | Amino acids | $^{14}$C d.p.m. x $10^{-3}$/g brain | | |
| --- | --- | --- | --- | --- | --- | --- |
| | | | | Glutamate | Glutamine | Aspartate |
| 9 sec | 33 | 38 | 12 | 7.6 | 2.1 | .36 |
| 50 sec | 60 | 43 | 32 | 13.2 | 17.5 | .9 |
| μmol/g brain | | | | 11.3 | 4.5 | 2.8 |

The injection solution, 0.2 ml, contained 1 μCi [1-$^{14}$C]butyrate, specific activity 25 μCi/μmol and 2.9 μCi $^{3}$H$_2$O. BUI is defined in Table I.

TABLE VI. INCORPORATION OF LABEL INTO BRAIN METABOLITES FOLLOWING A CAROTID INJECTION OF [2-$^{14}$C]PYRUVATE

| Time after injection | BUI | Total | Lactate | Amino acids | $^{14}$C d.p.m. x $10^{-3}$/g brain | | |
| --- | --- | --- | --- | --- | --- | --- | --- |
| | | | | | Glutamate | Glutamine | Aspartate |
| 10 sec | 28 | 65 | 27 | 7.6 | 5.3 | .35 | .74 |
| 50 sec | 35 | 56 | 13 | 29.6 | 23.6 | 2.2 | 1.9 |

The injection solution, 0.2 ml, contained 2 μCi [2-$^{14}$C]pyruvate, specific activity 8.8 μCi/μmol and 3.8 μCi $^{3}$H$_2$O.

Although both butyrate and pyruvate are probably transported into brain by the same carrier system their metabolic
fate within the CNS is completely different.   This is obvious
from a comparison of the labelling of brain glutamine relative
to glutamate (Table VII).

With either precursor, for the amino acids to be labelled
metabolism must have occurred via acetyl-CoA formation and the
necessary enzymes for this are located in mitochondria.
Pyruvate enters mitochondria by a transport system (Papa et al.,
1971; Land and Clark, 1974) some properties of which resemble
those of the monocarboxylic carrier of the blood-brain barrier.
Whether butyrate shares the same transport system as pyruvate
in brain mitochondria has not been tested.   What has been shown,
however, is that the enzymes for butyrate metabolism are enriched in some populations of brain mitochondria (Reijnierse
et al., 1975) although where these mitochondria might be in the
intact tissue is not known.   We suggest that, based on the
information in Tables V and VI the application of suitable
techniques of autoradiography might delineate a difference in
the localization of the pools of amino acids labelled from
either [$^{14}$C]-butyrate or [$^{14}$C]-pyruvate given as a bolus injection into the carotid artery.   If brains were fixed within
1 to 2 min after injection label in the original precursor
would be low and at least 70 per cent would be in the amino
acids.

In an earlier attempt to localize the site of metabolism
of different precursors use was made of a pathological situation in which astroglia show a selective, watery swelling.

TABLE VII. RELATIVE SPECIFIC ACTIVITIES OF BRAIN AMINO ACIDS
AFTER CAROTID INJECTION OF [1-$^{14}$C]BUTYRATE OR [2-$^{14}$C]PYRUVATE

| Time after injection | $\dfrac{\text{SA Glutamine}}{\text{SA Glutamate}}$ | | $\dfrac{\text{SA Aspartate}}{\text{SA Glutamate}}$ | |
|---|---|---|---|---|
| | after Butyrate | after Pyruvate | after Butyrate | after Pyruvate |
| 9-10 sec | ·69 | ·16 | ·19 | ·5 |
| 50 sec | 3·33 | ·23 | ·27 | ·33 |

Experiments were as described in Tables V and VI.

This occurs in animals given a portocaval anastomosis (Zamora et al., 1973). A summary of the metabolic findings were given by Cremer et al.,(1975b). It was shown that with $[^{14}C]$-acetate or $[^{14}C]$-butyrate there was a marked reduction in the labelling of brain amino acids whereas with $[^{14}C]$-glucose there were few differences from control animals. These results were thought to lend support to the suggestion that the oxidation of short chain fatty acids normally occurred mainly in glial cells (Balázs et al., 1973).

More recent studies on this animal model have shown that the primary cause for the reduction in brain labelling from acetate and butyrate is an alteration to the transport carrier system of the brain capillary endothelial cells (Cremer et al., 1977b). There was a marked decrease in the total capacity of the transport system, $V_{max}$, with no change in the $K_m$ values. Transport of glucose was unaffected, but transport of pyruvate, butyrate and acetate was decreased.

Experiments with rats given a portocaval anastomosis comparable to those described in Tables V and VI after a carotid injection of either $[1-^{14}C]$butyrate or $[2-^{14}C]$pyruvate showed that if the distribution of label in various brain metabolites was expressed as a percentage of the total radioactivity in the brain then the values were very similar to those for control animals (Cremer et al., 1977b). The rate-determining step was therefore at the level of transport across brain capillary endothelial cells. The factors influencing the transport carrier during a chronic liver bypass are not known but the decrease was a gradual process taking several days, but once reached it remained for many weeks.

In contrast to the decrease in the capacity of the monocarboxylic acid carrier there was an increase in the transport of the amino acids, tyrosine and tryptophan. In control animals the BUI values for tyrosine and tryptophan were 25 and 30 whereas they were 37 and 46 in rats three weeks after a portocaval anastomosis (Sarna, 1977). Other amino acids remain to be tested.

The various findings described in this and the preceding section show that changes can occur in the properties of the carrier systems of the blood-brain barrier which will have a direct bearing on quantitative aspects of brain metabolism.

III   EFFECTS OF THE ANTICONVULSANT DI-n-PROPYL
ACETATE ON BRAIN METABOLISM

The anticonvulsant properties of di-n-propyl acetate (DPA)
were first reported by Meunier et al., (1963).  This compound
is now used in the treatment of epilepsy.   Animal studies have
shown a correlation between the amount of DPA in the brain, the
protection against audiogenic seizures and an increase in GABA
concentration (Ciesielski et al., 1975).   The latter is probably due to the inhibition by DPA of succinic semialdehyde dehydrogenase (Harvey et al., 1975; Anlezark et al., 1976) and is
though to account for the anticonvulsant action.   However,
some alternative possibilities were considered by Anlezark et
al., (1976).   These were that DPA acted directly on receptors
for GABA or other amino acids,or that it acted on carriers
involved in transport of GABA and related compounds.

We have recently carried out some investigations on various
aspects of the action of DPA in vivo which we report here for
the first time.

We tested the effect of DPA on transport carrier systems
of brain capillary endothelial cells using the carotid artery
bolus injection technique.   From its chemical structure it
seemed possible that DPA might itself be transported into the
CNS via the monocarboxylic acid carrier.   We have not shown
this directly but DPA was found to inhibit the transport of
several other monocarboxylic acids;  data for butyrate and
pyruvate are given in Table VII.   DPA was without effect on
glucose transport.

TABLE VII   DI-n-PROPYL ACETATE ON BLOOD-BRAIN TRANSPORT

| Di-n-propyl acetate concentration (mM): | Brain Uptake Index | | | |
|---|---|---|---|---|
| | O | 5 | 7.5 | 20 |
| $[1-^{14}C]$Butyrate, ·02 mM | 42 | 27 | – | 23 |
| $[2-^{14}C]$Pyruvate,. ·08 mM | 40 | 25 | 20 | 17 |
| $[2-^{14}C]$Glucose,  ·2  mM | 26 | – | – | 26 |

BUI is defined in Table I.

   To test the effect of DPA on brain metabolism the dose
chosen was that which prevented seizures induced by pentylenetetrazol.   In our rats this was 350 mg/kg given by intraperitoneal injection.   In addition to the increase in GABA
there was a significant increase in the concentration of blood
and brain glucose (Table VIII).   The overall rate of glucose
utilization by the brain of rats given DPA was estimated by the
procedure of Hawkins et al., (1974) based on plasma glucose
specific radioactivity as the precursor and also by the modification of Borgström et al., (1976) using brain glucose as the
precursor.   Typical curves for plasma and brain glucose labelling in control and DPA treated rats, injected intravenously
with $[2-^{14}C]$glucose, are shown in Figure 2.   In both groups of
animals isotopic equilibrium between plasma and brain glucose
was reached by 2 minutes.   Rates of utilization, estimated
from the quantity of label accumulated in non-glucose brain
metabolites, are given in Table IX.   DPA lowered glucose
utilization by about 20%.

TABLE VIII   METABOLITE CHANGES AFTER DI-n-PROPYL ACETATE

|                | μmol per g or ml | |
|                | Control | Di-n-propyl acetate |
|----------------|---------|---------------------|
| Blood glucose  | 6.7     | 8.2 *               |
| Brain glucose  | 2.0     | 2.7 *               |
| Brain glutamate| 13.6    | 13.9                |
| Brain GABA     | 2.0     | 2.9 *               |

* Significantly different from control.
  Rats were given 350 mg/kg of DPA by intraperitoneal injection and 15 minutes later brains were removed by the "blow-
  freeze" technique.

TABLE IX    RATE OF GLUCOSE UTILIZATION BY RAT BRAIN

|                | μmol/g.min | |
| Precursor:     | Plasma[a] Glucose | Brain[b] Glucose |
|----------------|-------------------|------------------|
| Control        | ·73               | ·81              |
| Di-n-propylacetate 350 mg/kg | ·67 | ·68           |

Rates were estimated by the procedure of (a) Hawkins et al.,
1974; (b) Borgström et al., (1976).

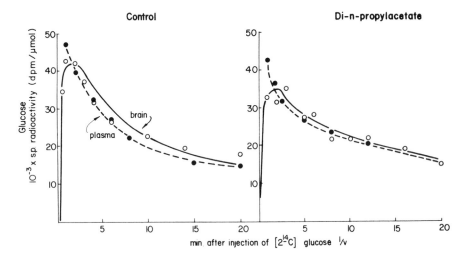

FIGURE 2. Glucose specific radioactivities in plasma and brain.
Rats were injected intravenously with [2-¹⁴C]glucose, 5 μCi per
100 g body wt; one group received 350 mg/kg of di-n-propylacetate 15 min earlier. Brains were removed by the blow-freeze
technique of Veech et al., (1973).

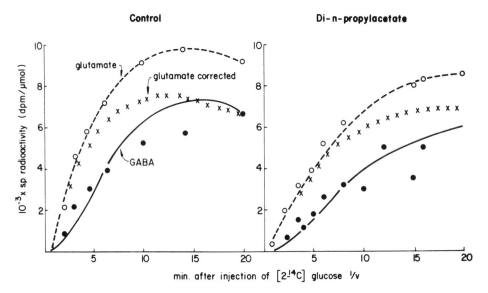

FIGURE 3.Specific radioactivities of glutamate and GABA. Experimental details are as given in the legend to Figure 2. Curves
were fitted to the data as described in the text. The corrected
specific radioactivity of glutamate=observed specific radioactivity $\times(2/3 + 1/3\,e^{-kt})$ where k is chosen such that the corrected
specific radioactivity is 80% of the observed after 10 min.

We were interested whether it was possible to detect changes in the turnover of amino acids, particularly glutamate and
GABA.  With $[2\text{-}^{14}C]$glucose the rise in specific radioactivity
of glutamate was slowed by DPA treatment (Figure 3).  This
could be due to a slowed rate of glutamate formation or to a
reduced rate of isotopic $^{14}C$ exchange between 2-oxoglutarate
and glutamate.

GABA formation was estimated by assuming a simple precursor-
product relationship between labelled glutamate and GABA.
Fitting of precursor curves and estimation of the rate of product formation was essentially as described by Cremer et al.,
(1975a).  A correction was made to the specific radioactivity
of glutamate to allow for label present in C-1, which would be
lost during decarboxylation to form GABA.  The correction term
used was based on data from O'Neal and Koeppe, (1966) showing
that 20% of label was in C-1 of glutamate at 10 minutes after
an intra-venous injection of $[2\text{-}^{14}C]$glucose.  The corrected
curves for glutamate and the calculated curves for GABA are
shown in Figure 3 for control and DPA treated rats.

On the assumption that the size of the glutamate and GABA
pools labelled were the same as those determined experimentally
(Table VIII) the estimated rates of GABA formation were 0.76
and 0.56 μmol/g.min in control and DPA treated rats, respectively.  The k values for GABA were 0.38 and 0.23 min$^{-1}$.

However, it is obvious that the calculated GABA curves are
a poor fit to the data, indicating that treating glutamate and
GABA as metabolically homogenous pools is an over-simplifica-
tion.  It seems more probable that part of the GABA is formed
from a small pool of more highly labelled glutamate.  This has
been proposed by Patel et al., (1974) based on evidence from
post-mortem changes in GABA labelling.  These authors suggested
that the more rapidly labelled GABA might represent the portion
formed in synaptic terminals.  From the data in Figure 3, if
the early time points for the specific radioactivity of GABA
represent this portion then it appears to be less affected by
DPA than the more slowly labelled GABA.  Godin et al., (1969)
using $[U\text{-}^{14}C]$glucose stated that the labelling of brain amino
acids was not changed by DPA, but their data were confined to
the late time point of 30 minutes.

Experiments were also carried out with $[1\text{-}^{14}C]$butyrate as
the precursor.  Rather surprisingly, in rats dosed with 350
mg/kg of DPA 15 minutes prior to the injection of $[1\text{-}^{14}C]$
butyrate there was no decrease in the total radioactivity in

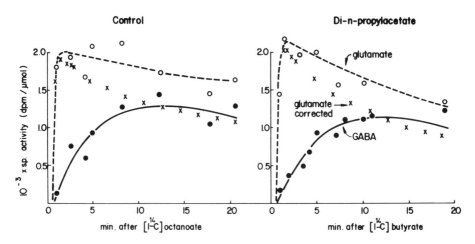

FIGURE 4. Specific radioactivities of glutamate and GABA.
Rats were injected intravenously with either $[1-^{14}C]$octanoate
or $[1-^{14}C]$butyrate, 5 μCi per 100 g body wt; one group
received 350 mg/kg of di-n-propylacetate 15 min earlier.
Curves were fitted to the data as described in the text.
Elsewhere, (Cremer et al., 1977) butyrate and octanoate have
been shown to be identical as precursors of brain glutamate
and glutamine.   The corrected specific radioactivity is 74%
of the observed after 10 min (see Legend to Figure 3).

the brain.   Presumably the concentration of DPA in the plasma
was too low to inhibit the monocarboxylic acid carrier.   The
labelling of brain glutamine was typically high and was unaffected by DPA treatment.   The rates of formation of GABA were
estimated in the same way as in the $[^{14}C]$glucose experiments.
The specific radioactivity-time curves for glutamate and GABA
are shown in Figure 4. When glutamate was labelled from short
chain fatty acids the label in GABA was consistent with a
simple precursor-product relationship between the two amino
acids in both the control and the DPA treated animals.   The
estimated rates of GABA formation were 0.36 and 0.34 μmol/g.min
giving a turnover coefficient for GABA of 0.18 and 0.14 $min^{-1}$
in controls and DPA treated animals respectively.

Our findings with DPA are consistent with it having a
direct effect on the degradation of a pool of GABA labelled
from glucose and also indicate other, more general changes to
glucose metabolism.   The lack of effect on the labelling of
brain amino acids when other precursors, such as short chain
fatty acids are used, puts DPA into the class of compounds

discussed previously by Cremer (1973) and Möhler et al.(1975).

The rates of GABA formation estimated from labelling data
with either glucose or butyrate as precursors are high.    If,
as seems likely, the glutamate pools from which GABA is formed
are only a fraction of the total but contain a high proportion
of the counts, then the rates of GABA formation will be lower.
The difficulty still remains of how to obtain sufficient information to allow more accurate estimates of the size and turnover rates of different pools of amino acids in the functioning
brain.

## REFERENCES

Albers, R.W., Koval, G., McKhann G. and Ricks, D., 1961.
     Quantitative studies of in vivo γ-aminobutyrate metabolism,
     in "Regional Neurochemistry" (S.S.Kety and J.Elkes, eds.),
     pp. 340-347, Pergamon Press, Oxford.
Anlezark, G., Horton, R.W., Meldrum, B.S. and Saiwaya, M.C.B.,
     1976, Anticonvulsant action of ethanolamine-O-sulphate and
     di-n-propylacetate and the metabolism of γ-aminobutyric
     acid (GABA) in mice with audiogenic seizures, Biochem.
     Pharmacol., 25: 413-417.
Aprison, M.H., Daly, E.C., Shank, R.P. and McBride, W.J.,1975,
     Neurochemical evidence for glycine as a transmitter and a
     model for its intrasynaptosomal compartmentation, in
     "Metabolic Compartmentation and Neurotransmission" (S.Berl,
     D.D. Clarke and D.Schneider, eds.), pp.37-63, Plenum Press,
     New York and London.
Bachelard, H.S., Daniel, P.M. Love, E.R. and Pratt, O.E., 1973,
     The transport of glucose into the brain of the rat in vivo.
     Proc.Roy.Soc.London B. 183: 71-82.
Balázs, R., Patel, A.J. and Richter, D., 1973, Metabolic com-
     partments in the brain: their properties and relation to
     morphological structures, in "Metabolic Compartmentation
     in the Brain" (R. Balázs and J.E. Cremer, eds.), pp.
     167-184, Macmillan, London.
Baños, G., Daniel, P.M. Moorhouse, S.R. and Pratt, O.E., 1973,
     The influx of amino acids into the brain of the rat in vivo:
     the essential compared with the non-essential amino acids,
     Proc.Roy.Soc.London B., 183: 59-70.
Berl, S., 1973, Biochemical consequences of compartmentation
     of glutamate and associated metabolites, in "Metabolic
     Compartmentation in the Brain" (R. Balázs and J.E. Cremer,
     eds.), pp.3-17, Macmillan, London.
Berl, S., Clarke, D.D. and Schneider, D.(eds.), 1975, in
     "Metabolic Compartmentation and Neurotransmission", Plenum
     Press, New York and London.

Betz, A.L., Gilboe, D.D. and Drewes, L.R., 1975, Kinetics of
    unidirectional leucine transport into brain:  effects
    of isoleucine, valine and anoxia, Am.J.Physiol. 228:
    895-900.
Borgström, L.K., Norberg, K. and Siesjo, B.K., 1976, Acta
    physiol.Scand. 96: 569-574.
Ciesielski, L., Maitre, M., Cash, C. and Mandel, P., 1975,
    Regional distribution in brain and effect on cerebral
    mitochondrial respiration of the anticonvulsive drug
    n-dipropylacetate, Biochem.Pharmacol. 24: 1055-1058.
Costa, E., Carenzi, A., Cheney, D., Guidotti, A., Racagni, G.
    and Zivkovic, B., 1975, Compartmentation of striatal
    dopamine: problems in assessing the dynamics of func-
    tional and storage pools of transmitters, in "Metabolic
    Compartmentation and Neurotransmission" (S. Berl, D.D.
    Clarke and D. Schneider, eds.), pp.167-186, Plenum Press,
    New York and London.
Costa, E. and Neff, N.H., 1970, Estimation of turnover rates
    to study the metabolic regulation of the steady-state
    level of neuronal monoamines, in "Handbook of Neuro-
    chemistry", (A. Lajtha, ed.), 4: pp. 45-90, Plenum Press,
    New York.
Cremer, J.E., 1964, Amino acid metabolism in rat brain studied
    with $^{14}$C-labelled glucose, J.Neurochem, 11: 165-185.
Cremer, J.E., 1971, Incorporation of label from D-β-hydroxy-
    [$^{14}$C]butyrate and [3-14C]acetoacetate into amino acids in
    rat brain in vivo, Biochem.J., 122: 135-138.
Cremer, J.E., 1973, Changes within metabolic compartments
    related to the functional state and the action of drugs
    on the whole brain, in "Metabolic Compartmentation in the
    Brain" (R. Balázs and J.E. Cremer, eds.), pp.81-93,
    Macmillan, London.
Cremer, J.E., Braun, L.D. and Oldendorf, W.H., 1976, Changes
    during development in transport processes of the blood-
    brain barrier, Biochim.Biophys.Acta, 448: 633-637.
Cremer, J.E. and Heath, D.F., 1974, The estimation of rates
    of utilization of glucose and ketone bodies in the brain
    of the suckling rat using compartmental analysis of
    isotopic data, Biochem.J., 142: 527-544.
Cremer, J.E. and Heath, D.F., 1975, Glucose and ketone-body
    utilization in young rats: a compartmental analysis of
    isotopic data, in "Metabolic Compartmentation and
    Neurotransmission" (S. Berl, D.D. Clarke and D.Schneider,
    eds.), pp. 545-558, Plenum Press, New York and London.
Cremer, J.E. Heath, D.F., Teal, H.M., Woods, M.S. and Cavanagh,
    J.B., 1975a, Some dynamic aspects of brain metabolism in
    rats given a portocaval anastomosis, Neuropath.and Appl.
    Neurobiol., 3: 293-311.

Cremer, J.E., Heath, D.F., Patel, A.J., Balázs, R. and
    Cavanagh, J.B., 1975b, An experimental model of CNS
    changes associated with chronic liver disease: porto-
    caval anastomosis in the rat, in "Metabolic Compart-
    mentation and Neurotransmission" (S. Berl, D.D. Clarke
    and D. Schneider, eds.), pp. 461-478, Plenum Press, New
    York and London.
Cremer, J.E., Lai, J.C.K. and Sarna, G.S. 1977b, Rapid blood-
    brain transport and metabolism of butyrate and pyruvate
    in the rat after portocaval anastomosis, J.Physiol.
    266: 70-71P.
Cremer, J.E., Teal, H.M., Heath, D.F. and Cavanagh, J.B.,
    1977a, The influence of portocaval anastomosis on the
    metabolism of labelled octanoate, butyrate and leucine
    in rat brain, J.Neurochem., 28: 215-222.
Crone, C., 1965, Facilitated transfer of glucose from blood
    into brain tissue, J.Physiol.(Lond.) 181: 103-113.
Gibson, G.E. and Blass, J.P., 1976, Impaired synthesis of
    acetylcholine in brain accompanying mild hypoxia and
    hypoglycemia, J.Neurochem.27: 37-42.
Gibson, G.E., Jope, R. and Blass, J.P., 1975, Decreased
    synthesis of acetylcholine accompanying impaired oxida-
    tion of pyruvic acid in rat brain minces, Biochem.J.
    148: 17-23.
Gjedde, A. and Crone, C., 1975, Induction processes in blood-
    brain transfer of ketone bodies during starvation, Am.J.
    Physiol.229: 1165-1169.
Godin, Y., Heiner, L., Mark, J. and Mandel, P., 1969, Effects
    of di-n-propylacetate, an anticonvulsive compound, on
    GABA metabolism, J.Neurochem.16: 869-873.
Harvey, P.K.P., Bradford, H.F. and Davison, A.N., 1975, The
    inhibitory effect of sodium n-dipropyl acetate on the
    degradative enzymes of the GABA shunt, FEBS Letters, 52:
    251-254.
Hawkins, R.A., Miller, A.L., Cremer, J.E. and Veech, R.L.,
    1974, Measurement of the rate of glucose utilization by
    rat brain in vivo, J.Neurochem.23: 917-923.
Hawkins, R.A., Williamson, D.H. and Krebs, H.A., 1971, Ketone-
    body utilization by adult and suckling rat brain in vivo,
    Biochem.J. 122: 13-18.
Kraus, H., Schlenker, S. and Schwedesky, D., 1974, Developmental
    changes of cerebral ketone body utilization in human
    infants, Hoppe-Seyler's Z.Physiol.Chem. 355: 164-170.
Lajtha, A., Lahiri, S. and Toth, J., 1963, The brain barrier
    system-IV, J.Neurochem.10: 773-765.
Land, J.M. and Clark, J.B., 1974, Inhibition of pyruvate and
    β-hydroxybutyrate oxidation in rat brain mitochondria by
    phenyl pyruvate and α-ketoisocaproate, FEBS Letters, 44:
    348-351.

Meunier, H., Carraz, G., Meunier, Y., Eymard, P. and Aimard, M., 1963, Propriétés pharmacodynamiques de l'acide n-dipropylacétique, Thérapie 18: 435-438.

Möhler, H.P., Patel, A.J. and Balázs, R., 1975, Effect of 1-hydroxy-3-aminopyrrolidone-2 and other CNS depressants on metabolic compartmentation in the brain, in "Metabolic Compartmentation and Neurotransmission" (S. Berl, D.D. Clarke and D. Schneider, eds.), pp.385-395, Plenum Press, New York and London.

Moore, T.J., Lione, A.P., Sugden, M.C. and Regen, D.M., 1976, β-Hydroxybutyrate transport in rat brain: developmental and dietary modulations, Am.J.Physiol., 230: 619-630.

Oldendorf, W.H., 1970, Measurement of brain uptake of radio-labeled substances using a tritiated water internal standard, Brain.Res. 24: 372-376.

Oldendorf, W.H., 1971, Brain uptake of radiolabelled amino acids, amines, and hexoses after arterial injection, Am.J.Physiol. 221: 1629-1639.

Oldendorf, W.H., 1973, Carrier mediated blood-brain barrier transport of short-chain monocarboxylic organic acids, Am.J.Physiol. 224: 1450-1453.

Oldendorf, W.H. and Braun, L.D., 1976, [3H]Tryptamine and 3H-water as diffusable internal standards for measuring brain extraction of radio-labeled substances following carotid injection, Brain Res., 113: 219-224.

Oldendorf, W.H. and Szabo, J., 1976, Amino acid assignment to one of three blood-brain barrier amino acid carriers, Am.J.Physiol. 230: 94-98.

O'Neal, R.M. and Koeppe, R.E., 1966, Precursors in vivo of glutamate, aspartate and their derivatives of rat brain, J.Neurochem., 13: 835-847.

Owen, O.E., Morgan, A.P., Kemp, H.G., Sullivan, J.M. Herrera, M.G. and Cahill, G.F., 1967, Brain metabolism during fasting, J.Clin.Invest. 46(10): 1589-1595.

Papa, S., Francavilla, A., Paradies, G. and Meduri, B., 1971, The transport of pyruvate in rat liver mitochondria, FEBS Letters, 12: 285-288.

Pardridge, W.M., 1977, Kinetics of competitive inhibition of neutral amino acid transport across the blood-brain barrier, J.Neurochem. 28: 103-108.

Pardridge, W.M. and Oldendorf, W.H., 1975, Kinetics of blood-brain barrier transport of hexoses, Biochim.Biophys.Acta 382: 377-392.

Patel, A.J., Johnson, A.L. and Balázs, R., 1974, Metabolic compartmentation of glutamate associated with the formation of γ-aminobutyrate, J.Neurochem. 23: 1271-1279.

Persson, B., Settergren, G. and Dahlquist, G., 1972, Cerebral arterio-venous difference of acetoacetate and D-β-hydroxy-butyrate in children, Acta Paediatr.Scand. 61: 273-278.

Reijnierse, G.L.A., Veldstra, H. and Van den Berg, C.J., 1975, Short-chain fatty acid synthases in brain, Biochem.J. 152: 477-484.

Sarna, G.S., 1977, Ph.D. Thesis, University of London.

Sershen, H. and Lajtha, A., 1976, Capillary transport of amino acids in the developing brain, Exp.Neurol.53: 465-474.

Shank, R.P. and Aprison, M.H., 1970, The metabolism in vivo of glycine and serine in eight areas of the rat central nervous system, J.Neurochem. 17: 1461-1475.

Van den Berg, C.J., 1973, The tricarboxylic acid cycle in the developing brain.  Its function in energy production, amino acid synthesis and lipid synthesis, in "Inborn Errors of Metabolism" (F.Hommes and C.J. Van den Berg, eds.), pp.69-77, Academic Press, London.

Veech, R.L., Harris, R.L., Veloso, D. and Veech, E.H., 1973, Freeze-blowing: a new technique for the study of brain in vivo, J.Neurochem., 20: 183-188.

Yudilevich, D.L., de Rose, N. and Sepulveda, F.V., 1972, Facilitated transport of amino acids through the blood-brain barrier of the dog studied in a single capillary circulation, Brain.Res. 44: 569-578.

Yudilevich, D.L. and Sepulveda, F.V., 1976, The specificity of amino acid and sugar carriers in the capillaries of the dog brain studied in vivo by rapid indicator dilution, Adv.in Exp.Med.and Biol. 69: 77-87.

Zamora, A.J., Cavanagh, J.B. and Kyu, M.H., 1973, Ultra-structural responses of the astrocytes to portocaval anastomosis in the rat, J.Neurol.Sci. 18: 25-45.

METABOLIC COMPARTMENTATION OF THE GLUTAMATE - GLUTAMINE SYSTEM:

GLIAL CONTRIBUTION

S. Berl and D.D. Clarke

Department of Neurology, Mount Sinai School of Medicine
New York, New York, 10029, and Department of Chemistry
Fordham University, Bronx, New York, 10458

## INTRODUCTION

In the two previous symposia on Metabolic Compartmentation in Brain (Balazs and Cremer, 1973; Berl et al., 1975) it had been suggested by several of the participants that the several pools of glutamate and related metabolites revealed by the use of labelled tracers are probably localized in different cell types, namely neurons and glia. The nerve endings were suggested as a possible third compartment although in a two compartment model they were included with the neurons and dendrites. The two compartment model has been relatively successful in fitting most of the experimental data probably because the focus has been on the relationship of glutamate to glutamine metabolism. Since the nerve endings do not appear to be particularly active in glutamine formation their consideration as a separate pool could be neglected in the interpretation of the experimental data. However, when the formation of GABA from a variety of different labelled precursors such as acetate (Berl et al., 1970), glucose (Gaitonde, 1965; Cremer 1973) and glutamine (Berl et al., 1961; Shank and Aprison, 1977) as well as the location of glutamate decarboxylase in nerve endings (Saito et al., 1974) is considered it as evident that a separate pool of glutamate for GABA formation is required.

Differential Effects of Inhibition on the Labelling of Glutamine and GABA.

Confirmation of the idea that glutamine and GABA formation occurred in different compartments was obtained by the study of the effects of metabolic inhibitors on the labelling of these amino

acids by different radioactive precursors. Although glutamic acid
is the immediate precursor of both glutamine and GABA the ratios
of the specific activities of these two substances to that of
glutamic acid were considerably different and were differently
affected by these inhibitors (Tables I, III). The specific activity
of glutamine was approximately 15-30 times greater than that of
GABA for substrates which yielded glutamine with a relative specific
activity (RSA, glutamate = 1) >1 and only approximately twice that
of GABA for glucose, a substrate which yielded glutamine of RSA <1
(Table I ). Inhibitors which did not affect directly the activity
of glutamine synthetase or glutamate decarboxylase but rather enzymes on the pathway to glutamate formation did differentially influence the flux of label into glutamine and GABA. Fluoroacetate
(1mM) decreased the RSA of glutamine by 60-90% from radioactive
glutamate, aspartate and acetate. The RSA of GABA was decreased
20-40% under the same conditions. Fluorocitrate (1mM) decreased
the RSA of glutamine 99% while the RSA of GABA was lowered by 40%.
On the other hand, elevation of the $K^+$ concentrations in the medium from 5mM to 27mM decreased the RSA of GABA to a greater extent
than that of glutamine. This affect was most marked with [1-$^{14}$C]
acetate as the precursor in which case the RSA of GABA was decreased by 99% whereas the RSA of glutamine was decreased by approximately 50%. Elevation of [$K^+$] in the medium seems to have inhibited
label from the acetate from entering that pool of glutamate which
labels GABA. This pool of glutamate is presumably in the nerve
endings. In studies on the effects of tetrodotoxin on the metabolism of acetate added to brain slices (Chan and Quastel, 1970) a
similar conclusion was reached, namely, that part of the acetate is
probably metabolized in nerve endings.

Table I.  Guinea Pig Brain Slices:  Relative Specific Activity
(Glutamic Acid = 1)

|  |  | [U-$^{14}$C]Glutamate | | [U-$^{14}$C]Aspartate | | [1-$^{14}$C]Acetate | |
| --- | --- | --- | --- | --- | --- | --- | --- |
|  |  | Gm | GABA | Gm | GABA | Gm | GABA |
| Control |  | 1.7 | 0.11 | 3.4 | 0.10 | 6.3 | 0.25 |
| FAc | 1mM | 0.7 | 0.06 | 0.4 | 0.08 | 0.4 | 0.15 |
| FCit | 1mM | - | - | - | - | 0.04 | 0.15 |
| AOAA | 1mM | 0.7 | <0.01 | 1.1 | < 0.01 | 9.5 | <0.01 |
| $K^+$ | 27mM | 1.6 | 0.05 | 1.0 | 0.06 | 3.3 | <0.01 |
| -Ca$^{++}$ |  | 0.2 | 0.05 | 0.2 | 0.06 | 2.0 | 0.20 |
| Ouabain | 0.01mM | - | - | - | - | 0.3 | 0.07 |

2.5 ml Krebs-Ringer phosphate, 55mM glucose, 0.5 μCi glutamate or
aspartate (>200uCi/μmole) or 2.0 μCi acetate (58 μCi/umole); 10
min at 37°.  Gm = glutamine; FAc = fluoroacetate; FCit = fluorocitrate; AOAA = aminooxyacetic acid. (From Berl, et al., 1970;
Clarke, et al., 1970).

Omission of $Ca^{2+}$ from the incubation medium also caused differential inhibition of the labelling of glutamine and GABA relative to that of glutamate. The RSA of glutamine was lowered to a much greater extent than was that of GABA particularly from radioactive acetate. The pool of glutamate that forms GABA appears to be less affected by lowering the $[Ca^{2+}]$ than is the pool of glutamate that forms glutamine. Ouabain, an inhibitor of the membrane $Na^+/K^+$ pump, also inhibited glutamine formation from labelled acetate much more than that of GABA. The pool of glutamate that labels GABA is different from the pool of glutamate that labels glutamine.

In contrast to the other inhibitors discussed above, ouabain caused significant leakage of amino acid into the incubation medium (Table II). In the absence of ouabain, glutamine accumulated in the medium to a far greater extent than did glutamate, aspartate or GABA. The presence of ouabain did not increase the leakage of glutamine but did increase markedly the accumulation in the medium of glutamate, in particular, as well as aspartate and GABA. Similar leakage of amino acids caused by ouabain was described by Quastel (1975). In addition, since the leakage of glutamate and GABA was blocked by tetrodotoxin, Quastel suggested that this leakage was from the neuron. Since glutamine leakage was not blocked by this toxin the implication was that its leakage was from nonneuronal cells, probably glia. However, since glutamine efflux was not affected by ouabain, an inhibitor of the $Na^+/K^+$ ATPase it was concluded that its confinement to the cell is not sodium dependent. It also follows that glutamine can diffuse readily from any cells where it is formed.

The measurement of the specific activities of these amino acids labelled with $[1-^{14}C]$acetate in the slice and medium under these conditions supplied additional interesting information. Without ouabain in the medium the specific activity of the glutamate was slightly higher in the medium than in the slice (Fig. 1). In the presence of ouabain the specific activity of the glutamate in the medium was increased considerably without affecting the specific activity of the glutmate in the slice, except at 30 min when it was somewhat decreased. It would appear that the newly formed glutamate leaked in the medium faster than it was able to mix with the total glutamate in the slice. On the other hand, in control experiments, the specific activity of the glutamine was up to 3 times greater in the medium than in the slice (Fig. 2). Thus, newly formed glutamine entered the medium more rapidly than it mixed with the total tissue pool. The presence of ouabain depressed the specific activities of the glutamine in both the medium and slice although that in the medium remained much higher than that in the slice. It would appear that a pool of glutamate that served as the precursor for glutamine had selectively leaked into the medium in the presence of ouabain and thus decreased the for-

Table II.  Guinea Pig Brain Slice Media:  Effect of Ouabain on
Amino Acid Levels.

|  | Min. | μmoles/g tissue | | | |
|---|---|---|---|---|---|
|  |  | Glutamic Acid | Glutamine | Aspartic Acid | GABA |
| Control | 10 | 0.06 | 0.20 | < 0.01 | < 0.01 |
|  | 20 | 0.06 | 0.40 | < 0.01 | 0.16 |
|  | 30 | 0.08 | 0.61 | 0.05 | 0.11 |
| Ouabain 10−5M | 10 | 0.12 | 0.26 | 0.06 | 0.10 |
|  | 20 | 1.04 | 0.58 | 0.26 | 0.46 |
|  | 30 | 2.63 | 0.71 | 0.45 | 0.67 |

See Table 1 for experimental details (From Berl et al., 1970).

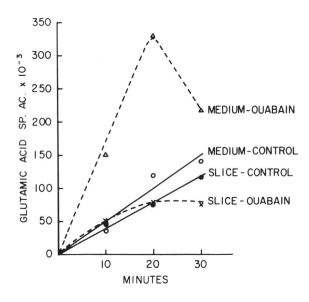

Figure 1.  Specific activity of glutamate from [1−14C]acetate in
brain slice and incubation medium in the presence and absence of
10−5M ouabain.  See Table 1 for other details.  (From Berl et al.,
1970).

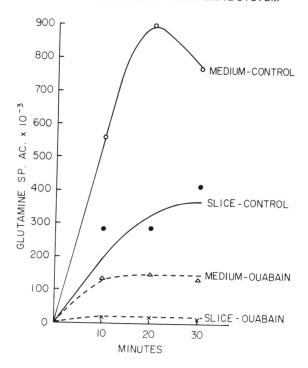

Figure 2. Specific activity of glutamine from [1-$^{14}$C]acetate in brain slice and incubation medium in the presence and absence of 10$^{-5}$M ouabain. See Table 1 for other details. (From Berl et al., 1970).

mation of glutamine of high specific activity. The RSA's of the glutamine reflected these changes in specific activities (Fig. 3). Under control conditons, at 10 minutes, the RSA of glutamine in the slice was approxiamtely 6 and that in the medium 15. The presence of ouabain depressed the RSA of glutamine to <1 in both the slice and medium but the former was affected even more than the latter.

It is not entirely clear whether the glutamate that leaked into medium in the presence of ouabain originated exclusively from neurons, glia or both. The studies of Quastel (1975) showed that tetrodotoxin blocked the ouabain induced leakage and suggested

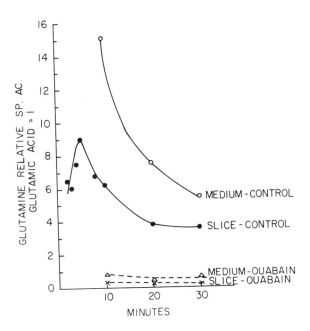

Figure 3. Relative specific activity of glutamine (glutamate = 1) from [1-$^{14}$C]acetate in brain slice and incubation medium in the presence and absence of $10^{-5}$M ouabain. See Table I for the details (From Berl et al., 1970).

that the glutamate efflux in the presence of ouabain was largely from neurons. In addition, uptake of glutamate into non-neuronal sites (such as glia) for conversion to glutamine may also be inhibited (Berl et al., 1970). It was also found in the latter studies that the influx of [1-$^{14}$C]acetate into the slice was decreased by 1/3 to 1/2 in the presence of ouabain. If this effect was mainly on glia, where it is thought that acetate is normally in large part metabolized, the data may reflect an overemphasis on neuronal metabolism of the acetate in the presence of ouabain. However, it is most likely that glutamate is leaking from both neurons and glia in the presence of ouabain.

Another point which we would like to underline is that the glutamine did not appear to be retained in cells by an active uptake process and, therefore, may diffuse from one cell to another and thus serve as a means of communication between cells, namely, glia and neurons. This concept was first suggested by the finding that radioactive glutamine can readily enter brain cells and more effectively label GABA than glutamate or its precursors (Berl et al., 1961). Van den Berg and Garfinkel (1971) developed the hypothesis that glutamine may conserve metabolic products of the Krebs cycle by shuttling between glutamate at one site and GABA at another. The reports of Bradford and Cotman in this volume provide further evidence for this hypothesis.

Additional support for this idea derives from evidence that synaptosomal preparations can take up $[^{14}C]$ glutamine and rapidly convert it to glutamate and GABA (Baldessarini and Yorke, 1974; Bradford and Ward, 1976; Siegel, Nicklas, Berl and Clarke, unpublished observations). More detailed studies by Shank and Aprison (1977) using toad brain preparations have confirmed and extended these observations that glutamine can form GABA more effectively than other precursors including glucose.

In some respects fluoroacetate and fluorocitrate resemble ouabain in their effects on $[1-^{14}C]$acetate metabolism in brain slices. Thus, these inhibitors decreased the influx of labelled acetate into the tissue, decreased the specific activity of glutamic acid and had an even greater effect on the RSA of glutamine (Clarke et al., 1970). Both sets of inhibitors did not affect oxygen utilization, or the production of $^{14}CO_2$ from $[6-^{14}C]$ glucose, but did inhibit the production of $^{14}CO_2$ from $[1-^{14}C]$acetate and the labelling of glutamine from both precursors (Gonda and Quastel, 1966). However, these fluorinated inhibitors did not decrease the levels of the amino acids in the tissue or increase their efflux into the medium. Therefore, these inhibitors are not entirely similar to ouabain in their modes of action although they do appear to be particularly effective against that small pool of glutamate active in glutamine formation.

Inhibition of the influx of $[1-^{14}C]$acetate into the slice by fluoroacetate (Table III) might be explained by competitive inhibition because of similarity of structure. This explanation would be more difficult to apply to fluorocitrate which had similar effects on the entry of labelled acetate. On the other hand, fluoroacetate did not limit the entry of labelled glutamate, aspartate or GABA into the slice nor did it effect the specific activity of glutamate' from any of these labelled compounds; the RSA of glutamine was markedly reduced in all cases (Table III). Since this inhibition of glutamine labelling occurred with both $[U-^{14}C]$ and $[1-^{14}C]$ glutamate as added tracers, and purified brain gluta-

Table III.   Guinea Pig Brain Slices:   Metabolic Inhibition By
            Fluoroacetate and Fluorocitrate (1mM)

| | Total cpm/μmole x $10^{-6}$ | Glutamic Acid cpm/μmole x $10^{-4}$ | Glutamine RSA |
|---|---|---|---|
| [1-$^{14}$C]Acetate | | | |
| Control | 1.95 | 4.69 | 5.87 |
| FAc | 0.85 | 1.36 | 0.40 |
| FCit | 0.85 | 1.45 | 0.04 |
| [U-$^{14}$C]Glutamate | | | |
| Control | 2.02 | 20.1 | 1.32 |
| FAc | 2.18 | 20.8 | 0.70 |
| [1-$^{14}$C]Glutamate | | | |
| Control | 2.92 | 27.2 | 0.97 |
| FAc | 2.98 | 33.8 | 0.49 |
| [U-$^{14}$C]Aspartate | | | |
| Control | 1.58 | 2.90 | 3.45 |
| FAc | 1.53 | 2.66 | 0.38 |
| [1-$^{14}$C]GABA | | | |
| Control | 1.36 | 0.20 | 4.45 |
| FAc | 1.73 | 0.21 | 0.60 |

10 min incubation
RSA = Relative Specific Activity (glutamate = 1).
See Table 1 for experimental details (From Clarke, et al.,
1970).

mine synthetase was not affected by either fluoroacetate (Lahiri
and Quastel, 1963; Clarke et al., 1970) or fluorocitrate (Clarke
et al., 1970),  a likely explanation would be that the Krebs cycle
that supplied the ATP for glutamine synthesis is the one most
affected by these inhibitors, although the total tissue level of
ATP was not decreased (Gonda and Quastel, 1966; Goldberg et al.,
1966).   We have explained this in the past by fluoroacetate inhibition of a Krebs cycle associated with a small pool of glutamate
active in glutamine formation.

It is particularly striking, however, that the specific activity of glutamate from labelled aspartate or GABA was not inhibited
by fluoroacetate whereas the labelling of glutamine was inhibited
in both cases approximately 90%.   It would appear, therefore, that
the Krebs cycle involved in the formation of glutamate from these
precursors is separate from the Krebs cycle related to the pool of
ATP utilized for glutamine formation.   A possibility which merits
further consideration is that the glutamate is formed at one site
(nerve endings), released at these synapses and taken up at another
site (glia) for inactivation by amidation to glutamine.

Glutamate Dehydrogenase and Ammonia Metabolism.

The two enzymes that are important in the formation of glutamic acid are glutamate aminotransferase (transaminase) and glutamate dehydrogenase. Since $NH_4^+$ can be incorporated directly into
glutamate only via the glutamate dehydrogenase pathway studies with
$^{15}NH_4^+$ focused on the contribution of this enzyme to the compartmentation of the glutamate-glutamine system (Berl, et al., 1962).
In in vivo studies with the cat, $^{15}N$-ammonium acetate was infused
via the carotid artery. In the brain, the $\alpha$-amino group of the
glutamine contained as much as 10 times the quantity of $^{15}N$ as
that found in the $\alpha$-amino group of the glutamate. The data suggested that glutamate dehydrogenase must be associated with a pool
of glutamate which is closely associated with glutamine synthesis.

In vitro studies with aminooxyacetic acid (AOAA), a potent
inhibitor of both transaminases and decarboxylases, complemented
these results (Berl et al., 1970; (Table IV). The AOAA (1 mM in
the incubation medium) inhibited the conversion of [U-$^{14}$C]glutamate
to aspartate 88%, of [U-$^{14}$C]aspartate to glutamate 96%, and of
[1-$^{14}$C]acetate to aspartate 90%. The entry into the Krebs cycle
of labelled aspartate added to the medium was almost completely
inhibited by AOAA since 99.5% (not shown in the table) of the
label remained in aspartate. The metabolism of the glutamate was
also retarded and radioactivity remained in glutamate and glutamine.
The labelling of GABA from the three precursors was inhibited by
at least 95% by the AOAA. The distribution of radioactivity from
[1-$^{14}$C]acetate was affected somewhat differently by the AOAA. The
percent radioactivity in the glutamate was decreased by 54% while
that in glutamine increased by 11% (Berl et al., 1970). This was
reflected in an increased in the RSA of glutamine over the control
values with labelled acetate (Table IV). Thus the glutamate dehydrogenase pathway must be contributing significantly to the labelling of glutamate and glutamine from radioactive acetate since the
transaminases were effectively inhibited by the AOAA. All of these
observations are consistent with the interpretation that the large
pool or pools of glutamate which are not active in glutamine formation are associated in large part with transaminase. On the
other hand, a smaller pool of glutamate is associated with glutamate dehydrogenase and glutamine synthetase and is readily available for glutamine formation.

Whereas, $^{15}NH_4^+$ can enter glutamate only via the dehydrogenase
pathway exclusively, $\alpha$ ketoglutarate can be converted to glutamate
via both the dehydrogenase and the transaminase pathways. A further
effort to evaluate the contribution of each of these pathways was
attempted by a study of the incorporation of labelled $\alpha$ketoglutarate
into glutamate and glutamine in the presence of AOAA and $NH_4^+$.

As reported by many others, incubation of guinea pig brain

Table IV.   Guinea Pig Brain Slices: Effect of Aminooxyacetic Acid

|  | cpm/umole x $10^{-3}$ | | Relative Specific Activity | |
|---|---|---|---|---|
|  | Control | AOAA, 1mM | Control | AOAA, 1mM |
| $[U\text{-}^{14}C]$Glutamate | | | | |
| GA | 167 | 321 | 1 | 1 |
| Gm | 284 | 225 ( 21) | 1.7 | 0.7 |
| GABA | 18 | $<$1 (>95) | 0.11 | $<$0.01 |
| AA | 62.5 | 7.4 ( 88) | 0.37 | 0.02 |
| $[U\text{-}^{14}C]$Aspartate | | | | |
| GA | 41 | 1.7 ( 96) | 1 | 1 |
| Gm | 130.5 | 1.8 ( 98) | 3.4 | 1.1 |
| GABA | 4.1 | $<$0.02 (>99) | 0.10 | $<$ 0.01 |
| AA | 1,337 | 1,266 | 32.6 | 745 |
| $[1\text{-}^{14}C]$Acetate | | | | |
| GA | 45.2 | 17.2 ( 62) | 1 | 1 |
| Gm | 301.6 | 152.5 ( 50) | 6.3 | 9.5 |
| GABA | 11.3 | $<$ 0.17 (>98) | 0.25 | $<$0.01 |
| AA | 26.7 | 2.7 ( 90) | 0.59 | 0.16 |

( ) = % inhibition
See Table 1 for experimental details.  (From Berl et al., 1970).

slices in the presence of 1mM $NH_4^+$ significantly increased the levels of glutamine in the tissue (Table V).  Addition of AOAA (1mM) to the medium also increased the level of glutamine in the brain slice and the combination of both AOAA and $NH_4^+$ were approximately additive.

   As demonstrated above with other labelled precursors, glutamate-aminotransferase and glutamate decarboxylase were effectively inhibited by AOAA in these experiments since the specific activity of aspartate was decreased by 97% and that of GABA by 99% (Table VI). Under the conditions of these experiments (1mM AOAA) the specific activity of glutamate was approximately 10%, and that of glutamine was approximately 25% of the control values; therefore, the RSA of glutamine was increased approximately 2.5 times the value obtained from control experiments (Table VII).  In the presence of ammonium acetate (1mM), the specific activity of glutamate was decreased to approximately 30% of control values and the RSA of glutamine was increased approximately 2.5-fold.  Although the trends were similar with both the AOAA and $NH_4^+$, the depressed specific activity of glutamate occurred for different reasons.  In the former case the flux of label into glutamate was depressed by inhibition of transaminase, whereas, in  the latter case, the RSA of aspartate indica-

Table V.   Guinea Pig Brain Slices: Levels of Amino Acids

| Addition 1mM | Glutamate | Glutamine | Aspartate | GABA |
|---|---|---|---|---|
| None | 8.5 | 2.3 | 1.7 | 2.6 |
| NH$_4^+$ | 7.5* | 3.0* | 1.6 | 2.6 |
| AOAA | 7.1* | 2.6** | 2.6* | 2.0* |
| AOAA + NH$_4^+$ | 6.6*+ | 3.2*+ | 2.3* | 1.8* |

*p$<$0.01;   **p$<$0.05 as compared to none.   +p$<$0.01 as compared to AOAA addition.   See Table 1 for experimental details.

Table VI.   Guinea Pig Brain Slices: Radioactivity

| Precursor [5-$^{14}$C]$_\alpha$KG | Specific Activity x 10$^{-4}$ | | | |
|---|---|---|---|---|
| | GA | Gm | AA | GABA |
| Control | 8.86 | 36.53 | 4.34 | 1.23 |
| NH$_4^+$ | 2.64 | 27.78 | 1.82 | 0.73 |
| AOAA | 0.92 | 8.68 | 0.12 | 0.007 |
| AOAA + NH$_4^+$ | 1.02 | 14.44 | 0.27 | 0.017 |
| [2-$^{14}$C]Glucose | | | | |
| Control | 0.94 | 0.32 | 0.31 | 0.155 |
| NH$_4^+$ | 1.37 | 0.39 | 0.79 | 0.23 |

Krebs-Ringer bicarbonate.   [5-$^{14}$C]$_\alpha$KG = 1 μCi ketoglutarate
(10 μCi/μmole); [2-$^{14}$C]Glucose = 2 μCi glucose, 5.5 mM; NH$_4^+$ =
1 mM ammonium acetate.   GA = glutamate; Gm = glutamine. AA =
aspartate.
Incubation time 10 min at 37°.
Each result is the average from 2 or more slices.

ted no inhibition of transaminase.   In contrast, in presence of
NH$_4^+$, when [2-$^{14}$C]glucose was the precursor, the specific
activity of glutamate increased and that of glutamine
did not change significantly (Table VI).   This resulted
in a decrease in the RSA of glutamine (Table VII).   Therefore, the
decreased specific activity of the glutamate formed from ketoglutarate in the presence of ammonia was due to stimulation of the
flux of unlabelled glucose into ketoglutarate and thus into glutamate.   In vivo experiments also demonstrated an increased flux
of glucose into the Krebs cycle in brain of rats acutely intoxicated
with NH$_4^+$ (Hawkins et al., 1973).   In the presence of both AOAA and
NH$_4^+$, although   transaminase was inhibited, glutamine formation was
stimulated as shown by increased level of specific activity above
that obtained with AOAA alone.   Thus the RSA of glutamine was raised

Table VII.   Guinea Pig Brain Slices.

| Precursor | Relative Specific Activity | | |
|---|---|---|---|
| [5-$^{14}$C] $\alpha$KG | Gm | AA | GABA |
| Control | 4.04 | 0.50 | 0.14 |
| NH$_4$$^+$ | 10.60 | 0.69 | 0.28 |
| AOAA | 9.44 | 0.14 | 0.01 |
| AOAA + NH$_4$$^+$ | 14.15 | 0.26 | 0.02 |
| | | | |
| [2-$^{14}$C]Glucose | | | |
| Control | 0.43 | 0.43 | 0.17 |
| NH$_4$$^+$ | 0.24 | 0.49 | 0.17 |

Relative Specific Activity (GA = 1).   See Table VI for experimental details.

to a value of approximately 14.   Since both the specific activities as well as the levels of the amino acids were altered in these experiments, the percentage distribution of the radioactivity, which take both factors into account, presents a more accurate picture of the changes in the metabolism induced by these drugs (Table VIII).   With labelled ketoglutarate as the precursor ammonia decreased the amount of label in glutamate and increased that in glutamine.   AOAA depressed severely the amount of label in glutamate and increased that in glutamine to a lesser extent.   The addition of both AOAA and NH$_4$$^+$ had no additional affect on the labelling of glutamate but doubled the amount of label in the glutamine as compared to AOAA alone.   In contrast, with [2-$^{14}$C]glucose as the labelled compound, NH$_4$$^+$ stimulated the labelling of glutamate but decreased the percentage of label incorporated into glutamine. This stimulation of glutamine formation by NH$_4$$^+$ in the presence of transaminase inhibition by AOAA could only occur if glutamate dehydrogenase was active in glutamine formation.   Furthermore, since the RSA of glutamine was 14 under these conditions, that pool of glutamate that interacted with glutamate dehydrogenase and was active in glutamine formation was approximately 7% or less of the total tissue glutamate.   On the other hand, NH$_4$$^+$ stimulated the flux of glucose into glutamate but not into that pool of glutamate which is active in glutamine formation.

Table VIII.  Guinea Pig Brain Slices: % Distribution
of Radioactivity

| Precursor | $[5-^{14}C]$ Ketoglutarate | | | | $[2-^{14}C]$ Glucose | |
| --- | --- | --- | --- | --- | --- | --- |
| Addition | None | $NH_4^+$ | AOAA | AOAA $+NH_4^+$ | None | $NH_4^+$ |
| Glutamate | 38 | 14 | 6 | 6 | 7 | 12 |
| Glutamine | 38 | 54 | 21 | 41 | 1.0 | 0.5 |
| Aspartate | 4 | 2 | 0.3 | 0.6 | 0.8 | 1.6 |
| GABA | 1.4 | 1.2 | 0.01 | 0.05 | 0.4 | 0.6 |
| Total cpm/g tissue x $10^{-6}$ | 2.05 | 1.45 | 1.13 | 1.00 | 0.97 | 0.90 |

Data from trichloroacetic acid extract of the tissue.  See Table VI
for experimental details.


DISCUSSION

The differential effects of a variety of inhibitors on the
labelling of glutamine and GABA clearly indicate that the glutamate
pool that is closely related to GAD and hence to GABA formation
has a different locus than the glutamate pool related to glutamate
dehydrogenase and glutamine synthetase and hance to glutamine formation.  The localization of GAD largely in the nerve endings by
histochemical and chemical means places the site of GABA formation
and its precursor pool of glutamate in the nerve endings.  Consequently, glutamine and its precursor pool of glutamate must be at
another site.  That this latter locus is probably in glia has been
suggested by a number of different lines of evidence.

1.  In both experimental animals in which ammonia was infused
or hepatoportal shunt performed, as well as in humans with hepatic
encephalopathy the astrocytes were the cells most severely patho-
logically affected (Cavanagh, 1974).  This has been take to suggest
that the metabolic detoxification and toxic effects of ammonia
occurs in these cells.

2.  Histochemical studies have been reported to show increased
levels of glutamate dehydrogenase activity in the astrocytes of
rats with encephalopathy produced by portocaval shunt (Norenberg,
1976).  Immunohistochemical studies from the same laboratory indicated that glutamine synthetase was exclusively localized in
glial cells (Martinez-Hernandex, et al., 1977.  Neuronal cell bodies, endothelial cells  and choroid epithelium appeared to contain
no enzyme.  However,  the reliability of quantitative conclusions

as to enzyme activity and localization based on such staining techniques has not been clearly established.

3. Measurement of glutamine synthetase following retrograde neuronal degeneration in the CNS of cats has indicated that glutamine synthetase is probably only in the glial-capillary wall porttions of the brain (Utley, 1964).

These studies all support the theory that glutamine synthesis arises from a small pool of glutamate which is probably localized in the glia.

In addition, glutamate dehydrogenase and acetyl CoA synthetase have been demonstrated to be enriched in a fraction of brain mitochondria which sediments in a sucrose density gradient more rapidly than does the average of the total brain mitochondria (Reijnierse et al., 1975). It may be that the former mitochondria are derived from glial cells, but direct evidence for such a hypothesis has not yet been obtained. Another characteristic of the Krebs cycle associated with glutamate dehydrogenase and acetyl CoA synthase appears to be that citrate synthase in this cycle with small pools of intermediates is operating far from equilibrium, while in the Krebs cycle with larger pools of intermediates the citrate synthase would appear to be operating close to equilibrium. This is based on a kinetic isotope effect observed in the labelling of glutamate and glutamine with tritiated acetate but not with tritiated glucose (Van den Berg and Ronda, 1976a).

Since $CO_2$ fixation is also markedly increased in ammonia stressed animals (Berl, 1971), the enzymes involved in this process are probably also closely associated with glutamate dehydrogenase and glutamine synthetase and could be expected to be enriched in glia. However, direct experimental evidence for such localization has not been reported. On this basis the glia would appear to have a greater capacity than neurons for utilizing the Krebs cycle for biosynthetic purposes e.g., glutamine formation.

Another approach which provided indications for an anatomical basis of amino acid compartmentation was the comparison of the specific activities of glutamate and glutamine during maturation of the kitten (Berl, 1965), rat (Patel and Balazs, 1970) and mouse brain (Van den Berg and Ronda, 1976b). With maturation there appeared to be a contraction of the pool of glutamic acid available for glutamine formation and an expansion of the pool or pools of glutamic acid not immediately available for glutamine synthesis (Berl, 1965). Thus, there was an approximately 5-10-fold increase in the ratios of specific activities of glutamine and glutamate as a result of the growth and maturaton in various brain areas, while during the same period glutamate levels approximately doubled and glutamine levels were essentially unchanged in most brain areas. The maximal increase in glutamate (as well as aspartate and GABA) occurred in the neocortex during the period of maximal elaboration of dendritic systems of pyramidal neurons and further growth of cell bodies and axonal networks. This late postnatal maturation period correlated reasonably well with the tissue course of glutamate compartmentation. This would place the developing larger pool of glutamate in the cell bodies, axons and or dendrites. This again would be consistent with the localization of the small pool of glutamate active in glutamine formation primarily in the glia.

It was mentioned earlier that the RSA of glutamine approached values as high as 14 when $[5-^{14}C]$ ketoglutarate was the labelled precursor and AOAA + $NH_4^+$ were present in the incubation medium. Therefore the small pool of glutamate active in glutamine formation under these conditions could not be any larger than approximately 7% of the total glutamate. Such disparate distributions of glutamate have not been observed either in glial cultures or in isolated cellular preparations. Therefore, only a part of the glial glutamate would seem to constitute the small pool of glutamate involved in glutamine formation. Perhaps it is the glutamate formed in the astrocytic mitochondria which is metabolically close to glutamate dehydrogenase that consitutes this small pool. This newly formed glutamate must be released from the mitochondria as quickly as it is formed and converted to glutamine by glutamine synthetase (a non-mitochondrial enzyme) much more rapidly than it can mix with the glutamate in the cytosol.

The studies with ouabain indicated that this newly formed glutmaine readily diffused from the brain tissue into the incubation medium and its release and reuptake did not appear to be energy dependent. In contrast, much of the glutamate (newly formed from acetate) maybe in nerve endings from which it was released and taken up into glia and converted to glutamine. This pool of glutamate appeared to be associated with glutamine formation since in the presence of ouabain it accumulated in the medium and formation of glutamine was prevented. This effect of ouabain on glutamate may have been on its release, reuptake or both.

Along this line of reasoning the effects of fluoroacetate and fluorocitrate on the labelling of glutamate and glutamine from acetate, aspartate and GABA are of particular interest. The data supports the postulate that glutamate formed in nerve endings may be released and taken up by the glia and converted to glutamine. In agreement with Quastel (1975) it would appear that acetate may be metabolized in part in neurons and not exclusively in glia. Therefore labelled acetate may not be an adequate marker of glial metabolism.

Another point which should be emphasized is that the data on the effects of the inhibitors, e.g., fluoroacetate and ouabain on the labelling of glutamate and glutmaine from the various precursors would best be explained by the existence of at least two small pools of glutamate (Balazs et al., 1973) only one of which is closely related to glutamine synthetase, the other must be released from its site of synthesis before it can be converted to glutamine.

Finally, it should be pointed out that isolated glia and neurons need not be expected to demonstrate the classical picture of the specific activity of glutamine greater than that of glutamate. All the evidence presently available suggests that structural relationships are required for the demonstration of this phenomenon.

## ACKNOWLEDGEMENT

These studies were supported in part by NIMH Grant MH-25505 and the Clinical Center for Research in Parkinson's and Allied Disorders, NIH Grant NS-11631.

## REFERENCES

Balazs, R., and Cremer, J.E., 1973, (eds.) 1973, in "Metabolic Compartmentation in the Brain", Macmillan Press, London.

Balazs, R., Patel, A.J., and Richter, D., 1973, Metabolic compartments in the brain. Their properties and relation to morphological structures, in "Metabolic Compartmentation in Brain", (R. Balazs, and J.E. Cremer, eds), pp. 167-184, Macmillan Press, London.

Baldessarini, R.J., and Yorke, C., 1974, Uptake and release of possible false transmitter amino acids by rat brain tissue, J. Neurochem. 23:839-848.

Berl, S., 1965, Compartmentation of glutamic acid metabolism in developing cerebral cortex, J. Biol. Chem. 240:2047-2054.

Berl, S., 1971, Cerebral amino acid metabolism in hepatic coma, Exp. Biol. Med. 4:71-84.

Berl, S., Clarke, D.D. and Nicklas, W.J., 1970, Compartmentation of citric acid cycle metabolism in brain, J. Neurochem. 17:999-1007.

Berl, S., Clarke, D.D., and Schneider, D., (eds.), 1975, in "Metabolic Compartmentation and Neurotransmission, Plenum Press, New York.

Berl, S. Lajtha, A., and Waelsch, H., 1961, Amino Acid and protein metabolism - VI Cerebral compartments of glutamic acid metabolism, J. Neurochem. 7:186-197.

Berl, S., Takagaki, G., Clarke, D.D., and Waelsch, H., 1962, Metabolic compartments in vivo: Ammonia and glutamic acid metabolism in brain and liver, J. Biol. Chem., 237:2562-2569.

Bradford, H.F., and Ward, H.K., 1976, On glutaminase activity in mammalian synaptosomes, Brain Res. 110:115-125.

Cavanagh, J.B., 1974, Liver bypass and the glia, in "Brain Dysfunction in Metabolic Disorders," Vol. 53 (F. Plum, ed), pp. 13-38, Raven Press, N.Y.

Chan, S.L., and Quastel, J.H., 1970, Effects of neurotropic drugs on sodium influx into rat brain cortex in vitro, Biochem. Pharmacol. 19:1071-1085.

Clarke, D.D., Nicklas, W.J., and Berl, S., 1970, Tricarboxylic acid cycle metabolism in brain, Biochem. J. 120:345-351.

Cremer, J.E., 1973, Changes within metabolic compartments related to the functional state and the action of drugs on the whole brain, in "Metabolic Compartmentation in the Brain", (R. Balazs and J.E. Cremer eds.), pp. 81-93, Macmillan Press, London.

Gaitonde, M.K., 1965, Rate of utilization of glucose and compartmentation of $\alpha$oxoglutarate and glutamate in rat brain, Biochem. J. 95: 803-810.

Goldberg, N.D., Passonneau, J.V., and Lowry, O.H., 1966, Effects of changes in brain metabolism in the levels of citric acid cycle intermediates, J. Biol. Chem. 211:3997-4003.

Gonda, O., and Quastel, J.H., 1966, Transport and metabolism of acetate in rat brain cortex in vitro, Biochem. J. 100: 83-94.

Hawkins, R.A., Miller, A.L., Nielson, R.C., and Veech, R.L., 1973, The acute action of ammonia on rat brain metabolism in vivo, Biochem. J. 134:1001-1003.

Lahiri, S., and Quastel, J.H., 1963, Fluoroacetate and the metabolism of ammonia in brain, Biochem. J. 89:157-163.

Martinez-Hernandez, A., Bell, K.P., and Norenberg, M.D., 1977, Glutamine synthetase: Glial localization in brain, Science, 195: 1356-1358.

Norenberg, M.D., 1976, Histochemical studies in experimental portosystemic encephalopathy, Arch. Neurol. 33:265-269.

Patel, A.J., and Balazs, R., 1970, Manifestation of metabolic compartmentation of the rat brain, J. Neurochem. 17: 955-971.

Quastel, J.H., 1975, Metabolic compartmentation in the brain and effects of metabolic inhibitors, in "Metabolic Compartmentation and Neurotransmission," (S. Berl, D.D. Clarke and D. Schneider eds.), pp. 337-361, Plenum Press, N.Y.

Reijnierse, G.L.A., Veldstra, H., and Van den Berg, C.J., 1975, Short-chain fatty acid synthesis in brain, Biochem. J., 152: 477-484.

Saito, K., Barber, R., Jang-Yen, W., Matsuda, T., Roberts, E., and Vaughn, J.E., 1974, Immunohistochemical localization of glutamate decarboxylase in rat cerebellum, Proc. Nat. Acad. Sci., U.S.A. 71:269-273.

Shank, R.P., and Aprison, M.H., 1977, Glutamine uptake and metabo-
    lism by the isolated toad brain: Evidence pertaining to its
    proposed role as a transmitter precursor, J. Neurochem., 28:
    1189-1196.
Utley, J.D., 1964, Glutamine synthetase, glutamotransferase, and
    glutaminase in neurons and non-neural tissue in the medial
    geniculate body of the cat, Biochem. Pharmacol., 13:1383-1392.
Van den Berg, C.J., and Garfinkel, D., 1971, A simulation study
    of brain compartments, Biochem. J., 123:211-218.
Van den Berg, C.J., and Ronda, G., 1976a, The incorporation of
    double-labelled acetate into glutamate and related amino acids
    from adult mouse brain, J. Neurochem., 27:1443-1448.
Van den Berg, C.J., and Ronda, G., 1976b, Metabolism of glutamate
    and related amino acids in the 10-day old mouse, J. Neurochem.,
    27:1449-1453.

# COMPARTMENTATION OF AMINO ACIDS IN BRAIN: THE GABA-GLUTAMINE-GLUTAMATE CYCLE

C. J. Van den Berg, D. F. Matheson* and W. C. Nijenmanting

Studygroup Inborn Errors and Brain
Department of Psychiatry
Faculty of Medicine
University of Groningen, Netherlands

*Erindale College
University of Totonto
Missisauga, Canada

Almost immediately after it was observed that increases of ammonia in the brain resulted in an increase of glutamine, it was postulated that the conversion of glutamate into glutamine served to detoxify the toxic ammonia. It was assumed that this glutamine was not degraded within the brain, but left this structure. Krebs (1936) wrote: "There is evidence in favour of the assumption that 'glutaminase" is a fragment of the synthesizing systems and that under physiological conditions it is concerned only with synthesis (of glutamine)". Somewhat later, Weil-Malherbe (1950) summarized his position as follows: "The evidence is thus in favor of glutamine as the end product of the "ammonia-binding mechanism" and in accord with the conception of glutamine as the transport and storage form of ammonia, synthesized at the centers of ammonia formation and hydrolyzed at the centers of ammonia disposal or utilization" (pp.555).

In the fifties Bessman advocated at various occasions his conviction, conception or hypothesis that the toxicity of ammonia was the result of an inhibition of oxidative processes leading to a decrease of the production and utilization of ATP (Bessman and Bessman, 1955). Ammonia was supposed to remove $\alpha$-oxoglutarate from the tricarboxylic acid cycle by converting it via glutamate dehydrogenase and glutamine synthase, acting in tandem, into glutamine. Not only would this result in a depletion of the tricarboxylic acid cycle intermediates, there would also be a decrease in ATP, needed

to synthesize glutamine from glutamate and ammonia. Some evidence
was given showing a decrease in α-oxoglutarate upon repeated
injections of ammonia-salts.

In 1962 Weil-Malherbe (1962) summarized his position again:
"It thus appears that many of the effects that might be attributed
to a toxic action of ammonia are in reality the results of a
detoxification mechanism. This is not to deny the toxicity of
ammonia itself. Indeed, the fact that the synthesis of glutamine
has priority over many other energy-consuming reactions and the
further fact that the synthesis of glutamate proceeds in spite of
the risk of a depletion of dicarboxylic acids suggest that the intracellular accumulation of ammonia has to be prevented even through
a high price may have to be paid for it".(pp.328).Did the concept
that the toxic action of ammonia is caused by the same mechanism
as the detoxification of ammonia present a problem?

But, is there available solid evidence that ammonia leads to
a decreased formation of ATP or equivalent high-energy compounds?
And further, is there evidence that decreases in ATP production can
lead to the whole spectrum of neurological and other symptoms,
such as coma or convulsions, shown by ammonia? We will not try to
answer this last question; there is a vast and partly confusing
literature on the relation between energy conversions and brain
function, but the first question can be answered, as a number of
investigators have recently carried out careful investigations on
the effect of ammonia on energy conversion processes in the brain.
It might be noted in passing that interest in this field is
stimulated by the search for mechanisms explaining the neurological
sequelae from a number of liver diseases and from some inborn
errors of metabolism.

Bessman and Bessman (1955) presented, as already stated, some
evidence that repeated injections of ammonium salts did lead to a
decrease of α-oxoglutarate in the brain. A number of reports
followed in which decreases of α-oxoglutarate and ATP were found,
in accordance with Bessman's hypothesis (summarized by Schenker
et al.,1974). More recent work has, however, failed to confirm
those older findings; probably because methods have been used in
which post-mortem changes were avoided as much as possible (Hindfelt and Siesjö,1971; Hawkins et al.,1973). The latter authors
investigated the effect of high amounts of ammonium acetate on a
large number of compounds in the brain of rats. The animals were
killed just before the onset of convulsions; there is no doubt
that there was a "brain dysfunction". The authors conclude: "The results indicate that $NH_4^+$ stimulates metabolism but does not interfere with brain energy balance. The increased rate of oxidative
metabolism could not be accounted for only on the basis of
glutamine synthesis". (Hawkins et al.,1973,pp. 1001).

We seem, therefore, to be in a position where we have a
hypothesis without evidence to support it. In theory, it is still
possible that there are in a very small fraction of the brain

changes going on in energy conversion processes which serve as
initiators for the more general neurological dysfunctions, but the
observation that increases in glutamine upon administration of
ammonium salts are easily found in all brain parts makes such an
idea not very attractive at this moment. It seems better to search
for other mechanisms.

We have spend this space on this history as the Krebs/Weil-
Malherbe/Bessman ideas have been very popular and found a wide
circulation in textbooks etc. It should be admitted that the
mechanism proposed is simple and elegant, and that there were indeed some data which seemed to support the ammonia-energy-depletion
concept. It will certainly happen that some of the data we will
use further in this story also are to some extent artifactual;
the analysis of compounds in the brain which are part of complex
and dynamic metabolic networks is difficult and full of unexpected
pitfalls. Although a large mass of data has accumulated over the
last decades in the field of amino acid metabolism in brain, our
knowledge is still crude with respect to the metabolic fine-
structure of the brain. It is tempting to try to replace the old
ammonia-energy-depletion theory by a new one, for example an
ammonia-glutamate/GABA-neurotransmitter theory, but that seems
senseless and might even be misleading. From amino acids to brain
function is too large a jump; shortcuts by the mere combination of
words do not serve any purpose.

## I. GLUTAMINE FORMATION AND DEGRADATION

Krebs (1935) and Weil-Malherbe (1936) established in the
thirties very nicely and clearly that brain slices were capable
of forming large amounts of glutamine from ammonia and glutamate.
As already stated Krebs was convinced that this glutamine was not
broken down within the brain. *In vivo*, there are also increases of
glutamine upon administration of ammonium salts (see: Van den Berg,
1970).

While those data establish  some role for glutamine in
ammonia metabolism when ammonia levels are increased, they do not
allow conclusions about glutamine metabolism during normal conditions.
Without the use of labelled precursors it is very difficult to
study the dynamics of glutamine in normal conditions. If in those
normal conditions there is an active formation of glutamine without
degradation of this glutamine within the brain, the brain would
loose a fair amount of carbon- and nitrogen-atoms continuously. No
such losses have been found, however.

In the late fifties Waelsch and his colleagues started to use
labelled precursors for the study of the *in vivo* dynamics of amino
acid metabolism in the brain. It became immediately clear that
glutamine was metabolically a very active compound, even in conditions when no ammonia was given (see for review: Berl and Clarke,
1969). When labelled glutamine was injected intracisternally in the
rat, it was found to be rapidly metabolized into glutamate, GABA
and other amino acids (Berl et al.,1961).

At that time the glutamate-glutamine system was considered to be a sort of buffer for the control of ammonia. Ammonia itself was thought to be intimately related to "nervous activity". One of the mechanisms by which ammonia was supposed to play its role was as a donor of amide groups of proteins. It was thought that "nervous activity" would lead to the release of free ammonia from the amide groups of proteins. This ammonia would then be converted to glutamine,which would subsequently be used again, either for the synthesis or for the amidation of proteins. It was, in fact, to test this sort of ideas that Waelsch and his collaborators started to use $^{15}$N-labelled ammonium salts. Not much of the label, however, was found to enter the proteins. This disappointment was compensated for by the unexpected finding of a very large incorporation of $^{15}$N in the amino-group of glutamine, suggesting that this glutamine was formed from a small fraction of the total glutamate pool present in brain (Berl et al.,1962). Although in these experiments large amounts of $^{15}$N-ammonium salts had to be infused in order to be able to carry out the $^{15}$N determinations, experiments done at the time with labelled carbon dioxide with and without giving ammonium salts indicated clearly that extensive formation of glutamine took place even in the absence of added ammonium salts (Waelsch et al.,1964).

Extensive computer simulation of the data was performed by Garfinkel (1966). The model proposed consisted of two compartments; in one of the two there was a large pool of glutamate from which little glutamine was formed, while in the other there was a small pool of glutamate from which glutamine was formed at a high rate. Information on the sequence of reactions, was proposed by Berl and Clarke (1969). In these models the glutamate-glutamine system was represented as a reversible reaction, mainly as a buffer system for ammonia.

In the meantime, O'Neal and Koeppe (1966) published an extensive set of data on the incorporation of various specifically labelled precursors into the individual carbon atoms of glutamate and aspartate. They developed a scheme, consisting of two tricarboxylic acid cycles, which were connected with each other by movements of glutamate. The glutamate-glutamine system was in the established tradition considered as a reversible reaction, with some glutamine leaving the brain. Following O'Neal and Koeppe we did an extensive study on the rate of incorporation of specifically labelled glucose and acetate into brain amino acids (Van den Berg et al.,1966; Van den Berg et al.,1969). It was found that with acetate as a precursor glutamate was labelled later than glutamine, and from this we suggested that there was in brain an extensive conversion of glutamine into glutamate. This, of course, was known. From a comparison of the rate of incorporation of $(1-^{14}C)-$ and $(2-^{14}C)$ acetate into glutamine and glutamate with each other it appeared, however, that the glutamate formed from glutamine was located in another pool or compartment than the glutamate from which the glutamine was formed. Evidently, glutamine is transported from its site of synthesis to another site, where it is degraded into glutamate. A computer simulation of this model resulted after some manipulation of the various parameters in a reasonable fit of the observed and the calculated data (Van den Berg and Garfinkel, 1971). The model developed is certainly a gross oversimplification; refinements on the basis of more extensive data will be needed.

The model has two features which are relevant for this discussion: 1) a small pool of glutamate is converted into glutamine and this glutamine moves to a site where the glutamate is of a large-compartment-type and 2) from a pool of glutamate, which is of the large-compartment-type, GABA is formed; this GABA moves to a site, where the small glutamate pool is located and where it is converted into glutamine via a segment of the tricarboxylic acid cycle. In the model we assumed that the flow of GABA in one and the flow of glutamine in the opposite direction were equal; we will come back to this point further on. It has not been discussed extensively that when GABA and glutamine move in opposite directions there is a net transport of nitrogen in the direction of glutamine movement. In order for the system to be balanced, there should therefore be a movement of nitrogen, in one form or another in the direction opposite to that of glutamine movement.

## II. SOME FURTHER ARGUMENTS FOR THE TRANSPORT OF GLUTAMINE WITHIN THE BRAIN

When ammonia is given to experimental animals, there is, as has already been noted, a rapid rise of glutamine in the brain. From those findings it was concluded that this rise of glutamine was the result of an increased formation of glutamine. As ammonia ia a reaction partner of both glutamate dehydrogenase and glutamine synthase, one would hardly need more direct evidence (Matheson and Van den Berg, 1975). When we observed that ammonium chloride, given one minute before labelled acetate, did not result in an increase of glutamine labelling, we were at first surprised. We had expected an increase. Although we knew that the glutamate pool from which glutamine is formed was small and probably not large enough for all the glutamine to be formed from it, the glutamate dehydrogenase reaction could serve to supply more of this glutamate. That glutamate dehydrogenase was involved in the synthesis of glutamine seemed to follow directly from the observations of Berl et al.(1962) that $^{15}$N from ammonium salts was found to be incorporated into the $\alpha$-aminogroup of glutamine.

Puzzled by the lack of increase of acetate incorporation into glutamine in the ammoniated animals, we did an experiment in which the ammonium chloride was injected 5min after the labelled acetate had been given. The purpose of this experiment was to see whether ammonium chloride injections would influence the rate of disappearance of label from glutamine, once this glutamine was labelled. An advantage of this experimental procedure is that the effect of ammonia on a large pool of labelled glutamine is investigated; in

the experiments in which changes in the rate of labelled acetate
incorporation were investigated, trace amounts of the label were
injected. In those circumstances small changes in the distribution
of tracer in the body can easily lead to changes in the label
found in certain body constituents. Indeed, in a repetition of the
earlier experiments we have now observed an increased incorporation
of labelled acetate into glutamine under the influence of ammonium
chloride (Nijenmanting et al.,1977). The experiment in which we injected the ammonium chloride at a time when glutamine was highly
labelled is less liable to give data which cannot be interpreted
very easily.

    When the ammonium chloride was injected 5min after the labelled
acetate, there was no decrease of the label in glutamine, while in
the control animals there was the normally occurring decrease
(Fig. 1, Matheson and Van den Berg, 1975).

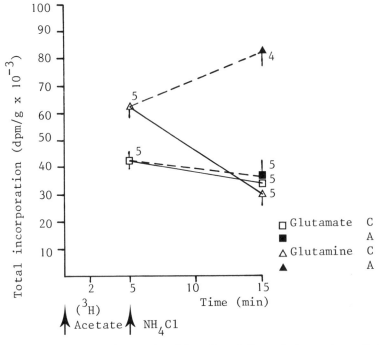

FIGURE 1. Effect of ammonium chloride, 7mmol/kg, injected at 5min
after labelled acetate on the rate of disappearance of label from
glutamine. C: control animals, A: ammoniated animals. From:
Matheson and Van den Berg (1975).

From this experiment we conclude that ammonium chloride injections
led to an inhibition of the rate of degradation of glutamine in
the brain. From our experiments nothing can be concluded about the
mechanism of this inhibition, but Bradford and Ward (1976) have
shown that addition of ammonia to synaptosomal preparations in-

hibited the conversion of labelled glutamine into glutamate,
probably by inhibiting glutaminase.

In the first five minutes after the injection of ammonium
chloride to mice in about 7mmol/kg, there was as noted an increase
of glutamine. At the same time we observed a decrease of glutamate
and aspartate (Table 1, Matheson and Van den Berg,1975)

TABLE 1. LEVELS OF GLUTAMATE AND GLUTAMINE IN ADULT
CONTROL AND AMMONIUM CHLORIDE-TREATED MOUSE BRAIN

| Time after injection (min) | Glutamate (μmol/g brain) | Glutamine | $\Sigma$ α-amino nitrogen |
|---|---|---|---|
| Control | 9.99 ± 0.69 (33) | 4.29 ± 0.53 (33) | 17.18 ± 0.64 (25) |
| 3 | 9.59 ± 0.54 ( 7) | 4.90 ± 1.36 ( 7) | 17.13 ± 0.67 ( 6) |
| 6 | 9.06 ± 0.54 ( 5) | 5.80 ± 0.93 (10) | 17.06 ± 0.42 ( 5) |
| 11 | 8.85 ± 0.54 ( 5) | 5.87 ± 0.90 ( 5) | 17.13 ± 0.58 ( 4) |
| 16 | 8.41 ± 0.94 ( 8) | 7.16 ± 0.50 ( 4) | 18.18 ± 0.46 ( 4) |

Mice were injected with 7mmol/kg of ammonium chloride. Data taken
from Van den Berg and Matheson (1975) and unpublished.

The sum of α-amino-groups in those three amino acids remained
constant. Those findings almost certainly prove that no increased
flux through glutamate dehydrogenase in the direction of glutamate
synthesis was taking place. The absence of an increased incorporation
of labelled β-hydroxybutyrate and acetate into brain amino acids
(data not given) also argue for a lack of increase of this reaction.
It is also to be noted that Hindfelt and Siesjö(1971) and Hawkins
et al.(1973) did not find decreases in α-oxoglutarate in animals
injected with ammonium salts. These findings combined suggest that
a few minutes after the injection of ammonium salts the rise of
glutamine is certainly not the result of a large divertment of α-
oxoglutarate from the tricarboxylic acid cycle.

Between 10 and 15min after the injection of ammonium chloride,
however, there was a clear rise in the combined amino groups in
glutamate, glutamine and aspartate (Table 1). This, then, would
indicate that at those later times there is an increased flux
through glutamate dehydrogenase. A small increase of this summated
α-amino-groups was found by Hawkins et al.(1973) at about 5-6min
after the injection of ammonium acetate to rats. These rats were
killed just before they would have shown convulsions. The amount
of ammonium chloride we injected in mice was such, 7mmol/kg, that
no convulsions would occur, although pronounced neurological dysfunctions were present. The effect of ammonium chloride on amino

acid metabolism seems, therefore, to be dependent very much on the amount injected and on the time the brain is exposed to ammonium chloride. The mechanism which leads to the inhibition of glutamine degradation comes into play very rapidly after the injection of relatively low amounts of ammonium chloride. Only at fairly high amounts of ammonium chloride or at longer times after the injection of ammonium chloride is there an increase in the flux through glutamate dehydrogenase and glutamine synthase in the direction of glutamine synthesis. It is to be noted that a decrease in the rate of degradation of glutamine in the brain does lead to a binding of ammonia, and is therefore as effective for the control of ammonia levels than changes in the rate of synthesis of glutamine.

### III. THE LINK BETWEEN GLUTAMINE AND GABA

Labelled GABA, when injected into the brain, is rapidly incorporated into glutamine (Roberts et al.,1958). Similar observations have been made in slices (Balázs et al.,1970). It was, therefore, natural to assume that in brain GABA is converted via a segment of the tricarboxylic acid cycle and glutamate into glutamine. In order to find more evidence for this sequence we carried out a few experiments with aminooxyacetic acid. This compound when given in doses of 20mg/kg or higher, is a powerful *in vivo* inhibitor of GABA-transaminase (Van Gelder, 1966). We firstly checked whether other transaminase reactions were inhibited by determining the incorporation of labelled $\beta$-hydroxybutyrate into glutamate and related amino acids in animals which had received 40mg/kg of aminooxyacetic acid for one hour. No changes were found (data not given).

TABLE 2. EFFECT OF AMMONIA ON GLUTAMATE AND
GLUTAMINE LEVELS

Ammonium chloride injected 1h after AOAA: time after ammonia 6min

| Treatment | Control | $NH_4Cl$-treated | Difference |
|-----------|---------|------------------|------------|
| Glutamine | | | |
| none | $4.20 \pm 0.43$ (10) | $5.80 \pm 0.83$ (10) | + 1.60 |
| AOAA 20mg/kg | $3.18 \pm 0.61$ ( 8) | $3.10 \pm 0.33$ ( 4) | − 0.08 |
| AOAA 80mg/kg | $3.44 \pm 0.33$ ( 3) | $2.43 \pm 0.58$ ( 4) | − 1.01 |
| Glutamate | | | |
| none | $9.78 \pm 0.61$ (11) | $9.06 \pm 0.54$ ( 4) | − 0.72 |
| AOAA 20mg/kg | $9.64 \pm 1.25$ ( 8) | $9.73 \pm 0.15$ ( 3) | + 0.09 |
| AOAA 80mg/kg | $7.60 \pm 0.09$ ( 3) | $6.22 \pm 0.16$ ( 3) | − 1.38 |

Values in $\mu$mol/g wet wt

The mice received 7mmol/kg of ammonium chloride. Data from Van den Berg and Matheson (1975).

Having established that GABA-transaminase is probably the only transaminase which was measurably inhibited, we injected ammonium chloride 1hr after 20 or 80mg/kg of aminooxyacetic acid was given. The animals were killed at 6min after the injection of ammonium chloride and the levels of glutamate, aspartate and glutamine measured.

In the controls there was the expected increase of glutamine, but this increase was absent in the animals pretreated with amino-oxyacetic acid. How to explain these findings? Let us assume that a few minutes after the injection of 7mmol/kg of ammonium chloride its major effect in the brain is to inhibit the degradation of glutamine. Then it follows that the rate of increase of glutamine, after the inhibition sets in, is related to the rate of synthesis of glutamine. If this is indeed the case then the absence of an increase of glutamine in animals which had received ammonium chloride 1hr after aminooxyacetic acid, indicates that there was a substantial decrease in the rate of synthesis of glutamine. As in these animals GABA degradation is inhibited, these results are consistent with the hypothesis that GABA degradation and glutamine synthesis are coupled to each other.

## IV. AMINOOXYACETIC ACID AND GABA

Van Gelder (1966) and Kuriyama et al.(1966) followed the changes in GABA in mice brain for several hours after the administration of aminooxyacetic acid. It was found that there was a steady increase in GABA up to 3-6hr; to about 17μmol/gram of wet weight at 3hr in the experiments reported by Van Gelder (1966) and to about 10μmol/gram of wet weight at 6hr in those reported by Kuriyama et al.(1966). The increase in GABA is far greater than the decrease observed in some of the other amino acids (Kuriyama et al.,1966; Van den Berg and Matheson, 1975).

What is the source of the carbon and the nitrogen which accumulates as GABA? If GABA degradation is linked to glutamine synthesis which in turn is used again for the synthesis of GABA, the blockade of GABA degradation should result in a decreased formation of glutamine-which it does see the preceding paragraph-and should then also lead to a reduction in the rate of synthesis of GABA, due to the lack of glutamate. This,however, does not occur. Evidently, glutamine is not an obligatory source of carbon and nitrogen for GABA synthesis.

Are these other sources only called upon when there is not enough glutamine to replenish the loss of tricarboxylic acid cycle intermediates, due to the synthesis and removal of GABA, or are they also very important in normal conditions? We have cited al-ready that labelled glutamine when injected into the brain is rapidly converted into glutamate and GABA. Recently, Shank and Aprison (1977) conducted an extensive kinetic analysis of glutamine metabolism in the toad brain and produced evidence for the role of glutamine as a precursor of GABA.

It is, of course, very hard to convert labelling data into rates. To calculate the contribution of glutamine to GABA synthesis would require much more extensive labelling data than are currently available. Still, most of the evidence available seems to be consistent with the role of glutamine in GABA synthesis. To explain the discrepancies between the conclusions drawn on the basis of the labelling data and on the continuous rise of GABA in the presence of aminooxyacetic acid, we will have to postulate that the presence of aminooxyacetic acid leads to the activation of other mechanisms. The nature of those mechanisms is completely unknown. It is possible that carbon dioxide fixation at the level of pyruvate becomes more active, or that amino acids released by the hydrolysis of proteins are being used, or that glutamine from the circulation starts entering the brain. It would be very worthwhile to get some more information.

We do not know very much on the mechanisms of control of GABA synthesis. It is very likely the amount of glutamate which reaches glutamate decarboxylase that controls the rate of GABA synthesis. But, what controls the amount of glutamate in the nerve-endings producing GABA? If glutamine is indeed an important source of glutamate for GABA production, what are the mechanisms by which the transport of glutamine to those sites of GABA is controlled? Our ignorance is almost absolute and it is very hard to device *in vivo* experiments that will give answers to those questions.

It is worthwhile to mention that when aminooxyacetic acid is given to mice, there is about 15min after its injection, a phase where the animals are a bit "excited". After a few minutes this phase is over and the animals become very quiet.At high doses of aminooxyacetic acid, convulsions might occur. It is possible, that this "excited" phase corresponds with a shift from glutamine as a source of GABA to other sources, but to draw such conclusions from changes in the behaviour of an animal can be extremely dangerous. This can be illustrated nicely by comparing the effects of ammonium chloride and aminooxyacetic acid. Their effects on the intact animals are strikingly different, while both these compounds interrupt the GABA-glutamine-glutamate cycle!

## V. THE GLUTAMATE-GLUTAMINE CYCLE

Earlier, as already emphasized, it was widely believed that the reversible glutamate-glutamine interconversion had a role in the control of ammonia levels in the brain. More recently, movements of glutamate and glutamine between cells have become part of this scheme. Benjamin and Quastel (1975) wrote: "The suggestion of the existence of a cycle of events linking the neurons and the glia, and involving the interconversion of glutamate and glutamine, gives the ammonium ion an important role in the maintenance of the steady state of glutamate in the nervous system as it is necessary for the return of glutamate to the neuron in the form of glutamine after its release from the neuron by excitation" (pp.205). Very

similar thoughts have been expressed by Bradford and Dodd (1976)
on the basis of experiments in which it was found that addition
of ammonia to synaptosomal preparations resulted in an inhibition
of the conversion of glutamine into glutamate (Bradford and Ward,
1976).

The rate of increase of glutamine in the mice brain after the
injection of ammonium chloride is about 0.25μmol/min per gram wet
weight. The rate of synthesis of GABA in mice brain is somewhere
between 0.1 and 0.15μmol/min per gram wet weight (see: Van den Berg
et al.,1975). Therefore, not all glutamine has a role as a precursor
of GABA; it is very likely that the difference in glutamine
synthesis, around 0.1μmol/min per gram wet weight, does have a
function in the glutamate-glutamine cycle, or in a glutamate-
aspartate-glutamine cycle.

## VI. THE LOCALIZATIONS OF THESE CYCLES

A large fraction of the glutamate decarboxylase, probably 60%
or more, is located in nerve-endings (Salganicoff and De Robertis,
1965; Van Kempen et al.,1965). Most of the GABA is formed in these
nerve-endings, one can suppose. As there is very little or no GABA-
transaminase in the glutamate decarboxylase nerve-endings,the
degradation of GABA, or the GABA to glutamine part of the cycle,
has to occur at another site than the synthesis of GABA. It has been
argued by many (see: Baláfzs and Cremer,1973; Berl et al.,1975) that
the small glutamate compartment and therefore the sites where GABA
is converted into glutamine, is located in glia-cells.

Some enzymes, eg. GABA-transaminase and glutamine synthase,
have critical functions in one or more of these amino acid-cycles.
Data on the cellular localization of these enzymes are of direct
importance for this localization problem. Evidence, previously
summarized (Van den Berg et al.,1975) suggested that GABA-trans-
aminaɾe was present in glia-cells as well as in neurons. Recent
evidence has supported this conclusion (Hyde and Robinson,1976).It
is to be noted that these authors found evidence for the presence
of GABA-transaminase in presynaptic terminals. This contrasts with
conclusions drawn from studies on the distribution of glutamate
decarboxylase and GABA-transaminase in sucrose-density gradients.
The curves found have such a form that it does seem unlikely that
there is a measurable amount of GABA-transaminase in nerve-endings
which contain glutamate decarboxylase (see: Van den Berg et al.,
1975). If there is no GABA-transaminase present in the glutamate
decarboxylase terminals, then the proposals that some GABA-transaminase inhibitors have anticonvulsive properties because they
elevate GABA presynaptically, have not much support.

From the distribution of GABA-transaminase one can conclude
that the small compartment , in so far as it  converts GABA into
glutamine is present both in neurons and in glia-cells. Those cells
are presumably located near the sites where GABA is acting as neurotransmitter. If so, then glutamine synthase should also be present

both in neurons and glia-cells. The conversion of glutamate into glutamine is so basic for cellular metabolism, for example for the synthesis of glutamine for protein synthesis, that one would assume this enzyme to be present everywhere. Recent histochemical evidence, however, seems to indicate that this enzyme is mainly present in glia-cells (Martinez-Hernandez et al.,1977). This is fully in accordance with the models in which the small glutamate compartment is present in glia-cells, but presents some problem for the models in which at least part of the small compartment is also present in neurons. It is possible that the techniques used for the histochemical investigations were such that the neuronal glutamine synthase was lost or did not become visible.

In discussing the role of enzymes in the compartmentation of amino acids we have assumed without going into details that GABA-transaminase, glutamate dehydrogenase and glutamine synthase are markers for the small glutamate compartment. We have shown, however, that GABA-transaminase and glutamate dehydrogenase were not in the same proportion to each other present in the same mitochondria (Reijnierse et al.,1975). The small compartment is certainly heterogeneous; previously we have suggested that there may exist at least 5 or more different types of small compartments. In the absence of new relevant data we will not discuss this matter here further (Van den Berg et al.,1975). In the context of this paper, however, it may be suggested that the dual action of ammonia on amino metabolism (see earlier) is related to an action of ammonia on the metabolic sequence, or metabolic space, in which GABA-transaminase and glutamine synthase are present and to an action of ammonia on the metabolic space in which glutamate dehydrogenase and glutamine synthase are present. The first metabolic space is part of the GABA-glutamine-glutamate cycle, while the latter metabolic space may be a part of the glutamate-glutamine cycle.

Finally, we would like to emphasize that no definite proof is available for the assumption that all the GABA, which is degraded by GABA-transaminase, is converted into glutamine; only a part might follow this route, while another part might follow another route. This could explain the discrepancies found for the localization of GABA-transaminase and glutamine synthase.

## VII. SUMMARY

Amino acid metabolism in brain can be affected by ammonium salts in a number of ways. At low doses and short times after the injection of ammonium chloride in mice, its main effect is to decrease the degradation of glutamine within the brain. At higher doses and at longer time intervals ammonium chloride is capable of increasing the rate of synthesis of glutamate plus glutamine. There is no evidence available that this increase in the rate of synthesis of glutamate, plus glutamine, results in a depletion of tricarboxylic acid cycle intermediates and that this depletion is one of the main factors causing brain dysfunction.

The energy-depletion theory seems not any more to be founded on solid experimental observations; it does,however, not seem to be very useful to replace this theory by one in which changes in neurotransmitters are held to be causative for the brain dysfunction. Although it is certainly possible that changes in amino acid neurotransmitters, affected by ammonia, play an important role in causing the brain dysfunction, it is currently impossible to support such a suggestion by solid data.

The data obtained with ammonium chloride with and without aminooxyacetic acid are most easily explained in terms of a GABA-glutamine-glutamate cycle. Earlier proposals for the existence of such a cycle were mainly based on an interpretation of complex kinetic isotope data. Although such a cycle does exist it is very likely that different types or forms of this cycle do occur in brain. Glutamine does not only play a role in this GABA-glutamine-glutamate cycle, but also in glutamine-glutamate cycles, postulated by other authors.

## REFERENCES

Balázs,R., and Cremer,J.E.(Eds) 1973, Metabolic Compartmentation in the Brain, MacMillan,London.

Balázs,R., Machiyama,Y., Hammond,B.J., Julian,T., and Richter,D., 1970, The operation of the $\gamma$-aminobutyrate bypath of the tricarboxylic acid cycle in brain tissue *in vitro*, Biochem.J.116: 445-467.

Benjamin,A.M., and Quastel,J.H., 1975, Metabolism of amino acids and ammonia in rat brain cortex slices *in vitro*: a possible role of ammonia in brain function, *J.Neurochem*. 25: 197-206.

Berl,S., and Clarke,D.D., 1969, Compartmentation of amino acid metabolism, *in* "Handbook of Neurochemistry" Vol.2 (A.Lajtha, ed),Plenum Press,New York.

Berl,S., Clarke,D.D., and Schneider,D., (Eds),1975, Metabolic Compartmentation and Neurotransmission, Plenum Press,New York.

Berl,S., Lajtha,A., and Waelsch,H., 1961, Amino acid and protein metabolism. VI.Cerebral compartments of glutamic acid metabolism, *J.Neurochem*. 7: 186-197.

Berl,S., Takagaki,G., Clarke,D.D., and Waelsch,H., 1962, Metabolic compartments *in vivo*. Ammonia and glutamic acid metabolism in brain and liver, *J.Biol.Chem*. 237: 2562-2569.

Bessman,S.P., and Bessman,A.N., 1955, The cerebral and peripheral uptake of ammonia in liver disease with an hypothesis for the mechanism of hepatic coma, *J.Clin.Invest*. 34: 622-628.

Bradford,H.F., and Dodd,P.R., 1976, Biochemistry and basic mechanisms in epilepsy, *in* "Biochemistry and Neurological Disease", (A.N.Davison,ed), Blackwell Scientific Publishers, London.

Bradford,H.F., and Ward, H.K., 1976, On glutaminase activity in mammalian synaptosomes, *Brain Res*. 110: 115-125.

Garfinkel,D., 1966, A simulation study of the metabolism and com-
     partmentation in brain of glutamate, aspartate, the Krebs cycle
     and related metabolites, *J.Biol.Chem*. 241: 3918-3929.
Hawkins,R.A., Miller,A.L., Nielsen,R.C., and Veech,R.L., 1973, The
     acute action of ammonia on rat brain metabolism *in vivo*, *Bio-
     chem.J*. 134: 1001-1008.
Hindfelt,B., and Siesjö,B.K., 1971, Cerebral effects of acute
     ammonia intoxication. II. The effect upon energy metabolism,
     *Scand.J.Clin.Lab.Invest*. 28: 365-374.
Hyde,J.C., and Robinson,N., 1976, Electron cytochemical localization
     of gamma-aminobutyric acid catabolism in rat cerebellar cortex,
     *Histochem*. 49: 51-65.
Krebs,H.A., 1935, Metabolism of amino acids. IV.The synthesis of
     glutamine from glutamic acid and ammonia, and the enzymic hydro-
     lysis of glutamine in animal tissue, *Biochem.J*. 29: 1951-1969.
Krebs,H.A., 1936, Metabolism of amino acids and related substances,
     *Ann.Rev.Biochem*. 5: 247-270.
Kuriyama,K., Roberts,E., and Rubinstein,M.K., 1966, Elevation of
     $\gamma$-aminobutyric acid in brain with amino-oxyacetic acid and
     susceptibility to convulsive seizures in mice: a quantitative
     re-evaluation, *Biochem.Pharmacol*. 15: 221-236.
Martinez-Hernandez,A., Bell,K.P., and Norenberg,M.D., 1977, Glutamine
     synthetase: glial localization in brain, *Science*,195: 1356-1358.
Matheson,D.F., and Van den Berg,C.J., 1975, Ammonia and brain
     glutamine: inhibition of glutamine degradation by ammonia,
     *Biochem.Soc.Trans*. 3: 525-528.
Nijenmanting,W.C., Matheson,D.F., and Van den Berg,C.J., 1977,
     Glutamate-glutamine compartmentation in brain; effects of site
     of injection of the precursor and effects of ammonia, Abstracts
     6th Meeting ISN,Copenhagen.
O'Neal,R.M., and Koeppe,R.E., 1966, Precursors *in vivo* of glutamate,
     aspartate and their derivatives of rat brain, *J.Neurochem*. 13:
     835-847.
Reijnierse,G.L.A., Veldstra,H., and Van den Berg,C.J., 1975, Sub-
     cellular localization of $\gamma$-aminobutyrate transaminase and
     glutamate dehydrogenase in adult rat brain, *Biochem.J*. 152:
     469-475.
Roberts,E., Rothstein,M., and Baxter,C.F., 1958, Some metabolic
     studies of $\gamma$-aminobutyric acid, *Proc.Soc.Exp.Biol.Med*. 97:
     796-802.
Salganicoff,L., and De Robertis,E., 1965, Subcellular distribution
     of the enzymes of the glutamic, glutamine and $\gamma$-aminobutyric acid
     cycles in rat brain, *J.Neurochem*. 12: 287-309.
Schenker,S., Breen,K.J., and Hoyumpa,A.M., 1974, Hepatic encephalo-
     pathy: current status, *Gastroenterology* 66: 121-151.
Shank,R.P., and Aprison,M.H., 1977, Glutamine uptake and metabolism
     by the isolated toad brain: evidence pertaining to its proposed
     role as a transmitter precursor, *J.Neurochem*. 28: 1189-1196.
Van den Berg,C.J., 1970, Glutamate and glutamine, *in* "Handbook of
     Neurochemistry", Vol.3 (A.Lajtha,ed), Plenum Press, New York.

Van den Berg,C.J., and Garfinkel,D.,1971, A simulation study of
    brain compartments. Metabolism of glutamate and related sub-
    stances in mouse brain, *Biochem.J*. 123: 211-218.
Van den Berg,C.J., and Matheson,D.F., 1975, The formation of
    glutamine in mouse brain: effect of aminooxyacetic acid and
    ammonia, *Biochem.Soc.Trans*. 3: 528-530.
Van den Berg,C.J., Mela,P.,and Waelsch,H., 1966, On the contribution
    of the tricarboxylic acid cycle to the synthesis of glutamate,
    glutamine and aspartate in brain, *Biochem.Biophys.Res.Commun*.
    23: 479-484.
Van den Berg,C.J., Kržalić,Lj., Mela,P.,and Waelsch,H., 1969, Com-
    partmentation of glutamate metabolism in brain. Evidence for
    the existence of two different tricarboxylic acid cycles in
    brain, *Biochem.J*. 113: 281-290.
Van den Berg,C.J.,Matheson,D.F., Ronda,G.,Reijnierse,G.L.A.,Blok-
    huis,G.G.D.,Kroon,M.C.,Clarke,D.D.,and Garfinkel,D., 1975, A
    model of glutamate metabolism in brain; a biochemical analysis
    of a heterogeneous structure, *in* "Metabolic Compartmentation and
    Neurotransmission",(S.Berl, D.D.Clarke and D.Schneider,eds),
    Plenum Press,New York.
Van Gelder,N.M.,1966, The effect of aminooxyacetic acid on the
    metabolism of γ-aminobutyric acid in brain, *Biochem.Pharmacol*.
    15: 533-539.
Van Kempen,G.M.J., Van den Berg,C.J.,Van der Helm,H.J.,and Veldstra,
    H.,1965, Intracellular localization of glutamate decarboxylase,
    γ-aminobutyrate transaminase and some other enzymes in brain
    tissue, *J.Neurochem*. 12: 581-588.
Waelsch,H.,Berl,S.,Rossi,C.A.,Clarke,D.D., and Purpura,D.P., 1964,
    Quantitative aspects of $CO_2$ fixation in mammalian brain *in vivo*,
    *J.Neurochem*. 11: 717-728.
Weil-Malherbe,H.,1936, Studies on brain metabolism. 1.The metabolism
    of glutamic acid in brain, *Biochem.J*. 30: 665-676.
Weil-Malherbe,H.,1950, Significance of glutamic acid for the
    metabolism of nervous tissue, *Physiol.Rev*. 30: 549-568.
Weil-Malherbe,H.,1962, Ammonia metabolism in the brain, *in* "Neuro-
    chemistry",2$^e$ ed.(K.A.C.Eliot, I.H.Page and J.H.Quastel,eds)
    Charles C.Thomas,Springfield,USA.

COMPUTER MODELING AS AN AID TO UNDERSTANDING METABOLIC

COMPARTMENTATION OF THE KREBS CYCLE IN BRAIN TISSUE

D. D. Clarke[1], J. London[2] and D. Garfinkel[3]

Department of Chemistry, Fordham University, N.Y.(1),
and Moore School of Engineering, Univ. of Pennsylvania,
Philadelphia, PA., USA (2,3).

The basic observation which lead to the postulate of the
metabolic compartmentation of glutamate metabolism in
brain, as well as of the related Krebs cycles, has been
the subject of two previous symposia in this series(
Balazs and Cremer, 1973; Berl et al.,1975) and is well
known to most of the members of this Advanced Study Institute. In taking an overview of the field we can summarize by saying that labeled substrates fall into two
classes, those yielding brain glutamine with a specific
activity greater than glutamate and those giving the
opposite behavior. Hence the two cycle models have been
considered as the simplest possible ones which can lead
to a reasonable fit to both sets of experimental data.
By following other indices, e.g. the specific activity of
aspartate relative to glutamate or the distribution of
label between C-1 of glutamine and the rest of the molecule further sub-classifications can be made and these
point to the need for further subdivision of the two
cycle models. On the other hand, models with three to
five cycles and associated pools of amino acids related
to these Krebs cycles are extremely underdetermined with
the experimental data currently available (van den Berg et
al.,1975). Furthermore, it seems to be getting more difficult to generate the masses of data needed to refine
such models. Accordingly we have been setting our sights
lower as far as developing multicycle models and rather
have been trying to examine pieces of existing models in
more detail with a view to refining these sub-models further before tackling the bigger problems.

In general our two compartment Krebs cycle models
have been relatively successful in fitting most of the
experimental data on the labeling of glutamate, glutamine, GABA and aspartate generated in a number of labor-
atories(van den Berg and Garfinkel,1971). Of these substances aspartate still is the most difficult to fit properly i.e. the model clearly has deficiencies in that
area. A high point in the success of our models was reported at the last NATO ASI of this series when the Carshalton group and ourselves reported on the simulation
of an experiment still in progress with reasonably good
predictions (Mohler et al.,1974). Here labeled succinate
was administered to rats and the labeling of glutamate
and related amino acids followed with time. We have nothing as dramatic as this to report here. Rather we have
been going back over older data and concentrating on those
aspects which were conveniently ignored to get the model
working.

This approach of building sub-models has been used
extensively by Cremer and Heath (1974). A word of caution
must be sounded about this approach viz. that one must
always be cognizant that it is quite easy to achieve limited solutions to parts of the model but these may be
invalid because they introduce inconsistencies in the
total model.

One area which has been underemphasized in our models
is the compartmentation of glutamine metabolism. Compart-
menting glutamine metabolism gives a better fit to experimental data than if this is left out. However, leaving it
out does not ruin the model, thus we have not paid much
attention generally to this aspect of our models. This is
particularly true when the relative specific activity
(RSA) of glutamine is the index monitored. It is less
true with other indices. One of the latter indices is the
ratio of the labeling of C-1 to C-5 of glutamate after
the administration of $[1-^{14}C]$acetate. When such specifically labeled acetate enters the Krebs cycle only C-5 of
glutamate is labeled immediately and C-1 doesn't acquire
any label until after the cycle has rotated once. On the
next turn of the cycle C-1 is lost as $[^{14}CO]$. In agreement with this picture guinea pig brain slices incubated
with $[1-^{14}C]$acetate for various time periods show a rapid
increase in the percentage of label in C-1 of glutamate
and glutamine (Nicklas et al.,1969).

The fact that glutamine acquires label in this position faster than glutamate clearly points to the fact
that glutamine is being made from a pool of glutamate
which is a small part of the total tissue glutamate and
which is communicating with the Krebs cycle more rapidly

than the total tissue glutamate. This was the point emphasized in the original publication of this data. The
fact that glutamine was also compartmented was pointed
out but not emphasized (Nicklas et al.,1969).
      Recently we reexamined this data using the clearly
oversimplified model of two pools each of glutamate and
glutamine which were not communicating. Such simple models
(fig. 1) allow derivation of analytical expressions as
described by Cremer and Heath (1974) and one can use
optimization techniques to find the best fit of the analytical curve to the experimental data. Such a best fit
curve is shown in Fig. 2 for the data of Nicklas et al.
(1969) on the percentage of label in C-1 of glutamine.
The fit is clearly excellent. The assumption used here
is that labeled acetate labels C-5 of glutamine and that
half of this label is lost in the rotation of the Krebs
cycle to yield C-1 of glutamine. In the next rotation of
the cycle all of the label in C-1 of glutamine is lost.
Arbitrarily the radioactivity was divided into pools of
equal size. These did not communicate as that would have
complicated the analytical solution considerably. We
performed these operations on the DEC-10 computer at the
Medical School Computer Facility of the University of
Pennsylvania.  However they could be handled on a modern
desk calculator as is done by Cremer and Heath. The use
of the computer made it much easier to dissect the curves
describing the two different pools of glutamine as shown
in Fig. 3. These pools of glutamine clearly have very
different turnover times.
      The same type of analysis (Fig. 1) was done on the
data for glutamate and the best fit curve is shown in
Fig. 4. Again the fit of the analytically specified
curve to the data is excellent. The individual curves
describing the separate pools of glutamate as generated
by the computer are shown in Fig. 5

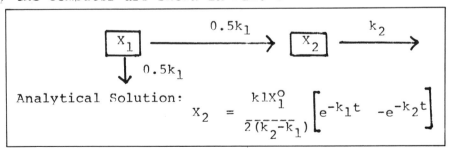

Figure 1.   Simplified Model for Distribution of Label
            between C-5 and C-1 of Glutamine and/or
            Glutamate.

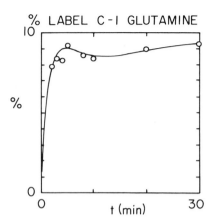

Figure 2. Two Independent Compartments for Cycling of
Label in Glutamine. Experimental points from
Nicklas et al. (1969).

% label in C-1 of glutamine = $12.50\left[e^{-0.1348t}-e^{-0.6738t}\right]$

$+23.21\left[e^{-0.01437t}\pm e^{-0.04533t}\right]$

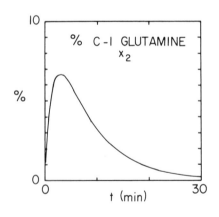

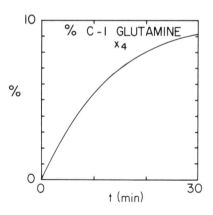

Figure 3. Computer Generated Separate Pools to fit data
in Fig. 2. Left, pool 1; Right pool 2.

Pool 1. % label = $12.50\left[e^{-0.1348t}-e^{-0.6738t}\right]$

Pool 2. % label = $23.21\left[e^{-0.01437t}-e^{-0.04533t}\right]$

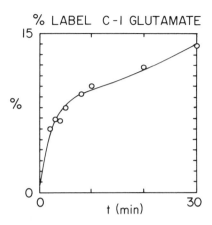

Figure 4. Two Independent Compartments for Cycling of Label in Glutamate. Experimental points from Nicklas et al. (1969).

% label in C-1 = $10.14 \left[ e^{-0.06694t} - e^{-0.3790t} \right]$

$\qquad -52.68 \left[ e^{-0.009833t} - e^{-0.0005t} \right]$

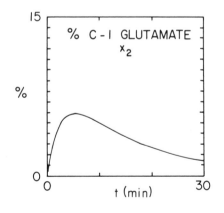

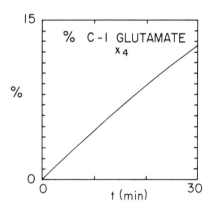

Figure 5. Computer Generated Separate Pools to fit data in Fig. 4. Left, pool 1; Right, pool 2.

Pool 1. % label = $10.14 \left[ e^{-0.06694t} - e^{-0.3970t} \right]$

Pool 2. % label = $-52.68 \left[ e^{-0.009833t} - e^{-0.0005t} \right]$

The interpretation of these curves in terms of the overall
model is problematical. The ratio of the pool sizes of
glutamate and of glutamine were arbitrarily taken as
unity. However these could be varied over wide ranges of
ratios and still be made to fit the data. The rate constants change with the pool sizes but we have found no way
to arrive at a unique solution for this set of data using
this oversimplified model.  There is no doubt that glutamate and glutamine communicate with each other via glutamine synthetase and glutaminase but introduction of such
reactions into the oversimplified model makes it almost
impossible to use the analytical approach and forces one
back to simulation models. To date it has not proved
practical to simulate even a simple model which pictures
two separate pools of glutamate and glutamine communicating with each other on a desk calculator; one is forced
back to the large computer. We have been making some
attempts to obtain a unique or a more limited set of
solutions for this problem but have not focussed much
effort in that direction to date.

Rather we have been focussing on the data reported
by Cremer at the last ASI in this series (Cremer et al.,
1975a) and elsewhere (Cremer et al.,1975b).  The analytical approach described above was employed by these
workers to analyse their data on rats which were made
encephalopathic by producing a porto-caval shunt. The
glutamine levels in the brains of such animals increase
threefold over controls and the animals were examined some
six weeks after being operated on so that they were close
to steady state conditions.  All previous workers have
studied ammonia intoxication under acute conditions of
ammonia treatment where glutamine levels were changing
during the experiment. Presently available simulation
methods do not handle such situations well.

Cremer found that the labeling of glutamate after
injection of labeled glucose could be treated quite
accurately as a single pool system both in control and
experimental animals. The analytical expression so developed was used to derive the labeling of glutamine.
When the labeling of glutamine by $[2-^{14}C]$ -glucose and
$[1-^{14}C]$ -butyrate were compared, these authors concluded
that there was no overlap of the pools of glutamine labeled by glucose and by butyrate or by acetate which
behaves similarly to butyrate (Cremer et al.,1975b). This
puzzled us because our models show all labeling of glutamine to come from a small pool of glutamate which is more
heavily labeled by acetate than by glucose. This model,
first developed by van den Berg and Garfinkel (1971) and
later modified by us accounted very well for the experi-

mental observations from Quastel's laboratory (Lahiri and Quastel, 1963) that fluoroacetate at 1mM inhibits the labeling of glutamine from labeled glucose as well as from labeled acetate. At the same time oxygen uptake by the tissue or $[^{14}CO_2]$ production from $[^{14}C]$-glucose were not affected by this concentration of fluoroacetate but $[^{14}CO_2]$ production from labeled acetate was affected (Gonda and Quastel, 1966). This would imply that all glutamine is labeled via a small pool of glutamate which communicates with a Krebs cycle containing small pools of intermediates which is selectively labeled by acetate and inhibited by fluoroacetate and fluorocitrate. It appeared to us that the model proposed by the Carshalton group was contrary to this postulate.

Glutamine is known to leak from brain slices into the incubation medium readily and inhibitors such as ouabain do not affect this leakage significantly (Quastel, 1975). $[^{14}C]$-glutamine added to brain slices also is readily taken up into the tissue and labels GABA even more effectively than does exogenous glutamate (Berl and Lajtha, 1961; Shank and Aprison, 1977). Thus glutamine would seem to be taken up appreciably at nerve endings. Glutaminase appears to be enriched in nerve endings and presumably hydrolyzes glutamine to glutamate there. This glutamate probably constitutes a pool of glutamate more accessible to glutamate decarboxylase than that located elsewhere in the tissue. Thus a basis for glutamine compartmentation is that glutamine does not remain where it is synthesized (i.e. in contact with glutamine synthetase) but migrates to other sites.

Since the meaning of the non-overlap of pools of glutamine labeled by $[2-^{14}C]$-glucose and $[1-^{14}C]$-butyrate, suggested by Cremer et al. (1975a,b), was unclear to us we attempted to fit their data for the control animals to the current model for mouse brain. Since glucose was administered intravenously rather than intraperitoneally, as in most previous work, the forcing function for feeding glucose into the brain model was modified from that of van den Berg and Garfinkel (1971) to one corresponding to the data on the specific activity of brain glucose at different times after injection (Cremer et al.,1975b). The specific activity of glutamate calculated from the model is compared with the data of Cremer et al. in Table I. A scaling factor (2.5) was employed to match the specific activities calculated from the model with the experimental values. The fit of the experimental points up to thirty minutes is excellent and at least as good as that derived by Cremer et al. assuming a single compartment system for glutamate labeling by glucose. On

TABLE I.

Specific Activity of Glutamate in Normal Rats

Comparison of Experimental with Predicted Values.

| Time minutes | Experimental c.p.m.x10$^{-3}$ | Calculated c.p.m.x10$^{-3}$ | (Error)$^2$ |
|---|---|---|---|
| 1 | 0.33 | 0.75 | 0.1739 |
| 2 | 1.67 | 2.18 | 0.2601 |
| 4 | 4.20 | 5.25 | 1.1025 |
| 5 | 5.80 | 6.53 | 0.5256 |
| 9 | 8.50 | 9.13 | 0.3906 |
| 10 | 10.50 | 9.55 | 0.9025 |
| 20 | 8.70 | 8.30 | 0.1600 |
| 30 | 6.70 | 5.60 | 1.2100 |
| | Sum of the squares = | | 4.7252 |
| | | | |
| 40 | 9.00 | 3.05 | 35.4025 |
| | Sum of the squares = | | 40.1277 |

F statistic = 8.49

Experimental values were read from curves published by Cremer et al. (1975b). Calculated values are from the model of van den Berg and Garfinkel (1971) modified by Clarke (in preparation). The values generated by the model were multiplied by a scaling factor of 2.50 for this comparison.

this basis we thought that the elevated value for the forty minute time point was due to secondary labeling of brain amino acids by recycling of label from the liver. If Cremer et al.'s analytical curve were recalculated dropping the forty minute time point there was a dramatic decline in the sum of the squares of the errors suggesting that this assumption was justified. The fact that the forty minute time point is well above the calculated curve also in the operated animals increases the probability that this assumption is valid. We were quite surprised that our model fit the data of Cremer et al. so well without modification.

The specific activity of glutamine calculated in the model did not match the experimental data as well as did that for glutamate. The major discrepancy was that the predicted specific activity of glutamine increased much more rapidly than was observed experimentally. This

lead to a peak in the curve of the specific activity of
glutamine vs. time at 15 minutes in the model instead of
at 20 minutes as observed experimentally. The peak could
be altered by manipulating glutamine compartments but
we chose not to focus on this aspect of the data. Rather
we were concerned to see what changes were necessary in
the model to simulate the data for the operated animals.
If the model were simply altered to increase the total
pool size of glutamine threefold - as observed experimentally - far too much radioactivity accumulated in
glutamine i.e. three times as much as in controls while
in the experimental animals the increase was closer to
twofold (Cremer et al.,1975b).

The relative specific activity of glutamine after
injection of $[1-^{14}C]$-butyrate into the operated animals
was considerably less than in controls (Cremer et al.,
1975b). This suggested to us that part of the butyrate
in the operated animals was entering the pool of glutamate labeled primarily by glucose. Further support of
this idea came from the observations of these authors
that the labeling of amino acids increased quite markedly as compared to lipids the operated animals over controls. Since acetoacetate labels pools of glutamate
labeled by glucose more heavily than those labeled by
acetate (Cremer and Heath, 1974) we postulated that part
of the butyrate is converted to acetoacetate which enters
the pools of glutamate labeled by glucose in greater
quantities in operated animals than in controls. It would
be a formidable problem in the absence of any experimental
data to calculate the rate at which acetoacetate should
be fed to the brain in our model to test this hypothesis.
A device which bypassed this problem with a minimum of
modification of the model was to introduce a "leak" of
radioactivity from the small pool of glutamate which is
very active in making glutamine to the large pool of glutamate which is primarily labeled by glucose. By varying
the rate of this new reaction or "leak" it was possible
to match the specific activity of glutamate in the operated animals while keeping the labeling of glutamine
within the same range as experimentally observed (Table
II). This modification also lowers the RSA of glutamine
after injection of labeled acetate (or butyrate) to
bring these values into line with the experimentally observed values.

The data of Cremer et al.(1975b) thus can be matched,
at least to a first approximation, by the model of brain
metabolism developed by van den Berg and Garfinkel and
modified by Clarke. It does not require separate pools
of glutamine labeled by glucose and by acetate as postu-

TABLE II.

Specific Activity of Glutamate in Operated Rats.

Comparison of Experimental with Predicted Values.

| Time minutes | Experimental c.p.m.x10$^{-3}$ | Calculated c.p.m.x10$^{-3}$ | (Error)$^2$ |
|---|---|---|---|
| 3 | 6.0 | 4.02 | 3.9204 |
| 5 | 7.0 | 7.10 | 0.0100 |
| 6 | 10.0 | 7.68 | 5.3824 |
| 9.5 | 12.0 | 10.00 | 4.0000 |
| 10.4 | 10.8 | 10.00 | 0.6400 |
| 24.0 | 10.5 | 7.50 | 9.0000 |
| 30.0 | 6.67 | 6.73 | 0.0036 |
|  | Sum of the squares = | | 22.9604 |
| 40.0 | 7.40 | 5.00 | 5.7600 |
|  | Sum of the squares = | | 28.6664 |

Experimental values were read from curves published by
Cremer et al. (1975b). Calculated values from the model
of van den Berg and Garfinkel (1971) modified by Clarke
(in preparation). The values generated by the model were
multiplied by a scaling factor of 2.50 for this comparison.

lated by Cremer et al. This does not mean that glutamine
pools are not present in the brain but rather that they
are not neccessarily related as described by those workers. Thus the strategy of Cremer et al. to develop an
oversimplified model works well to predict the labeling
of glutamate. The relationship of glutamate to glutamine
predicted by their model, however, would seem to provide
some problems with fitting other types of experimental
data mentioned earlier.
       The interpretation of the "leak" in our model is
somewhat of a problem because animals with a deficiency
of liver function cannot be expected to excrete increased
quantities of ketone bodies from the liver. Besides, Dr.
Cremer has checked this point in her animals and there is
no increase of circulating ketone bodies (private communication). It may be that the brain can convert acetate
or butyrate, in part, to ketone bodies and that this is
increased in animals which are chronically exposed to
increased levels of ammonia in the circulation due to
the porto-caval shunt. This of course raises the question of whether the leak should be set at zero in the

model for normal animals as we have done up to now.

Such a diversion of acetate from the small to the large pool of glutamate could, if true, also explain some of the data mentioned earlier on the inhibition of glutamine labeling but not that of glutamate by fluoroacetate and fluorocitrate in guinea pig brain slices. It also raises questions as to the validity of the assumption that acetate labels glial pools of glutamate exclusively which many workers in the field now seem to be making.

Another piece of information which may be related to this idea is the report that injection of short chain fatty acids into rats acts synergistically with ammonia to produce coma in these animals (Zieve et al.,1974). These animals have intact livers and so may be feeding ketone bodies to the brain under such experimental conditions. Cremer and Heath (1974) have shown that in the suckling rat ketone bodies contribute significantly to the fuels taken up by the brain from the blood.

As mentioned earlier the RSA of glutamine is not very sensitive to the compartmentation of glutamine. An index which is more sensitive to the compartmentation of glutamine is the distribution of label between C-1 and C-5 of glutamate and glutamine. Unfortunately that set of data was not available in the set of experiments analyzed above. While the example at the beginning of this paper was from an in vitro situation, evidence for the compartmentation of glutamate and glutamine based on labeling of C-1 and C-5 of glutamate can be seen in the data published for certain in vivo experiments. One example of this is seen in the work of Cremer and Heath (1974) in which young rats were injected with $[2-^{14}C]$-glucose. These authors could not fit their data on the percentage of label in C-1 of glutamate at the early time points i.e. less than five minutes, to a single compartment model and suggested that the results were probably erroneous. Rather they can be fitted to a model of the type described at the beginning of this paper. Evidence of this type is also to be seen in the data of Gaitonde (1965). However in that set of experiments $[U-^{14}C]$-glucose was used and this makes mathematical analysis of the data particularly difficult. Both the methyl and carboxyl groups of acetyl coenzymeA become labeled in such experiments and these labels are lost at different rates during the rotation of the Krebs cycle (Clarke et al.,1975).

Another set of data that is extremely useful in specifying models of this type is that for the specific activity of GABA. Unfortunately that set of data was not

available in the experiments on the rats with the portocaval anastomosis.

Large models of the type with which we have been
working seem to be the best approach to date to keep
track of the multitude of variables which even simple
experiments can generate. They require numerical integration rather than analytical integration and are still
relatively expensive to run despite the many improvements in the technology of running them. They are more
difficult to comprehend than the simpler analytically
soluble models which can be handled on a desk calculator and which are intuitively much easier to grasp. However we think these complex models are still essential
at our present stage of development to handle reasonable
neurochemical models of the labeling of the labeling of
amino acids related to the Krebs cycle.

While we have focussed on our successes we would
not wish to leave you with the idea that we have solved
all of our problems. In general aspartate remains the
most difficult amino acid to fit to the model. This is
in part related to the very low levels of oxalacetate
in brain as well as in other tissues. That too is the
major source of the difficulties in the numerical integration procedures. No attempts to date have come even
close to approximating the uneven labeling of the carboxyl groups of brain aspartate described by Nicklas et al.
(1969). We do continue to progress slowly and I hope I
have convinced you that modeling is a useful exercise
in trying to gain further insights into the interpretation of our experimental data.

ACKNOWLEDGMENT

This work was supported in part by grant GM-16501
from the National Institutes of Health, USA and by a
Faculty Research grant from Fordham University.

REFERENCES

Balazs, R., and Cremer, J.E. (eds.), 1973, "Metabolic
        Compartmentation in the Brain", MacMillan Press,
        London.
Berl, S., Clarke, D.D., and Schneider, D. (eds) "Metabolic
        Compartmentation and Neurotransmission", Plenum
        Press, New York.
Berl, S., and Lajtha, A., 1961, Amino acid and protein
        metabolism VI-Cerebral compartments of glutamic
        acid metabolism. J. Neurochem. 7, 186-197.
Clarke, D.D., Ronan, F.J., Dicker, E., and Tirri, L.,

1975, Ethanol and its relation to amino acid metabol-
ism in brain, in "Metabolic Compartmentation and
Neurotransmission" (S. Berl, D.D.Clarke and D.
Schneider, eds.) Plenum Press, N. Y. pp. 449-460.

Cremer, J.F., and Heath, D.F., 1974, The estimation of
rates of utilization of glucose and ketone bodies
using compartmental analysis of isotopic data.
Biochem. J., 142, 527-544.

Cremer, J. F., and Heath, D.F., 1975, Glucose and ketone
body utilization in young rat brain: A compartmental
analysis of isotopic data, in "Metabolic Compartmentation and Neurotransmission" (S. Berl, D. D. Clarke
and D. Schneider, eds.) Plenum Press, N. Y. pp.
545-558

Cremer, J.F., Heath, D.F., Patel, A.J., Balazs, R., and
Cavanagh, J.B., 1975a, An experimental model of CNS
changes associated with chronic liver disease: Portocaval anastomosis in the rat, in "Metabolic Compartmentation and Neurotransmission" (S.Berl, D.D.Clarke,
and D. Schneider, eds.) Plenum Press, N.Y. pp.
461-478

Cremer, J.F., Heath, D.F., Teal, H.M., Woods, M.S., and
Cavanagh, J.B., 1975b, Some dynamic aspects of brain
metabolism in rats given a portocaval anastomosis,
Neuropath. and Appl. Neurobiol. 1, 293-311

Gaitonde, M.K., 1965, Rate of utilization of glucose and
compartmentation of $\alpha$-oxoglutarate and glutamate in
rat brain, Biochem. J. 95, 803-810

Gonda, O., and Quastel, J.H., 1966, Transport and metabolism of acetate in rat brain cortex in vitro,
Biochem. J. 100, 83-94

Lahiri, S. and Quastel, J.H., 1963, Fluoroacetate and the
metabolism of ammonia in brain, Biochem. J. 89,
157-163

Mohler,H., Patel, A. J., and Balazs, R., 1974, Metabolic
compartmentation in the brain:Metabolism of a tricarboxylic cycle intermediate [1,4-$^{14}$C]-succinate
after intracranial administration, J. Neurochem.
23, 285-289

Nicklas, W.J., Clarke, D.D., and Berl, S., 1969, Decarboxylation studies of glutamate, glutamine and aspartate
from brain labeled with [1-$^{14}$C]-acetate and L-[U-
$^{14}$C]-aspartate and L-[U-$^{14}$C]-glutamate, J. Neurochem.
549-558

Quastel, J.H., 1975, Metabolic compartmentation in the
brain and effects of metabolic Inhibitors, in "Metabolic compartmentation and Neurotransmission" (S.
Berl, D.D.Clarke and D. Schneider, eds.) Plenum
Press, N. Y. pp. 337-361

Shank, R.P., and Aprison, M.H., 1977, Glutamine uptake
    and metabolism by isolated toad brain: evidence per-
    taining to its proposed role as a transmitter pre-
    cursor, J. Neurochem. 28, 1189-1196
van den Berg, C.J., and Garfinkel, D., 1971, A simulation
    study of brain compartments: metabolism of glutama-
    te and related substances in mouse brain, Biochem.
    J. 123, 211-218
van den Berg, C.J., Reynierse, G.L.A., Blockuis, G.G.D.,
    Kroon, M.C., Ronda. G., Clarke, D.D., and Garfinkel,
    D., 1975, A model of glutamate metabolism in brain:
    A biochemical analysis of a heterogeneous structure
    in "Metabolic Compartmentation and Neurotransmission"
(S. Berl, D.D.Clarke and D. Schneider, eds.)Plenum Press,
    N. Y. pp. 515-543.
Zieve, F.J., Zieve, L., Doizaki, W.M., and Gilsdorf, R.B.
    1974, Synergism between ammonia and fatty acids in
    the production of coma: Implications for hepatic
    coma. J. Pharmacol. & Exptl. Therap. 191, 10-16

# INDEX